Human Perception of Objects

Early Visual Processing of Spatial Form
Defined by Luminance, Color, Texture,
Motion, and Binocular Disparity

David Regan

York University, Toronto
University of Toronto

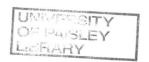
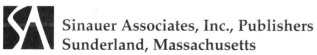

Sinauer Associates, Inc., Publishers
Sunderland, Massachusetts

About the Cover:

Front: The prey of both large and small predators have evolved remarkably effective natural camouflage. An important driving force in the evolution of the visual systems of predators is the necessity to break the camouflage of their prey. Many predators can move at great speed, but only over a short distance. This lioness illustrates how many predators use their natural camouflage to maximize the chance of a kill by stationing themselves close to their unsuspecting prey. Photograph © Heather Angel.

Back: Stimulus used by Regan and Hong (1995) to test detection of texture-defined letters in patients (see pp. 284–288).

Human Perception of Objects:
Early Visual Processing of Spatial Form
Defined by Luminance, Color,
Texture, Motion, and Binocular Disparity

© Copyright 2000 by Sinauer Associates, Inc.
All rights reserved.

This book may not be reproduced in whole or in part for any purpose whatever without permission from the publisher. For information or to order, address:

Sinauer Associates, Inc., P.O. Box 407
Sunderland, Massachusetts, 01375-0407 U.S.A.
Fax: 413-549-1118. E-mail: publish@sinauer.com

Library of Congress Cataloging-in-Publication Data

Regan, D. (David), 1935–
  Human perception of objects : early visual processing of spatial form defined by luminance, color, texture, motion, and binocular disparity / David Regan.
    p. cm.
  Includes bibliographical references and index.
  ISBN 0-87893-753-6
  1. Space perception. 2. Visual perception. I. Title.
QP491 .R445 1999
152.14'2--dc21

99-057028

Printed in U.S.A.

5 4 3 2 1

Contents

CHAPTER 4
Texture-Defined Form 267

CHAPTER 5
Motion-Defined Form   295

CHAPTER 6
Disparity-Defined Form   343

CHAPTER 7
Integration of the Five Kinds of Spatial Information: Speculation 375

APPENDIX A
Systems Science and Systems Analysis 385

APPENDIX B
Outline of Fourier Methods and Related Topics 405

Preface

Science and technology have advanced in more than direct ratio to the ability of men to contrive methods by which phenomena which otherwise could be known only through the senses of touch, hearing, taste, and smell have been brought within the range of visual recognition and measurement and thus become subjects to that logical symbolization without which rational thought and analysis are impossible.

William N. Ivins, Jr., *On the Rationalization of Sight* (1938; quoted in Crosby, 1997)

The eye is the master of astronomy. It makes cosmography. It advises and corrects all human arts. . . . The eye carries men to different parts of the world. It is the prince of mathematics. . . . It has created architecture, and perspective, and divine painting. . . . It has discovered navigation.

Leonardo da Vinci (1452–1519; quoted in Crosby, 1997)

There are many reasons for carrying out research in visual psychophysics. Clinical psychophysicists seek to contribute to neurology, ophthalmology, or optometry by devising noninvasive procedures for strengthening differential diagnoses or for monitoring therapy. Human-factors specialists address such issues as highway safety by improving visual aspects of highway design and highway lighting, and by designing visual screening tests. They also seek to improve the training of commercial airline pilots by improving the visual displays in flight simulators. Some visual psychophysicists seek to improve the quality of displays such as the familiar TV by better interfacing the display to the human eye. And in recent years the designers of visually guided machines have looked to the human visual system, realizing that it embodies solutions to the severe problems that they encounter.

In the hope that it may help students to read between the lines of this book, I will say that none of the above is the reason for my fascination with vision research. My interest in sensory perception was implanted through an accidental exposure during the susceptible midteens to Immanuel Kant's *Critique of Pure*

Reason. Although the immediate effect was a motivation to study physics, after many years I moved on to human brain electrophysiology and sensory psychophysics as offering more direct approaches to the study of the perceived physical world in which we live.

In the writing of this book I have made a considerable effort to give a fair presentation of conflicting viewpoints. I am not alone in finding tendentiousness to be a mighty irritation. But, realizing that too much detachment can be almost as irritating, and with the intent of maintaining a coherent line of narration, I have not hesitated to state my opinion. At the worst, I hope that I have provided something to argue about.

Many books on visual psychophysics are collections of chapters, each of which is written by a different author. This format can provide a uniformly high and up-to-date level of scholarship over a broad research area when the individual authors are authorities on their various topics and the editing is careful and firm. However, it is often difficult to integrate different viewpoints and approaches, and a systematic comparison of methods is often lacking. A coherent overview is, in principle, more easily approximated in a monograph written by a single author, but the disadvantage of this more traditional format is the difficulty of ensuring an adequate standard of discussion in areas outside one author's expertise. A single author depends on the critical advice of fellow scientists. In writing this book over the last eight years, I was fortunate that many colleagues generously gave their time to criticize successive drafts. They removed many misconceptions and errors. The errors and misconceptions that remain are all my own, and the following acknowledgment of valuable advice and comments does not imply agreement with any of the views expressed in this book. I thank A. Bradley, J. Enright, J. Foley, I. Howard, L. Kaufman, S. Klein, M. J. Morgan, H. C. Nothdurft, A. Reeves, M. P. Regan, A. Smith, R. M. Steinman, E. Switkes, M. Treisman, C. W. Tyler, J. D. Victor, R. J. Watt, L. Wilcox, and H. Wilson.

Douglas Regan typed the first thirty or so drafts when this book was in the form of a review paper. Without Derek Harnanansingh's wizardry with the computer and cheerful good humor this book would have been very much harder to complete in more ways than one. I thank Marian Regan for her unfailingly cheerful support through the writing of this book, for mathematical advice, and for hilarity at my less well-founded ideas. I am indebted to Dr. Hua Hong for brilliantly creative software over the last ten years. And finally, I thank big, handsome Ginger who, after patrolling his territory each morning, settled down on my desk at 4–5 A.M. to act as my overseer through most of the two thousand or so hours that it took during the last eight months to convert a journal article into a book.

The initial stage of this writing was made possible by a fellowship from the I. W. Killam Trust. The research of my laboratory was sponsored by the U.S. Air Force Office for Scientific Research and supported by the National Sciences and Engineering Research Council of Canada and by CRESTech. I would be grateful for comments from readers on errors and omissions, and suggestions as to how the book might be improved. My e-mail address is dregan@yorku.ca.

A Note to Research Students

Through the first thirty or so drafts, written over more than five years, of what became this book, I was writing a research monograph intended for publication in a journal, and only at a very late stage was it suggested that, because of copyright problems when making multiple photocopies of a journal article, it would better serve the interests of students to publish it as a book. During the last eight months I have added many sections in an attempt to convert to textbook format. I hope that the joints are not too jarringly evident.

Over the last ten to twenty years, many of the papers published in such journals as *Vision Research* and the *Journal of the Optical Society of America* demanded more than a nodding acquaintance with certain areas of undergraduate-level and postgraduate-level physics and mathematics if they were to be fully understood. When teaching graduate courses in psychology, I have found that this demand can create problems for the large numbers of psychology students who have little or no formal training in physics or mathematics. These students face the further problem that accurate texts on these topics are written for B.Sc. and Ph.D. students of physics and mathematics, so that the level of treatment renders the material almost inaccessible to them. Furthermore, advanced physics and mathematics textbooks contain an enormous amount of material, only a tiny fraction of which the psychophysics student needs to understand. Bearing this in mind, I added Appendixes A–I. In these appendixes, I have done my utmost to explain the relevant topics in physics and mathematics in such a way as to place them (without misleading oversimplification) within the intuitive grasp of a student with little experience of physics or mathematics. To clarify some difficult points I have explained several misconceptions. Since my aim is to ease the problems faced by student researchers, I ask them for feedback on the deficiencies of the appendixes, and suggestions as to how they might be improved. My e-mail address is dregan@yorku.ca.

In an attempt to inject some life into the narrative, I have scattered the text with footnotes intended to set the content of the book in a variety of more general contexts and to bring out larger issues. Whenever possible I explain hypotheses and experimental findings in terms of everyday experience.

I return time and time again to two major themes: how the characteristics of the human visual system support visually guided, goal-directed motor action; and how the functional characteristics of our visual system can be understood in terms of evolutionary pressures in the remote past.

Another major theme is that research is done by individual researchers. Although the scientific *method* is dispassionate, the *doing* of research is highly personal. That is my reason for including footnotes that outline the life and (often difficult) circumstances in which individual researchers laid down the foundations of our field of research.

How good at book learning must you be?

In recent years it seems to be more and more the case that research students are selected on the basis of their ability to score high marks at the undergraduate level.* My impression, however, is that high marks in undergraduate courses are by no means an infallible predictor of an individual's future contributions to research. Of at least equal importance is a hunger to understand, combined with a disposition to think about a problem night and day over a long period. Questioning the correctness of received opinion and the views of your elders (be discreet!) and self-demandingly setting your own standard are important, as is whatever it takes to keep going in the face of disappointment and lack of encouragement (more on that later).

I was fortunate to read physics at a small college and to be taught by eminent scientists, several of whom, including P. M. S. Blackett and D. Gabor, received Nobel Prizes—though in 1953 I was so ignorant that I had no idea what that meant. My good fortune was that these individuals did not attempt to impress and overwhelm their students with their verbal dexterity and speed of thought; they did not seem aggressively "clever" (in the English sense of the word); even

---

* Many graduate students are left to "find their own feet." Some do, some don't. Among the ones who don't are a few students who have been uncommonly successful at undergraduate level. Not understanding that being a researcher is quite different from being an undergraduate (see pp. 501–502)—and why that is—they may fall back on approaches and mental attitudes that have served them so well in the past. Such students have been disadvantaged by being told that they are clever. It is important to realize that a good undergraduate record is what gets you into graduate school (just as being very good at Rugby football helped to get you into London University medical school in the 1940s and 1950s), and gives you the opportunity to enter an exhilarating and entirely different new world. The formerly high-achieving student who found coursework and examinations easy and who now is struggling with research should not assume that he or she is personally lacking. It means that you are now in the real, the serious, game. And that it is time to play it with full visceral commitment if you have the desire to do research.

their day-to-day work in the laboratory did not seem dramatic to me. When I started to do research I encountered many individuals who thought far more quickly than I, who were far more adept with words and arguments, and who presented their research with much drama. I was intimidated by such individuals and my self-confidence was shaken. I might well not have persisted in research had it not been for memories of those, such as Blackett, whose demeanor was so different but whose achievements were so much greater.

"Positive feedback" from others is less valuable than sharp criticism. Sharp criticism is a compliment to you. By criticizing your work or your attitude, the criticizer takes your work or yourself seriously enough to offer help while taking the risk that you may react in an embarrassing manner.

The nature of psychophysics

It was Fechner who, in 1860, provided the insight that allowed the methods of experimental physics to be applied to the study of sensory perception. Rather than grapple with the problem of quantifying something so insubstantial as a sensation, he sidestepped the problem by proposing that a motor response could be used as a measure of the output of a sensory system. In this way he reduced the experimental study of sensory perception to a procedure familiar to experimental physicists, i.e., comparing the quantified output of a system with the quantified input to the system (the stimulus in this case). He devised the following methods for the new science of *psychophysics*: the method of adjustments; the method of limits; the method of constant stimuli. Fechner's innovation allowed the methods of *experimental* physics to be applied to the study of sensation. A more subtle point concerns the nature of *theoretical* physics.

It can be argued that our understanding of physical phenomena lies not in the so-called facts of physics, but rather in those hypotheses or theories that not only provide a systematic mathematical relationship between experimental observations, but also succeed best in predicting new phenomena. These hypotheses or theories are insubstantial things of the mind rather than being concrete entities or facts. They are subject to experimental refutation at any time. Indeed, during the last 100 years very many well-respected theories have been refuted, including some ways of looking at the world that had seemingly attained the status of self-evident truths. (However, their historical importance as conceptual stepping-stones will always remain.)

Theories are framed in terms of abstract concepts (including mathematical relationships) rather than in terms of concrete entities. When teaching physics I found that some students who had never been confronted with this reality experienced growing unease as their studies progressed to a level where confrontation could no longer be avoided. They struggled despairingly to visualize in concrete terms such abstractions as the field vectors **E**, **H**, and **B**, trying to treat them as physical entities rather than as theoretical constructs. Vision research students sometimes show a similar unease when they confuse a hypothesis with an observation. (Some authors do not help when they present hypotheses as though they were facts.) I find it helpful when reading a paper, and especially the introduction, to keep at the front of my mind the question: Is that an observation or is that a hypothesis?

Another source of puzzlement is that light is sometimes described as a wave— e.g., when explaining the refraction of light, the imaging properties of lenses and the interference of light (see pp. 430–434), and is sometimes described in terms of localized packets of energy called photons (e.g., when explaining the emission of absorption of light—see footnote on page 198 and pp. 436–439). Some students try to visualize how light can be both a wave and a particle. This problem can be eased by realizing that the wave description and the particle description are just that: *descriptions*. They are the stuff of hypotheses rather than of concrete entities. In some situations the behavior of light is most easily described in terms of a wave hypothesis. In other situations the behavior of light is most easily described in terms of a particle hypothesis.

Why it should be necessary to perform such mental gymnastics to explain light remains a profound mystery. Some think it is because the act of observation (i.e., making a measurement) determines what is observed. It is also possible that the complementarity of the wave/particle descriptions reflects a limitation of human thought processes that has only recently been revealed by experimental physicists, a limitation that was not evident in human tool-making endeavors.

The status of psychophysics

I caution students trained in psychology not to be overimpressed by physics, a discipline many of whose practitioners are expert in public relations. The fact that physicists have made enormous advances in our understanding of the natural world does not necessarily imply that their methods would be equally successful in brain research or in psychology. Psychology students are advised to take from physics and mathematics what is useful for their field and leave what is not. For example, the very high quantitative and statistical exactitude that characterizes many models in physics is often inappropriate in psychophysics. W. D. Wright (1970) underlined this last point in an informal presentation to the Colour Group. "The C.I.E. Colorimetry Committee recently in their wisdom have been looking at the old 1930 observer data and have been smoothing the data to obtain more consistent calculations with computers. This has also involved some extrapolation and, in smoothing, they have added some additional decimal places. When I look at the revised table of the $\bar{x}$, $\bar{y}$, $\bar{z}$ functions, I am rather surprised to say the least. You see, I know how inaccurate the actual measurements really were. . . . Guild did not take any observations below 400 nm and neither did I, and neither did Gibson and Tyndal on the V_λ curve, and yet at a wavelength of 362 nm, for example, we find a value $\bar{y}$ of 0.00000492604! This, in spite of the fact that at 400 nm the value of $\bar{y}$ may be in error by a factor of 10. . . . I know we can put the blame on the computer but we must not abdicate our common sense altogether."

Physicists commonly reduce a problem to its empirical essence. Brain researchers cannot sidestep empirical complexity with such lordly ease. And the saying "God is a mathematician" is a shorthand for the eyebrow-raising exactitude with which the predictions of theoretical physicists correspond to empirical observation. Although there is general agreement that top physicists play the scientific game superbly well, their achievements are, nevertheless, astonishing. It is as though they pushed an open door. The precision with which the human mind can describe and predict the physical world has suggested to some that theoretical physics is not so much a description of an external reality, but rather a description of the process of observation. Brain researchers should not assume that their door will also be unlocked.

Research students in psychophysics should not feel that their chosen field is inferior to physics, mathematics, or physiology. Psychophysics has no reason to defer to any other science.

Reading a journal article

Some journal articles are written in a curious way—in the passive voice, perhaps to give the impression that, rather than being a personal creation, the research just happened by itself, untouched by human hand. But, as I discuss on pages 505–506, essentially all journal articles are written in a way that gives a misleading impression of how science is actually done.*

Sometimes when reading a journal article I cannot understand why certain experiments were done in a certain way while others were not done at all, and why some previously published papers were discussed in detail while others were not mentioned. In subsequent discussions with colleagues I not infrequently find that my failure to understand was caused by insufficient brainpower. But this is not always the case. I was very slow to learn (and, having learnt, very slow to accept) that a cautious and suspicious attitude to the written word, seeking always to "read between the lines," is as necessary when reading a journal article as when reading a newspaper. For example, when reading a journal article I find it helpful to ask myself why the article was written.

---

* In 1968 Henk van der Tweel invited me to visit Amsterdam to carry out an experiment with him and Henk Spekreijse. They had prepared well for the hypothesis I wished to test, and had provided equipment for recording human brain responses, building a visual stimulator and purchasing many large and expensive color filters. I was the first subject. By midday on the first morning of a two- to three-week visit, recordings of my brain responses indicated that the hypothesis was a total failure. I secretly feared that I had abused the hospitality of my generous hosts. So when Henk Spekreijse suggested going out for a *Warm Vlees Tosti* (a delicious Dutch invention), I leapt to my feet, eager for a diversion. In my haste I clumsily knocked the stimulator optics. Peering into it to check whether it was broken, I saw an astonishing phenomenon: constant visual suppression of part of the image in one eye. We all looked at it. Now we had an experiment. Lunch was a celebration. But the formal report bore little relation to the way in which this piece of research came to be (Spekreijse, van der Tweel & Regan, 1972).

Why are there not more successful research scientists?

I have already hinted that some successful researchers were not outstanding undergraduates. I even knew one who had no undergraduate degree at all and had to be appointed as Associate Professor because there is no such title in England and, therefore, no job description. Some successful research scientists are quick-thinking, articulate, bright, and what the English call "clever." Many are not. What does it take to be a research scientist?

Desire

The most important requirement is an overwhelming desire to do research—to find things out for yourself to your own satisfaction. With this desire, other things become secondary.

In short, desire must overcome natural lethargy and that particular softness of character that shows up as a deficiency in fortitude. In this respect students today are badly served by exposure to the current North American outbreak of whining, whingeing, self-pitying victimhood.

I know that research often brings me great exhilaration and joy, and I believe that to be a common experience. The joy of research does not seem to diminish with age. At 64, I have never been so excited and exhilarated with scientific speculation and experimental research.

Keeping going and self-motivation

I play a man who the world got wrong. You know, it's not his fault, it's never his fault. I went through all that when I was in the theatre, "I can't get on because I'm working class," "I can't get on because they're all poofs and I'm not." You can always make an excuse for losing.

Maurice Micklewhite (a.k.a. Michael Caine),
interviewed about his role in the movie *Little Voice*,
Sunday Times (London), 13 December 1998

It is not all exhilaration and joy. In striving to find a job that allows the time, the space, and the equipment to do research, one may come close to despair, especially when the striving extends over years. And even when that striving is (for the time being) over, in almost any experiment there comes a time when one grimly recognizes that much time and energy have been wasted going up blind alleys; when one cannot see how to break out of the problem; and when one is physically tired, mentally tired, overworked, and feeling down. And I have long grown accustomed to the fact that a proper understanding of a topic that I need to understand is beyond me. So just as in sport, where the strength and speed to carry out some action was only acquired through hundreds of hours of effort, I must struggle to strengthen my conceptual grasp of some principle of method, of physics, or of mathematics—until I can use it. And this is just as frustratingly slow, and just as demanding of the determination to "stay with it," as it was during my athletic years.

Different people have different ways of digging deep for the will to keep trying. In the hope that it may be of help to some students I will end by describing my line of thought on this.

To be in a position that, with luck, one might extend human understanding of the physical and mental world in which we live is a rare privilege. Vast numbers of people with equal or greater capability, intelligence, and desire never were, or never will be, in such a position. Some are unable to do so because they live in underdeveloped countries. Others may live in a wealthy country, but their government makes no provision for the children of poor parents to experience a highly academic education that stretches them and allows them to develop their talents.* Others do not become researchers because they were born in the wrong place at the wrong time. This point is sharply illustrated by the following extract: "Scientists themselves were presently shocked by the deaths of some of the most talented young scientists, such as H. G. J. Moseley in 1915, who were killed in routine military operations in which no use at all was being made of their special scientific gifts" (Crowther, 1974, p.171).

Rutherford's student Chadwick was more fortunate. He was spared because he was in Berlin at the outbreak of hostilities, having been awarded a studentship in 1913 to study under Professor Geiger (he of the Geiger counter). Chadwick was promptly interned in Ruhleben Camp. With generous help from German scientific colleagues, he and other prisoners organized a little research laboratory. In 1918 Rutherford found him a university position: if he could run a lab in Ruhleben, he could run one anywhere. In 1935 Chadwick was awarded the Nobel Prize in physics for his discovery of the neutron.

The 25-year-old W. L. Bragg was working in the front-line trenches using Helmholtz resonators tuned to very low frequencies to triangulate onto the sites of German heavy guns when he received a message from his father, W. H. Bragg, to tell him that they had been awarded jointly the Nobel Prize in physics. The message was greeted with little interest by Bragg's platoon until they found that W. H. Bragg had, thoughtfully, included a crate of Scotch with his letter of congratulation.

At afternoon tea at Imperial College I once asked P. M. S. Blackett the kind of question that naïve and ignorant young men ask: "What was the thing in your life that you remember most clearly?"

"The smell of burning flesh on the lower deck at the Battle of Jutland" was his immediate response before he strode off. He had been in the Royal Navy for ten

---

* Such a provision was in force in England through the 1940s and 1950s in the form of an examination taken at 11 years of age that gave entry to the selective so-called Grammar Schools.

years, and commanded a destroyer during the First World War.* In 1918 the Admiralty arranged for selected officers to attend Cambridge University for "holiday courses." Three weeks after arriving, and having attended lectures given by Rutherford, he resigned from the Navy (thereby losing his gratuity) and became an undergraduate. He graduated in 1921. By 1933 he and Occialini had, using the Wilson cloud chamber, visually demonstrated showers of positive and negative electrons, thus confirming Dirac's conception of antimatter.† In 1948 Blackett was awarded the Nobel Prize for physics.

So here we have three individuals who, by chance, escaped death and went on to win the Nobel Prize in physics—and one who might well have done so, but was killed. Similar accounts could, no doubt, be told about the young physicists in all the other nations who fought in the 1914–1918 war, and also about the young chemists, the young biologists, and so on. And what of the many, many more who had no time to realize and develop their scientific skills before they were killed, mutilated, or driven insane?

And what of the young women of that generation? Following the slaughter of young males,‡ many millions of young women would find themselves unencumbered by husbands or children, free to pursue their métier with less distraction than the young women of today. But things were different then. It was very

---

* Perhaps it was those experiences that made him a lifelong and outspoken communist—a political commitment that, no doubt, raised eyebrows when he was appointed advisor on nuclear warfare to NATO in the 1950s at the height of the Cold War.

† Nowadays the conception of antimatter is commonplace currency. It was used to power the warp drive in the starship *Enterprise* in the original "Star Trek" series.

‡ Approximately 10 million European soldiers were killed or died of wounds, and about 20 million were wounded or driven insane. Most were between 19 and 25 years of age, though Billy Cotton (later an entertainment impresario) was only 14 when he waded ashore under machine-gun fire at Cape Helles on the Gallipoli peninsula, and more than one 55-year-old lies in the somber Tyn Cot cemetery in front of Passchendaele village.

difficult for a woman to gain even undergraduate status in a science faculty, and even more difficult to become a research student and then go on and pursue her own independent research.

When I feel disheartened I think of those with far greater ability than I who had no chance to use it, and imagine them looking at me sadly: "Look, he can't endure a bit of disappointment. What a feeble fellow! What a delicate flower! If only I were in his place."

> Nick retreated to a curved stone bench, ignoring the damp seeping through the seat of his pants, and staring at the inscription: TO THE MISSING OF THE SOMME.* He was repelled by it. The monument towered over the landscape but it didn't soar as a cathedral does. The arches found the sky empty and returned to earth; they opened on to emptiness. It reminded Nick, appropriately enough, of a warrior's helmet with no head inside. No, worse than that: Golgotha, the place of skulls. If, as Nick believed, you should go to the past, looking not for messages of warning, but simply to be humbled by the weight of human experience that has preceded the brief flicker of your own few days, then Thiepval succeeded brilliantly.

> Pat Barker, *Another World*, 1998

---

* A stone plaque explains that on the surface of the monument "is recorded the names of the 73,077 men who disappeared here and near this place between July and December of 1916 and have no known grave." And this is a British Commonwealth memorial. After the first few days, the Battle of the Somme was not one-sided; the German Army also lost some 600,000 killed and wounded.

CHAPTER 1

How Do We See Objects? Conceptualizing the Question and Tackling It

As many more individuals of each species are born than can possibly survive; and as, consequently, there is a frequently recurring struggle for existence, it follows that any being, if it varies however slightly in any manner profitable to itself, under the complex and sometimes varying conditions of life, will have a better chance of surviving, and thus be naturally selected.

C. Darwin, *The Origin of Species*, 1859

For as long as there had been human moth collectors, the peppered moth *Biston betuleria* had been known as a light-coloured creature, and there was no specimen of the mutant black-winged form (the aptly-named *Biston carbonaria*) in any collection: its rarity was maintained by birds which found *carbonaria* easy to see on the pale lichen-covered tree branches on which it rested during the day. The first specimen of *carbonaria* was captured in 1848, and by 1855 the black form had multiplied to comprise 98% of populations in the Manchester area of Northern England, the previously-common pale form having decreased from near-100% to 2%. The start of the Industrial Revolution and the associated pollution of the air had killed the light-coloured tree lichen and blackened the trees. Birds now found *betuleria* far easier than *carbonaria* to see against the tree bark. (The birds, as agents of natural selection, presumably did not change their preference as to the visual presentation of their food: they simply caught the moths that they saw.) The smoke abatement laws of recent years resulted in the re-establishment of light coloured tree lichens in the Industrial North of England after a gap of more than 100 years. And the percentage of the peppered moth population that is pale-coloured has started to increase in the Manchester area, while the percentage of the black form is, correspondingly, decreasing year-by-year.

C. O'Toole, *Alien Empire*, 1995

Figure 1.1 shows the effective camouflage of the pale-colored and dark forms of the peppered moth.

Was the Evolution of Our Visual System Driven by the Evolution of Natural Camouflage?

There is no single design of eye. It is not only that there are many kinds of eye: differences can be gross (Land & Fernald, 1992; Walls, 1942). Some eyes differ exceedingly from what we can too easily assume to be the norm, that is, the organ of sight of *Homo sapiens*. But in spite of their widely differing physical structures, all eyes have a common function, one that presumably is of high significance for evolutionary success. They allow their owners to detect and recognize distant objects immediately and confidently, and to judge ahead of time whether the motion of these objects relative to the observing eye will result in a future collision.

Animals who are subject to the attention of predators, and especially those who lack the equipment to fight back, have evolved a variety of countermeasures,

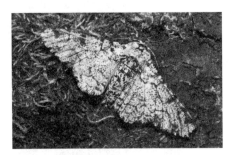

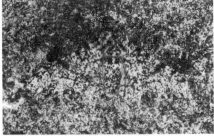

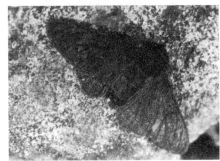

1.1 A species adapts to environmental pollution. Against pale lichen the light-colored moth is well camouflaged (top right), but the black form is not (bottom right). On blackened trees the light-colored moth is easily seen (top left). From O'Toole (1995).

including the ability to merge into their surroundings. Driven by evolutionary pressure, animals who eat other animals have developed visual systems that can use any one of five means to break the camouflage of their prey so that they can be seen from a distance. Since one of these means is to detect an object via relative motion, an animal who senses the proximity of a predator must remain absolutely still. The sand grouse chick in Color Plate 1 merges fairly well into its surroundings, though it would be seen from a few meters by a predator with binocular depth perception, and from a still greater distance if it threw a shadow. (Some animals conceal their shadow with camouflaged wing covers.) The flounder fish merges with its surroundings in terms of mean luminance, color, and texture; furthermore, when it flattens itself against the seabed, it renders its camouflage tolerably secure against predators with binocular depth perception (Color Plate 2). Another way of achieving camouflage against binocular stereopsis is to merge into a natural three-dimensional structure, as illustrated by the crab spider in Color Plate 3 and by the leaf katydid in Color Plate 4 (which has the misfortune to be the main source of food for many birds and several species of monkey in the forests of Peru). In both cases, however, the animals' clearly visible legs detract from otherwise excellent camouflage. Some animals solve this problem by developing ragged extensions to their legs that seem to form part of the plants whose coloring they assume.

Effective though these adaptations are, these animals are only camouflaged against a background of quite specific color, texture, and reflectance. To allow for changes in their surroundings, some animals change their color with the seasons. The weasel, for example, has a white winter coat and a darker one for summer. More remarkably, some animals can change their coloration within a short time period. The chameleon is proverbial, but other less exotic species, including some reptiles and amphibians and many species of fish, can also change color. For example, some minnows sense (through their eyes) changes in the color and texture of the stream bed, and change their skin pigmentation accordingly. In some species, the color change may take minutes or hours, but the cuttlefish can change color within seconds (von Frisch, 1973).

A necessary condition for perceiving objects and the relations between them is that an observer's visual system should segregate the objects' retinal images from their surroundings. That is self-evident. But it is not intuitively obvious what kinds of visual difference between an object and its surroundings can render that object visible to an observing eye. Laboratory experiments have shown empirically that any one of the following five kinds of visual difference can support image segregation: luminance, texture, motion, color, or binocular disparity. When an object matches its surroundings in all five respects, it cannot be seen and is said to be *perfectly camouflaged*.

Although the five kinds of spatial contrast are handled differently during the earliest stages of processing, the survival interests of the organism dictate their rapid and reliable integration at a stage of visual information processing that precedes the initiation of motor action.* From the viewpoint of the organism, an object is an object; where and what the object is, and whether it will come into contact with the organism are the critical concerns; from the viewpoint of the organism details of *how* the organism's visual system segregates the object from its surroundings are irrelevant, so long as the job is done effectively and quickly.†

The Organization of This Book

MacKay (1965) noted that there are at least three ways in which scientists try to understand a machine or a biological organism.

1. Study it as a whole.
2. Take it to pieces and try to understand the parts and how they might work together.
3. Try to reassemble the parts we understand and test whether the synthesis performs like the original.

In the context of the human visual system, experimental method (1) covers the following three kinds of psychophysical investigation: baseline experiments on normally sighted observers, experimental studies carried out on normally sighted observers while disturbing the visual system nondestructively (e.g., adaptation experiments), and experimental studies of abnormal (e.g., color-defective) visual systems. Experimental method (2) takes the form of anatomical investigations of the human visual system and certain physiological investigations of the visual systems of nonhuman animals including nonhuman primates. Experimental method (3) includes the assembly of artificial parts in an attempt

---

* Similar ecological surmises are inserted at many points in this book. But the experiments I review are almost entirely restricted to the laboratory. They use visual stimuli that are much simpler than the everyday visual environment. Some readers may see this as a failure to deliver on the promise of discussing our understanding of the perceived visual world, pointing, perhaps, to the work of Gibson and his colleagues as a more direct route to such understanding (Gibson, 1966, 1979). To these readers, I say that I agree as to the ultimate objective, but I think it is reasonable to break down a challenge that is far beyond one's capability into a sequence of challenges, each of which is within one's capability. According to this strategy, when the results of laboratory experiments that used a given set of simplified stimuli are understood (in the sense that they are predicted by a mathematical model), then stimulus complexity can be increased a little and a more comprehensive model developed, step by step. (The history of research on color vision illustrates this kind of conceptual development.) It is only within the last few years that systematic quantitative studies of the visual processing of natural images have been combined with mathematical modeling (e.g., Schaaf & Hateren, 1996; Pelah, 1997).

† When the captain of a 1942 fighting ship signaled "full speed ahead" after he had sighted an enemy submarine, he did not need to know and probably did not even wish to know how the seamen on the lower deck would work together to carry out his order. That the fastest reliable method for carrying out the order had been practiced to perfection was a level of micromanagement for which petty officers carried responsibility. The captain required only that the order be carried out as quickly and effectively as possible—whatever the means adopted.

to synthesize something that functions sufficiently like the human visual system to allow the device to serve as a model. Attempts to synthesize the whole from its parts can also be entirely theoretical. For example, an assembly of theoretical constructs can be represented abstractly within a computer.

In this book I provide a critical review of psychophysical data on the five kinds of spatial contrast that can support image segregation and attempt to integrate those data. The intent is to define what will be required to attain an understanding of image segregation, an understanding that incorporates the early processing *of luminance-defined* (*LD*), *texture-defined* (*TD*), *motion-defined* (*MD*), *color-defined* (*CD*), and *disparity-defined* (*DD*) spatial form. I will focus on the following three early processes: detecting spatial contrast in the retinal image, assigning a unique location to a boundary defined by spatial contrast, and discriminating the spatial characteristics of an object's retinal image (e.g., location, size, shape, and orientation).

Although each is requisite for object perception, these early processes are of course only part of the story. Among the major questions outside the scope of this monograph are the nature of visual experience, visual memory, and attention (see Nakayama, 1990). Spatial vision within the peripheral visual field is discussed only when relevant to foveal function. A number of specific questions that are closer to the focus of this book have not been discussed for reasons of brevity. These include the early processing of shape in the third (depth) dimension, and the question of how a three-dimensional object can be recognized from a single view even though the shape of its retinal image can vary exceedingly with the observer's viewpoint (see Richards et al., 1987; Hildreth, 1998).

The organization of this book is as follows. After noting that this is a book about human vision rather than machine vision, I review in Chapter 1 some of the concepts and methods that are key to all that follows. On pages 25–26, I set out the rationale for psychophysical research that I adopt in this book. Students should be aware that this rationale is quite different from that adopted by some other authors. Both sides of this disagreement have strong and valid arguments. It is a real disagreement that, in my view, is not best dealt with by looking for some consensus. I have contrasted the different rationales as plainly as I can to help readers more easily make up their own minds.

In Chapters 2–6 I discuss, in turn, spatial vision for LD form, CD form, TD form, MD form, and DD form. The organization of Chapters 3–6 is similar to that of Chapter 2. In Chapter 7 I discuss the convergence of spatial information carried by the five kinds of contrast and suggest ways in which data on all five kinds of spatial contrast might be viewed as a whole.

My sympathies lie with the graduate student whose reason for signing on to graduate school was a fervent desire to *do experimental research*; who feels that so-called "library research" is no substitute at all; who has had enough of sitting in class being talked at; and who suspects that too much time and effort can be spent on learning about the scientific literature, believing that these efforts leave less time for empirical research, and might blunt the edge of one's ability to do it. To such students I apologize for the absence of "how to do" in this book and for what might seem its overly academic tone. In the hope of redressing the balance to some small extent I added Appendix J and "A note to students." I shall say no more at this point except to suggest that Platt (1964), Chamberlin (1965), and Woodford (1967) provide useful hints.

Visually Guided Goal-Directed Action

If we assume that the purpose of the visual system is knowable, we might then go on to explore the assumption that this purpose is to provide visual guidance for goal-directed motor action.*

In 1965 Donald MacKay published a formal discussion of goal-directed motor action in which he contrasted conscious action with reflexive reaction. He pointed out that some low-level neurophysiological arrangements have been modeled in terms of a simple human-designed feedback control loop. For example, according to the *servo theory* of the skeletal muscle control system, muscle spindles that discharge into the spinal cord serve as combined indicators and evaluators of muscle length in a control loop similar to Figure 1.2, in which "E" is the main muscle fiber system and "S" is the spinal neuron pool. The resulting tendency is to maintain the muscle at a given equilibrium length, actively resisting the effects of changes in load. In a further analogy, control signals from higher centers act as the "indication of goal" (Matthews, 1964).

In the simple system shown in Figure 1.2, whenever the goal signal (I_G) changes, the signal to evoke the response from E must come entirely by way of

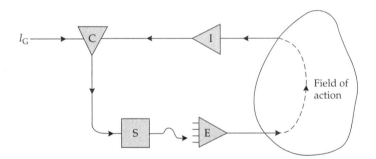

1.2 Simple feedback control loop. Key: I_G: signal that indicates the goal. E: An effector system capable of a range of activities (e.g., heating or cooling), S: A selector that determines the form of activity selected from E's repertoire, according to information received from I. I: An indicator of the variable under control (e.g., temperature), C: A means of calculating the (positive or negative) error signal (e.g., the difference between the desired temperature and the actual temperature). After MacKay (1965).

*Given that the primate visual system evolved over geological time and is (in early life) developed in concert with the motor system, then it might be profitable to bear in mind the characteristics of the motor system when thinking about vision. For example, there may be properties of the visual system that make better sense when considered in the light of motor action and the organization of the motor cortices. On pages 211–215 of Regan (1989a), I provided a brief introduction to the motor cortices with references for further reading.

subsystem C. MacKay pointed out that it is often possible to increase speed and accuracy by arranging that, in addition to the *feedback* signal from C, the selector system S receives an input computed directly from I_G. Even if this *feedforward* only roughly approximates the signal required for E to achieve the desired goal, it will reduce the demands on C, leaving subsystem C free to concentrate on fine adjustment with a consequent enhancement of efficiency (Figure 1.3).

Over 30 years later this concept of MacKay's resurfaced in the proposal that the human cerebellum contains an internal model of the human motor apparatus that allows the motor signals required to achieve a desired goal to be precomputed and delivered in feedforward mode rather than via an error-correcting feedback loop, thus allowing humans to perform actions more quickly than would be required for feedback signals to traverse the feedback loop (Wolpert et al., 1998). The memorable catches that have been achieved by the very few outstanding close-to-the-wicket fielders in cricket, and the astonishing responses of the top goaltenders in ice hockey, are prime contenders for such an explanation.

MacKay noted that a simple servo loop similar to those shown in Figures 1.2 or 1.3 can be used in its turn as the effector in another, higher-order, control system. His example was power-assisted steering in automobiles (Figure 1.4). The driver, steering by information received visually from the road, can be regarded as the evaluator in a second-order control loop in which the entire steering servo acts as an effector. In this example there is scope for action of a new kind: *intelligent action.* Intelligent action makes use of the regularities and redundancies (predictability) in the pattern of demand, so that a given level of performance can be achieved with a smaller amount of incoming information (or a higher level of performance with the same amount).

It is the feedforward system in Figure 1.4 that can be used to profit from predictability. This kind of intelligent adaptation falls under the headings of learning and cognition.

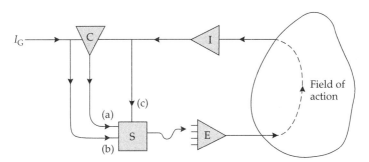

1.3 Simple loop with feedforward. Key: (a): Feedback; (b): feedforward from indication of goal (IG); (c): feedforward from indication of field state. After MacKay (1965).

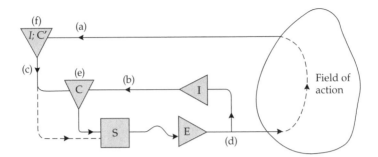

1.4 Second-order control of steering. Key: (a): Information from road; (b): indication of road wheel angle; (c): angle of steering wheel (dashed line shows optional feedforward); (d): angle of road wheels; (e): mechanical comparator; (f): driver (combining functions of second-order indicator, comparator, and goal-setter). After MacKay (1965)

For the reader who wishes to pursue this topic of servo systems and control, Di Stefano et al. (1967) provide an introductory text.

Psychophysical Methods and Psychophysical Models

Psychophysical models are based on psychophysical data, and to understand the nature of psychophysical data, it is necessary to understand how the data are obtained.

Psychophysical methods and data

There are several excellent textbooks on psychophysical methods and psychophysical theory, but most, if not all, are hard going for the beginning graduate student, and are stronger on theory than on practical advice. In the following section I have provided the minimum theoretical background necessary to understand modern psychophysics as well as notes on experimental design and pitfalls.

Standard methods for adult observers.

> Psychophysical models are based on a comparison of the information presented to an observer's eye and the observer's response to that information.

This statement is not as vague as it might seem. In psychophysics, an observer's "response" has a meaning that is far more specific than the everyday meaning of the word. In the wider world of science, the word "information" has a special meaning also. In this section I will review the concept of *psychophysical threshold* at an introductory level that will be sufficient to understand what follows, and I leave for a later section a discussion of the scientific concept of "information."

The psychometric function is central to modern quantitative psychophysics. The basic idea can be understood in terms of the following example (Figure 1.5). Suppose that four small dim lights (called fixation marks) are arranged in the form of a square at one end of a dark room (F1, F2, F3, and F4 in Figure 1.5A). These lights are always switched on. An observer sitting at the other end of the room is instructed to maintain gaze at the center of the square. (If the observer follows this instruction, the experimenter will be able to place stimuli at known retinal locations.) At the center of the square is a stimulator (display D in Figure 1.5A) that, when switched on, displays a homogeneous patch of light whose luminance can be preset to one of, for example, five possible values. One of these values (L_R) is the reference, and the other four ($[L_T]_1, \ldots, [L_T]_4$) are test values, all of which are brighter than the reference. The observer is told that each *trial* will consist of two test intervals that will be designated by two tones, and that the two test intervals will be separated by an intertest interval (see Figure 1.5B). The observer is told that a light will be presented at the center of the fixation area during each of the two test intervals. He or she is instructed to signal whether the brighter light was presented in the first interval or the second interval by pressing one of two buttons labeled "first" and "second." Alternatively, and more commonly, the observer is instructed to signal whether the light presented during the second interval was brighter than the light presented during the first interval.* Some time after the observer responds, a second trial is initiated (see Figure 1.5B), and so on until the required number of trials have been completed.

The trials are organized as follows. In any given trial the reference stimulus is presented during one of the two intervals, and one of the four test stimuli (selected randomly) is presented during the other interval. The reference stimulus is presented first or second on a random basis.

Figure 1.5C shows typical response data. The percentage of "second presentation was brighter than the first" responses is plotted versus the difference between the luminances of the test and reference stimuli in a way that takes into account whether the test stimulus was presented during the first or second interval of a trial. Figure 1.5C shows that when the highest test luminance ($[L_T]_4$) was presented first, the observer never responded "second presentation was brighter," and when test luminance $(L_T)_4$ was presented second, the observer always responded "second presentation was brighter." For progressively lower test luminances ($[L_T]_3$, $[L_T]_2$, and $[L_T]_1$), the observer made progressively more errors.

In order to estimate† the observer's psychophysical threshold, the experimenter fits some function to the data points. The particular function that the experimenter fits to the data points in Figure 1.5C depends on the particular

---

* This signal can take many forms including pressing one button labeled "yes." This kind of response data is not usually plotted in the way depicted in Figure 1.5C.

† Estimation is used here in the sense of approximating a population parameter from data.

(A)

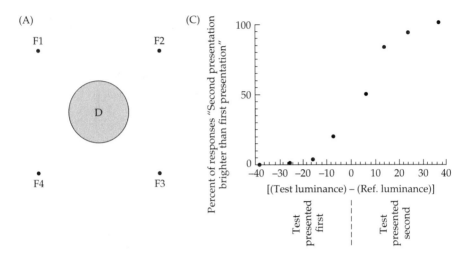

(C)

(B)

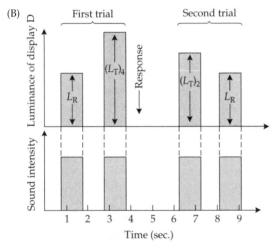

1.5 Psychophysical methods and psychophysical data. Typical optical arrangement (A) and temporal design (B) for the method of temporal two-alternative forced
choice (2AFC). (C) Examples of psychophysical data are shown, while part (D)[fac-
ing page]) shows a curve fitted to the data in (C). (E) The fitted curve in (D) plotted
on probability paper, showing the data points in (C) re-plotted; (ΔL)Th is the 75%
threshold. The typical stimulus arrangement for the method of spatial 2AFC is
shown in (F).

model of the sensory discrimination process favored by the experimenter. One
model calls for the response data to be fitted by a cumulative normal distribution
(Finney, 1971; Macmillan & Creelman, 1991). *Probit analysis* is a procedure for fitting a best-fitting cumulative normal distribution to the response data (see the
continuous line in Figure 1.5D; see also Finney [1971]). The procedure can be

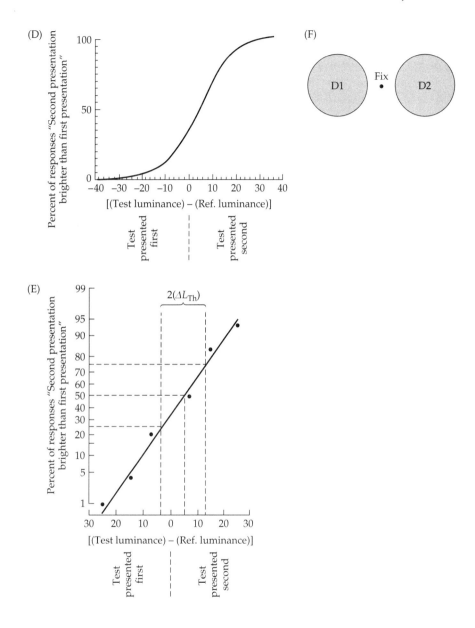

visualized in terms of Figure 1.5E, where the data from part C are plotted on *probability paper*. The best-fitting straight line in part E is the best-fitting cumulative normal distribution in part D.

Parts D and E of Figure 1.5 highlight the point that psychophysical threshold is not a sharp discontinuity. In parts D and E it is not the case that the observer's responses are 100% correct for all values of $(L_T - L_R)$ above a certain level, and 100% wrong for all values below that level. Rather, the observer's performance changes smoothly from chance (50% correct) to nearly 100% correct as the value of $(L_T - L_R)$ is progressively increased.*

Where, then, is the "threshold?"

The location of the threshold is the choice of the experimenter, and different experimenters use different definitions.

Threshold $(\Delta L)_{Th}$ in the case of Figure1.5D and E could be defined as half the distance along the abscissa between the 20% and 80% points on the ordinate. This choice has the advantage that, according to signal detection theory, threshold corresponds to one standard deviation (SD) of the underlying noise distribution. Other authors prefer to define threshold as half the distance along the abscissa between the 25% and 75% points on the abscissa, i.e., the stimulus level that gives a response accuracy halfway between chance and 100% correct. This is the choice illustrated in Figure 1.5E. The 92% correct point (two standard deviations of the underlying noise function) has even been defined as threshold (Bown, 1990). These different choices, of course, give different threshold estimates from the same response data, and this should be borne in mind when comparing thresholds reported by different authors. Fortunately, it is straightforward to convert thresholds based on different points on the psychometric function to a common format (Macmillan & Creelman, 1991).

In Figure 1.5E the 50% point does not fall at zero on the abscissa. In our present case the location on the abscissa of the 50% point is of little interest, but in some of the experiments whose design allows it to be labeled the *point of subjective equality*, adaptation-induced changes in its location can be the main item of interest (see Figure 2.62).

I have found the way of handling psychophysical data that is illustrated in Figure 1.5C–E to be convenient. It has the advantage that bias (the location of the 50% point) is dissociated from the threshold.

An alternative way of plotting a psychometric function is to convert the ordinate to percent correct responses, so that the response level varies between chance (50% correct) and 100% rather than 0% to 100% as in Figure 1.5C. (This is one way to handle an observer's responses to the question, "Was the second presentation brighter than the first?") When fitting a curve to such data, the chosen function must be modified to the 50%–100% format (see Macmillan & Creelman, 1991, p. 190). Detection threshold data obtained by means of the yes–no procedure can be plotted in this way (or in a "corrected for guessing" format; see McKee et al.,

---

* Many—even recent—discussions of so-called subliminal perception are undermined by this point. An observer whose behavior is affected by a stimulus may claim that he or she cannot detect a stimulus even though detection performance is well above chance. This is a potential source of serious embarrassment that can be avoided by measuring the psychometric function for detecting the stimulus in question.

1985). According to McKee et al. (1985), the 0%–100% format leads to more precise estimates of thresholds than does the 50%–100% format.

An alternative model of the sensory discrimination process requires the response data to be fitted to a logistic function rather than a cumulative normal distribution. Berkson (1951, 1953, 1955a,b, 1957, 1960) describes a procedure for fitting a *logistic function* to response data. According to Finney (1971, pp. 94–97) this choice has little effect on threshold estimates, though the threshold is more easily computed because no iteration is required.

A third possibility is the *Weibull function*. It has valuable theoretical properties (Green and Luce, 1975; Quick, 1974), and has often been used in vision research (Graham, 1989; Nachmias, 1981). The choice of theoretical approach is now more consequent: the shapes of the Weibull function and the cumulative normal distribution differ considerably (see Figure 8.2 on p. 189 of Macmillan & Creelman, 1991). The choice of 0%–100% versus 50%–100% ordinate, linear versus logarithmic abscissa, and cumulative normal versus logistic versus Weibull function is discussed succinctly by Macmillan and Creelman (1991, pp. 186–190).

Figure 1.5E brings out the importance of choice of stimulus levels. It is self-evident that the smaller the error in the slope of the line, the higher the precision of the threshold estimate. Points near the midpoint of the line have little effect on the slope of the best-fitting line. For greatest efficiency in estimating the slope of the line, Levitt (1971) and Finney (1971) advise that it is better to err in selecting stimulus levels that give response probabilities that lie further from the midpoint of the curve than by selecting levels that give response probabilities closer to the midpoint of the curve. When probit analysis is to be used, Levitt (1971) recommends that the experimenter should select the stimulus levels so that responses cluster around 80% and 20% in Figure 1.5E. Such points strongly constrain the slope of the line: their errors produce a lower error in the slope estimation than do points closer to the midpoint of the line.

In practice, however, it can be advantageous to choose the highest of the several stimulus levels so that it gives responses that are 100% correct. This has been done in Figure 1.5C. Although the 100% correct points contribute little to the process of estimating threshold (they are lost in part E because there is no 0% or 100% level on probability paper), they serve the purpose of helping to maintain the observer's morale. Some observers who are naive as to the purpose of an experiment (and, in the author's experience, most patients) lose heart and may stop trying when they receive too much "response incorrect" feedback or (when no feedback is provided) are uncertain on too many trials.

> A disheartened observer is prone to generate noisy data, and even the most ingenious method of analysis cannot extract meaning from noise. It is far better to attend closely to the observer's mental (and physical) comfort and thereby obtain less noisy data.

In selecting the test stimulus levels the experimenter treads a fine line. If the proportion of trials that produce a 100%-correct response is too great, some observers become a little careless, and the resulting threshold estimate is a little too high. But an estimate that is "a little too high" is better than rubbishy data.

A detailed discussion of errors in estimating threshold, especially when the total number of responses is low (as is, unavoidably, the case in many clinical and infant studies), is provided by McKee et al. (1985).

Achieving the optimal placement of points is akin to hitting a moving target. In addition to the everyday circadian variations of threshold (for example, Barlow et al. [1997] note that the circadian variation of contrast threshold is about three-fold; see also Bassi and Powers [1986]), and the effects of possible overindulgence during the previous 24 hours or so, threshold progressively falls as the observer learns the task. For the most reliable thresholds, it is usual to plot threshold estimates through the learning period until an asymptotic level has been reached (McKee & Westheimer, 1978; Fahle, 1997; Herzog & Fahle, 1997) and, according to my experience, carry out the measurement at the same time of the day. However, there is no avoiding the fact that the method of constant stimuli is a clumsy instrument when one is attempting to hit a rapidly moving target (e.g., when sensitivity is changing due to adaptation). Tracking procedures, described later in this section are more convenient in that regard.

The threshold described on pp. 9–12 is called luminance increment threshold or luminance discrimination threshold. If the luminance of the reference stimulus had been zero, the threshold could have been labeled a luminance detection threshold (the two tones are essential only in this case.)

Westheimer and McKee (1977) showed that the reference stimulus is not really necessary. It can be omitted, and the observer instructed to signal whether the test luminance is higher or lower than the mean of the stimulus set. After sufficient trials have been presented to ensure that the observer has learned the task, the response data collected using no reference stimulus and the data collected using a reference stimulus usually support similar threshold estimates. The explanation for this finding is controversial (see pp. 184–191).

In the procedure described we combined the method of constant stimuli with *temporal two-alternative forced choice* (temporal 2AFC; see below for a definition of *forced choice*).

Figure 1.5F illustrates a typical optical setup for a second kind of forced choice procedure called *spatial 2AFC*. In spatial 2AFC, there is a single fixation mark (FIX) and two displays (D1 and D2). One display is the reference and the other is one of the test stimuli. The reference is randomly presented by D1 or D2 and the test stimulus in any given trial is a random selection from the test stimulus set. The observer is instructed to signal whether D2 is brighter or dimmer than D1 (or vice versa). The response data are treated as for temporal 2AFC. The observer may be instructed to fixate the mark continuously or, alternatively, be allowed to look from one display to the other.

The label "forced choice" is misleading insofar as the choices made by observers in forced choice procedures are no more constrained than in many other procedures in which "I don't know" is not an acceptable response. As in many other procedures there are two possible classes of stimuli. The defining feature of 2AFC is that *both classes are presented on every trial* (in a random temporal or random spatial order). The observer is not required to indicate which class of stimuli was presented (since both were presented), but rather the order of presentation (e.g., first/second or left/right). Note that forced choice designs always employ two stimulus classes, but the number of possible responses need not necessarily be two (i.e., more generally, *m* AFC).

Methods that do not fit this description are, by definition, not forced choice methods. For example, in one *reminder* experimental design, the reference stimulus is always presented first using the method of constant stimuli. This may improve the performance of unpracticed observers and can, therefore, be useful, especially when the task is unusually difficult; but it is not a forced choice procedure (Macmillan & Creelman, 1991, pp. 134–143). See Figure 1.7 for an example of data collected using this "reminder" procedure.

One reason for using 2AFC is that 2AFC discourages bias. This does not mean, however, that bias is necessarily absent. For example, in spatial 2AFC some observers may be biased towards the item presented on the right (for a telling example, see Macmillan & Creelman, 1991, p. 137). And if the observer uses different hands to press two different buttons, a hand preference (or even a sore thumb) can cause one button to be favored over the other. This kind of bias is indicated by a bodily shift of the psychometric function (as in Figure 1.5C). Also, in temporal 2AFC, a briefly lived adaptation effect can cause the sensory effect of a stimulus to depend on whether it is presented first or second.

Forced choice procedures are commonly used by investigators who focus on sensory processing, and wish to measure the observer's sensitivity without having to allow for the observer's criterion. The concept of psychophysical criterion, important in itself, is discussed in Green and Swets (1974, pp. 43–45), Macmillan and Creelman (1991, pp. 5–55), and by Swets (1973).

One method for quantifying criterion (as well as sensitivity) is by analyzing the results of a *yes–no* experiment. In the *one-interval yes–no* design, for example, a single stimulus drawn from one of two stimulus classes is presented on each trial, and the observer is instructed to signal from which class it is drawn. This yes–no experiment measures *discrimination,* i.e., the ability to tell two stimuli apart. If one of the two stimulus classes is a stimulus intensity of zero, the experiment measures detection sensitivity. Suppose that 50 presentations of stimulus A and 50 presentations of stimulus B are interleaved randomly, and that the observer correctly identifies stimulus A forty times. The *hit rate* (*H*) is 0.8. Suppose further that on 20 of the 50 presentations of stimulus B the observer incorrectly responds "stimulus A." The *false alarm rate* (*F*) is 0.4. The sensitivity measure (*d'*) is defined in terms of *z*, the inverse of the normal distribution function

$$d' = z(H) - z(F) \tag{1.1}$$

By consulting a table of *z* values (e.g., Macmillan & Creelman, 1991, p. 318) it can be seen that in our example (where *H* = 0.8 and *F* = 0.4) that the value of *d'* is

1.095. A d' of 1.0 is equal to one SD of the underlying normal distribution. The value of d' has considerable theoretical significance in the context of signal detection theory and can be converted into a location on the psychometric function.

In many experiments it is the observer's criterion that is of interest. The observer's criterion can be quantified in several ways including the *likelihood ratio* (β), defined by the following equation

$$\log (\beta) = -0.5[z(H)^2 - z(F)^2] \qquad (1.2)$$

(Swets, 1973; Macmillan & Creelman, 1971, 40).

Rating experiments differ from yes–no experiments only in the response set available to the observer. For example, the observer may use a numerical scale (e.g., 1 to 10) to express great confidence in one alternative (e.g., 10) through uncertainty (e.g., 5) to great confidence in the other alternative (e.g., 1). This method is discussed in Macmillan and Creelman (1991, pp. 58–62). Rating procedures have been favored by several authors. For example, a *maximum likelihood* procedure* described by Dorfman and Alf (1969) has been used both by Levi and by Klein in many of their investigations of spatial vision (e.g., Levi & Klein, 1982, 1983; Klein, 1985a,b).

The method of constant stimuli requires the experimenter to choose the set of stimulus levels in advance and, because only a narrow range of the psychometric function is useful (near-chance or near-perfect responses are almost useless for the purpose of estimating threshold), the experimenter must first locate this critical range—a task that can be frustrated by day-to-day changes in its location. In contrast, when an adaptive method is used, any given stimulus is selected on the basis of the observer's previous responses. The adaptive procedure itself "homes on to" the critical range of the psychometric function; because its purpose is to locate a point on the psychometric function, an adaptive procedure, by its nature, concentrates the test stimuli into a range of levels close to the desired point.

Experimenters whose primary interest is the observer's sensitivity can choose to combine forced choice methods with *adaptive tracking procedures*.

The simplest adaptive procedure (the up–down method) is to increase the stimulus level by some fixed amount (the *step size*) if the observer responds correctly and to decrease the stimulus level by the same amount if the observer responds incorrectly until the *staircase* (i.e., successive responses) oscillates about the 50% point on the psychometric function (Békésy, 1947; Wetherill, 1966; Wetherill & Levitt, 1965).

A problem that was soon encountered by the early users of staircase methods is that the observer can anticipate the next stimulus if only one staircase is used. To avoid this problem it is usual to interleave (randomly) two or more staircases.

---

* To make a maximum-likelihood estimation is to estimate a parameter by finding the value for which the observed data are most likely.

More efficient adaptive tracking procedures start with a large step size and reduce it by a predetermined amount at a predetermined stage of the staircase.

Levitt (1971) has documented tracking rules that cause a staircase to converge onto a point of the psychometric function other than the 50% point. He drew attention to two important features of this *"transformed up-down method"*:

> The threshold estimate does not depend on the experimenter's model of sensory discrimination. That is, the estimate is not obtained by fitting some function (e.g., cumulative normal distribution, logistic, Weibull) to the response data. A second feature is that it is possible to track gradual drifts of visual sensitivity.

So far we have assumed that successive responses are statistically independent. Levitt (1967) gives a procedure for testing that assumption and revealing any *sequential dependencies*.

Macmillan and Creelman (1991, pp. 190–208) discuss the relative advantages of different adaptive packages including PEST (Taylor & Creelman, 1967), Best PEST (Penland, 1980; Liberman & Penland, 1982), QUEST (Watson & Pelli, 1983), APE (Watt & Andrews, 1981), and Hall's hybrid procedure (Hall, 1981).

PEST's computation of the next stimulus level to be presented depends on the past history of the run, *but only on recent history*. In maximum-likelihood procedures, a best estimate is calculated after each trial but this estimate is *based on the entire history of the run*. The next level is set to that estimate, and the run continues. The maximum-likelihood computation assumes that the underlying psychometric function follows some particular equation such as cumulative normal distribution, logistic, or Weibull (Madigan & Williams, 1987). The maximum-likelihood approach is used in BestPEST, QUEST, APE, and Hall's hybrid procedure. As an aid to experimental design, Macmillan and Creelman (1991, pp. 305–312) provide a useful flow chart to help experimenters choose the most appropriate procedure.

It should be noted, however, that adaptive tracking methods are not necessarily faster than the method of constant stimuli. According to McKee et al. (1985, p. 286): "The variability of staircase estimates of threshold cannot be less than the variability of threshold estimates derived from the method of constant stimuli given an optimum placement of trials."

A psychophysical pitfall.

> No animal intelligence so captured the imagination of layman and scholar alike as that attributed to Clever Hans, the horse of Mr. von Osten. Hans gave every evidence of being able to add and subtract, multiply and divide—operations performed with equal accuracy upon integers or fractions. He was also able to read and spell, to identify musical tones, and to state the relationship of tones to one another. His preferred mode of communication was by means of converting all his answers to a number and tapping out these numbers with his foot. . . . [O]n September 12, 1904, thirteen men risked their professional reputations by certifying that Hans was receiving no intentional cues from his owner or from

any other questioner. Furthermore, these men including in their number a psychologist, a physiologist, a veterinarian, a director of the Berlin Zoo, and a circus manager, certified that their investigations revealed no presence of signs or cues of even an unintentional nature.

"This is a case," the investigating committee wrote, "which appears in principle to differ from any hitherto discovered." A "serious and incisive" inquiry into the cleverness of Hans was recommended, and subsequently conducted. Oskar Pfungst and Carl Strumf, who conducted the inquiry concluded that: "the slight forward inclination of the questioner's head, to better see Hans' hoof tapping was the signal for Hans to start tapping" and that, "Hans was sensitive to tiny upward motions of the head, even to the raising of eyebrows or the dilation of nostrils, any of which was sufficient to stop his tapping." Most interesting was the finding that, even after he had learnt the cueing system very well, Pfungst still cued Hans unintentionally, though he was consciously trying to suppress sending the crucial visual messages. (Pfungst, 1911/1965, pp. ix–xii)

Figure 1.6 shows Clever Hans and notes of his correct answers.

Although the psychophysical methods described earlier allow an observer's sensitivity to be quantified rigorously, the methods offer only partial protection from extreme embarrassment. A question arises: "Have I quantified the sensitivity that I thought I was quantifying?"

One might obtain a good-looking psychometric function using, say, temporal 2AFC. But what if the variable that you have plotted along the x-axis is not the

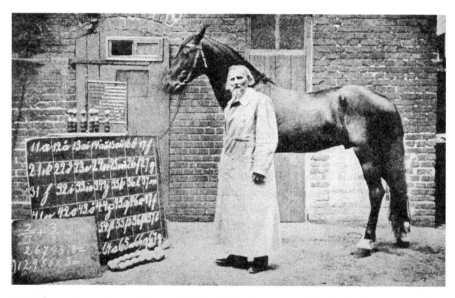

1.6 Clever Hans. From Pfungst (1911/1965). Copyright Holt & Co. Reproduced by permission.

variable on which the observer based his or her responses? What if the observer's responses were based on some other variable that co-varied with your target variable? How would you know?

The following anecdote illustrates the degree of unfriendliness that this problem can assume. While measuring contrast sensitivity functions of juveniles, I encountered a young gentleman (aged 8 years) whose contrast thresholds were many times lower than any in the literature. This result was repeatable, and I was using the well-accepted psychophysical method of temporal 2AFC. I carefully recalibrated the equipment using several methods. The young gentleman continued to generate excellent psychometric functions, responding with 100% accuracy to gratings for which my responses were at chance. Several sessions later I had run control experiments for every artifact that I could think of, even putting the monitor in one room and all the other equipment in the next room but two. Finally, I placed the monitor inside an insulated box with a small window on one side and, somewhat desperately, even placed the box within a Faraday cage made of chicken-wire netting. Contrast detection threshold rose at once to the level of a rather ordinary 8-year-old.

To test the obvious explanation I equipped myself with a microphone and oscilloscope, took the monitor from its box, and found that the sinusoidal voltage I was applying to the monitor in order to create the grating caused the monitor to produce a sound whose frequency was higher than I could hear but was not, evidently, beyond the hearing range of the young gentleman who, even when confronted with the sound recordings, still continued to smile enigmatically when I asked how he decided whether the grating was presented first or second.

This was in 1979, and ever since I have felt unease at the fact that it is not possible to be 100% certain as to whether the observer followed the instruction to base his or her responses on the task-relevant variables and to ignore all task-irrelevant variables, because it is not possible to be 100% certain that you have identified all the task-irrelevant variables that co-vary with the task-relevant variable.

> In principle, however, it is possible to establish that an observer's responses were not based on any of several known task-irrelevant variables.

One popular way of addressing this problem is to impose a random trial-to-trial variation on one or more task-irrelevant variables. For example, when measuring the Weber fraction for discriminating a grating's spatial frequency, it is possible that an observer might be influenced by changes in perceived contrast associated with changes in spatial frequency and not base his or her responses entirely on the task-relevant variable (spatial frequency in this case). Here, we might introduce random trial-to-trial variations of contrast in an attempt to render perceived contrast a less-reliable cue to spatial frequency. The effectiveness of this stratagem is, however, often limited. It is often the case that only a small range of random variation is possible. And it is difficult to be certain that the stratagem has succeeded.

An alternative approach to this problem that I have found to be useful (Regan & Hamstra, 1993), is to adopt a variant of the "concurrent paradigm" (Graham, 1989, pp. 337–379). For example, Vincent and Regan (1995) arranged a stimulus set that can be visualized as a 6 × 6 × 6 cube of test stimulus cells. The 216 cells corresponded to 216 test gratings that had different combination of spatial frequency, orientation, and contrast. Spatial frequency varied along one edge of the cube, but orientation and contrast were constant along that edge. Orientation varied along a second edge of the cube, but spatial frequency and contrast were constant along that edge. Contrast varied along the third edge of the cube, but spatial frequency and orientation were constant along that edge. In other words, spatial frequency, orientation, and contrast were orthogonal within the set of 216 test stimuli. The spatial frequency, orientation, and contrast of the reference stimulus were equal to the corresponding means for the set of 216 test stimuli.

Consider the case in which the observer was instructed to discriminate spatial frequency only. The response data contained in the 216 response cells could be analyzed in three ways so as to give three psychometric functions, all of which had the same ordinate but had either spatial frequency, orientation, or contrast plotted along the abscissa. If the slope of the first psychometric function was steep while the other two were perfectly flat, we could conclude that the observer totally ignored trial-to-trial variations in both orientation and contrast.

Figure 1.7A–I shows the results of a three-task experiment in which, after each trial, the observer was required to discriminate spatial frequency, orientation, and contrast. Figure 1.7A–I indicates that, when carrying out each of the three tasks, the observer ignored almost completely trial-to-trial variations in the two task-irrelevant variables. I will not discuss multitask procedures further. Readers who wish to pursue this topic are referred to Graham (1989) and to Pohlman and Sorkin (1976).

The experimental design just described is simple in that the three relevant variables could be rendered orthogonal within the entire set of test stimuli. In such a situation, stepwise regression is an alternative method of analysis. In some experimental situations, however, it is not possible to render all the task-relevant and task-irrelevant variables orthogonal within the entire set of test stimuli. Regression analysis can be unsatisfactory in such cases; because of the intercor-

1.7 Nine psychometric functions obtained simultaneously. The 216 trial stimuli ▶ were presented in random order. The stimuli were gratings whose six possible orientations, six possible spatial frequencies, and six possible contrasts were combined in many different ways. These three variables were orthogonal within the stimulus set. The observers' task was to signal, after each trial, whether the grating's orientation was clockwise or anticlockwise of the mean for the stimulus set, and also whether its spatial frequency and contrast were higher or lower than the mean for the stimulus set (3 tasks). Thus, for each of the three tasks, the observer was required to unconfound variations in the task-relevant variable from simultaneous trial-to-trial variations in the two task-irrelevant variables. These psychometric functions show that the observer performed the tasks almost perfectly. From Vincent and Regan (1995).

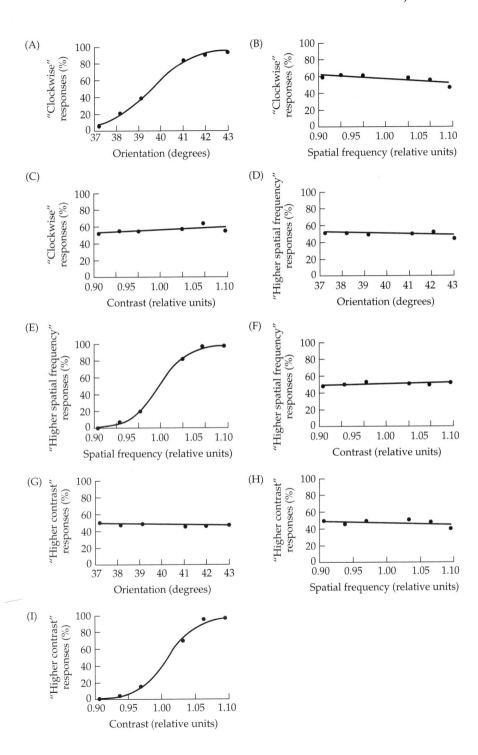

relations between variables, the partial regression coefficients can be disappointingly low for an experimenter who feels confident that the observer's performance was better than the statistical analysis seems to indicate.

An approach that I have found useful is to divide the set of test stimuli into subsets, and to render the task-relevant variable orthogonal with respect to one (or more) task-irrelevant variables within each subset. If the subsets are organized so that the observer is unable to tell from which subset any given stimulus is drawn, then we can assume that the observer will use the same response strategy for the entire set of test stimuli. (And this can be confirmed by checking that the task-relevant variable gives the same psychometric function for every one of the subsets.) An example of this approach was described by Kohly and Regan (1998, 1999a) in the context of measuring the Weber fraction for discriminating the speed of a cyclopean grating. In this example, there were no less than five task-irrelevant variables (namely, distance moved during the presentation, spatial frequency, temporal frequency, presentation duration, and perceived depth of the corrugation) so that five subsets were required. Within each subset, speed was rendered orthogonal to one or more of the task-irrelevant variables. The response data gave a total of 10 psychometric functions in which the five with speed plotted as abscissa had the same (steep) slope, while the other five had much shallower slopes. The fact that the speed psychometric functions were far steeper than the other five psychometric functions meant that the observer's responses were much more strongly influenced by trial-to-trial variation in speed than by trial-to-trial variations in any of the five task-irrelevant variables.

To deal with the problem that the slopes of the task-irrelevant functions, though shallow, were not perfectly flat, Kohly and Regan (1998, 1999a) defined a *confidence ratio*. They calculated this ratio as follows: From the first subset, calculate the ratio between the Weber fraction for the psychometric function in which distance moved was plotted along the abscissae and the Weber fraction for the psychometric function in which speed was plotted along the abscissa. Then repeat this calculation for the remaining four subsets. The lowest of these five ratios is the confidence ratio.

The confidence ratio quantified the degree to which we may be confident that the observer based his or her responses on trial-to-trial variations of the task-relevant variable while ignoring trial-to-trial variations in all five task-irrelevant variables.

Infant psychophysics. One kind of problem that the experimenter can encounter with young observers was brought out by my anecdote about the enigmatic young gentleman who *would not* speak. A second kind of problem is faced by experimenters whose subjects are infants who *cannot* speak—nor do very much at all except sleep, feed, and develop their brains at an astonishing rate.

It is difficult to overstate the importance of infant psychophysics. First, it is of great scientific importance to understand how the sensory (and cognitive) systems develop to normal adult levels, and the degree to which sensory experience and interpersonal interactions with the mother (e.g., being talked at) are essential for attaining the analytic capabilities of the visual (and auditory) systems that are necessary for adult-level skills of eye–hand coordination and communication.

Also, early detection of abnormal development can allow better management of the developmental disorder. The early treatment of amblyopia to prevent permanent visual loss is a case in point (see, for example, Levi, 1991, and Regan, 1989a, pp. 524–531 and pp. 465–470, respectively). A second illustration of this general point is the importance of early detection of hearing loss in low-birth-weight "at risk" neonates, so that hearing aids can be provided to allow normal language development.*

Psychophysical procedures that are suitable for adults are usually not suitable for infants. But there is an alternative that works well with infants younger than about 10 to18 months. *Preferential looking* methods are based on the observation that, given a choice, an infant prefers to look at a patterned stimulus rather than an unpatterned stimulus. Davida Teller (1979) converted this observation into a refined forced choice psychophysical procedure that quantifies the infant's preference. In Teller's method, called *forced choice preferential looking* (FPL), an infant is presented with a patterned stimulus that is either to the left or to the right of the center of a large unpatterned screen. The mean luminances of the screen and the pattern are matched so that, if an infant's visual acuity is too low to resolve the pattern, it will see the entire screen as patternless. An observer stationed behind the screen looks through a small peephole at the center of the screen and, on each trial, judges whether the infant looks to the left or right of the peephole. Above-chance performance *on the part of the observer* indicates that the infant can resolve the grating. For rigorous measurements, the psychophysical method of constant stimuli can be combined with FPL (Teller, 1979; Gwiazda et al., 1980, 1986; Held, 1991; Teller & Movshon, 1986; Mohn & Van Hof–Van Duin, 1991).

Brain recording techniques that are of value in testing the sensory function of neonates and infants are reviewed in Regan (1989a) and Regan and Spekreijse (1986).

Information

Within the context of communication or information theory the term *information* has a more restricted and precise definition than in everyday usage and, subject

---

* "As the human brain develops during the first year of life, the words and sentences others utter supply an auditory input that interacts somehow with gene-directed maturational processes to initiate permanent brain changes and the ability to speak one's native language. No one knows how early in life this interaction begins, so the conservative audiological program aimed at preventing delay in language-learning will identify the deaf baby and eliminate his handicap as soon as possible after birth." Galambos (1986) thus identifies the prevention of a potentially devastating consequence of ear disease in babies as a major role of techniques for recording brain responses to auditory stimulation in newborns. I provide a summary of this topic, the cost/benefit analysis, and the identification of "at risk babies" in Regan (1989a, pp. 487–491).

to this severe restriction of meaning, information can be measured quantitatively in a way that does not depend on the physical units of the stimulus and response.

> Information is something we gain when an event tells us something we did not already know. The amount of information gained is measured by the amount of uncertainty that is lost and is quantified on a log scale in, for example, bits (i.e., binary digits).

This can be understood as follows. Suppose that one wishes to find a book in a library, and knows already that the book is located on one of two shelves. If the librarian points out which of the two alternative shelves it is on, the two alternatives (2^1) are reduced to one (2^0) and one bit of information has been transmitted. If there had been four possible shelves to choose from, the librarian would have transmitted two bits of information (2^2) in pointing out the correct shelf. In general, N bits of information are transmitted when 2^N equally likely alternatives are reduced to one. A slightly more complex formula is required when all alternatives are not equally likely (Attneave, 1959; Allusi, 1970).

The scientific definition of information is closely related to the definition of entropy in statistical thermodynamics. (Heat flows from high to low temperatures, never from low to high; a ball rolls down and never up a slope; the state of the physical world progresses towards a higher and higher probability [i.e., entropy increases]: everything is slowly degrading and running down and, eventually, the "clock will stop.") A thorough discussion of this and related issues is available in Brillouin (1962).

The *communication theory* of Shannon and Weaver (1949) and the *information theories* of Gabor (1946) and of MacKay (1950, 1956) were developed in the context of radio and telephonic communication, but were subsequently applied to a remarkably broad range of different areas. Communication theory provided a quantitative definition of information and rate of flow of information along a *"passive communication channel,"* which is defined as shown in Figure 1.8.

According to Shannon and Weaver's communication theory, a message is selected from a "source" and coded for transmission over a "communication channel" for subsequent decoding into a form appropriate for its final "destina-

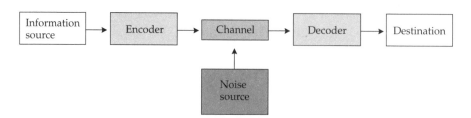

1.8 Schematic diagram of the flow of information through a communication channel. After Shannon and Weaver (1949).

tion" (see Figure 1.8). In the process of transmission, undesirable changes ("noise") may be introduced that distort or degrade the signal. This, in essence, is the idea that has been borrowed from engineering to serve as a conceptual tool in sensory psychophysics, cognitive psychology, and neuroscience.

Some caution is called for when applying the concepts of communication theory (such as, for example, channel capacity) to human perception. As already stated, the communication theory of Shannon and Weaver was originally formulated in the context of a passive communication channel. But a passive channel is not always a good model of human information processing. For example, what corresponds to the *destination* in the human visual system? Information theory presupposes the existence of someone to receive the information. Again, the classic definition of information does not allow for the subjective importance of a communication. If there are two equally likely possibilities—you will/you will not be shot at dawn tomorrow—from a communication theory point of view, these two possibilities are not weighted differently; the announcement of your fate transmits one bit of information, whatever the outcome.

Class A and Class B observations

As to how psychophysical data may be interpreted in terms of neural mechanisms, I can do no better than refer to G. S. Brindley. He noted that the main function of science is the formulation and testing of hypotheses, and went on to say that although "it would seem that no physiological hypothesis that is also stated in physical, chemical and anatomical terms can ever predict the result of a sensory experiment, in which a report of sensations is concerned" one exception should be made. It is difficult to doubt the hypothesis that "whenever two stimuli cause physically indistinguishable signals to be sent from the sense organs to the brain, the sensations produced by these stimuli, as reported by the subject in words, symbols or actions, must also be indistinguishable." He defined Class A observations as those "that assert merely that 'the stimuli α and β under conditions X, Y produce the same sensation' or 'the stimuli α and β under conditions X, Y produce different sensations." Any observation that cannot be expressed as the identity or non-identity of two sensations he termed a Class B observation.

Noting that the use of Class A observations as a basis for analyzing the function of the eye and visual pathway is generally accepted, he stated that the value of Class B observations in this context is quite controversial. Citing the report of the Committee on Vision of the Optical Society of America (1933–1934) and the "admirable papers on visual subjects of Dr. W. S. Stiles" as expressing (explicitly or implicitly) a "Class A only" viewpoint, Brindley contrasted this with the "extreme liberal opinion" of Dr. S. S. Stevens, who makes "no distinction between Class A and Class B, nor any similar division of sensory experiments, and holds that all sensory observations that can be made consistently, and upon which different subjects agree, should be equally admissible as means of analyzing the function of sensory pathways." Taking the middle ground, Brindley concluded that "Class B observations can sometimes provide valuably suggestive evidence."

Brindley added that: "If a physiological hypothesis, i.e., a hypothesis about function that is stated in physical, chemical and anatomical terms, is to imply a given result for a sensory experiment, the background of theory assumed in conjunction with it must be enlarged to include hypotheses containing psychological terms as well as physicochemical and anatomical. These may be called *psychophysical linking hypotheses*" (Brindley, 1970, pp. 132–135).

Psychophysics is not physiology: Mathematical versus structural models of a system

We begin by considering the nature of a psychophysical model. As already mentioned, quantitative psychophysical models of visual perception are based on a comparison of the information presented to an observer's eye and the observer's responses to that information. Therefore, they model the activity of the visual system as a whole.*

A psychophysical model that is framed entirely in terms of sequential stages of processing lumps together the consequences of feedforward, feedback, and lateral neural connections within the visual system; efferent as well as afferent signals; interactions between widely distributed systems of the cortex; and interactions between the cortex and the (at least) 20 subcortical nuclei that are reciprocally connected to the cortex (Mountcastle, 1979, 1995; Tigges & Tigges, 1985). The finding that the lateral geniculate body receives perhaps 10 fibers that originate in primary visual cortex for every one that originates in the retina (Gilbert & Kelly, 1975) conveys some feel for the magnitude of information feedback within the visual system. Even retinal function cannot be regarded as a series of sequential processes with no feedback (Figure 1.9). Readers who seek to understand the anatomy and physiology that underlie visual perception could do no better than read *Perceptual Neuroscience* by Vernon Mountcastle.

The nature of a psychophysical model can be understood in terms of the distinction made in *systems analysis* between the functional (i.e., mathematical) model of a system that enables the system's output for any arbitrary input to be predicted, versus the structural model of the same system (i.e., a description of the system's physical parts, and their interconnections) (Marmarelis & Marmarelis, 1978; White & Tauber, 1969). A psychophysical model is an example of what is meant by a functional or mathematical model in the context of systems

---

* Many definitions of "system" are current in science and engineering. Furthermore, the term is also used somewhat casually in the news media. Formal definitions usually include the notion of purpose or goal. For example, a system is a "collection of interacting functional units that are combined to achieve purposive behaviour" or "an integrated assembly of interacting elements designed to carry out cooperatively a predetermined function" (White & Tauber, 1969, p. 3). Among the many human-made systems that have been studied thoroughly by means of quantitative mathematical methods of linear and nonlinear systems analysis are the following: a system for supplying electrical power to an entire country; the servo-control systems of a heavy jet aircraft; the control system of a nuclear reactor; the sewage system of a city treated as a whole.

Direction of incoming light

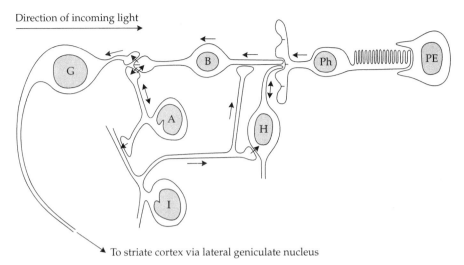

To striate cortex via lateral geniculate nucleus

1.9 Signal feedback and lateral interactions within the retina. Light enters from the left and passes through the retina before reaching the photoreceptors (Ph) and produces an electrochemical signal that flows against the direction of the incoming light to the ganglion cells (G); from there it passes (via the lateral geniculate nucleus) to primary visual cortex. The neural network consists of horizontal (H), bipolar (B), amacrine (A), and interlexiform (I) cells. Arrows indicate signal flow. PE indicates pigment epithelium. After Ehinger (1985).

analysis. The force of this distinction is that, for a system composed of multiple interconnected nonlinear parts, the system as a whole may have *system properties*—functional properties that are created by the interconnections between the parts—that do not necessarily exist at the level of the individual parts (Marmarelis & Marmarelis, 1978; Mountcastle, 1979).* In other words, such a system may be *qualitatively* different from any of its parts. In this sense, psychophysical and structural models of the visual system are complementary descriptions of the same nonlinear system. Thus, my focus is different, and in a sense less ambitious, than the aim of psychophysicists who seek to explain vision in terms of known physiological entities. Relevant here is Westheimer's (1986)

---

* Our understanding of the points just mentioned is usually attributed to the development of systems science. According to White and Tauber (1969, p. 1), "The power and utility of systems concepts and methods in technology, management, economics and other fields, although clearly traceable to classical mathematics and science and more dramatically to the complex technical and scientific development of World War II, have become generally recognized only since the mid 1950s." It is intriguing that even before the publication of his 1926 book, the philosopher Jan Smuts had coined the word "holism," which he defined as "a unity of parts which is so close and intense as to be more than the sums of its parts . . . . There is a progressive grading of this holistic synthesis from (a) mere physical mixtures, where the structure is almost negligible, and the parts largely preserve their separate characters

statement that such writings portray "the preoccupation of current psychologists with the interim findings of physiology instead of concentrating on their birthright."

An exchange of opinions that bears on the general problems of relating the properties of brain cells to the behavior of the organism as a whole focused on the comparatively simple issue of *central pattern generators* (Selverston et al., 1980). (A central pattern generator is a neural mechanism that is responsible for generating repetitive motor actions [Kaneko, 1980].) The exchange of opinions exposed, for discussion, an implicit assumption of those who conceive the physical structure of the brain in terms of "compartments," "mechanisms," or "modules." This assumption is that the group of neurons in question is an independent functional unit rather than a group of neurons whose population properties are influenced by the rest of the central nervous system. Or, putting this another way: To what extent are the properties of one's putative neural mechanism a laboratory artifact created by designing one's experiment on the assumption that the group of neurons is an independent unit?

Selverston (p. 561) stated that "the central pattern generator is a machine—a complex operating system made up of interrelated parts" and, crucially, went on to assert: "To understand its operation we must know the number of parts it contains and as much as possible about the characteristics of each part." He emphasized the technical difficulty of identifying all the neurons involved in a central pattern generator (CPG), and drew attention to the large number of variables that must be known in order to specify the operation of each neuron. (Bullock [1976] listed 46 properties with which integration of signals and neural states may be accomplished.)

The reductionist assumption was strongly challenged in this exchange of opinions—even in the context of understanding a central pattern generator consisting of only a few dozen neurons. It was asserted that understanding a group of as few as 30 brain cells verges on the impossible. In response to Selverston's statement, Kaneko (1980, p. 54) commented that if the minimum requirement for "understanding" a CPG is indeed to know the membrane properties, synaptic properties, and all the connections of all the individual neurons that constitute the CPG, then the task is (at the least) overwhelming. "After all, it is quite unusu-

---

and activities or functions, to (b) chemical compounds where the structure is more synthetic and the activities and functions of the parts are strongly influenced by the new structure and can only with difficulty be traced to the individual parts; and, again, to (c) organisms, where a still more intense synthesis of elements has been effected, which impresses the parts or organs far more intimately with a unified character, and a system of central control, regulation and co–ordination of all the parts, and organs arises." (Smuts, 1926). (In earlier lives, the philosopher Jan Smuts had been General Jan Smuts, Commander of Boer Forces in the Cape, during the Anglo–Boer War of 1899–1902, had been appointed by his former enemy to the British War Cabinet during the desperate months of 1917, and had exerted his utmost efforts—though with tragically insufficient effect—to soften the terms of the Versailles Peace Treaty which, as Plenipotentiary for South Africa, he signed in 1919 [Smuts, Jr., 1952]).

al to hold the opinion that to understand the operation of a digital computer one must understand the critical variables of every individual circuit element. Nevertheless, very many people understand computers well enough to use them." And, echoing Kaneko's comment, several others preferred that the title of Selverston's target article ("Are central pattern generators understandable?") would have been more optimistic—along the lines of "At what level will central pattern generators be understood?"—adding that "philosophy leads to pessimism, research to understanding" (Selverston, 1980, p. 561).

Summarizing this section:

1. The mathematical level of description may be exceedingly difficult to relate to the structural level of description, even for nonlinear systems that are vastly simpler than the human visual system.*
2. The sequence of processing stages in a psychophysical model of visual information processing may have little relation to the peripheral-to-central sequence of cortical areas.
3. The question of where in the visual system a particular process is carried out may not be meaningful: The physical basis of a system property cannot be assigned any discrete location within the system.†

Appendix A provides a more detailed discussion of the distinctions between psychophysical and structural models of the visual system.

I have heard it asserted that psychophysics is unnecessary; that physiology is the basic brain science; and that the psychophysics can be inferred from the physiology. Psychophysics students who feel intimidated by the astonishing achievements of physiologists should realize that, as we stand today, the above statement is not so much wrong as nonsensical.

Arguably, it is not necessarily the case that a useful psychophysical model would be "physiologically plausible" in the sense that each stage of the model corresponds to some kind of neuron or cortical area that is known at the present time. It might even be counterproductive to emphasize physiological plausibility in the absence of either a sufficiently detailed knowledge of all the physiological subunits within the visual system, or a sufficient understanding of the mathematical

---

* Although the neocortex of humans is only 3 to 4 mm thick it has, because of its convolutions, an area of approximately 2600 cm^2. It contains up to 28×10^9 neurons and approximately the same number of glial cells. Cortical neurons are connected with each other and with subcortical nuclei through a vast number (about 10^{12}) of synapses (Mountcastle, 1997). Roughly half the cells in the cortex receive visual inputs. Mountcastle (1999) provides a fascinating account of perceptual neuroscience.

† In the context of brain imaging using techniques such as fMRI, this point implies that unless some given brain function is shown not to be a system property, then the finding that some location within the brain shows greater activity when this particular function is being exercised than when it is not cannot be taken to indicate that the physiological basis for the particular function has any particular location within the brain.

principles that underlie their cooperative functioning. A mathematical understanding of the physical principles of the cooperative operation of visual-system
neurons is a different and, perhaps, more remote goal than a successful psychophysical model of the operation of the visual system as a whole. And
although it may well be interesting to speculate on possible physiological bases
for one's psychophysical findings, it is by no means necessary to do so. The
search for physiological "relevance" at single-cell level inserted into many otherwise excellent psychophysical reports sometimes has an air of desperation akin to
the sight of a heavyweight boxer trying to fit into an airline seat.

> As a science, psychophysics is self-sufficient. It has a long and distin-
> guished history. Psychophysics is not some poor relation of physiolo-
> gy. Indeed, much of modern visual physiology has been driven by
> psychophysical discoveries.

By restricting myself to the functional analysis of the visual system as a whole I
have chosen a relatively simple topic. This implies no disrespect for those researchers
who combine physiology with the psychophysics of nonhuman primates. Their
combination of astonishing technical and scientific ingenuity is advancing our
knowledge of the physiological basis of perception at an accelerating rate.
Mountcastle (1998) provides an inspiring overview of this area of research.

The "sets of filters" hypothesis

According to Craik (1960):

> Now in mathematics it is legitimate to seek transformations through which cer-
> tain quantities (such as the physical laws of nature and the velocity of light)
> remain invariant. In fact, the action of certain physical devices which 'recog-
> nize' or respond identically to certain simple objects can be treated in terms of
> such transformations. Thus the essential part of physical 'recognising' instru-
> ments is usually a filter whether it be a mechanical sieve, an optical filter, or a
> tuned electrical circuit which 'passes' only quantities of the kind it is required to
> identify and rejects all others. Mathematically, the situation here is that, in a per-
> fect filter, the transformation leaves the desired quantity unaltered, but reduces
> all others to zero. (Craik, 1960)

I suggested that the working hypothesis illustrated in Figure 1.10 might prove
useful in attempting to model functionally the early stages of visual processing
(Regan, 1982).

Figure 1.10 is a much-reduced schematic of a general system. In a general system, any given output is a function of all the inputs and there may be nonlinear
crosstalk between responses to some or all of the inputs. If we started from a general system model, a rationally advancing science of psychophysics would verge
on the impossible because the output produced by any given input would depend,
not only on that input, but also on the particular values of every other input. Figure
1.10 illustrates the assumption that the early processing of at least some kinds of

visual information is, to a first approximation, independent and also free from crosstalk. The background to this approach is discussed in Chapter 8.

I suppose that retinal image information passes through a limited number of parallel visual information processors *sets of filters,* each of which is selectively sensitive to either a visual submodality or to an abstract feature of the retinal image (e.g., a ratio), labeled A, B, C, and so on, in Figure 1.10.

For the purpose of illustration, suppose that A in Figure 1.10 is the submodality of wavelength. The uppermost set of filters, therefore, is selectively sensitive to wavelength. According to the well-established trichromatic theory of color vision, the *set* consists of three filters whose peak sensitivities are at different wavelengths, and these three filters have broad overlapping sensitivity curves that are not affected by cognitive variables (Wright, 1946; see Color Plate 6). Over a broad range of visual environments the sensitivity profile of any given one of the three filters is (almost) independent of the nature of the retinal image including its luminance. Major breakdown occurs only under extreme conditions.

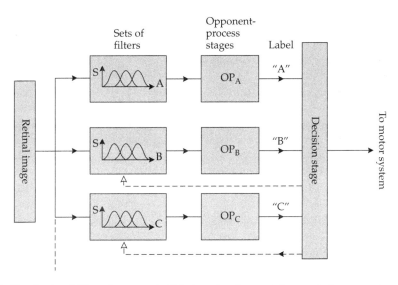

1.10 The "sets of filters" concept. This is a simple special case of the general non-linear system depicted in Figure A.1 illustrating the hypothesis that, to a good approximation, any given *set of filters* is sensitive to only one visual submodality or abstract feature, and it processes visual information independently of all other sets of filters. Fine-grain information represented by the relative activity of filters within any given set is recovered at an opponent stage of processing. Variable *A* is wavelength. The dashed lines with arrowheads indicate a possibility that descending task-dependent signals might affect the properties of some sets of filters.

In the conditions that the basic data of trichromatic theory were collected (a 2 × 1.5 degree, bipartite, foveally viewed patch; see Wright, 1991), stimulus luminance is represented by the sum of the outputs of three filters (though the contribution of the short-wavelength filter is very small), while wavelength is represented by the pattern of activity among the three filters. To a good approximation these representations are orthogonal (Wright, 1946, 1991).

It has been firmly established that, although the initial filtering of wavelength is coarse, very small differences in wavelength can be discriminated. Although a filter's full bandwidth at half-height is about 100 nanometers (nm), wavelength discrimination threshold can approach 1 nm. According to the classical model of color vision, this fine-grain information is recovered from the filter outputs at an *opponent stage of processing* (OP$_A$ in Figure 1.10). (See pp. 211–219 for a discussion of the distinction between the processing of achromatic contrast and that of chromatic contrast [Hering, 1920; Hurvich, 1981].) The reason why wavelength discrimination threshold is so remarkably low is that the three filters have low output noise and stable sensitivity profiles.

> The output of stage OP$_A$ carries a *label* for variable A that determines the perceived hue of a small patch with dark surround.

By analogy with the classical theory of color vision, I proposed that there are corresponding sets of filters for B, C, and so on. In particular, the set of filters for B is insensitive to A, C, and so on (Regan, 1982).

The number of filters in any given set may be other than three. For example, it seems that there are eight filters for stereomotion, each of which prefers a different value of the ratio $(d\phi/dt)/(d\delta/dt)$ (where $d\phi/dt$ is the approaching object's angular velocity parallel to the frontal plane, and $d\delta/dt$ is its rate of change of disparity) (Beverley & Regan, 1973; Regan et al., 1998). Now the crucial point:

> To a close approximation, sets of filters operate independently of each other.

We represent the outputs of the N sets of filters in an abstract space of N dimensions. The output of any given set of filters is a vector along one of the dimensions of this vector space. I assume that the vector space is *orthogonal*, i.e., the scalar product of any two unit vectors is zero (Schey, 1973). This crucial orthogonality concept is emphasized by Westheimer (1981) in an incisive review of the channeling hypothesis. Orthogonality can be understood intuitively in terms of our familiar Euclidian space: in the case of simple geometric vectors in Euclidean space, orthogonal vectors are perpendicular. Recollect that we are discussing a mathematical (functional) rather than a structural model. How this orthogonality of representation might be achieved physiologically is discussed on pp. 35 and 377–378.

The orthogonality of visual representation imposed by the operation of sets of filters is much more general than the orthogonality described by the trichromatic theory, and it does not necessarily correspond to an orthogonality in the external world (Regan, 1982).

In Figure 1.10 each submodality or abstract feature is depicted as having a separate discrimination stage (OP), but this is not necessary for the present argument: some convergence of information from different "sets of filters" may occur before the discrimination stage. In Figure 1.10, information as to *A*, *B*, *C*, and so on is carried on separate labeled lines. A physiological realization of this arrangement would require a larger amount of neural machinery than if several qualitatively different kinds of information were carried along one line. Surprisingly little attention has been paid to this fundamental and important problem by physiologists.*

The arrowed dashed lines directed "against the current" that start at later levels of processing and terminate at the sets of filters B, C, and so forth, indicate that sets of filters (other than submodality *A*) might be modified or even created by task-dependent descending signals. This would reconcile economy of resources with the well-known finding that the progressive reduction of threshold that occurs as the observer learns the task can be specific for eye, stimulus location, and stimulus orientation, implying that the plasticity necessary for learning exists at an early stage of visual processing (Karni & Sagi, 1991; Poggio et al., 1992; Polat & Sagi, 1994). Furthermore, the finding that practice effects can be remarkably specific to the task being learned in that the learning often does not transfer to other tasks (Poggio et al., 1992; Ahissar & Hochstein, 1993; Fahle & Morgan, 1996; Fahle, 1997) implies that passive viewing is not enough: high-level cognitive (task-driven stimulus evaluation) processes are necessary. Among the models that have been proposed for modification of early processing by descending signals are those of Anderson and Van Essen (1987) and Tsotsos (1993).

Finally, I should note that it is irrelevant to this discussion whether or not the classical spatial-frequency channels are independent (see pp. 75–91). A *set of filters* is a quite different concept from a spatial-frequency channel.

Rationale for the sets of filters hypothesis

The rationale for the hypothesis illustrated in Figure 1.10 is as follows:

> For the organism, one possible advantage of passing retinal image information through selectively sensitive and independently functioning *sets of filters* is that the same process of early visual analysis can be accurately and reliably carried out, not only when the visual environment is simple, but also when it is complex. If different sets of filters have nonoverlapping sensitivities, then indifference to visual scene complexity would be, in principle, established at the level of the *sets of filters* (Regan, 1982).

---

* Chung, Raymond, and Lettvin (1970, p. 72) noted that, "The meaning of the message in a neuron has usually been guessed by observing the relations between a stimulus and a change in the number of impulses discharged by the neuron per unit time." They went on

And just as a change in the pattern of activity among the short-, medium-, and long-wavelength filters represents a change in light wavelength, while a change in the summed activity of the filters represents a change in light intensity, so do the eight binocular filters for motion in depth provide orthogonal representations of the direction of motion in depth and the rate of change of binocular disparity (Beverley & Regan, 1973; Portfors & Regan, 1996; Regan et al., 1998). I suppose that all the sets of filters similarly represent orthogonally both a qualitative and an intensive variable.

In principle, orthogonal processing has the further advantage of conciseness in representing those informational features of the visual environment that are important for purposive motor activity. (The role of visual codes in reducing redundancy has been discussed by Attneave [1954, 1959] and Barlow [1972, 1974].) Brillouin (1962) provides a thorough and formal treatment of coding and the representation of information.

Finally, consider how a new skill of eye–limb coordination might be acquired. I assume that, during training, the decision stage in Figure 1.10 is progressively modified so as to convert inputs from several sets of filters into the appropriate motor actions (Regan, 1982). For example, in the case of learning how to catch a ball, these inputs will include monocular and binocular indications of the time of arrival [$\theta/(d\theta/dt)$ and $I/D(d\delta/dt)$, respectively] and of the direction of motion [$(d\phi/dt)/(d\theta/dt)$ and $(d\phi/dt)/(d\delta/dt)$, respectively] of the approaching ball. If, to a good approximation, the relevant sets of filters operate independently of each other, the skill, once learned, will transfer from the visual environment in which it was learned to quite different visual environments. It is known that this is the case, at least to a first approximation. It is not the case that a skill such as catching a ball must be reacquired when the visual environment is changed, as it would be if the sets of filters that provide the required visual information did not operate independently of each other and of all other sets of filters (Regan, 1982). (This implies that individuals whose sets of filters have overlapping sensitivities, or that interact when simultaneously active might, in complex visual environments, find difficulty in using eye–hand skills learned in simpler visual environments. There is some supporting evidence for this prediction [Beverley & Regan, 1980c; Kruk et al., 1981, 1983; Kruk & Regan, 1983].)

---

to suggest that information might be encoded in terms of the temporal pattern of firing, and that a temporal pattern of firing might be transformed into a spatial pattern of activation. More recently, it has been suggested that the principal components of the firing pattern encode information (Optican & Richmond, 1987; Richmond et al., 1987). A minimally mathematical introduction to principal component analysis, with caveats, is provided in Regan, 1989a, pp. 61–64. It has also been proposed that information that is not encoded in terms of the activity of any individual neuron may be encoded in terms of the relative activity within a population of neurons (Mountcastle, 1979; Victor, Purpura, & Mao, 1994). And it may also be the case that slow-wave activity encodes information that is incompletely represented, or even not represented, in spike firing (reviewed in Regan, 1972).

Modularity

Modularity of processing has recently become a popular concept in vision research, and the simplification illustrated in Figure 1.10 falls under this heading. However, the defining features of the sets of filters proposal are described as follows: the proposal applies specifically to functional (psychophysical) as distinct from structural (physiological) analyses of the visual system; nonoverlapping sensitivities and independence of processing are key to the definition of a set of filters; no assertion is made as to independence at later stages of processing.

Evidence for quasi-independent processing

Evidence for quasi-independent early processing (of at least small changes) has been reported for several pairs or triplets of submodalities and abstract features, including the following:

1. Wavelength and radiance (Wright, 1928, 1946, 1991)
2. Spatial frequency and orientation (Blakemore & Campbell, 1969; Blakemore & Nachmias, 1971)
3. Spatial frequency, orientation, and contrast (Vincent & Regan, 1995)
4. The rate of increase of an object's angular subtense and the component of its velocity parallel to the frontal plane (Regan & Beverley, 1978, 1980)
5. The rate of change of an object's disparity and the component of its velocity parallel to the frontal plane (Beverley & Regan, 1973; Richards & Regan, 1973; Regan et al., 1998; Hong & Regan, 1989)
6. The speed and direction of the component of a target's velocity parallel to the frontal plane (Levinson & Sekular, 1980)
7. The ratio $\theta/(d\theta/dt)$, $d\theta/dt$ and θ, where $\theta/(d\theta/dt)$ is the time to collision with a rigid sphere approaching the eye at constant speed, θ is its instantaneous angular subtense, and $d\theta/dt$ is its instantaneous rate of increase of subtense (Regan & Hamstra, 1993; Regan & Vincent, 1995)
8. The ratio $(d\phi/dt)/(d\delta/dt)$, $d\phi/dt$ and $d\delta/dt$, where $(d\phi/dt)/(d\delta/dt)$ is a binocular correlate of the direction of motion in depth of an approaching object, $d\phi/dt$ is the component of the object's velocity parallel to the frontal plane, and $d\delta/dt$ is its rate of change or horizontal binocular disparity (Portfors-Yeomans & Regan, 1996)
9. The ratio $(d\phi/dt)/(d\theta/dt)$, $d\phi/dt$ and $d\theta/dt$, where $(d\phi/dt)/(d\theta/dt)$ is a monocularly available correlate of the direction of motion in depth of an approaching object, $d\phi/dt$ is the component of the object's velocity parallel to the frontal plane, and $d\theta/dt$ is its rate of increase of angular subtense (Regan & Kaushal, 1994)
10. Rate of change of disparity and total change of disparity (Portfors & Regan, 1997)
11. The speed, change of position, and temporal frequency of a cyclopean grating (Kohly & Regan, 1998, 1999a)

Opponent processing

A piece of recent history brings out, not only the general principle of opponent processing, but also the deceptively difficult and deep nature of the basic idea.

One of my more vivid childhood memories is the awe-inspiring and strangely beautiful sight of moonlit German bombers, floating, seemingly aimlessly, high above my home in a blacked-out town. But, unknown to my awed and fascinated self, the presence of the beautiful flying machines had an implication more threatening than their individual bomb loads. After the bombing of blacked-out Coventry on the night of November 14–15, 1940, no member of the British public could doubt the Luftwaffe's ability to find their targets at night. In late 1940, the Luftwaffe could place one of their aircraft to within 400 m over England and drop bombs with high accuracy at night on a blacked-out city (Jones, 1978). It seems probable that the general population would have been even more annoyed than they already were, had it been generally known that this feat was not only far beyond the capability of the Royal Air Force, but was greeted with incredulous astonishment by the eminent scientists of British Scientific Intelligence.

R. V. Jones (1978) related that, as a 28-year-old junior member of Scientific Intelligence, he put forward the hypothesis that the Luftwaffe had developed a guidance method that used radio waves. This hypothesis was dismissed by scientists far more senior than he. For example, P. M. S. Blackett stated that he did not see how a radio beam could possibly be used to achieve such a high precision of navigation at large distances from the radio transmitter. Blackett, a man of formidable intelligence and wide knowledge, who was soon to be awarded the Nobel Prize for physics, based his rejection on the fact that a radio beam grows wider as the distance from the transmitter increases, and to achieve the accuracy demonstrated by the Luftwaffe night bombers, the width of the transmitting antenna would have to be impractically large.* Also, the signal strength of a radio beam fluctuates strongly after it has traveled several hundred miles, so the pilot would not be able to locate the center of the beam with the required accuracy.

Yet R. V. Jones was correct, though it required the personal intervention of Churchill to ensure that empirical proof was obtained. It is tempting to speculate that the principle used by the Luftwaffe might have been intuitively obvious to a perceptual psychologist of even modest attainment *who had been told about opponent processing in the context of the psychophysical theory of color vision*, a topic which,

---

* Jones (1978, p. 124) framed the problem in terms of a question: How can one define the direction of a beam generated by an aperture which is a given number of wavelengths wide? "At first sight this may appear to be the resolving power as calculated by Lord Rayleigh—and indeed Rayleigh thought it was. But the Rayleigh criterion applies properly to the closeness to which two sources can approach before they appear to merge into one when viewed through the aperture, i.e., of establishing that two separate diffraction patterns are involved. By contrast, the precision with which the direction of a single source can be defined is the precision with which the central direction of a single diffraction pattern can be established when no other pattern is present, and this precision may be a million or more times greater than the resolving power." See pp. 44–48 for the relevance of this statement to the problem of spatial localization.

to judge from P. M. S. Blackett's response, had little relevance for subatomic physics (but see pp. 154–155 and the footnote on page 157).

The fact that opponent processing is a feature not only of human color vision, but also of color vision in many species including shallow-water fish, who may well have been exploiting its advantages for several hundred million years, is worth some reflection. This thought has implications for the analysis of biological systems in general that are discussed on pp 400–402.

The principle of opponency is shown in Figure 1.11. Two antennae are placed side by side, one of which (A1) broadcasts dots while the other (A2) broadcasts dashes. (It is essential that the beams overlap.) A pilot flying exactly along the center of the overlap region hears a continuous tone, but a slight deviation to the left unbalances the signals and the pilot hears dots, while if the pilot deviates to the right, he hears dashes. The angular accuracy of navigation can be very much higher than with one beam alone, and much less than the angular width of either beam.

It will be useful to consider the factors that limit the smallest angular deviation ($\Delta\theta$) that can be distinguished from noise (i.e., the angular threshold). In the first instance let us suppose that, for either antenna, signal power (S) varies with direction (θ) according to $\cos^2\theta$ (see Figure 1.11B). Clearly, the rate of change of S with respect to θ will be zero along the center of the beam near the locally flat top of the $(\cos\theta)^2$ lobe in Figure 1.11B, but is positive for directions to the left of center and negative for directions to the right of center, being given by $\partial S/\partial\theta = -2\cos\theta \sin\theta$ for a $(\cos\theta)^2$ lobe. Depending on the shape of the lobe, the magnitude of $\partial S/\partial\theta$ may be maximal at some intermediate value of θ (as is the case for the Figure 1.11B lobe shape), or may asymptote to a ceiling value, or may progressively increase as θ departs from zero.

If we ignore all factors other than $\partial S/\partial\theta$, directional discrimination will be best for the line of flight that gives the greatest difference in $\partial S/\partial\theta$ between the two beams. In the case of the Figure 1.11B lobe shape, beam A1 should be directed to the left of the intended line of flight so that $\partial S/\partial\theta$ is maximal along the line of flight, and beam A2 should be similarly directed to the right of the line of flight. This idealized situation is illustrated in Figure 1.11C.

There is, however, an additional factor. In all cases of interest to us, the signal power S declines monotonically as the magnitude of θ increases. In Figure 1.11D, for example, where $\partial S/\partial\theta$ is shown progressively increasing with θ, there will be some point (θ_M) beyond which any potential reduction of angular discrimination threshold will be more than offset by the decline of power S. In part D, the region beyond this point is shown dotted. In practice, the optimal beam separation will be $2\theta_M$ as illustrated in Figure 1.11D.

The third factor that limits directional discrimination is as follows: Even if the pilot flies exactly along the midline, faint dots or faint dashes will be heard from time to time because of irregular fluctuations in the *relative* signal strengths of the two beams. Errors in the direction of flight cannot be detected unless they produce dots or dashes that are appreciably louder than these random fluctuations in relative signal strength.

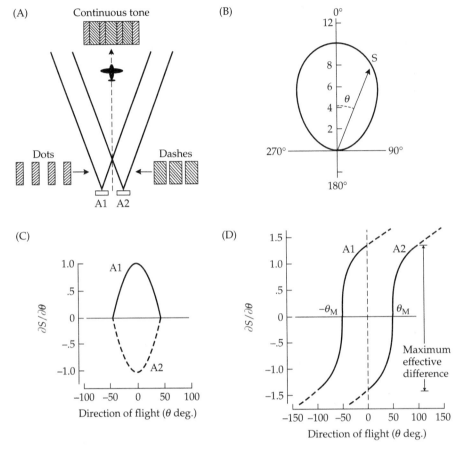

1.11 The concept of opponent processing. (A) Radio antenna A1 broadcasts dots, while A2 broadcasts dashes. The pilot hears a continuous tone only if the line of flight is exactly along the center of the overlapping beams. (B) Variation of signal power (S) with direction (θ). (C) Variation of $\partial S/\partial \theta$ with θ for beams 1 and 2. The two beams are shown not parallel, but diverging at an angle of 90 degrees. (D) Variation of $\partial S/\partial \theta$ for lobes different in shape from the $\cos^2$ shape shown in part B. Part D also illustrates that, beyond a certain point (θ_M), any potential reduction of angular discrimination threshold is more than offset by decline of signal power. After Regan (1986a).

Noisy variations of receiver gain in the frequency range of the dots and dashes will also limit directional discrimination. Note, though, that:

> Directional discrimination threshold is quite unaffected by fluctuations in signal strength that are common to both beams, even when these fluctuations are large. Compare the situation when only one beam is used. Large fluctuations of absolute signal strength produce a correspondingly large increase of directional discrimination threshold.

As an example of biological opponency, let us consider stimulus orientation. Suppose we have a population of cortical neurons, each of which is sensitive to orientation, spatial frequency, contrast, velocity, color, luminance, temporal frequency, and so on (though the pattern of sensitivities is quite different for different neurons in the population). The following discussion parallels the discussion of Figure 1.11, except that grating orientation or line orientation rather than direction is represented by θ, signal power (S) is replaced by neural sensitivity, and the two lobes, one of which is shown in Figure 1.11B, are neural orientation tuning curves.

We select a pair of neurons that prefer different orientations. A change of stimulus orientation will alter the *relative* activities of the two neurons. In this way, a more central neural mechanism that was sensitive to the relative activity of the two more peripheral neurons could discriminate a clockwise from an anticlockwise change of orientation that was much less than the orientation-tuning bandwidth of either neuron because, as illustrated in Figure 1.11, orientation discrimination threshold would be limited by the difference in the slopes of the sensitivity curves of the two peripheral neurons, by uncorrelated noise in the two neurons' outputs, and possibly also by noise in the more central mechanism, rather than by the orientation-tuning bandwidths of the two peripheral neurons. (This property would be rather independent of the form of opponency. For example, it would hold for both subtractive and ratio opponency.) Which pair of neurons would be most important for orientation discrimination can also be understood in terms of Figure 1.11: it would be the pair whose $\partial S/\partial\theta$ differed most, allowing for the decline of signal strength with stimulus orientation (θ) (Regan & Beverley, 1985; see Figure 2.26 and pp. 115–123).

We suppose that each restricted area of the visual field drives a limited number of such neurons. Only 4 to 8 neural elements that are narrowly tuned to orientation are required to account for orientation discrimination, a minimum requirement being two that prefer orientations placed at about 15 to 20 degrees to either side of vertical and two that prefer orientations placed at about 15 to 20 degrees to either side of horizontal (see Figure 2.31).

"Regional binding" and "boundary detection" models

I will discuss two general kinds of psychophysical object-detector models. Consider, for example, the situation that retinal image segregation is based on a difference in texture. One kind of model of segregation involves a comparison of any given texture element with its neighbors to find whether they are the same, so as to identify an area of relatively homogenous texture (e.g., Caelli, 1985). This area will be processed as though it is an object's retinal image. This is a *grouping for similarity* or *regional binding* type of model and dates back to the Gestaltists. A second kind of model, *boundary detection*, involves a comparison that identifies a relatively large difference between neighboring texture elements (Nothdurft, 1985a,b, 1990, 1991a; Landy & Bergen, 1991). This sharp spatial gradient will be processed as though it defines the outer boundary of an object's retinal image. We will see how the two modeling approaches have usually been used on an either/or basis. A subset of the available data on image segregation and object perception is explained by one kind of model, while a different subset of the data is explained by the other kind of model. I will integrate the two kinds of models in an attempt to explain why people can discriminate and recognize with similar facility solid luminance-defined (LD) shapes and line drawings of those shapes.*

Inter-Observer Variability and Classification Schemes

> Statistics are slippery things, however, beloved by people who don't generally "see" shape very well but understand numbers. Statistics always involve assumptions about the nature of the underlying reality from which you have selected a sample; if those assumptions are incorrect, they can warp the results into something that is biologically meaningless. For me the anatomy and morphology were quite clear: gracile and robust australopithecines were different sorts of animal from each other, and early *Homo* was a third type. (Walker & Shipman, 1996, p. 111)

Many human-made systems have functions that can be realized by several different physical structures,† so that interindividual variability may well be greater for the structural organization than for the functional organization of the human visual system. Having offered that speculation, I should add that intersubject differences in psychophysical data are greater (and, perhaps, much greater) than would be revealed by a cursory glance over the psychophysical literature.

Because the problem of neuron-to-neuron variability confronts the electrophysiologist more starkly and unavoidably than the problem of intersubject variability confronts the psychophysicist, it will be useful to discuss the problem in the context of electrophysiology before turning to psychophysics. It would be laughably unacceptable (though, perhaps, not completely incorrect) to start a paper with the words: "We recorded from 250 cells. No two cells had exactly the same properties. We propose 250 categories of firing behavior." Rather, the electrophysiologist must attempt to distinguish a multimodal (e.g., a bimodal or trimodal) from a continuous variation of any given neural behavior, while striving to impose order on the data by means of some classification scheme—an order that may or may not eventually prove to exist. Classification schemes are central to conceptual ordering, both as a precursor of hypotheses and as an integral part of hypotheses.

---

* This is an old problem. Kaufman (personal communication, 1997) stated: "The Gestaltists (Koffka, 1935) took their very name from the fact that we may 'recognize with similar facility line drawings of shapes and solid LD shapes.' Such phenomena suggest that the forms (Gestalten) are other than the mere sum of their parts, thus anticipating the idea that the perceptual system is essentially nonlinear."

† For example, the functional plan of a 1940 AM radio whose active circuit elements were vacuum tubes ("valves" in the U.K.) might be similar to the functional plan of a 1970 AM radio whose active circuit elements were transistors. But the physical principles of vacuum-tube technology and solid-state technology are completely different.

> The degree of violence to be done to empirical data by the conceptual process of classification calls for delicate judgment on the part of the experimenter, who must steer a course between hallucinating an imaginary order within random variation and failing to see a pattern that will be obvious to later researchers—in hindsight.

Stone's book on the classification of retinal ganglion cells (e.g., the distinction between X-cells and Y-cells) goes far beyond its nominal topic and contains a number of illuminating remarks on the role of classification schemes in general, and on how they are used by practicing scientists (Stone, 1983, pp. 79–81, 135–145). For example,

> the classification of retinal ganglion cells is not a straightforward, objective task, but is as much a product of the observer's presuppositions as any other scientific proposition. . . . Yet it is a fair and relevant criticism of neurobiologists (including myself) that we have been largely unaware of the problems of methodology inherent in classification, and of the substantial literature that exists on those problems. There has been little awareness either of the central part played by classification (whether of nerve cells, plants, animals, aphasias, or rocks) in the organization of bodies of knowledge. Perhaps, as a consequence, much of the variety and inconsistency found among neuronal classification stems from differences between scientists in our presuppositions. (Stone, 1983, p. 123)

In what follows it will become evident that Stone's words apply equally well to psychophysics as to single-cell studies. Electrophysiologists have little control over the nature of the cell they encounter with their electrode tip. The extent of neuron-to-neuron variability is so blatantly obvious that it is difficult to ignore. In contrast, psychophysicists have a great deal of control in selecting their observers. Some psychophysical conclusions are based on data collected from very few observers, and these observers are commonly drawn from a sharply restricted population: graduate students and faculty, often with extensive experience of psychophysical procedures, detailed knowledge of the field, and expectations about the results of an experiment. It is temptingly easy to accept that, if data collected from naive observers support the conclusions less firmly, it is because these observers have inferior motivation or inferior psychophysical skills. And, a report of the number of observers who were rejected because their data were unsatisfactory in some way is often lacking.*

---

* The primary goal of Wright's (1929) report was to provide, for industrial users, a standard basis for the CIE specification of color. To achieve the primary goal it was necessary to arrive at a procedure that minimized intersubject variations in the color matching data. But even when the only visible target inside a dark room was a 1.5 × 2.0 degree stimulus field centered on the relatively homogeneous, rod-free fovea, a field that was devoid of spatial structure when the two halves were matched, considerable intersubject variability remained. Some observers gave unreliable or aberrant data. These observers were rejected from the study (Wright, personal communication, 1957). For this reason an important

Even if it were shown that intersubject variability in psychophysical data was far less than neuron-to-neuron variability (as it presumably is), the psychophysicist is faced with the same challenge as the electrophysiologist in trying to impose order on variable data by sorting the data into a small number of (preferably meaningful) classifications.

It might help me as a reader of the psychophysical literature (and, perhaps, others too) to compare and evaluate competing classifications and models if we were better informed about intersubject variability of the relevant psychophysical data. Although conclusions might lose a little of their intellectual edge and their weight, the consequent improvement in their longevity might well be beneficial to all in the long run.

Disordered Vision

As mentioned above in the section on the sets of filters hypothesis, the orthogonality with which the outputs of the sets of filters represent the retinal image is, by definition, created by the selectivity of their sensitivities and the independence with which they operate in parallel; it is by no means necessarily the case that this orthogonality is a property of the external world. How then, can we identify the submodalities or abstract features designated B, C, and so on, in Figure 1.10? This is not a trivial problem and not one, I think, that can be solved theoretically or computationally.

One approach to identifying B, C, and so on, is to assume that each correlates with some feature of the physical three-dimensional world that is important to the organism. For example, there is evidence for one monocular and one binocular set of filters that signal the direction of an approaching object's motion in depth, and one monocular and one binocular set of filters that signals the time remaining before the approaching object will reach the observer (see p. 35).

---

1. The astonishing feat of eye–limb coordination demonstrated by top sports players can—by exaggeration—draw attention to visual functions that may escape notice in everyday life (e.g., Beverley & Regan, 1973, 1975; Regan et al., 1979).
2. A second possibility is that studies of disordered vision might help to identify B, C, and so forth. Suppose that some visual disorder causes failure in only one filter or set of filters. By collecting data on the consequent psychophysical abnormalities, we can define

---

phenomenon of retinal image stabilization remained undiscovered for many decades. In 1956, K. J. McCree had traveled from New Zealand to undertake Ph.D. thesis work on color matching under Wright's supervision. He soon found that he was unable to collect reliable color-matching data, and that the harder he tried, the worse was his performance: he would certainly have been rejected from the 1929 study. His short-term fixation was so steady that the subjective difference in hue between the two halves of the field fluctuated exceedingly while he looked at the target. His dismay was short-lived: he investigated and wrote his

the nature of what has been lost. We may then assume that normally sighted individuals possess whatever has been lost. Whether this candidate functional subunit processes its preferred submodality or abstract feature independently of all others can then be established by studies on normally sighted individuals. The congenital deuteranopic and protanopic defects of color vision are a classical example of this line of argument. Figure 2.67 shows a more recent example of this approach. Stereomotion blindness is a third example (Richards & Regan, 1973; Regan et al., 1986; Hong & Regan, 1989).

We will see that the following questions can be addressed by carrying out psychophysical studies on patients. Can a central lesion abolish the ability to *detect* one of the five kinds of spatial contrast while sparing the ability to detect any of the remaining four kinds? Can a central lesion abolish the ability to *recognize* objects defined by one of the five kinds of spatial contrast while sparing the ability to recognize any of the remaining four kinds? And, more generally, can a central lesion *dissociate* the following: sensitivity to differences in successively inspected targets; sensitivity to local spatial contrast; spatial discriminations; the ability to recognize shapes?

I will distinguish between the results of four classes of tests when discussing data obtained from patients. Consider, for example, texture-defined form. The first class of test assesses the ability to discriminate different textures by inspecting them in succession using the same retinal region (usually the fovea). The second class of test assesses the ability to detect the spatial structure of a pattern composed of two or more textures (see pp. 274–277). This capacity can either be referred to as the ability to detect texture-defined spatial contrast or texture-defined form. (An illustration of the distinction between the two kinds of tests is discriminating a texture difference by successively inspecting two differently textured areas versus detecting a boundary between two contiguous but differently textured areas [as discussed in Chapter 4 and illustrated in Figure 4.1]. The results of a successive inspection test do not necessarily predict the result of a spatial contrast test, presumably because certain lateral interactions are involved in a spatial contrast test that are not involved in a successive inspection test).

The third class of test requires observers to perform spatial discrimination on texture-defined form. For example, they must judge which of two texture-defined spatial forms has a larger area or which is longer (see Chapter 4 and Figure 4.7). The fourth class of test requires observers to recognize and name a texture-

Ph.D. thesis on the phenomenon. In 1957, I was a participant in his experiment. By voluntary fixation, both McCree and I were able to eliminate the perceived difference in hue between wavelengths spaced as far apart in the spectrum as blue and red. Other observers were able to eliminate the perceived difference between wavelengths on one or the other side of yellow. Such observers seem not to be uncommon (McCree, 1960). In this case, the results of rejecting observers who gave aberrant results did not compromise the conclusions of Wright's 1929 study. But a benign outcome is not assured in all cases.

defined object or shape (see Figure 4.10). This kind of test demands long-term visual memory (see the section on short-term memory and attention in Chapter 2 and Klatzky, 1980).

These four kinds of tests exist for texture, luminance, color, motion, and disparity. Examples of form-detection and form-recognition tests for texture-defined and motion-defined form (the particular spatial forms being letters of the alphabet) are given in Regan et al. (1991, 1992b); Regan and Hong (1990, 1994, 1995); Regan and Simpson (1995); Simpson and Regan (1995).

Spatial Discriminations, Hyperacuities, and Impostors

As background to this section, students are recommended to read two reviews by Westheimer (1979, 1981). The subtle concepts that are the topic of these reviews are discussed with such clarity that they seem simple. These reviews refresh the reader's mind and, as has been said, gratefully, by more than one well-known current researcher, can stimulate and "kick start" the reader's thinking so that he or she goes on to develop original ideas.*

First we will discuss some visual tasks that are not spatial discriminations, though they masquerade as such. Citing Hecht and Mintz (1939), Westheimer (1981) noted that a black line can be detected against a bright background when its width is only about 2 seconds of arc (in particular, a wire 1 cm thick can be seen against the sky from about 1 km).† But, he points out, this tells us little about spatial vision. The retinal image of the blue sky is a uniformly illuminated area and the black line causes a local dip in the luminance of this image (ΔL_1 in Figure 1.12). For a very narrow black line, the width of the dip is determined by the eye's optics rather than by the width of the line (see the section on diffraction and the Airey disc in Appendix B). Thus, for example, if the thickness of the black line is increased threefold, the width of the dip remains approximately the same, though the amplitude of the dip increases to ΔL_2 (dashed line in Figure 1.12). An observ-

---

* Students soon find that this is not the case for all papers on visual psychophysics. My experience is that because a paper is difficult, it does not necessarily follow that it contains new concepts of depth and subtlety. After struggling with mind-deadening formalism, excessively tendentious discussion, and misleadingly selective choice of citations until the "take home" message was at last revealed, I have too often found that the resulting disappointment called for a brisk walk in the open air.

† Vision scientists specify an object's size in terms of the angle it subtends at the eye (its angular subtense) rather than in terms of the size of its retinal image. To specify the size of any given object's retinal image would call for some exceedingly precise measurements of the dimensions and optical properties of the eye of the observer. And, because the eyes of different people vary in size and optical properties (not to mention the effect of wearing spectacles), the retinal image size of an object of any given angular subtense would vary from observer to observer.

It is helpful to remember that a length x cm viewed at a distance D subtends approximately $(57x)/D$ degrees if $x \ll D$, so that a grating of spatial S cycles/cm, viewed from D cm would have a spatial frequency of $S*D/57$ cycles/degree. A useful rule of thumb is that 1 cm viewed at 57 cm (or 1 inch viewed at 57 inches) subtends approximately one degree.

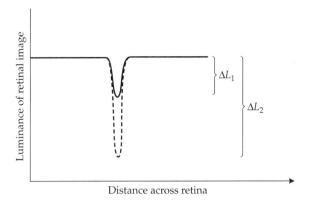

1.12 Retinal image of a very narrow black line. The solid curve shows the image of a very narrow line. The dashed curve shows the image of a line about three times thicker. Because the image of either line is determined entirely by the eye's optics, the retinal images of the two lines have the same width. But the light decrement in the image of the thicker line (ΔL_2) is almost three times as large as the decrement in the image of the thinner line (ΔL_1).

er's ability to detect the black line depends on whether ΔL exceeds the luminance different threshold of the eye in its prevailing state of light adaptation.

So, although at first sight the 2 seconds of arc might seem to be a spatial acuity, black line detection is not a spatial task. Rather, it is a contrast or incremental luminance task. Black line detection can be regarded as equivalent to an incremental luminance threshold of about 1%.

Another way of bringing out this point is to consider what decides whether we can see a particular star. The angular subtense of stars other than our sun is so small that their apparent size is determined by the eye's optics (see pp. 439–440). Whether or not a particular star is visible will be determined by the total light energy in its retinal image relative to the luminance of the retinal image of the neighboring sky. Thus, the sky over a city seems to contain very few stars because the atmosphere backscatters city light. But in remote areas such as the high Arctic (and even sometimes in urban regions as, for example, in blacked-out, wartime Britain), the multitude of stars visible on a clear night is awe-inspiring.

Figure 1.13A shows the distribution of light across the retinal image of a distant star. When the target is a very narrow line, this distribution is called the eye's *line-spread function.** Several authors have measured line-spread functions in the fovea and periphery of individual eyes (Flamant, 1955; Westheimer & Campbell 1962; Krauskopf, 1962; Campbell & Gubisch, 1966; Jennings & Charman, 1981).

---

* The line-spread function is the line integral of the point spread function. And the optical transfer (OTF) of the eye (regarded as the imaging device) is the Fourier transform of the line-spread function. This means that, given an empirical measurement of any one of the three, the other two can be calculated. See Appendix B, pp. 416–420 and 435–436, Appendix C, pp. 445–446.

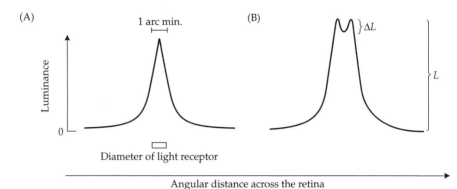

1.13 Visual resolution. (A) The line-spread function for the human eye. The foveal image of a very narrow line is a luminance distribution whose width at half-height is considerably greater than the distance between photoreceptors in the fovea. (B) The image of two very narrow lines that are close together. Unless the lines are sufficiently far apart that the decrement DL can be detected, the observer cannot tell whether there are two lines or only one. After Westheimer (1981).

Figure 1.13A shows that the width at half-height of the line-spread function in the foveal region of a well-corrected eye is at least twice the diameter of a foveal cone (photoreceptor). The width of this distribution is one of the important major determinants of the eye's *minimum angle of resolution* (i.e., the angular separation of two lines that can just be detected as separate).

Figure 1.13B shows the retinal image of two closely adjacent lines. The two lines will be resolved when the contrast of the dip (i.e., $\Delta L/L$) reaches contrast detection threshold for the eye's prevailing state of adaptation. And for any given line separation, the values of ΔL will be determined by the width of the line-spread function. A typical best value of minimum angle of resolution is one minute of arc.

Westheimer (1979, 1981) reminded the vision research community that it had long been known (since the 1860s) that several true spatial discrimination tasks give discrimination thresholds that are considerably (up to 10 times) finer that the minimum angle of resolution, and that by the 1890s it was realized the these discrimination thresholds were many times lower than the 25 seconds of arc separation between the most tightly packed foveal photoreceptors. For example, the just-noticeable spatial displacement of a single point or line can be as low as 10 seconds of arc, the just noticeable change in the separation of two parallel lines can be as low as 6 seconds of arc (see pp. 107–108), and step Vernier threshold (Vernier acuity) can be as low as a few seconds of arc (see pp. 98–106). It was already clear to Hering in 1899 that the neural processing underlying a Vernier acuity response depended on more than resolution.

Looking back over more than a century of research into spatial vision, Westheimer (1975) listed the many spatial tasks that gave angular thresholds considerably less than the shortest distance between foveal cones, and labeled such thresholds "hyperacuities."

In an early attempt to account for Vernier acuities of a few arc seconds, Hering proposed in 1899 that local sign is averaged along the length of each of the lines of a two-line Vernier target (Figure 2.17). This hypothesis went out of favor when it was shown that Vernier threshold for point stimuli is only a few seconds of arc (Ludvigh, 1953; Sullivan et al., 1972; Westheimer & McKee, 1977). More recent theoretical approaches to hyperacuities are covered on pp. 140–171.

A curious property of positional hyperacuities is that, in principle, they would be degraded if the eye's optics were *improved*. An explanation for this oddity is illustrated in Figure 1.14. If the point spread function were greatly narrower than the separation between photoreceptor centers, the retinal image of a star would have to move from position P1 to position P2 or to position P3 in Figure 1.14A before the change in location was signaled reliably. But, because light from the star spreads over several photoreceptors (see Figure 1.14B), a considerably smaller change in location can be signaled reliably in terms of the *relative activation* of photoreceptors R1–R7.

This argument implies that it should be possible to change the perceived location of a target without changing the location of its edges, and indeed this effect has been demonstrated (see pp. 98–106). However, the finding that the perceived location of

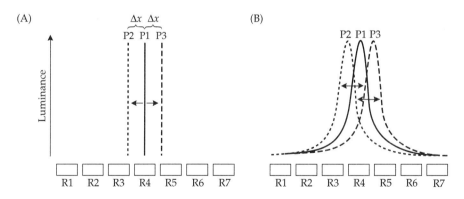

1.14 High acuity requires a blurred image. (A) If the image of a very thin line were considerably more narrow than the shortest distance between foveal photoreceptors (i.e., less than about 25 seconds of arc), the line would have to move distance Δx before the movement could be detected. (B) Because the light distribution in the image of a line spreads across several photoreceptors, a change in its position that is considerably less than Δx in (A) can be signaled reliably by a change in the pattern of activation across several photoreceptors.

a bar can be changed by shifting the centroid of the luminance distribution of its retinal image without changing the location of the bar's edges does not necessary imply that the location of the centroid is the *only* factor that determines the bar's perceived location. For example, what determines the perceived location of the bar's edges? Further to this point, how does information about the interior of the bar (e.g., centroid and texturing) combine with information about the boundary of the bar to determine perception of the location, width, and orientation of the bar? We will leave discussion of these issues to Chapter 2.

Figural Aftereffects

According to Graham (1965, p. 555) *figural aftereffects* are "effects due to viewing an inspection figure on later responses to a test figure." Some of the earliest reports were published by Gibson. He found that after inspecting a curved line for some time, a straight line appeared to be curved in the opposite direction. The aftereffect died away rapidly (Gibson, 1933). He also found that after inspecting for some time a line tilted anticlockwise of vertical, a vertical line appeared to be tilted clockwise of vertical, and that adapting to a line tilted clockwise of vertical produced the converse, briefly lived, negative aftereffect.

A proposed explanation for the tilt aftereffect (Sutherland, 1961) runs as follows. The orientation of a line is neurally represented by some average of all the responses of orientation-tuned cortical cells that respond to the line. Before adaptation, a vertical line would look vertical because it most strongly stimulated neurons that preferred the vertical orientation, and produced no overall bias in the responses from neurons that preferred other orientations. After adaptation to a line tilted through, for example, 7 degrees clockwise, neurons that preferred this orientation would become temporarily less responsive. In particular, neurons that preferred lines oriented clockwise of vertical would become less responsive than neurons that preferred lines tilted anticlockwise of vertical. When the observer looked at a vertical test line, the balance of neural activity would now be shifted temporarily towards neurons that preferred lines tilted anticlockwise of vertical so that the vertical line would appear to be tilted anticlockwise of vertical (see also Ganz, 1966; Ganz & Day, 1965).

In a series of experiments, Köhler and Wallach (1944) showed that the perceived location of a line or contour could be briefly changed following prolonged inspection of a line or contour in a nearby location. They called the effect *contour repulsion* or *displacement*. One of Köhler and Wallach's demonstrations of contour repulsion is illustrated in Figure 1.15. The observer was instructed to fixate the mark F_1 in Figure 1.15A. This caused the left visual field to adapt locally to the outlined rectangle, R. After some considerable time, the observer shifted fixation to F_2 in part B. Observers reported that the separation of lines L_1 and L'_1 was less than the separation of lines L_2 and L'_2, even though the two separations were physically equal. The previous retinal location of the rectangle is shown with dotted lines in Figure 1.15B.

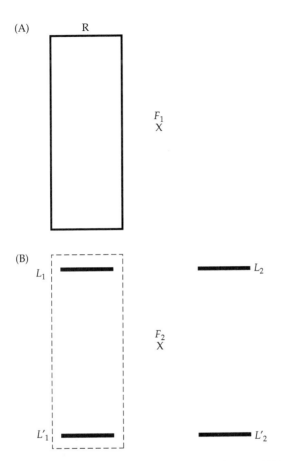

1.15 The contour repulsion effect. After fixating the mark F_1 in (A) for some time, quickly shift your gaze to F_2 in (B). Adapting to the rectangle in (A) causes the separation of lines $L_1L'_1$ to appear less than the separation of line $L_2L'_2$, even though the two separations are physically equal. After Köhler and Wallach (1944).

The older literature on figural aftereffects is reviewed in Kling and Riggs (1971, pp. 465–474) and Kaufman (1974, pp. 511–515).

Blakemore and Sutton (1969) described a figural aftereffect produced by adapting to a grating. If you move your eyes back and forth along the horizontal black bar at the center of the adapting pattern shown in Figure 1.16A for one or two minutes, then rapidly shift your gaze to the black dot at the center of the test pattern, the lower test grating will appear to have lower spatial frequency than the upper test grating, even though their spatial frequencies are physically identical.

The explanation proposed by Blakemore and Sutton for the aftereffect shown in Figure 1.16C was framed in terms of a parallel array of mechanisms, the output of each of which they supposed to carry a spatial-frequency label. (They assumed

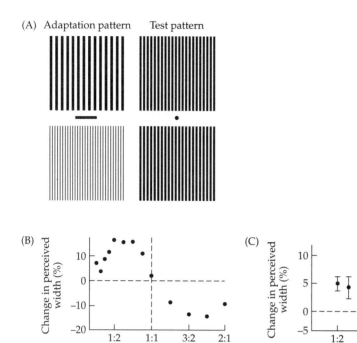

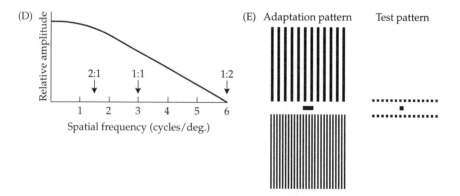

1.16 The Blakemore–Sutton aftereffect. (A) Run your eyes back and forth along the horizontal bar in the adapting pattern for one or two minutes. Now rapidly switch your gaze to the black spot in the test pattern. The upper gratings in the test pattern appear to have a higher spatial frequency than the lower grating, even though the two gratings are identical. (B) The spatial-frequency aftereffect quantified. (C) The perceived widening of a single test rectangle caused by adapting to a sinusoidal grating. (D) The low-frequency end of the amplitude spectrum of a rectangle whose width is 10 minutes of arc. The arrows indicate the spatial frequencies of some of the adapting gratings. (E) The Blakemore–Sutton aftereffect with short test gratings. A after Blakemore and Sutton, 1969; B–D after Frome et al. (1979); E from Levinson and Frome (1979).

that the receptive field of any one of these mechanisms was considerably wider than one grating bar.) Some of these hypothetical mechanisms would be maximally sensitive to low spatial frequencies, while others would prefer intermediate spatial frequencies, and still others, high spatial frequencies, along the lines of those shown in Figure 2.11. The crux of this hypothesis is that the perceived spatial frequency of any given grating is determined, not by its actual spatial frequency, but rather by the pattern of activity across the mechanisms within the array. (See Figure 2.28A for an illustration of this concept in the context of orientation-labeled outputs.) So, if adaptation to a grating of spatial frequency S cycles/degree exerts its largest desensitizing effect on mechanisms that are most sensitive to (and whose outputs carry the labels of) spatial frequencies close to S cycles/degree, this desensitization will cause a temporary shift in the balance across the outputs of the mechanisms within the array when subsequently stimulated by a grating whose spatial frequency is higher or lower than S cycles/degree.

Klein, Stromeyer, and Ganz (1974) challenged Blakemore and Sutton's proposal by showing that the detection threshold elevation caused by adaptation could be dissociated from the shift in perceived spatial frequency caused by the same adaptation. Using a center-surround stimulus configuration, they found a shift but no elevation. Similarly, they noted that Blakemore and Sutton's proposal predicted a shift that was of broader bandwidth than the shift observed. They suggested a two-stage model to explain the shift.

Frome et al. (1979) drew attention to an alternative explanation for the aftereffect. Their proposal was framed in terms of an array of mechanisms, the output of each of which carries a size (i.e., width) label rather than a spatial-frequency label. In this case, the receptive field of any given mechanism need be no wider than a single bar. According to this argument, the perceived spatial frequency of any given grating is determined by the balance of activity across the width-labeled outputs of mechanisms within the array. This proposal explains the data shown in Figure 1.16B quite as well as Blakemore and Sutton's proposal. The distinction between the two explanations is as follows. According to Blakemore and Sutton, the aftereffect is an altered perception of the spatial frequency of the grating as a whole, while Frome et al. attributed the aftereffect to an altered perception in the width of individual bars.

After pointing out that Blakemore and Sutton's experiment could not distinguish between these two candidate explanations for the aftereffect (because they used only a single bar width and corresponding single spatial frequency), Frome et al. proposed that the distinction could be made by substituting for the test grating a single solid bar or rectangle, because a single bar has broad spatial-frequency distribution (see Figure B.6). "If bar width is what matters psychophysically, adapting to a sinusoidal grating will have the same effect on a single bar as on a grating. But if spatial frequency is the determining variable, the effect on a bar and on a grating should be different" (Frome et al., 1979, p. 1328).

Their rationale can be understood in terms of Figure 1.16D (see also Figure B.6). The wider the test rectangle, the farther to the left is the first zero in its spectrum.

If the adapting effect is explained in terms of the spatial-frequency spectrum of the test bar, an adapting grating whose spatial frequency places it at or a little below the first zero in the spectrum of the test rectangle will, by rendering the visual system less sensitive to that spatial frequency, effectively shift the first zero leftwards, thus mimicking the effect of a widening of the test rectangle.

Rather than measuring the aftereffect by means of a test *grating* (as in Figure 1.16A,B), Frome et al. used a single solid vertically elongated test *rectangle*. Its width was fixed, but its height was adjustable. After adapting to a vertical grating, observers were instructed to adjust the *height* of the test rectangle until it appeared to be square. This "make a square" procedure, though indirect, provided a very sensitive measure of perceived *width* (for reasons explained on pp. 174–184). Frome et al. quantified the effect of grating adaptation on the perceived width of the test rectangle. She used the ratio between the height setting *before* adapting to the grating and the height setting *after* adapting to the grating.

Frome et al. reported what they described as a paradox. As shown in Figure 1.16C, the same adaptation process that caused the perceived spatial frequency of a grating of bar width W degrees to increase made a single rectangle of width W appear *wider*.

Reasoning that this effect would be geometrically impossible for a test grating with bright and dark bars of equal width, they replaced their single test rectangle with a test grating made of many small rectangles—in other words, they used a grating with very short bars (see Figure 1.16E). Once again, they quantified the change in perceived bar width by adjusting bar height until the short bars appeared to be square.

Levinson and Frome (1979) found that the perceived width of the short test bars was increased after adapting to a grating, and they showed that was the case whether the bar width of the adapting grating was narrower, equal to, or wider than the width of the short test bars. They confirmed that adapting to a grating of lower spatial frequency than the test grating increased the perceived spatial frequency of the test grating. They added that this paradox cannot be explained in terms of a difference in the spectra of the test and adapt stimuli. Nor can it be explained in terms of a perceived change in the relative widths of bright and dark bars.

The explanation that they offered was framed in terms of the Fourier analysis model of spatial vision (see pp. 143–144). They proposed that, under attentional control, observers can vary the width of visual field that is subjected to spatial-frequency analysis according to the psychophysical task being carried out. A larger area of the visual field would be subjected to spatial-frequency analysis when matching the spatial frequencies of test and reference gratings than when adjusting a single test rectangle to squareness.

I propose the following alternative possibility: (1) the visual system contains mechanisms whose outputs carry a periodicity (spatial frequency) label as well as mechanisms whose outputs carry a local size (width) label; (2) both kinds of output are always available to an observer, who can pay selective attention to one or the other set of labeled signals. The geometrical impossibility of an aftereffect in which perceived spatial frequency increases while the perceived width of grating bars also increases could then be explained by analogy with the standard explanation for the classical Waterfall illusion, where a test target appears to be in motion even though its location does not change. Levinson and Frome's (1979) finding is not, as they stated, "paradoxical" if we assume that size (width) and periodicity are signaled simultaneously and independently.

This possibility might be tested by requiring observers to judge, after every test presentation, both the postadaptation perceived spatial frequency of the short-barred grating illustrated in Figure 1.16E and the postadaptation perceived aspect ratio of individual bars, and by ensuring that each test presentation was sufficiently brief (and followed by a masker pattern) as to render unlikely an attention-driven switch of spatial-frequency analysis from small field to larger field analysis.

The generality of Blakemore and Sutton's aftereffect was questioned by Regan and Beverley (unpublished data, 1983). They repeated the Blakemore and Sutton experiment using the same kind of displays (Tektronix model 604 monitors) and procedures, and obtained closely similar results. However, they were unable to replicate the result when brighter displays were used (Tektronix model 608 monitors), and there was marked intersubject variation in the data obtained. Regan and Beverley also argued that, if one adopts a "relative activity" model of spatial-frequency discrimination (see Figure 2.25), Blakemore and Sutton's spatial-frequency repulsion effect should be accompanied by corresponding changes in spatial-frequency discrimination threshold. They found that adaptation did indeed produce considerable elevations of spatial-frequency discrimination threshold, but the plot of threshold elevation versus test spatial frequency had a quite different form from that predicted from the shape of a plot of perceived spatial frequency versus test spatial frequency.

Contrast Sensitivity Functions of Human Observers, and the Description of a Stimulus Pattern in Terms of Its Power Spectrum and Its Phase Spectrum

The contrast sensitivity function

Although contrast sensitivity functions are commonly used when employing Fourier methods in the design of linear optical systems such as, for example, camera lenses, it is important to be aware that Fourier methods are far less powerful when dealing with nonlinear systems such as the human visual system. Perhaps the chief merit of the human contrast sensitivity function is that it provides considerably more information than visual acuity: the contrast sensitivity function is a description of the visual systems's sensitivity to course-scale detail and medium-scale detail as well as to fine detail, while visual acuity quantifies sensitivity to fine detail only.

The following comments on contrast sensitivity functions apply to all the following five sections, each of which contains an account of the contrast sensitivity function for the particular type of spatial contrast discussed in that section. (The *contrast sensitivity function* is a plot of the reciprocal of the contrast detection threshold for a grating versus the spatial frequency of that grating.)

First I will review what is meant by the contrast sensitivity function for a luminance-defined grating (also called the contrast sensitivity characteristic or the contrast sensitivity curve, but not the modulation transfer function because the term "transfer function" is used only for linear systems).

A sinusoidal luminance grating looks like a blurred grill (upper half of Figure 1.17 and Figure 2.17A). A *sinusoidal waveform* is depicted in Figure 1.18A. Part B shows the luminance profile of a *sinusoidal grating*: a sinusoidal waveform added to a constant mean luminance (L_{mean}) (see pp. 420–422). The distance between adjacent bright or dim bars (i.e., one grating cycle) is the *spatial period* of the grating (P), and its reciprocal is the *spatial frequency*. In physics, spatial frequency is often expressed in cycles per mm distance perpendicular to the bars of the grating, but in vision research, spatial frequency is usually expressed in cycles per degree of angle subtended at the eye (see second footnote on page 44).

The grating's position (relative to some reference mark) can also be expressed in terms of grating periods. For example, a change in spatial phase of 180 degrees corresponds to a spatial displacement of one half-cycle that places bright bars exactly where dark bars used to be.

The *modulation* of a grating is equal to ($L_{max} - L_{min}$). This variable is commonly used in optical physics but seldom in psychophysics; there it is more common to use *spatial contrast*, usually defined as ($L_{max} - L_{min}$)/($L_{max} + L_{min}$), where L_{max} and L_{min} are, respectively, the maximum and minimum local luminances within the grating. (This formula is also called Michaelson contrast, see Appendix B, pp. 436–439). Spatial contrast can be expressed as a ratio or as a percentage. Thus, for example, the contrasts of the gratings whose luminance profile are

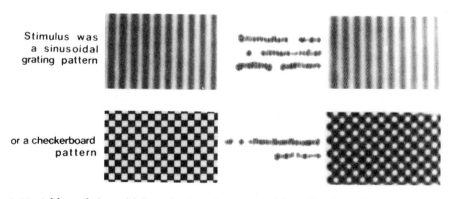

1.17 A blurred sinusoidal grating is still a sinusoidal grating, but a blurred checkerboard is not a checkerboard. From Bodis-Wollner et al. (1986).

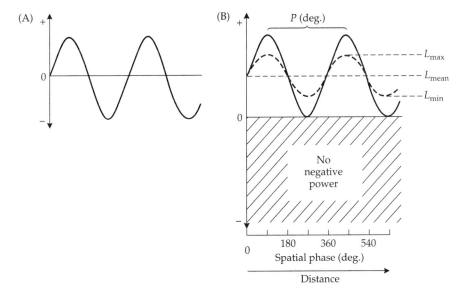

1.18 The profile of a sinusoidal grating is not a sinusoid. (A) A sinusoidal function of distance assumes both positive and negative values. (B) Because light energy
is never negative, the luminance profile of a sinusoidal grating is always positive.
Consequently, it is not correct to say that any arbitrary pattern or scene can be synthesized by superimposing sinusoidal gratings.

shown as a continuous line and a dashed line in Figure 1.18B are, respectively,
1.0 (or 100%) and 0.5 (or 50%).

For any given spatial frequency, contrast sensitivity is the reciprocal of contrast detection threshold. It can be measured in the manner described on pp. 8–17
and in Figure 1.5, but instead of using homogeneous stimulus displays, the displays would be gratings of different contrasts. If the reference grating has zero
contrast (i.e., it is an area of uniform luminance) we obtain a *grating detection
threshold*. (If the reference grating has a finite contrast we obtain a *contrast increment threshold*).

To obtain an observer's contrast sensitivity curve for luminance-defined gratings we would measure the observer's grating detection threshold for many spatial frequencies and plot the reciprocal of threshold as a function of spatial frequency (e.g., the open circles in Figure 1.19). The lowest detection threshold is
about 0.5% (i.e., the highest sensitivity is about 200), and this obtains at a spatial
frequency that depends on field size, and is about 5 cycles/deg. in Figure 1.19.

Two important points:

1. When interpreting the shape of the low-frequency segment of a contrast sensitivity function, it is important to bear in mind how many
   complete grating cycles (i.e., complete periods) are in the display. As
   the total number of cycles falls progressively below about five, the

grating's spatial frequency power spectrum is no longer narrow, but progressively spreads over a wider and wider band that may include considerable power at 0 cycles/degree (i.e., at zero spatial contrast), so that the interpretation of threshold measures, and even the concept of the grating's spatial frequency grows equivocal (see pp. 416–420).

2. When interpreting the shape of the high-frequency segment of a grating contrast sensitivity function, it is important to bear in mind how many independent spatial samples there are per grating cycle in the stimulus. It is possible to create continuous LD gratings that have a very large number of spatial samples per degree of visual angle, and contrast detection threshold can be measured up to spatial frequencies higher than 50 cycles/degree using such gratings. On the other hand, for texture-defined (TD), motion-defined (MD), and disparity-defined (DD) gratings, the number of spatial samples per degree has an upper limit. As discussed on pp. 470–476 it is known that grating detection threshold for LD and TD gratings can be limited by spatial sampling rather than the properties of the human visual system when the number of spatial samples per grating cycle falls below a number considerably higher than two.

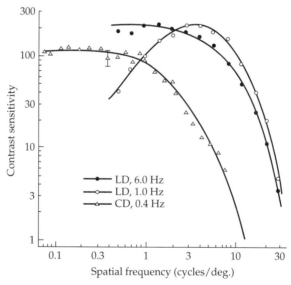

1.19 Contrast sensitivity functions for luminance and chromatic gratings. Open and filled circles indicate a luminance-defined grating that was counterphase-modulated at 1.0 Hz or 6.0 Hz. Field size was 2.5 × 2.5 degrees. Open triangles represent a color-defined (CD) grating (in this case, an equiluminant red–green grating) that was counterphase-modulated at a low frequency (0.4 Hz). Maximum field size was 23.5 degrees. Data from Robson (1966) and Mullen (1985).

The motivation for developing the formidable mathematical method called Fourier optics was the remarkable fact that, equipped with this method, a single measurement of the amplitude and phase characteristic of a linear optical imaging system (such as, for example, a camera lens or the optics of the eye) allows the image of any arbitrary spatial pattern to be obtained theoretically *knowing no more about the system than that it is linear* (Duffieux, 1946; Hopkins, 1955, 1956, 1962; Schade, 1948, 1958); see Appendix C. Unfortunately, this valuable mathematical property of the Fourier optics approach does not in general hold true for nonlinear optical systems (see Appendix B). This does not imply, however, that Fourier analysis cannot be a useful tool in the analysis of nonlinear systems (Hayashi, 1964; Blaquière, 1966; Hagedorn, 1982). Second-and higher-order harmonic components or subharmonic components in the response to a sinusoidal input are an immediate indicator of nonlinearity, and the particular components observed can provide clues to the kind of nonlinearity one has encountered. For example, M. P. Regan and D. Regan (1988, 1989a) describe a method for analyzing multistage nonlinear biological systems that is based on the Fourier transform.

The original motivation for measuring contrast sensitivity functions for the human visual system was that:

> If the system behaves linearly, the visual sensitivity to any arbitrary pattern can be predicted from a single measurement of the amplitude and phase characteristics of the system.

However, the value of the Fourier optics approach is limited by the fact that the human visual system is nonlinear, especially for contrasts well above grating detection threshold. And the retina is spatially inhomogeneous. Quite apart from these important limitations, it is often the case in experimental visual psychophysics that little or no information is obtained about the system's *phase characteristic*.

This takes us to an important issue. Because it is a difficult and often-misunderstood issue I will make a light pass over it at this point, and dig deeper in later sections, reserving a more formal outline for the Appendixes.

Two alternative (and complementary) ways of describing a spatial pattern

If the average person were shown a black and white photograph of a face and told, "have a go at specifying this picture scientifically so as to give a complete description," he or she might eventually reply "by measuring the brightness at every point on the picture." And this is (more or less) correct. Any pattern, whether as simple as a bright line or as complex as a black and white photograph of a face, can be specified fully by measuring the luminance at very many locations within the pattern. Indeed, the kind of newspaper picture that is composed of many tiny dots is based on this fact.

For the time being I ask the reader to accept that, rather than describing the pattern by assigning a number to every location within the pattern, it can be described in terms of the pattern as a whole, throwing away all location information and assigning two numbers to every spatial frequency of the pattern as a whole. These two numbers are a magnitude and a phase. For the present, that is all we need in order to understand the importance of the phase spectrum.

The importance of information carried by the phase spectrum is brought out dramatically in Figure 1.20.* Figure 1.20 illustrates that in face recognition, the phase spectrum can be more important than the magnitude spectrum (see Oppenhein & Lim, 1981; Field, 1987; Morgan et al., 1991; Tadmore & Tolhurst, 1992).

The phase spectrum is crucial, even for a pattern as simple as a line. The spatial frequency power spectrum of a single long thin bright line is the same as the power spectrum of a random one-dimensional variation of luminance that extends over a large distance. These two spatial waveforms differ only in their phase spectra: nevertheless, they look very different.

In the spatial-frequency description of a pattern as a whole, the phase spectrum carries important information about the distribution of light within the pattern.

This demonstration that spatial phase is important for face recognition can be taken together with the finding that human faces can be recognized even after spatial filtering removes all spatial frequencies higher than three to four cycles per face width (Ginsburg, 1978). Together they imply that, if they are to play a role in object recognition, hypothetical local mechanisms that analyze any given patch into the first three (Robson, 1975) harmonics must retain the information carried by the phase spectrum of the stimulus along the lines of Nachmias and Weber's (1975) hypothesis (see also Lawden [1983]).

However, the fact that the phase spectrum of the stimulus carries important information does not necessarily imply that the visual system encodes explicitly the phase spectrum of the stimulus.

---

* Geoffrey Arden, a past editor of *Vision Research*, has made many important contributions to electrodiagnosis and to vision research. Henk van der Tweel (1915–1997) made important contributions to cardiology in the Netherlands by designing and personally constructing the instruments that allowed advanced research on the electrical activity of the heart. He also made important contributions to human brain electrophysiology and, by no means the least of his accomplishments, he influenced greatly the scientific training of ophthalmologists. During the war he and his wife Liese helped others to safety at severe risk to their own lives. Although I had known and admired him since 1965, when he first invited me to visit his Department of Medical Physics at the University of Amsterdam to work with Henk Spekreijse and himself, it was not until after his death that I learned that he was not born Henk van der Tweel. That was his nom de guerre, his Resistance name, and the Dutch Government had allowed him to use it as his legal name when peace finally came to his country. His great skills as a forger, developed during the war, served him well in peace time. He became a noted restorer of Rembrandt etchings.

The English-language proceedings of a meeting organized by the Royal Academy of the Netherlands to celebrate the life of Henk van der Tweel (entitled *Van Hoofd en Hart: Henk van der Tweel 1915–1997*) is available from the Stichting Van Hoofd en Hart, P.O. Box 12011, 1100 AA Amsterdam–Zuidoost, The Netherlands.

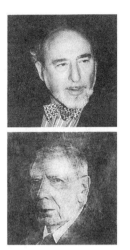 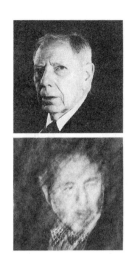

1.20 The phase spectrum is essential for face recognition. Digitized photographs of Geoffrey Arden (top left) and Henk van der Tweel (top right). When the power spectrum of Arden is combined with the phase spectrum of van der Tweel (bottom left), Arden is unrecognizable. When the power spectrum of van der Tweel is combined with the phase spectrum of Arden (bottom right), van der Tweel cannot be recognized. From van der Tweel and Reits (1998); courtesy of Henk Spekreijse.

Although this point puzzles many students, it is a pseudo-problem rather than a problem. The basic question is whether the early processing of, for example, a face, is based on (1) large filters that analyze either the face as a whole or patches of the face into a rough version of a power spectrum and a phase spectrum (in which case the relative spatial phases of the frequency components must be preserved), or (2) is based on the parallel analysis at many points over the face of the variation of local luminance across the face (in which case the phase spectrum does not enter the discussion).

> There is experimental evidence that the visual system does not encode explicitly the relative phases of a pattern's spatial-frequency components.

The evidence is as follows. First, if, in the spatial-frequency domain description of a nonsinusoidal grating pattern, the phase of a spatial-frequency component is changed by as much as 30 to 70 degrees, this change cannot be detected unless the associated changes in the local contrast within the target are sufficiently large (Burr, 1980; Badcock, 1984a,b).

And second, in a series of experiments, Badcock (1984a,b, 1988) dissociated differences in the phase spectrum of his stimulus pattern as a whole from the associated changes in the distribution of local contrast within the pattern. He concluded that the visual system is sensitive to the spatial distribution of local contrast within a pattern rather than to the relative phases of the spatial-frequency components of the pattern as a whole (see also Westheimer, 1977). Badcock (1988) noted that local contrast could be extracted by local filters with *Mexican-hat profiles* (Field, 1984; Rentschler & Treutwein, 1985; Hess & Pointer, 1987). Badcock's conclusion is consistent with data on visual sensitivity to spatial beat patterns, data that could not be explained in terms of phase signals provided by local-contrast detectors. Such signals could not have supported the measured visual sensitivity to displacement of the beats. On the other hand, the beat data could be explained straightforwardly in terms of local-contrast detectors whose outputs carried a position label (Badcock & Derrington, 1985, 1987, 1988; Derrington & Badcock, 1985, 1986).

Badcock (1988) pointed out that, when attempting to distinguish between visual system sensitivities to location and to spatial phase, it is important to use stimuli that do not confound these two quantities. To illustrate the fact that a change in the relative phases of spatial-frequency components in the spatial-frequency domain is not necessarily associated with any change of location in the spatial domain, he gave the following example. Consider two bars, some distance apart, whose locations are fixed. Now change the contrast of one of the bars. The phase spectrum of the pair of bars as a whole changes, but their locations remain fixed. Badcock then noted that Morgan and Regan (1987) had shown that this manipulation did not change the just-noticeable difference in the separation between the two bars.

Badcock drew attention to the point that experimental designs based on a simple sinusoidal grating (e.g., Nakayama & Silverman, 1985; Burgess & Ghanderian, 1984; Howard & Richardson, 1988) cannot distinguish between spatial phase and location, because the two quantities are totally confounded. (Another way of putting this is that spatial phase and location are different things only for patterns that contain two or more frequency components. With two frequency components, for example, we have the possibility that the phase of one component can vary relative to the phase of the other component.)

All of the authors cited so far used stimuli such as nonsinusoidal gratings whose luminance varied along only one dimension. Victor and Conte (1991) explored the role of the phase spectrum in discriminating between different two-dimensional textures. They concluded that there is no need to postulate that the visual system contains mechanisms that are specifically sensitive to spatial phase. Rather, they proposed, the visual system contains an array of parallel processors of local retinal image information that extracts edges independently of whether the edges are bright-dim or dim-bright (see Figure 7 of Victor and Conte [1991]). The essential features of this processor are "(i) local subunits whose outputs are independently rectified; and (ii) a second nonlinearity which pools these outputs along a line. Elimination of either of the two nonlinearities collapses the model to more standard models of cortical cells and edge detectors" (Victor & Conte, 1996, p. 1628).

"Mexican-Hat" Receptive Fields

Because the surfaces of different objects commonly have different reflectancies, an important retinal image indicator of a boundary between two objects is a spatially abrupt change of luminance. Although it may be low, the *percentage* change of luminance will be unaffected by very large changes in the intensity of illumination. Consider, for example, the spatial variation of luminance within the retinal image of a given scene that is viewed from a particular location. The spatial variation can be expressed in such a way that the expression is the same when the scene is illuminated by the midday sun and by the moon (providing that the sun and moon occupy the same position in the sky).

One way of describing the spatial variation of retinal image luminance so that it corresponds closely to the variation of reflectance in the scene under observation is in terms of spatial (luminance) contrast. There are, however, several alternative definitions of the contrast of an object's retinal image. Suppose that the object's retinal image is of uniform luminance L_1 and the surrounding areas of the retinal image are of uniform luminance L_2. As already mentioned, Michaelson contrast (defined as $[L_1 - L_2]/[L_1 + L_2]$) is commonly used for spatially periodic targets such as, for example, gratings. But there are at least two other definitions of contrast. The following two definitions are often used to express the contrast of an isolated object: the Weber contrast, $(L_1 - L_2)/L_2$; and $(L_1 - L_2)/L_1$—a definition proposed by Burr, Ross, and Morrone (1985). Weber contrast has the peculiarity that it can reach indefinitely high positive values, and in that sense does not correspond well with perception. The definition proposed by Burr et al. does not suffer from this drawback. Its highest possible value is 1.0 in accord with the Michaelson definition. But Burr and his colleagues have reported evidence that their definition of contrast has an even more important advantage over the Weber definition—namely, that the luminance that sets the local *gain* (L_1) is also the normalization factor for contrast. Appendix F, pp. 470–476, sets out the argument of Burr et al. in detail.

Pelli (1996) has pointed out that it is surprisingly difficult to quantify the contrast in a complex image, even for a complex image as simple as a Gaussian-weighted patch of a sinusoidal grating. He and others have argued that it is inappropriate to describe complex images such as natural scenes as having a single contrast value, and that global measures such as root mean square (RMS) contrast have little relation to the physiology of contrast coding (Pelli, 1990; Tadmore & Tolhurst, 1994, 1995; Tolhurst et al., 1996). Lillestæter (1993) offers a quantitative definition of *complex contrast*.

How the visual system extracts subtle spatial variations of luminance from the retinal image of any given scene in a way that is almost independent of the scene's level of illumination is a question that has attracted much discussion.

One hypothesis is that the retinal image is analyzed by a parallel array of receptive fields, each of which has an excitatory center and an inhibitory surround (or an inhibitory center and an excitatory surround), so that its sensitivity profile resembles a Mexican hat (Figure 1.21). A difference of Gaussians (DOG) sensitivity profile is conveniently computable and widely used (Rodieck & Stone, 1965a,b). Elongated (and hence orientation-selective) DOGs (Figure 1.22A) have been used in some models of spatial vision and circularly symmetric DOGs (Figure 1.22B) have been used in others.

If the areas under the excitatory and inhibitory sections of the sensitivity profile are equal (as in Figure 1.21), then the receptive field will be insensitive to a uniform luminance, and will respond only to a *spatial variation of luminance* (see Figure 2.46 for an explanation). An array of wide DOGs will analyze the retinal image at a coarse spatial scale, being selectively sensitive to large objects, while an array of narrow DOGs will analyze the retinal image at a fine spatial scale, being selectively sensitive to small objects (and sharp edges).

By using pieces of paper it is easy to demonstrate that a target whose reflectance is only a few percent higher than its surrounding can be almost as easily seen at midday under an overcast sky as at an illumination level more than 100,000 times higher under midday sun. Furthermore, the contrast of the target does not look greatly different at these low and high levels of illumination. How this observation can be explained has attracted a good deal of discussion. Suppose, for example, that the response of a Mexican-hat receptive field is given by $R = k(R_E - R_I)$, where the excitatory (R_E) and inhibitory (R_I) responses are obtained by multiplying the local luminance by the local sensitivity. If the excitatory and inhibitory responses are both linear functions of luminance then, if we increase the illumination level 100,000 times, the response of the receptive field will increase 100,000 times. (The concept of *contrast gain control* is discussed on pp. 83–85 and 394.) If, on the other hand, the excitatory and inhibitory responses

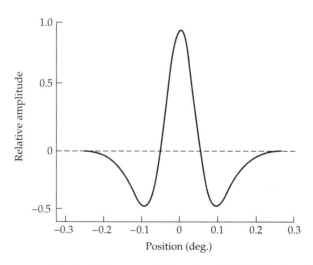

1.21 Luminance profile of a difference of Gaussians (DOG) Mexican-hat stimulus. Courtesy of Hugh Wilson.

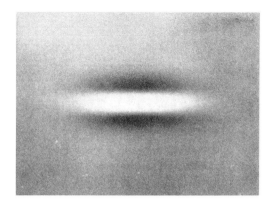 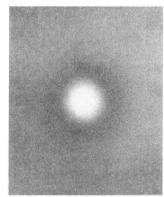

1.22 Difference of Gaussians (DOG) stimuli. Elongated stimulus. (B) Circularly symmetric DOG stimulus. Photographs courtesy of Hugh Wilson.

are different, nonlinear (e.g., compressive) functions of luminance, then the DOG might signal that the bright target was brighter than its surrounding, that it was the same brightness as its surroundings, and that it was dimmer than its surroundings as the illumination level was progressively raised. To further elaborate on this point, when discussing the effect of illumination level on a DOG's effectiveness as a contrast detector, it is necessary to specify which of the (at least) three definitions of contrast is to be used.

CHAPTER 2

Luminance-Defined Form

By relying on second-hand evidence one is bound to lose something of the truth and much of the human atmosphere. But no man exists who can claim to have witnessed everything at first-hand, or to have had all the knowledge available. The most we can ask is that each shall say frankly what he has to say. From a comparison of particular sincerities, truth will eventually emerge.

> From *Strange Defeat* by Marc Bloch ("Narbonne" in the French Resistance); born 1886; Medieval Historian and Professor of Economic History, Sorbonne Faculty of the University of Paris; executed by firing squad at Trévoux on the 16th of June 1944. Written in 1940 and hidden. Published posthumously in French. English edition 1968, New York, W.W. Norton & Co.

Preamble

Over the last 30 years a theoretical framework has been developed whose aim is to account for the visual detection and spatial discrimination of luminance-defined (LD) form. The basic idea is that LD spatial information from any small area of the retinal image passes through an array of parallel linear spatial filters. The current consensus is that any given filter responds most strongly to a target (such as a bar) of specific width and orientation, and that different filters prefer different widths and orientations. Because the spatial characteristics of a bar can be described either in terms of its width and height or in terms of spatial frequency, the filters are alternatively described as being either tuned to size (i.e., width) and orientation, or as being tuned to spatial frequency and orientation. In the early literature, the focus of Thomas was on width selectivity, while the focus of the Cambridge group was on spatial-frequency selectivity (Campbell & Kulikowski, 1966; Campbell & Robson, 1968; Thomas, 1968, 1970; Blakemore & Campbell, 1969; Blakemore & Nachmias, 1971).

As mentioned earlier, although the effects of spatial frequency and width on contrast sensitivity are equivalent descriptions and have an invariant relationship for a linear imaging system (such as a lens), in a nonlinear system, one description cannot in general be predicted from the other without a knowledge of the system equations; and the human visual system is strongly nonlinear especially when contrast is well above detection threshold (see Appendixes A & E and pp. 93–98).

Much of the evidence for spatial-frequency channels is based on psychophysical measurements carried out at contrast levels near detection threshold. The extent to which the theoretical position has to be modified to account for vision in the everyday environment is unclear: in everyday vision, contrast levels are commonly well above threshold, thus giving rise to the possibility of interactions between the filters and a consequent breakdown of their independence. And, indeed, there is psychophysical (Tolhurst & Thompson, 1985; DeValois, 1978; Olzak & Thomas, 1992; Wilson, 1991a) and objective (D. Regan & M. P. Regan, 1986, 1987, 1988; M. P. Regan & D. Regan, 1989b) evidence that, at suprathreshold levels of contrast, nonlinear interactions between differently tuned spatial filters are by no means negligible in human observers.

Because they are treated very thoroughly by Graham (1989), I have devoted less space than I otherwise would have done to a number of issues including probability summation, methodology, attention, and spatial-frequency channels. I refer the interested reader to Graham's book.

Detection of Luminance Spatial Contrast and the Contrast Sensitivity Function for Luminance-Defined Form

In this section I discuss the visual processing of two kinds of luminance-defined spatial form: a nonrepetitive form such as a single bar, and a repetitive form such as an extended grating.

Detection of a nonrepetitive local stimulus

Small circularly symmetrical targets might be expected to emphasize retinal processing (because the receptive fields of retinal ganglion cells are approximately circular; see Westheimer, 1967), but line targets might be expected to emphasize cortical processing (because many cortical cells have elongated receptive fields). Using that line of reasoning, several authors have measured visual sensitivity to a pattern of three bright lines (Thomas, 1968; Rentschler & Fiorentini, 1974; Hines,

1976; Wilson, 1978). All found that a three-line pattern is least visible when the two outer lines lie at a certain distance from either side of the central line. This finding can be explained by assuming that the three-line pattern was detected by a local neural mechanism, the center of whose elongated receptive field was excited by a bright line, while the outer regions of its elongated receptive field were inhibited when stimulated by a bright line. For example, the data points in Figure 2.1 show that, when the flanking lines were within about 0.05 degrees of the test line, sensitivity to the lines was increased, but when the flanking lines were 0.05 to 0.20 degrees from the central line, sensitivity to the lines was reduced. Wilson and Bergen (1979) subsequently explained their data by assuming that any given point in the fovea is served by *not less than* four such local receptive fields (though they did not exclude a number greater than four).

Detection of the spatial periodicity of a static grating

In this section I discuss research on the contrast required to render just visible the periodic structure of a grating. This kind of research is called *threshold psychophysics*. I also discuss research on the visual processing of gratings whose contrasts are sufficiently high to render them clearly visible, a kind of research called *suprathreshold psychophysics.*

The contrast sensitivity function at contrast detection threshold and the oblique effect for grating detection. Now we turn from the use of a nonrepetitive local

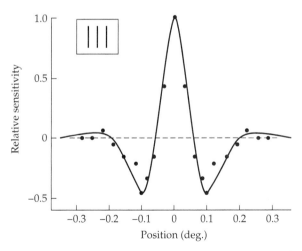

2.1 Data from an experiment measuring subthreshold summation between a center line and two flanking lines. The data show a central excitatory zone with inhibitory zones on either side. The solid curve is the inverse Fourier transform of the theoretical curve fit to the masking data in Figure 2.12D, which has a peak frequency of 4.0 cycles/deg. From Wilson (1991b).

stimulus to the use of a repetitive (i.e., spatially periodic) stimulus that extends over a considerable area. The human visual system's threshold contrast sensitivity function (CSF) for LD form has been described by plotting the reciprocal of contrast detection threshold for a sinusoidal grating versus the grating's spatial frequency. (The open circles in Figure 1.19 show that the shape of this threshold CSF is bandpass for a grating that is either static or modulated at a low temporal frequency [Schade, 1956; Robson, 1966].) The slope of the high-frequency segment of the CSF is approximately 1 dB per cycles per degree (i.e., a factor of two for every 6 cycles/deg.) for everyday photopic luminances (S. Klein, personal communication, January 1999).

Schade (1956) pointed out that the reduction of sensitivity at low spatial frequencies (shown by open circles in Figure 1.19) cannot be due to the optics of the eye.

Note, however, that the shape of the CSF depends on field size: peak sensitivity moves towards lower spatial frequencies as field size increases—the opposite effect to that produced by increasing grating luminance (Cohen et al., 1976, cited in Kelly, 1977, p. 119). The spatial frequency (obtained by extrapolation) at which contrast sensitivity falls to zero is called (sinewave) grating acuity.*

Grating detection can be regarded as being determined by a combination of two opposing factors: the contrast of the grating and the grating-induced variations of the local sensitivity of the retina. The sensitivity variation caused by a period of steady fixation can be rendered visible by abruptly reducing grating contrast to zero. The resulting negative afterimage of the grating is lowpass and does not extend to such high spatial frequencies as the CSF, consistent with the idea that the inhibitory surrounds of local receptive fields are insensitive to high spatial frequencies (Koenderink, 1972).

Contrast threshold is lowest in the fovea for all spatial frequencies over the range of 2 to 16 cycles/deg. that have been compared (Hiltz & Cavonius, 1974; Rijsdijk et al., 1980; Robson & Graham, 1981; Regan & Beverley, 1983b). A plot of log contrast sensitivity versus retinal eccentricity is approximately a straight line. Figure 2.2 illustrates this point for the particular case of the variation of sensitivity to a 2 cycles/deg. grating along a vertical line cutting through the fovea. Threshold is expressed as percent contrast on the left-hand ordinate in Figure 2.2 and in decibels (dB) on the right-hand ordinate.† Figure 2.3 illustrates that the

---

* Although grating acuity in Figure 1.19 is little higher than 35 cycles/deg., other authors have reported foveal acuities as high as 50 to 60 cycles/deg. and as low as 27 cycles/deg. (Campbell & Green, 1965; van Nes & Bouman, 1967; Leguire, 1991). Quite apart from inter-subject variability and the effect of luminance, a potent source of disagreement here is that different monitors have different spot sizes relative to the width of the display, so that if display contrast is not calibrated at high spatial frequencies, the measured high-frequency rolloff in sensitivity can include a substantial artifactual contribution from the display (Morgan & Watt, 1982; Hess & Baker, 1984; Regan, 1989a, p. 145).

† One decibel (dB) is equal to $10 \log_{10}$ (power ratio) = $20 \log_{10}$ (amplitude ratio). See Appendix H.

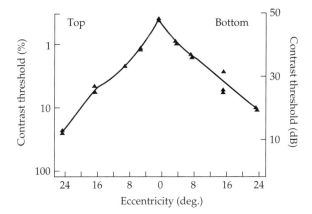

2.2 Log contrast sensitivity falls off approximately linearly with retinal eccentricity. Variation of contrast detection threshold along a vertical line cutting through the fovea (zero on the abscissa) for a grating of spatial frequency 2 cycles/deg. After Regan and Beverley (1983b).

rate of decrease of sensitivity with eccentricity is greater for high than for low spatial frequencies, so that the CSF is displaced more and more to lower spatial frequencies as eccentricity is increased (Koenderink et al., 1978a,b; Robson & Graham, 1981; Regan & Beverley, 1983b). Equal spacing of the *isocontrast contours* (shown as heavy lines in Figure 2.3A–C) means that contrast sensitivity fell off logarithmically with increasing eccentricity. For example, an increase from zero to

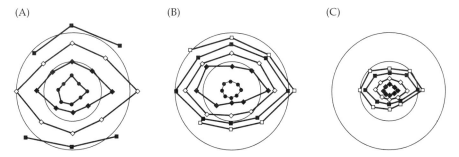

(A)   (B)   (C)

2.3 The rate of decrease of contrast sensitivity with eccentricity is greater for high spatial frequencies than for low spatial frequencies. (A) Data of Figure 2.2 replotted in the form of isocontrast contours. Isocontrast contours for gratings of 4 cycles/deg. and 8 cycles/deg., respectively, are shown in parts B and C. All test gratings were oriented vertically. Key: Filled circles, 39 dB; filled diamonds, 33 dB; open diamonds, 27 dB; filled squares, 21 dB; open squares, 15 dB. The dB values express threshold contrast relative to 100% contrast (100% contrast is 0 dB). After Regan and Beverley (1983b).

five degrees of eccentricity reduced contrast sensitivity by the same *fraction* as an increase from 20 to 25 degrees of eccentricity. The isocontrast contours grew progressively more crowded as the grating's spatial frequency was increased from 2 cycles/deg.(part A), through 4 cycles/deg. (part B), to 8 cycles/deg. (part C), indicating that the falloff of sensitivity became steeper as spatial frequency was increased.

For two of the three observers studied by Regan and Beverley (1983b), contrast sensitivity fell off more rapidly horizontally than vertically, producing the horizontally elongated closed isocontrast contours shown in Figure 2.3. On the other hand, the third observer's isocontrast contours were elongated vertically.

For many normally sighted observers, grating acuity is lower for oblique orientations than for gratings whose bars are vertical or horizontal (Taylor, 1963). This *oblique effect* averages about 1.5 dB for foveal vision (Timney & Muir, 1976), an effect equivalent to about 7 dB (i.e., about 2:1), for contrast sensitivity near the cutoff spatial frequency. (Candidate explanations of the oblique effect are discussed on pp. 115–123.)

Confirming the report of Berkeley et al. (1975), Figure 2.4 shows that the foveal oblique effect is restricted to high spatial frequencies. Regan and Beverley found the

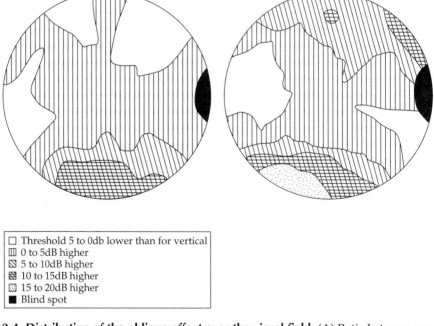

☐ Threshold 5 to 0db lower than for vertical
▥ 0 to 5dB higher
▧ 5 to 10dB higher
▨ 10 to 15dB higher
▤ 15 to 20dB higher
■ Blind spot

2.4 Distribution of the oblique effect over the visual field. (A) Ratio between contrast sensitivity for a grating oriented at 45 degrees and a grating with vertical bars. (B) Ratio between contrast sensitivity for a grating orientated at 135 degrees and a grating with vertical bars. Field diameter was 32 degrees of visual angle. Spatial frequency was 4 cycles/deg. After Regan and Beverley (1983b).

oblique effect to be negligible (in normally sighted observers), for a 4 cycles/deg. grating when viewed foveally.* But in peripheral vision the oblique effect could be as high as 15–20 dB (20 dB is a ratio of 10:1), with a repeatability of 2 to 3 dB.

Given that neurons with strong selectivity for orientation are not found peripheral to primary visual cortex, the visual fields shown in Figure 2.4 presumably reflect processing at or central to primary visual cortex.

The CSF at contrast levels above contrast detection threshold. It is not self-evident that models of the visual processing of small increments of contrast would necessarily provide a good description of everyday vision, because many everyday objects have high contrasts. (I will return to this point later when discussing orientation and spatial-frequency discrimination.) Here we should note that the suprathreshold CSF for a static grating has been measured by matching the perceived contrast of a test grating to the perceived contrast of a 5 cycles/deg. standard grating. When the contrast of the standard grating was only slightly above threshold, the suprathreshold sensitivity curve followed the inverted-U shape of the threshold CSF (see open circles in Figure 1.19). However, as the contrast of the standard was increased, the curve became progressively flatter over the entire 0.25 to 25 cycles/deg. range of spatial frequencies investigated. Relative adjustment of the *contrast gain* of cortical neurons tuned to spatial frequency has been proposed as a basis for this so-called contrast constancy (Georgeson & Sullivan, 1975; Georgeson, 1991; see pp. 83–85).

Effects of temporal frequency on grating contrast sensitivity I: Foveal vision

When a grating is presented for only a brief duration, is counterphase-modulated (Figure 2.5A), or is drifting, the shape of the contrast sensitivity function is changed. In particular, sensitivity at low spatial frequencies grows relatively higher, and the curve tends towards a lowpass rather than a bandpass shape (see Figure 1.19, filled circles). One proposed explanation for this finding is that the inhibitory surrounds of the local receptive fields prefer low spatial frequencies but are insensitive to high temporal frequencies. An alternative explanation is that the phase lag between center and surround does not remain at 180 degrees at high temporal frequencies so that, although the surround is still sensitive, it is no longer antagonistic (Hochstein & Shapley, 1976; Troy, 1983).

A different way of looking at the difference between the data shown as open and filled circles in Figure 1.19 is that the contrast sensitivity function is determined by two kinds of mechanisms whose temporal tuning curves are different. The evidence for this hypothesis is as follows.

If the contrast of a counterphase-modulated grating is slowly increased from zero until *something* is just visible, observers often say that the *something* looks more

---

* Figure 2.69 shows that the variation of foveal contrast sensitivity with grating orientation can be as high as 20:1 at low spatial frequencies in some patients with multiple sclerosis.

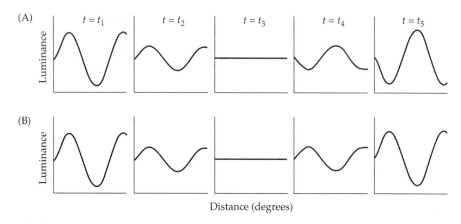

(A) $t = t_1$ | $t = t_2$ | $t = t_3$ | $t = t_4$ | $t = t_5$

Luminance

(B) Luminance

Distance (degrees)

2.5 Counterphase modulation and contrast modulation of a grating. (A) The time sequence $t = t_1$ to $t = t_5$ illustrates counterphase modulation of a grating. Local luminance is modulated as a function of time (in this case by a sinusoidal temporal waveform) at temporal frequency F Hz, adjacent bars being modulated in antiphase. Consequently, the grating's bright and dim bars exchange places $2F$ times per second. Thus, the sequence $t = t_1$ to $t = t_5$ shows one-half of a complete cycle of counterphase modulation. Counterphase modulation is sometimes called *pattern reversal*. (B) The *magnitude* of the grating's contrast is modulated as a function of time (in this case by a sinusoidal temporal waveform) at temporal frequency F Hz. The time sequence $t = t_1$ to $t = t_5$ illustrates that the bright and dim bars do not exchange places. Rather, the contrast oscillates at frequency F Hz between some maximum value (at $t = t_1$ and $t = t_5$) and zero (at $t = t_3$). One full cycle of modulation is shown.

like a static grating than a temporally modulated grating. This effect is especially clear when the grating's spatial frequency is greater than about 4 degrees (Kulikowski, 1971). Only if the contrast is increased some way above detection threshold does flicker or apparent movement become evident. The situation is quite different for gratings of low spatial frequency. As the contrast is slowly increased until *something* can just be detected, this *something* first detected is flicker or apparent movement. The spatial structure of this *something* is very indistinct. Only if contrast is increased some way above this *something* detection threshold can the position and width of the individual bars of the grating be clearly recognized (Van Nes et al., 1967).

Keesey (1972) found that these pattern-detection and flicker/movement thresholds are independent functions of temporal frequency. She proposed that they reveal the presence of two kinds of independent mechanisms. The output of one kind of mechanism carries a *flicker/movement label*. This kind of mechanism has poor spatial resolution. Although the second kind of mechanism is, like the first kind, selectively tuned to temporal frequency, activation does not result in any percept of temporal change because the output carries only one label: a *spatial structure label* (Tolhurst, 1973, 1975).

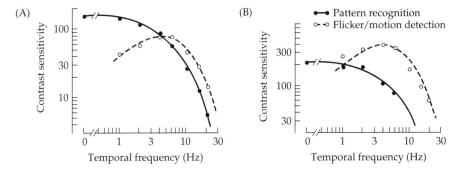

2.6 Filters that signal pattern and filters that signal flicker/motion. A grating whose contrast is sinusoidally modulated as a function of time can produce two percepts: spatial pattern and flicker/motion. (A) Thresholds for the two percepts for gratings of spatial frequency 12 cycles/deg. (B) Thresholds for the two percepts for gratings of spatial frequency 0.8 cycles/deg. After Kulikowski and Tolhurst (1973.)

Figure 2.6 compares the contrast sensitivities of two kinds of mechanism. The observer's experimental task was to adjust the contrast of a grating until flicker/motion could just be detected, then to repeat the adjustment until the grating's spatial structure (individual bars) could just be seen. The grating's contrast was modulated sinusoidally as a function of time, as illustrated in Figure 2.5B. In other words, at one instant the observer saw a uniform field (zero contrast), then contrast smoothly increased to a maximum, then smoothly returned to zero, and so on.

Figure 2.6A shows the results of this experiment for a grating of fairly high spatial frequency (12 cycles/deg.). Sensitivity to flicker/motion peaked at about 5 Hz and fell off steeply at low and high temporal frequencies (a *bandpass* temporal characteristic). Sensitivity to the grating's spatial structure was highest when the grating was static (i.e., temporally unmodulated, zero on the abscissa), and fell off as temporal frequency was progressively increased above about 4 Hz (a *lowpass* temporal characteristic). Figure 2.6B shows that, when the spatial frequency of the grating was reduced from 12 to 0.8 cycles/deg., the filters that signaled flicker/motion became about three times more sensitive while retaining the shape of their temporal tuning characteristic. In comparison, the increase of sensitivity for the filters that signaled the grating's spatial structure was considerably less than threefold.

> The filters that prefer high spatial frequencies and whose outputs carry a spatial-structure label respond equally well to stationary gratings and to drifting gratings, while the filters that prefer low spatial frequencies and whose outputs carry a flicker/movement label are very insensitive to stationary gratings, but respond well to drifting or counterphase-modulated gratings (Tolhurst, 1973).

This finding can account for the difference between the data shown as open and filled circles in Figure 1.19.

Effects of temporal frequency on grating contrast sensitivity II: Peripheral vision

The temporal characteristics shown in Figure 2.6 are for foveal vision. Figure 2.7 brings out the effect of eccentricity on the relative sensitivities of the two kinds of filter. The observers' task was the same as in Kulikowski and Tolhurst's experiment (though the grating was counterphase-modulated rather than contrast-modulated). For a grating whose spatial frequency was 2 cycles/deg. and whose temporal frequency was 8 Hz, the filters signaling flicker/motion were more sensitive than the filters signaling spatial structure when the grating was viewed foveally, but the relation reversed at large retinal eccentricities with a crossover point at about 14 degrees of eccentricity (Regan & Neima, 1984a).

Observers who carried out this experiment reported that, when the contrast of the counterphase-modulated, foveally viewed grating was slowly raised from zero until *something* was just visible, that *something* looked like flicker or apparent movement. But when the same grating was viewed in peripheral vision while

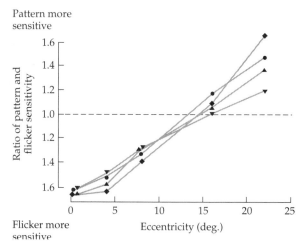

2.7 Effect of retinal eccentricity on contrast thresholds for perceiving pattern and flicker/motion. The ratio (threshold for perceiving pattern/threshold for perceiving flicker/motion) was plotted versus eccentricity in the visual field for the four oblique half-meridians. Pattern sensitivity was greater than flicker/motion sensitivity above the dotted line, and lower below the dotted line. The grating subtended 3.5 degrees, had a spatial frequency of 2.0 cycles/deg., and was counterphase-modulated at 8.0 Hz (so that bright and dim bars exchanged places 16 times per second). Data points are means for 10 normally sighted observers. Key: circles, upper left; diamonds, upper right; inverted triangles, lower left; triangles, lower right. From Regan and Neima (1984).

the same procedure was repeated, the *something* was a clearly visible grating whose clearly distinguishable bars appeared to be static, even though, when the observer looked straight at the grating, the bright and dim bars were clearly seen to be continually exchanging position.

Some observers expressed astonishment at this, and repeated the comparison several times to check that this was no trick, and had to be reassured that this was normal, and that there was nothing wrong with their vision. One interpretation of this effect is that:

When a stimulus pattern falls on peripheral retina, the visual system is less capable of recovering information carried by the phase spectrum of the pattern than when the same stimulus pattern is located on the fovea.

(See also Rentschler & Treutwein, 1985, and Bennett & Banks, 1987). This proposal lends additional significance to the point brought out in Figure 1.20. The finding that some kinds of moving stimuli that are perceived as stationary when viewed peripherally, but are clearly seen to be moving when viewed foveally (Pantle, 1992), may be related to this observation.

Channels for Luminance-Defined Form and Contrast Gain Control

The hypothesis that retinal information about luminance-defined form is processed through an array of parallel channels has driven much of the experimental research on human spatial vision carried out over the last 30 years.

Adaptation, masking, and other evidence for channels

Most of the early evidence for spatial channels was obtained psychophysically by measuring the contrast required to render a grating just visible (threshold psychophysics). The early psychophysically based models of spatial vision have, more recently, been forced to incorporate the concept of *contrast gain control* to allow for findings on the apparent contrast of a clearly visible grating. Adopting an experimental approach that is quite distinct from the psychophysical approach, some researchers have used electrical brain response recording techniques in human observers to investigate channeling in the processing of clearly visible gratings, and to investigate contrast gain control.

Psychophysical evidence for channels. Campbell and Robson (1968) concluded that the detection threshold for a squarewave grating was not consistent with the assumption that the contrast sensitivity curve (filled circles in Figure 1.19) represents a single visual channel. Their evidence was that detection threshold for a squarewave grating was only 1.3 times lower than detection threshold for a sinusoidal grating. They reasoned that, since the fundamental component in the frequency spectrum of a squarewave grating is 1.27 times larger than the fundamental component

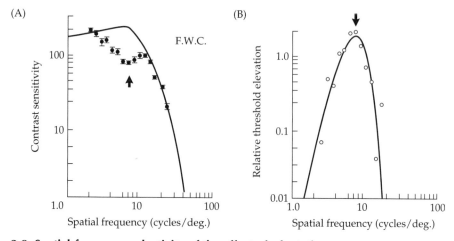

2.8 Spatial-frequency selectivity of the effect of adaptation on contrast sensitivity. (A) The continuous curve is the unadapted contrast sensitivity curve. The filled circles and vertical bars are the means and standard errors for redetermination of contrast sensitivity while the observer was continuously adapting to a high-contrast grating of spatial frequency 7.1 cycles/deg. (see arrow). (B) The vertical difference between each data point in (A) and the continuous curve in (A) was plotted as ordinate. The continuous curve is the function $[e^{-f^2} - e^{-(2f)^2}]^2$, where f is the spatial frequency. The observer was F. W. Campbell. After Blakemore and Campbell (1969).

in the frequency spectrum of a sinusoidal grating of the same peak-to-peak contrast (see Figure B.1), this finding implies that contrast detection threshold for the squarewave grating was determined entirely by its fundamental component. The third harmonic component (see Figure B.1D) had no effect. (See pp. 405–415.) They concluded that the first and third harmonics stimulated different channels, each of which had its own threshold, and that the responses to spatial frequencies separated by a factor of three were independent of one another (see also Graham & Nachmias, 1971).

> Thus, the visual system is nonlinear because the response to the squarewave grating was not equal to the sum of responses of the first and third harmonic components of the grating. (Linearity is defined on pp. 389–391.)

Refusing to abandon entirely the concept of linear processing, Campbell and Robson suggested that each individual channel behaves linearly (evidence reviewed in Klein, 1992) so that the visual system would be *piecewise* linear (defined in Appendix A, 389–391), a very different thing, though, from being linear. (As to whether any given channel can be regarded as being piecewise linear, see pp. 93–98.)

A different approach to uncovering spatial-frequency channels was adopted by Pantle and Sekuler (1968) and Blakemore and Campbell (1969). They found that, after inspecting a high-contrast grating for some minutes (a squarewave grating in the case of the first authors, a sinusoidal grating in the case of the second), contrast detection threshold was elevated for luminance gratings of similar orientation and spatial frequency, but was comparatively unaffected for gratings of very different orientations and spatial frequencies. In other words, adaptation produced a temporary notch in the CSF. The data points in Figure 2.8A show this temporary notch. Figure 2.8B shows the spatial-frequency selectivity of the threshold elevation shown in part A (see also Figure 2.9A). Figure 2.10A shows the orientation tuning of the threshold elevation. This contrast adaptation effect is distinct from light adaptation (Kelly & Burbeck, 1984).

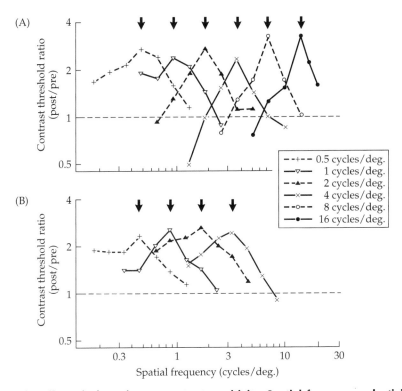

2.9 The effect of adaptation on contrast sensitivity: Spatial-frequency selectivity.
(A) Luminance contrast threshold elevations (post-/pre-) are plotted as a function of test grating spatial frequency. Arrows indicate adaptation spatial frequencies of 0.5, 1, 2, 4, 8, and 16 cycles/deg., respectively. (B) Similar to A except that adaptation and test stimuli were isoluminant red–green chromatic gratings. After Bradley et al. (1988).

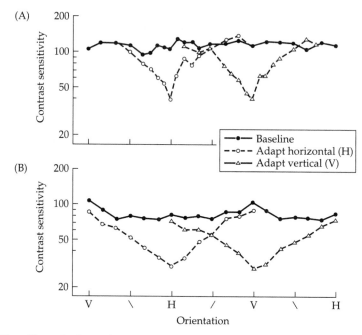

2.10 The effect of adaptation on contrast sensitivity: Orientation selectivity. (A) Luminance contrast sensitivities for a 2 cycles/deg. grating as a function of grating orientation after adapting to a uniformly illuminated screen (filled circles) and after adapting to a horizontal (open circles) and a vertical (open triangles) luminance grating. (B) Color contrast sensitivities for an isoluminant red–green grating as a function of orientation after adapting to a uniformly illuminated screen (filled circles) and after adapting to a horizontal (open circles) and a vertical (open triangles) red–green isoluminant grating. After Bradley et al. (1988).

The orientation-tuning bandwidth and the spatial-frequency tuning bandwidth of the detection threshold elevation are, respectively, about ±12 degrees and 1.4 octaves[*] (Gilinsky, 1968; Pantle & Sekuler, 1968; Campbell & Kulikowski, 1966; Blakemore & Campbell, 1969; Blakemore & Nachmias, 1971; Georgeson & Harris, 1984).

---

[*] In vision research, the sharpness of tuning is usually expressed as follows. Full bandwidth is defined as the ratio of the higher to the lower frequency at which sensitivity has declined to one-half peak sensitivity, the ratio being expressed in octaves, that is, the base 2 logarithm of the ratio. For example, a cell might give a maximum response for a grating of spatial frequency 7 cycles per degree (cpd) and half this response amplitude for gratings of 5 cycles/deg. and 10 cycles/deg. The full bandwidth would be 1.0 octave (1.0 octave is a 2:1 ratio, i. e., 10/5). A bandwidth of x octaves means a ratio of 2^x. For example, a 1.5 octave bandwidth is a ratio of $2^{1.5} = 2.8$. This conversion can be performed on a hand calculator.

To quantify temporal selectivity, the Q factor (defined as $Q = f_P/\Delta f$) has advantages over an octave measure (f_P is the temporal frequency of the peak, and Δf is the full bandwidth

A simple, though controversial, interpretation of these threshold elevations is as follows: (a) the filters that are most sensitive to the adapting stimulus determine both preadaptation and postadaptation thresholds; (b) these filters are excited by the adapting stimulus, and consequently their sensitivities are temporarily depressed; in other words, "response causes fatigue" (Braddick et al., 1978; Swift & Smith, 1982). On the basis of these assumptions, the postadaptation threshold elevations have, with other findings, been taken to indicate that luminance-contrast information is processed through multiple parallel spatial filters, each of which is sensitive to a limited range of orientations, and to a range of spatial frequencies considerably less than the bandwidth of the spatial-frequency filtering characteristic for luminance gratings (shown in Figure 1.19).

> As illustrated in Figure 2.11, the CSF is commonly regarded as being the envelope of many subunit sensitivity curves, each of which covers only a small fraction of the range of spatial frequencies encompassed by the complete function (the spatial-frequency channel or spatial filter hypothesis; Campbell & Robson, 1968).

Evidence that the contrast sensitivity curve lumps together the activities of two kinds of mechanism that differ in their *temporal tuning* (as distinct from spatial tuning) characteristics is shown in Figure 2.6.

To derive the bandwidth and sensitivity profiles of these spatial filters from adaptation and masking data is far from straightforward, and the results depend on the assumptions made (Klein et al., 1974; Georgeson & Harris, 1984; Kelly & Burbeck, 1984; Tyler et al., 1996). For example, the "response causes fatigue" hypothesis is called into question by the results of cross-masking between luminance and color gratings (see below) and by reports that adaptation can *reduce* contrast threshold (Tolhurst, 1972; Nachmias et al., 1973; Dealy & Tolhurst, 1974; DeValois, 1978). Again, it is not clear that adaptation is a desensitization caused by prolonged excitation. For example, Wilson (1975) developed a model in which adaptation was caused by long-lasting inhibition. It has also been suggested that adaptation involves *contrast gain control*, which changes the operating point to reduce the effect of response saturation (Greenlee et al., 1991; Wilson & Humanski, 1993; see pp. 83–85). It has also been argued that the bandwidth of a threshold elevation is not necessarily the same as the bandwidth of a channel, since different channels may determine threshold before and after adaptation

---

at half-power, i.e., the full bandwidth at $(1/\sqrt{2})$ of peak amplitude). When a periodic forcing function is applied to a resonant system, the system does not assume its steady-state response immediately. It takes several cycles to build up to the steady-state amplitude and phase. Again, if the forcing function is removed abruptly, the oscillations decay gradually. In the electrical case, for example, $Q = \pi/\delta$, where δ is the *logarithmic decrement*, defined by the equation $\delta = \ln(\theta_n/\theta_{n+1})$, where θ_n and θ_{n+1} are the amplitudes of successive deflections on the same side of zero. A demonstration that the human brain's response to flickering light shows this gradual buildup and gradual decay was provided by van der Tweel (1964). This illustration was reprinted as Figure 2.145 in Regan (1989a).

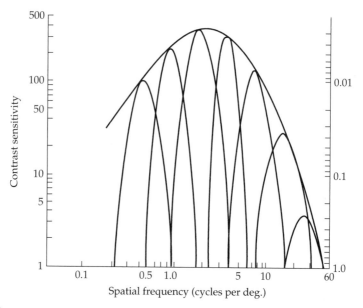

2.11 The contrast sensitivity function regarded as the envelope of multiple narrower-bandwidth channels. From Ginsburg (1981).

(Kelly & Burbeck, 1984). In any case, even if the same channels determine pre- and post-adaptation thresholds, the bandwidths will not be the same if the filter mechanisms are nonlinear (Foley, personal communication, June 1997). Tyler et al. (1996) have developed a simulation method for deriving filter bandwidths in which the assumptions are explicit.

Thomas (1968, 1970)was the first to suggest that the subunit sensitivity curves obtained psychophysically (Figure 2.8) correspond to cortical neurons whose receptive fields vary in size. This is now the consensus view. Further to this point, Patel (1966) showed theoretically that such a sensitivity curve can be modeled by viewing a grating through multiple, parallel, Mexican-hat receptive fields, each of which has an excitatory center and an inhibitory surround such as the local receptive field revealed by the data shown in Figure 2.1.

However, although cortical simple cells with Mexican-hat receptive fields are not uncommon, the receptive fields of other kinds of simple cell are quite different from the Mexican-hat shape that supposedly supports selectivity for bar width. For example, some simple cells are organized into two contiguous linear strips, one of which is excited while the other is inhibited by switching on a small spot of light (Hubel & Wiesel, 1962, 1968). Although a narrow Mexican-hat receptive field is not insensitive to an isolated light–dark edge (Thomas, 1970), it has been proposed that the human visual pathway contains filters that respond *best* to a single light–dark edge, and that homologues of edge-preferring cells are the physiological basis of such filters (Tolhurst, 1972a; Kulikowski & King-Smith, 1973; Shapley & Tolhurst, 1973; Tolhurst & Dealy, 1975). This proposal has been criticized on the grounds that the supporting evidence could also be explained by probability summation among analyzers sensitive to different spatial frequencies and positions (Graham, 1989, p. 239).

The finding that the spatial frequency of the peak threshold elevation always coincides with the spatial frequency of the adapting grating (represented by arrows in Figure 2.9A) has been taken to indicate that the human visual system contains an indefinitely large number of elemental spatial filters. In other words, it has been argued that there is a filter that prefers any given grating, whatever the grating's spatial frequency. However, it is not clear how this finding can be reconciled with the proposal that any given retinal location (in particular, the fovea) is served by filters that prefer only six spatial frequencies (Wilson, 1991b). Kelly (1977) suggested that, since the widths of the filters increase with retinal eccentricity, a grating that covers an extensive area of the retina will find optimally tuned filters at some eccentricity whatever the grating's spatial frequency. According to this argument, gratings of different spatial frequencies are detected by neurons that serve different retinal eccentricities: high spatial frequencies are detected by the central fovea, intermediate spatial frequencies by the parafovea, and low spatial frequencies by more peripheral retina. On the other hand, this proposal conflicts with the finding already mentioned that, for a grating of constant size, contrast sensitivity is highest in the fovea independently of spatial frequency (see Figures 2.2 and 2.3).

In their studies of spatial vision, Wilson et al. (1983) used a spatially localized test pattern. Because of the fit of this pattern to the data of the kind shown in Figure 2.12, they chose the sixth spatial derivative of a Gaussian function; see Figure 2.1. (Spatial derivatives are explained in Figures 2.44 and 2.45.) The spatial-frequency full bandwidth at half amplitude of this stimulus was 1.0 octave (i.e., 2:1). Wilson et al. used a masking technique to estimate the spatial-frequency tuning of the filters fed from the stimulated retinal region. The rationale of their technique was that if only one filter was effective at detection threshold, the contrast required to detect a fixed test grating would vary as a function of the spatial frequency of the masker grating. And this function would correspond to the sensitivity profile of the filter that determined test-grating detection.

The test and masker patterns differed slightly in orientation, so that the observer could be instructed to attend to the test pattern. (If the test and masker patterns had been parallel, the task would have changed to contrast increment detection when the two patterns had the same spatial frequency; see Figure 2.15.) As stated above, Wilson et al. explained their masking data by proposing that any given small area of the retina feeds *no less than* six filters that prefer the same orientation (this leaves open the possibility that the number is more than six). Tuning curves for Wilson's six filters fed by the fovea are shown in Figure 2.12. The spatial-frequency tuning bandwidth of the filters decreases from about 2.2 octaves at 0.8 cycles/deg. to about 1.3 octaves at 16 cycles/deg., and the orientation-tuning bandwidth falls from about ± 30 degrees at low spatial frequencies to about ± 15 degrees at high spatial frequencies (Phillips & Wilson, 1984). According to Wilson (1991b), this trend closely parallels a similar trend in single

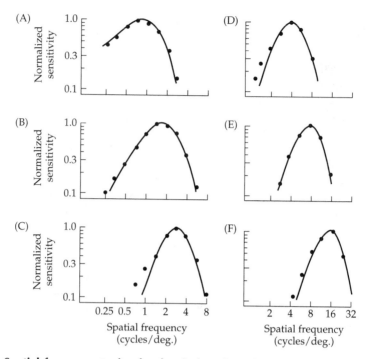

2.12 Spatial-frequency tuning for the six foveal mechanisms estimated by oblique masking. Note that the abscissae are different on the left and right. From Wilson, McFarlane, and Phillips (1983).

cells found in monkey visual cortex. Wilson's highest foveal filter prefers a spatial frequency of 16 cycles/deg., so that this filter alone would be responsible for processing all spatial frequencies from about 16 cycles/deg. up to the resolution limit of from 50 to 60 cycles/deg.

Smallman et al. (1996) have reported evidence for two additional foveal filters, one centered on 23 cycles/deg. and the other centered on 35 cycles/deg. The 35 cycles/deg. filter would have a receptive field center little wider than a single cone photoreceptor. (Smallman et al. used laser interface fringes to bypass the degrading effects of the eye's optics, as described on pp. 434–435, while Wilson's data were obtained with natural vision.)

As to the orientation tuning of spatial filters, Thomas and Gille (1979) found that two orientations can be discriminated perfectly at contrast detection threshold if their orientations differ by more than 20 to 30 degrees. If we assume that only the most sensitive orientation-tuned filter is excited at detection threshold, this important finding can be taken to indicate the following.

The outputs of the individual filters carry an orientation label.

This finding is a special case of the *labeled line* concept. The half-amplitude bandwidth of a vertically tuned filter ranged from 10 to 20 degrees for five observers.

Psychophysical evidence for contrast gain control. So far I have treated adaptation as though its only effect were to elevate contrast detection threshold. But if one stares at a high-contrast grating for some time, the grating's contrast appears to fade (Blakemore et al., 1971). Blakemore et al. (1973, p. 1929) suggested that the cause of both effects was a desensitization of "a particular population of feature-detecting neurons."

But what does *desensitization* mean? There is some physiological evidence that the effect of adaptation on neurons is to reduce their *contrast gain*, i.e., the ratio of neural firing to stimulus contrast (Ohzawa et al., 1985; Albrecht et al., 1984). On psychophysical grounds Georgeson (1985) concluded that the putative reduction of gain is subtractive when the test and adapting gratings have similar orientations.

Broad-band *inhibition* has been proposed as a mechanism to avoid saturation. Heeger (1992) argued that the inhibition should act in feedback mode. Feedback has also been invoked to account for disinhibition (Carpenter & Blakemore, 1973; Kurtenbach & Magnussen, 1981). Feedback of *excitation* has been offered as an explanation for the finding that the range of excitatory interactions increases with practice (Polat & Sagi, 1994). (Feedforward and feedback are discussed in outline form on pp. 6–8. Appendix A includes a quantitative illustration of feedback at pp. 391–393.)

Snowden and Hammett's (1992) measurements of the orientation-tuning bandwidth of the adaptation at suprathreshold rather than threshold levels of test contrast led to some surprising conclusions that were quite different from those of previous authors. Orientation-tuning bandwidth was considerably higher than at test grating threshold. When the test gratings had a very high contrast, the loss of perceived contrast showed little, if any, variation with test orientation; in other words, *orientation tuning was abolished*. (See also Li & Aslin [1992], Ross [1992], and Aslin & Lee [1993].) The spatial-frequency tuning of the adaptation also broadened as test contrast was progressively raised above detection threshold (Snowden & Hammett, 1996). This means that, for a given test frequency, there are some adapting frequencies that do not raise detection threshold, but do reduce perceived contrast.

Snowden and Hammett added: "When test and adapting gratings have the same spatial frequency, the loss of perceived contrast is well described by a subtractive effect; when they are radically different it can be described (to a first approximation) by a divisive (multiplicative) effect," suggesting that "One possibility is that there exist two mechanisms to adaptation—one whose effects appear as a subtractive process and is quite well tuned in the domains of orientation and spatial frequency, and another process which is divisive (multiplicative) and appears to have little tuning with respect to orientation and spatial frequency. Both subtractive and multiplicative adaptation processes have been suggested to occur in the domain of light adaptation (e.g., Hayhoe et al., 1987), which may have their counterparts in the domain of contrast adaptation." But "the notion of two separate processes receives little support from these studies." (Snowden & Hammett, 1996, pp. 1806, 1807.)

Estimates of the temporal and spatial characteristics of a hypothetical divisive gain control have been published by Wilson and Kim (1988). They reported that divisive gain control operates within the first 150 msec. after stimulus onset and is restricted to a region whose diameter is no more than 1.5 degrees. They compared their conclusions with the results of electrophysiological experiments on animals and humans. (Caveats as to the interpretation of some of the human data are discussed in the next section.)

Challenging Snowden and Hammett's conclusion, Ross and Speed (1996, p. 1816) found "no evidence that orthogonal and parallel gratings have different kinds of adapting effect." Furthermore, "a multiplicative hypothesis can be rejected as an explanation for any part of our data, but so too, can the subtractive hypothesis. . . . Ross and Speed (1991) suggested that contrast-response curves obey a form of the Naka–Rushton equation (Naka & Rushton, 1966), $R = C^n / (C^n + C^n_{50})$ and that adaptation both shifts the semi-saturation constant, C_{50} and changes the exponent n. This model of the effects of adaptation was developed to explain threshold elevation, but it can be applied to apparent contrast by assuming that apparent contrast is proportional to R, the response to input contrast C, in the model."

On the other hand, Ross and Speed added, "We cannot claim that Ross and Speed's (1991) model, as it stands, explains both threshold elevation and apparent contrast loss. To fit contrast loss data, different parameters are needed from those that were required to explain threshold elevation. And the model cannot explain why at 90% contrast parallel and orthogonal adaptors have identical effects, since it assumes greater effects for parallel adaptors at all contrasts" (Ross & Speed, 1996, p. 1817).

Intriguingly, Ross and Speed (1996, p. 1817) went on to say:

> In addition to the effects on apparent contrast discussed above, adaptation causes other, more subtle changes in the appearance of an affected grating. There are changes in the overall brightness of gratings and in the apparent size of bars, and slight changes in hue, towards yellow after parallel adaptation, and towards blue after orthogonal. Also, after both parallel adaptation and orthogonal adaptation, an affected grating looks more lustrous. Lustre is often a sign of rivalry within the visual system (Burr et al., 1986), and may be so here if the functional properties of some mechanisms are altered by adaptation but those of others are not. Evidently, much more happens in the visual system as a result of adaptation to a grating than can be captured by a model of lateral shifts of contrast transducer functions or a change in their response range. Presumably, it is to these wider effects, to the possibility of spatial spread of adaptation and to

interactions between adapting gratings side-by-side (see Cannon & Fullenkamp, 1991) that we must look to understand the anomalies in our results.

And as to the Victor–Conte hypothetical edge detector, "For this computational unit to retain its specificity over a wide contrast range, it is necessary that the effective setpoint of the second nonlinearity be adjusted based on some measure of stimulus contrast. Otherwise, setpoints which sufficed to detect edges at low contrasts would lose specificity at high contrasts, or setpoints which provided adequate specificity at high contrasts would fail to detect edges at low contrasts." (Victor & Conte, 1996, p. 1629.) To further investigate this proposed *contrast gain control* of their edge detector, Victor and Conte turned from human psychophysics to human brain recording. The results are described in the next section.

In the next section I describe how, in agreement with some of the behavioral findings just discussed but in conflict with others, objective (human brain recording) evidence indicates that, at high levels of contrast, the visual pathway contains mechanisms that are sharply tuned to both orientation and spatial frequency; and, though showing some features of divisive inhibition, the strong nonlinear interactions between these mechanisms are not simply divisive (see next section).

Objective evidence for channels and for contrast gain control. By exploiting nonlinearities in visual processing it has been possible to use electrical brain response recording in humans, not only to show that spatial filters exist at contrast levels well above detection threshold, but also to explore nonlinear interactions between mechanisms tuned to orientation and spatial frequency.

The suprathreshold brain response data shown in Figure 2.13 can be compared with the threshold psychophysical data shown in Figure 2.6. Figure 2.14A shows that for a fixed temporal counterphase-modulation frequency (10 Hz in this example), the spatial-frequency tuning curve of the brain response was, to a first approximation, invariant with grating contrast over contrast range between 15% and 100%.

Next, I asked whether plots such as those shown in Figures 2.13 and 2.14A lumped together the responses of multiple narrowly tuned subunits. I measured the spatial-frequency tuning of a masking effect as follows. The spatial frequency and orientation of the reference grating were held constant while it was counterphase-modulated at F_1 Hz. When a second (variable) grating was superimposed on the reference grating and counterphase-modulated at a slightly different frequency, F_2 Hz, the $2F_1$ Hz component of the brain response was strongly suppressed. Recognizing that this nonlinear interaction was a "signature" of neurons that "saw" both gratings, I varied the spatial frequency of the variable grating so as to measure the bandwidth of the nonlinear suppression effect. As shown in Figure 2.14B, the full bandwidth at half-height of the masking effect varied progressively from 0.4 to 1.0 octaves over the spatial-frequency range 5.2 to 1.6 cycles/deg. The suppression was always greatest at the spatial frequency tested.

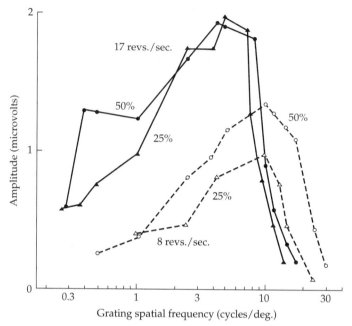

2.13 The spatial-frequency tuning of human brain responses to counterphase-modulated gratings depends on temporal frequency. The amplitude of the 2F Hz component of the brain response is plotted as ordinate versus the spatial frequency of the grating. Continuous lines are for gratings of 25% and 50% contrast that were counterphase-modulated at 8.5 Hz. Dashed lines are for gratings of 25% and 50% contrast that were counterphase-modulated at 4.0 Hz. The grating subtended 35 degrees (horizontal) × 22 degrees, and had a mean luminance of 103 cd/m². The subject fixated the center of the grating monocularly. After D. Regan (1983).

2.14 Spatially tuned submechanisms in the human visual system identified by ▶ recording brain responses. (A) Normalized brain response spatial tuning curves for a single grating of fixed 10 Hz counterphase-modulation frequency for grating contrasts of 15% (large solid squares, dotted line), 30% (open squares, broken line), 60% (solid circles, heavy continuous line), and 100% (stars, fine continuous line). (B) The amplitude of the 20 Hz component of the brain response to a reference grating whose spatial frequency was held constant while it was counterphase-modulated at a fixed temporal frequency of 10 Hz. Optically superimposed on the reference grating was a second grating whose spatial frequency was varied while being counterphase-modulated at a fixed temporal frequency of 9 Hz. The spatial frequency of this second grating is plotted as abscissa. The five plots show data for five experiments in which, as indicated by the vertical arrows, the spatial frequency of the reference grating was fixed at 1.6, 3.0, 3.7, 4.4, and 5.2 cycles/deg., respectively, in different experiments. After D. Regan (1983).

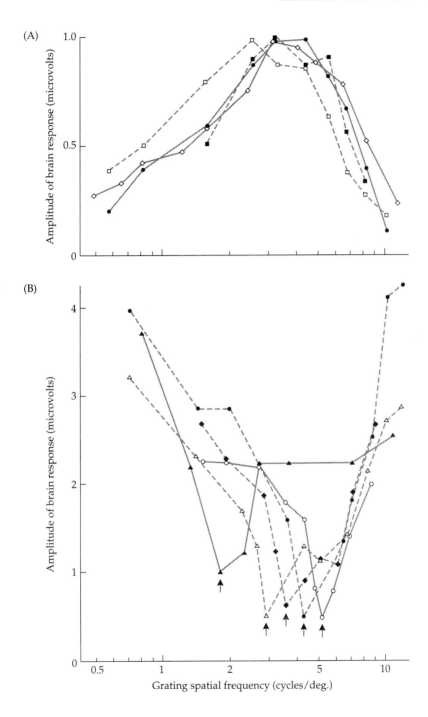

(A)

(B)

Grating spatial frequency (cycles/deg.)

A similar finding was reported by Fiorentini et al. (1983). (Field size was large in both studies.)

> This finding is consistent with the idea that, for any given spatial frequency, there is a neural mechanism most sensitive to that spatial frequency.

Findings were quite different when the spatial frequencies and orientations of the two gratings were the same and F_2 was varied. Masking was *not* always strongest when the two temporal frequencies were the same.

This finding can be understood if, at any given spatial frequency, there is only a small number of temporally tuned spatial filters, possibly only two, one of which is bandpass with respect to temporal frequency (i.e., phasic) while the other is lowpass (i.e., sustained).*

The orientation-tuning bandwidth of the electrophysiological masking effect was about 12 degrees (full bandwidth at half height), in good agreement with the most sharply tuned neurons in monkey area V1 and threshold psychophysical measurements in human (Regan & Regan, 1987).

By varying the relative phase of the two gratings we (D. Regan & M. P. Regan, 1988) distinguished between the following kinds of components.

1. Components of the brain response (e.g., $2F_1 + 2F_2$) that are sensitive to the spatial-frequency power content of the stimulus but not to the phase spectrum of the stimulus. That is, these components are insensitive to the pattern of luminance variation across the stimulus because when the phase difference between two superimposed gratings is varied through 360 degrees, the luminance distribution changes radically.
2. Components of the brain response (such as $F_1 + F_2$, $F_1 + 3F_2$, and $5F_2 - F_1$) that are affected when the spatial-frequency content is held constant while the phase spectrum (and, consequently, the luminance distribution) is changed.

> This finding can be understood if the visual system contains a mechanism that is selectively sensitive to the spatial-frequency content of a stimulus while being insensitive to the phase spectrum in addition to a mechanism that is sensitive to both the power spectrum and the phase spectrum of the stimulus.

There is minimal interaction between responses to gratings whose spatial frequencies are similar but whose orientations differ by 45 degrees (Regan & Regan, 1986, 1987), but there is a strong nonlinear interaction between responses to ver-

---

* Phasic (or transient) neurons respond to the onset and/or offset of a stimulus but not to its continued presence, while sustained neurons respond throughout a long presentation. In engineering terms, phasic neurons are AC-coupled and sustained neurons are DC-coupled.

tical and horizontal gratings (Morrone & Burr, 1986; Regan & Regan, 1986, 1987). The interaction is approximately as strong as the interaction between parallel gratings.

> This finding indicates that brain responses to two-dimensional patterns cannot, even roughly, be predicted on the basis of responses to single gratings.

Responses to gratings of widely different spatial frequencies also interact nonlinearly (M. P. Regan & D. Regan, 1989b). These interactions are different for parallel and orthogonal gratings. And when the gratings are orthogonal there is a marked asymmetry between the suppressive effect exerted by the high-frequency grating upon the low-frequency grating and the suppressive effect exerted by the low-frequency grating upon the high-frequency grating.

I will first describe the effect exerted by a high-frequency grating upon the brain responses produced by a low-frequency grating. The response to a vertical 1.0 cycles/deg. grating that was counterphase-modulated at F_1 Hz was suppressed by a second superimposed grating that was counterphase-modulated at F_2 Hz. (Both F_1 and F_2 were close to 8 Hz.) Suppression was strong (5- to 6-fold) when the second grating was vertical and its spatial frequency was between 1.5 and 13 cycles/deg. When the second grating was horizontal, suppression was strongest when the spatial frequency of the second grating was near 3 cycles/deg., but when its spatial frequency was between 5 and 10 cycles/deg., the suppression was weak.

Now to the effect exerted by a low-frequency grating upon the response to a high-frequency (13 cycles/deg.) grating. Whether the gratings were parallel or at right angles was comparatively unimportant; suppression was strong (5- to 20-fold) when the spatial frequency of the low-frequency grating was well below 6 cycles/deg., fell to zero near 6 cycles/deg., and was comparatively weak (about twofold) between 6 and 12 cycles/deg.

> The finding that simultaneous stimulation with two *parallel* gratings brought out strong violations of linearity indicates that the brain response to a complex one-dimensional pattern cannot fully be predicted from the responses to sinusoidal gratings used one at a time
> The finding that simultaneous stimulation with two *perpendicular* gratings brought out strong violations of linearity confirms that the brain response to a two-dimensional pattern cannot fully be predicted from the responses to individual sinusoidal gratings used one at a time.

Our finding for parallel gratings may be related to data on single cells in cat visual cortex. DeValois and Tootell (1983) reported widespread interactions between response to different spatial frequencies, and also that the interactions were asymmetric. In particular, they found that in many cells the response to a low-frequency grating was inhibited when they superimposed a high-frequency grating on the low-frequency grating. Additionally, the firing of single cortical cells showed nonlinear interactions between their responses to orthogonal gratings of differing spatial frequencies (Bonds, 1989).

I developed a rapid brain recording technique (first called *the method of averaging graphs*, later called the *sweep technique*) that can record an entire graph in 10 seconds—far faster than the conventional method of plotting a graph from individually recorded data points. And the method is considerably more resistant to certain kinds of noise (Regan, 1973a, 1975b). My purpose in developing this technique was to provide a very rapid means of assessing the visual (or auditory) status of infants from as young as a few days of age up to about seven years (see Regan, 1977),* and indeed the method has been skillfully exploited by Christopher Tyler, Anthony Norcia, and their colleagues in technically demanding studies of infant visual development (e.g., Norcia & Tyler, 1985; Norcia et al., 1986, 1988). But the sweep technique is also capable of documenting a rapid change in visual sensitivity (Regan, 1968, 1974). Nelson, Seiple, Kupersmith, and Carr (1984) exploited this feature in fine style when demonstrating the dynamics of the contrast gain control mechanism in humans (see also Bonds, 1991, and Geisler & Albrecht, 1992).

On the basis of their brain recordings in humans, Victor and Conte (1996, p. 1629) concluded that, "the neural measure of contrast is derived prior to the extraction of local features. That is, the gain control appears to act in a feedforward manner in which contrast (independent of the presence or absence of local features) adjusts the gain and dynamics of the feature-extracting stage." Their stimulus manipulation had been to jitter the relative spatial phase within the phase spectrum of a texture pattern as a whole so as to dissociate the salience of local features from contrast. (The distinction between feedforward and feedback is discussed on pp. 6–8.)

Some authors have argued that contrast gain control operates through divisive inhibition or is divisive (Morrone & Burr, 1986; Ross & Speed, 1991). But our finding that stimulation with two parallel superimposed gratings of the same spatial frequency produces cross-modulation terms other than $(F_1 + F_2)$ and $(F_1 - F_2)$, and that these terms are not only present in the brain response but can dominate the response, indicates that simple divisive gain control is not a sufficient explanation for the data (Regan & Regan, 1986, 1987, 1988; Regan, 1989a). (The first section in Appendix B explains why the only cross-modulation terms produced by pure divisive inhibition would be the $(F_1 + F_2)$ and $(F_1 - F_2)$ terms.)

---

* Any reader who chances across the 1973 reference will find that it describes a method for refracting an adult within a total recording time of about 30 seconds. The truth is that during a scientific discussion with a colleague, he mentioned that one of the five priorities set by the NEI for that five-year period was the development of a fast method for objective refraction. After a few moments of reflection I realized that a truly rapid technique that was sufficiently general to be used to measure several aspects of visual and auditory function would fill a recognized need in examining sensory functions in infants. So I agreed to try. It was an unwelcome diversion and at times, while trying to get the thing to work, I wished that I had kept my mouth shut.

In general, the output of a nonlinearity fed by the sum of two sinusoids may contain sinusoidal components whose frequencies are all the possible sum and difference combinations of the two input frequencies, i.e., frequencies $(nF_1 + mF_2)$ and $(nF_1 - mF_2)$ where F_1 and F_2 are the input frequencies, and n and m are integers or zero (when n or m is zero, the terms are called *harmonics* of F_1 and F_2). We developed a mathematical method for deriving these components for certain nonlinear systems composed of one or more (up to five) rectifier-like parts, and proposed that:

> The relative amplitudes of the various cross-modulation and harmonic components in the output of such a nonlinear system is characteristic of the particular system, i.e., is a "signature" of the system (M. P. Regan & D. Regan, 1988, 1989a).

In experimental studies, we have used this mathematical result to test computational models framed in terms of sequential monocular and binocular processing of a system composed of between one and five successive nonlinear stages (M. P. Regan & D. Regan, 1988, 1989a).

Marian P. Regan has also provided a mathematical analysis of the output of a rectifier-like nonlinearity when fed with either one or the sum of two amplitude-modulated or frequency-modulated sinusoids, and we have reported experimental data that are in tolerable accord with the theoretical predictions (M. P. Regan, 1994, 1996; M. P. Regan & D. Regan, 1993).

The "dipper" effect

In addition to the adaptation and oblique masking data just described, psychophysical models of spatial information processing must account for the parallel masking data shown by the filled symbols in Figure 2.15. On every trial a masker grating was presented in each of two successive time intervals. In one interval (selected randomly), a test grating was superimposed on the masker grating, and the observer's task was to identify which of the two intervals contained the test grating. This can be regarded as a contrast increment detection task, because both gratings had identical spatial frequencies, orientations, and spatial phases. Figure 2.15 shows the effect of the masker on the observer's ability to distinguish the test-grating-plus-masker-grating from the masker grating alone. For reasons explained later (pp. 250–253), in Figure 2.15 this masking effect is expressed relative to unmasked detection threshold for the test grating. Figure 2.15 shows that it is only a high-contrast masker that renders the test grating less detectable.

> A low-contrast masker grating makes the test grating more easily detectable—the remarkable "pedestal" or "dipper" effect.

This effect was discovered independently by Nachmias and Sansbury (1974) and Stromeyer and Klein (1974); see also Foley and Legge (1981).

Stimulus uncertainty is one proposed explanation for the dipper effect (Lasley & Cohn, 1981; Pelli, 1984). The basic idea is that the pedestal helps an observer

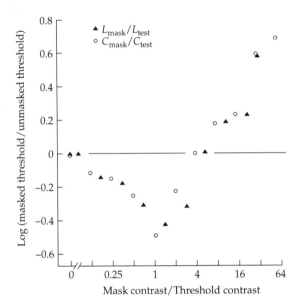

2.15 The dipper or pedestal effect. Detection threshold elevation for a test grating is plotted as ordinate versus the contrast of the masker grating (expressed as a multiple of detection threshold for the masker grating). For low masker contrasts, masking makes the test grating more detectable. Only when the masker contrasts are high does masking render the test grating less visible. Open circles: Both masker and test gratings are luminance-defined. Solid triangles: Both masker and test gratings are color-defined equiluminant red–green gratings. After Switkes, Bradley, and DeValois (1988).

to detect the test stimulus because it resembles the test stimulus and thus reduces stimulus uncertainty. Subsequently reported experimental evidence, however, seems to rule out this proposal (Eskew et al., 1991; Yang & Makous, 1995a,b).

Several authors have proposed models framed in terms of sequential processing stages in which any given processing stage lumps together one particular kind of processing. (Such models are distinct from the other extreme case of modeling that particular kind of processing as though it were distributed through the entire sequence of processing.) For example, according to the Legge and Foley (1980) model, the first stage (the receptive field) is linear spatiotemporal filtering. The second (nonlinear) stage has a fixed S-shaped input–output characteristic whose slope increases with contrast at low contrasts (to explain the facilitation in the left part of Figure 2.15) and decreases with contrast at high contrasts (to explain the attenuation in the right part of Figure 2.15). For an explanation of the reasoning behind this statement, see Figure 3.25; see also Nachmias and Sansbury (1974), Stromeyer and Klein (1974, 1975), Wilson (1980), and Foley and Legge (1981). Some authors have regarded this nonlinear curve as the input–output characteristic of a neural population that is located at some discrete site in the visual pathway. On the other hand, Switkes et al. (1988) pointed out that the accelerating and compressive components of the hypothetical nonlinearity need not necessarily be lumped at a single stage. Rather, they may be located at different stages in the sequence of processing, as illustrated in Figure 2.16D.

The receptive field and nonlinear stages just described are formally conceived as being noise-free; psychophysical modelers add the noise required to explain why contrast detection thresholds are not indefinitely low at the output of the nonlinearity (Legge & Foley, 1980; Watson & Robson, 1981; Watson, 1983; Nielson et al., 1985; Klein & Levi, 1985).

Foley (personal communication, June 1997) stated that "the class of static nonlinear model exemplified by the Legge and Foley (1980) model is rendered untenable by the results of subsequent studies (Ross & Speed, 1991; Ross et al., 1993; Foley 1994; Foley & Chen, 1997). A common factor in several more recent models is that the fixed S-shaped nonlinear stage has been removed, and a second broadly tuned stage operates in parallel with the linear receptive field. Later stages of processing receive, in addition to the input that originates in the linear receptive field, an input that has a divisive inhibitory effect on the signal from the linear receptive field."

Yang and Makous (1995a,b) have proposed an alternative explanation for at least part of the data shown in Figure 2.15 that they call "zero frequency masking." They draw attention to the point, discussed on pp. 416–420, that the Fourier spectrum of the test grating and pedestal as a whole is the sum of a spectrum similar to that shown in Figure B.7A and a spectrum similar to that shown in Figure B.6 (which has power at a spatial frequency of zero cycles/deg.). They then assume that low spatial frequencies in the test grating are masked by power at zero cycles/deg.

Another approach to explaining the dipper effect is described on pp. 174–184.

Demodulation

Experimental findings reported by Henning, Hertz, and Broadbent (1975) provided an early demonstration that the visual processing of spatial contrast is far from being linear. They used a sinusoidal grating of spatial frequency 9.5 cycles/deg. whose contrast was amplitude-modulated (AM) at a spatial frequency of 1.9 cycles/deg. The crucial point is that this grating contained no power at 1.9 cycles/deg. Figure 2.17B shows an amplitude-modulated grating.

By referring to Figure B.10F, it can be understood that the power was restricted to three narrow peaks centered on 7.6 (the *lower sideband*), 9.5 (the *carrier* frequency), and 11.4 cycles/deg. (the *upper sideband*).

Henning et al. used temporal two-alternative forced choice (see pp. 8–17 and Figure 1.5) in their three experiments. In Experiment (1), both test and reference intervals contained a high-contrast amplitude-modulated grating. During the test interval, a low-contrast sinusoidal grating of spatial frequency 1.9 cycles/deg.

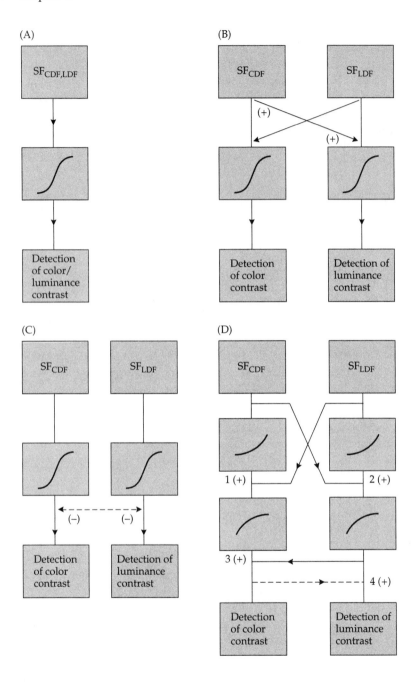

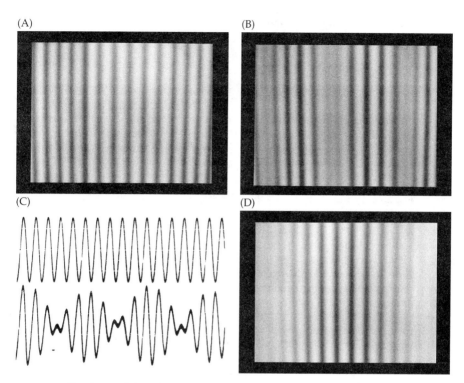

2.17 Amplitude-modulated gratings. (A) A sinusoidal grating of spatial frequency *S* cycles/deg. (B) The contrast of the grating in part A is amplitude-modulated along the *x*-axis by a sinusoid of spatial frequency 0.1 *S* cycles/deg. (C) The upper trace shows the sinusoid that created part A; the lower trace shows the AM waveform that created part B. (D) The contrast of a vertical sinusoidal grating is amplitude-modulated along the *x* axis by a half-sine of period 0.05*S* cycles/deg.

was superimposed on the AM grating. The observer's task was to signal whether the 1.9 cycles/deg. grating was presented in the first or the second interval. In Experiment (2), the AM grating was replaced by a high-contrast sinusoidal grating of spatial frequency 7.6 cycles/deg. (7.6 cycles/deg. was the frequency of the

◀ **2.16 Proposed interactions between the processing of luminance contrast and chromatic contrast.** Plus and minus signs indicate facilitation and inhibition, respectively. The S-shaped curve represents the nonlinear contrast transducer function. (A) Color-defined (CD) form and luminance-defined (LD) form share the same spatial filter. (B) Two-way excitatory interactions occur after the filtering stage, but before the transduction stage, and (C) two-way inhibitory interactions occur after the transduction stage. (D) The accelerating and compressive parts of the function are separate. Part B from Switkes, Bradley, and DeValois (1988). Part C from Mullen and Losada (1994).

AM grating's lower sideband, see Figure B.10F). In Experiment (3), the test interval contained only a 1.9 cycles/deg. sinusoidal grating, and the reference interval contained a uniform luminance. The mean luminances of all gratings were adjusted so that they provided no cue to the task.

Henning and his colleagues found that in Experiment (3), one observer could detect a 1.9 cycles/deg. grating of only 0.5% contrast, but required 3.8% contrast when the grating was superimposed on the AM grating. The effect of the 7.6 cycles/deg. masker was much smaller (0.9% contrast was required to detect the 1.9 cycles/deg. grating). Henning et al. concluded that the AM grating reduced the detectability of the 1.9 cycles/deg. test grating very considerably (more than 700% threshold elevation), and that this could not be attributed to the masking effect of either the 7.6 or the 9.5 cycles/deg. sidebands (which did have power in the spectrum of the AM grating).

It was as though the AM grating contained power near 1.9 cycles/deg. But, as already stated, there was no power at 1.9 cycles/deg. in the spectrum of the AM grating used by Henning et al. The AM grating contained no power anywhere near 1.9 cycles/deg.

Linear processing could not, by definition, give this result. (A *linear system* is defined on pp. 389–391). The unavoidable conclusion was that low-frequency power that caused the masking was extracted from the AM grating by a nonlinearity in the human visual system. This process is called *demodulation*, and is discussed in greater detail on pp. 426–427.*

An AM grating can be demodulated by either a *nonessential* or an *essential* nonlinearity (these terms are defined on p. 394). A second point: an AM grating can be demodulated by nonlinear processing of local *contrast* or (because eye movements are necessary to see a low-contrast grating) nonlinear processing of local *luminance* (see Appendix E).

It is known that the cone transducer characteristic is a nonessential nonlinearity (in particular, a compressive, approximately logarithmic function), and that, by creating harmonics that are not present in the stimulus, this causes high-contrast sinusoidal gratings to look nonsinusoidal (Davidson, 1968; Maudarbocus & Rudduck, 1973; Burton, 1973). Because of its high contrast, the AM masker grating would certainly be demodulated to some extent by the compressive photoreceptor characteristic. However, Henning et al. carried out control experiments

---

* Demodulation of an AM signal is a familiar concept. For example, an AM radio station amplitude modulates—at audio frequencies of up to 15,000 Hz or so—the high-frequency carrier signal it transmits. The carrier frequency is typically in the range 500,000 Hz to 1.5 million Hz. As illustrated in Figure B.10 (C,F,I), there is no audio frequency power in the signal received by a radio tuned to the AM station. The radio recovers the audio information by demodulating the AM signal it receives; see Figure B.11.

The input–output characteristics of some neurons can be modeled in terms of asymmetric rectifiers, whose arms can be described by a continuous function (e.g., linear, compressive,

and concluded that this early distortion of luminance signals was not sufficiently strong to account for their AM masking data.

Revisiting this question and using a quasi-FM masker grating (pp. 423–426) as well as an AM masker grating (whose 11 cycles/deg. carrier frequencies were modulated at 2.2 cycles/deg.), Nachmias and Rogowitz (1983) reported some findings that were in accord with the hypothesis that a nonessential nonlinearity was responsible for the low-frequency (2.2 cycles/deg.) masking effect of the modulated grating, and some findings that were not in accord with that hypothesis.

In discussing the findings of Henning et al., Wilson and Wilkinson (1997) suggested that the AM grating was demodulated by an essential nonlinearity (in particular, rectification) operating on the grating's local *contrast* (rather than on its local *luminance*), and proposed primary visual cortex as the site at which demodulation occurred. This proposal certainly has physiological plausibility. For example, as discussed in Appendix E, simple cortical cells have rectifier-like properties (because their resting discharge rate is low, and a cell cannot fire at a negative rate).

On the other hand, rectifier-like behavior is already established at retinal level (see Appendix E). As mentioned earlier, rectification of local light intensity might, in principle, have demodulated an AM grating already at retinal level.

What is the relative importance of rectification of temporal variation of local retinal luminance versus rectification of local spatial contrast? One possible approach to this question might take the following line. Consider first the finding (illustrated in Appendix E, Figure E.2), that adding noisy *temporal* variations to the visual input caused lateral geniculate cells to behave more linearly in their responses to a periodic time-varying signal (Spekreijse, 1969; Spekreijse et al., 1971). Suppose that demodulation of an AM grating is caused by rectification of temporal changes in local retinal luminance. Then if the amplitude-modulated grating in the Henning et al. experiment were subjected to a noisy variation of mean luminance (at constant spatial contrast), the threshold elevation for detecting the 1.9 cycles/deg. test grating would, presumably, be reduced. On the other hand, if demodulation was caused by rectification of local spatial contrast, then if a noisy variation of spatial contrast (that did not vary with time) were added to the amplitude-modulated grating in the Henning et al. experiment, the threshold elevation for detecting the 1.9 cycles/deg. test grating would, presumably, be reduced.

An indication of the relative importance of the two kinds of rectification might be obtained by comparing the effects of temporal noise and spatial noise on the threshold elevation for the 1.9 cycles/deg. test grating. I was unable to find any report on such an experiment.

---

accelerating, accelerating initially and compressive later). An analytic mathematical treatment of cascaded rectifiers is available in the case that the input is one sinewave of the sum of two sinewaves (M. P. Regan & D. Regan, 1988, 1989a). Mathematical treatments of the distortion produced by passing one (or two superimposed) amplitude-modulated or frequency-modulated sinusoids through a rectifier are also available (M. P. Regan & D. Regan, 1993; M. P. Regan, 1996).

The *sandwich system* (a biological sequence of linear filter–rectifier–linear filter) was conceived by Spekreijse (1966, 1969). He went on to use the two-sinewave technique of nonlinear systems analysis in applying sandwich-system analysis to both the human visual system (using a technique for recording electrical responses of the human brain) and the visual systems of animals (using microelectrodes to record single-unit activity). This way of modeling early processing has subsequently been used in modeling texture segregation (pp. 288–294) and the processing of "non-Fourier" motion (Chubb & Sperling, 1988, 1989).

A sandwich system has the feature that, because of the rectifier nonlinearity, the linear processing before and after rectification can be isolated experimentally and studied individually. The principle of this manipulation is described by Spekreijse (1966), Spekreijse and Oosting (1970), and Spekreijse and Reits (1982). An example of how a sandwich system can be disentangled psychophysically is given in Regan and Beverley (1980, 1981).

But according to Klein, the results of the Henning, Hertz, and Broadbent experiment is still a mystery. "It is clear that a simple rectification model doesn't work since that model would predict facilitation due to the dipper. However, clear facilitation isn't found" (S. Klein, personal communication, January 1999).

Positional Discrimination, Width Discrimination, Separation Discrimination, and Spatial Frequency Discrimination for Luminance-Defined Form

Since the time of the ancient Greeks, our ability to judge the absolute direction of an external object by means of vision has continued to attract speculation from philosophers and, in the modern era, hypotheses and experimental tests from scientists. Over the last 100 years, reliable quantitative measurements of the precision with which we can discriminate the *relative directions* of laboratory targets such as lines or edges has piled mystery upon mystery. In the following section I outline what is known about human visual sensitivity to absolute location and relative location, and I indicate why these findings are so surprising.

Positional discrimination: Vernier acuity and bisection acuity

Measuring a person's Vernier acuity, bisection acuity, width discrimination threshold, or line-separation discrimination threshold are widely employed procedures for estimating visual sensitivity to relative position. In addition, there is a sizeable literature on spatial-frequency discrimination, though there is controversy as to whether this discrimination is a measure of sensitivity to the separation between the bars of a grating or sensitivity to the gratings' spatial-frequency power spectrum.

Vernier acuity. According to Matin (1972), "Perhaps the most elementary fact of visual space perception is that the spatial order of stimulus points in the environment remains correctly preserved in perception. Around this central fact has developed the general viewpoint that the visual perception of direction is mediated in the visual neurosensory pathway by a system of local signs that topographically maps locations of retinal stimuli into values of perceived direction."

The idea that signals from any given point on the retina carry a *local sign* that is retained through later processing stages (Lotze, 1885) is basic to theories of spatial vision. Whether learned or innate, local sign fits the definition of a *primitive* "with its implication of being the result of an abstraction process distinguishable from that for all other visual attributes and one that is probably subserved by its own separate neural mechanism" (Westheimer, 1996).

Westheimer and McKee (1977) reported evidence that local sign can be assigned on the basis of pooled responses to stimulation that extends over several minutes of arc. More surprisingly, they also reported that

---

Pooling over several minutes of arc does not preclude the discrimination of differences of local sign as small as a few seconds of arc.

The evidence for this remarkable conclusion is described next. The target consisted of an array of nine bright, thin (0.25 arc min.) lines that were separated so closely that they could not be resolved. The observer's impression of the magnified version shown in Figure 2.18A was that of a solid bright bar. Any one of the lines could be made twice as bright as all the others, and the line selected could be different in the upper and lower halves of the target as, for example, in Figure 2.18A, where the brighter line is shown in bold. In the situation shown, the centroid of the luminance profile in the lower half was displaced with respect to the centroid in the upper half (arrows).*

Threshold for discriminating whether the displacement was leftwards or rightwards ranged from 4.3 to 5.5 seconds of arc for the three observers. Here, the very precise local sign is obtained by averaging across the width of the line rather than (as in Hering's view) by averaging along the length of the line (Watt & Morgan, 1983b); however, information along the length of the line may be used in some tasks (Watt et al., 1983; Badcock & Westheimer, 1985). In a further experiment, Westheimer and McKee (1977) used the target depicted in Figure 2.18B. The central line was the brightest in both the upper and the lower halves of the target, and the two halves were displaced bodily in the standard Vernier manner. Discrimination thresholds were the same as for the target shown in Figure 2.18A. This finding indicates that the spatial step along the edge of the standard Vernier target (Figure 2.19) is not essential for hyperacuity performance.† Westheimer and McKee pointed out that, although the very low hyperacuity thresholds may

---

* Centroid is defined as "The point in a geometrical figure whose coordinates are the arithmetical means of the coordinates of the points making up the figure. If the figure represents a body of uniform density, the centroid coincides with the center of mass" (Daintith & Nelson, 1989).

† The task of aligning two dots to the vertical can be carried out with a precision equal to the Vernier acuity for two long lines, when the dots are separated by 2 to 4 minutes of arc (Sullivan et al., 1972; Westheimer & McKee, 1977), and has the property that performance is

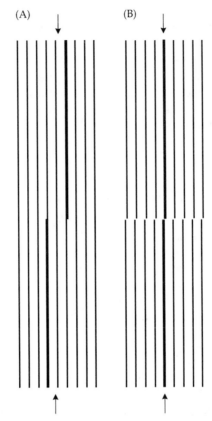

2.18 Discriminating the relative position of the centroid of a luminance distribution. (A) The nine very thin lines were so closely spaced that they looked like a solid bar of width 2 to 3 minutes of arc. Thick black lines indicate lines made twice as bright as all the others so as to displace the centroids of the light distribution in the upper and lower halves (arrows). This displacement was detected with 75% accuracy even though the edges of the bar were quite straight. (B) The Vernier displacement shown was detected with 75% accuracy. From Westheimer and McKee (1977b).

seem to suggest that visual system partitions space into extremely fine local-sign modules, hyperacuity responses can be based on the spatial pooling of light over distances at least order of magnitude larger than the difference signals that are subsequently extracted.

The visual system does not encode the absolute location of a local spatial feature with high accuracy. This is partly because of involuntary eye movements and

___

much less affected by blur than is Vernier acuity for two abutting lines. The two-dot task is sometimes classed as a Vernier acuity task, but may better be regarded as lining up two dots to match one's internal representation of the vertical (Morgan, 1991).

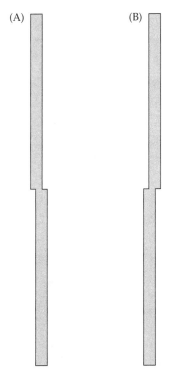

2.19 Standard Vernier line target. The observer's task is to signal whether the off-set of the lower line is to the right (A) or to the left (B). The just-noticeable offset can be as low as 2 to 5 seconds of arc, far less than the shortest distance between adjacent cones in the central fovea (approximately 25 seconds of arc).

partly because of an inaccurate sense of the direction of gaze. Figure 2.20 illustrates a test for assessing gaze control.*

Rather than attempting to measure the accuracy with which the absolute position of a local spatial feature can be estimated, it is common to take an indirect approach. One such approach is to measure the just-noticeable *temporal change* in the location of a single local spatial feature. A second example is to measure the just-noticeable *spatial difference* in the locations of two or more local spatial features,

* White et al. (1992) measured the ability to locate a target in the absence of any visual reference. They found that localization accuracy was proportional to target eccentricity; they proposed that accuracy was largely determined by cone position uncertainty and the spacing between ON–P_{beta} retinal ganglion cells. Hansen and Skavenski (1977) showed that subjects can return their eyes to a reference position following both saccades and slow phases of vestibular nystagmus, suggesting that eye position was signaled accurately during both kinds of eye movement and that this signal was closely time-locked to saccades. And subjects could strike blows within a few minutes of arc of a target localized only by

```
V Z N C S H R H V K D N C
H O R K O V S C N Z H V R
R K D S Z D N K S V N D H
D S V C C C C C C S K Z
N R Z C C C C C C R S N
O D R C C C C C C V O K
C Z R C C C C C C Z K D
R N K C C C C C C R N R
D S O C C C C C C K V Z
N C V C C C C C C S D O
S D R Z S D R Z K D V C R
H Z N K O V Z C N R K H D
V O S R N D H K V O C H K
```

2.20 High-contrast multiletter acuity chart. For this letter size, the central array consists of 49 identical letters. The central array is surrounded by three rows and three columns of randomly selected letters. There are 10 charts for letters of the size shown, and 10 charts for each of the 11 letter sizes in the acuity chart shown in Figure 2.66A. A few sets of low-contrast multiletter charts have also been printed.

for example, by means of the Vernier acuity procedure or the bisection acuity procedure (reviewed in Westheimer, 1979, 1981, and Morgan, 1991).

According to Westheimer and McKee (1977), it was already appreciated by Hering in 1899 that the just-detectable Vernier offset (2 to 5 seconds of arc) is considerably less than the shortest (25 seconds of arc) distance between retinal photoreceptors in the central fovea, and a great deal of effort has since been devoted to finding an explanation for this remarkable fact.

---

eye position, suggesting that motor systems detect eye position to better than 0.5 degrees and, furthermore, that the well-known large errors in controlling eye position in the dark can be attributed to poor spatial memory. But eye position control, though good, is far from perfect. Viewing a multiletter chart provides a convincing subjective demonstration of the unsteadiness of one's own gaze (Regan, 1988, Regan et al. 1992b). Figure 2.20 shows a multiletter chart. We used these charts in a study of 180 eyes of 90 children aged from 4 to 11 years (Kothe & Regan, 1990). We found that the development of gaze selection and control plays an important role in the development of Snellen acuity. Group mean decimal Snellen scores reached 1.45 by 10 to 11 years of age but, even for the two children with acuities of 1.8 and 1.9, acuity was not limited by ocular resolution but rather by small inadequacies of gaze selection and/or gaze control. (For such observers, the inaccuracy in gaze selection or control may be no more than 2.5 to 5 minutes of arc.) To measure an absolute error in gaze selection of 2.5 minutes of arc is far beyond the capability of the finest modern eye tracker. And the reduced visual acuity in some patients with the developmental disorder amblyopia is caused by tiny defects in the selection or control of gaze rather than abnormal lateral interaction within the visual system (Regan et al., 1992a).

Vernier offset judgment is not necessarily based on a comparison of the *absolute* locations of the two lines. Several other strategies are available for carrying out the task, and the relative effectiveness of the different strategies depends on the particular configuration of the Vernier target. One proposal is that the direction of Vernier offset correlates with the pattern of activity among multiple spatial filters that are driven from the same retinal location but prefer different orientations (Andrews, 1967; Findlay, 1973). A second proposal is that the direction of Vernier offset correlates with the pattern of activity among multiple spatial filters that prefer the same orientation but are driven from different spatial locations (Wilson, 1986, 1991b). A third proposal is that to detect a Vernier step is to detect a failure of co-linearity (Andrews et al. 1973; Watt et al., 1983; Watt, 1984a).

Evidence that Vernier acuity for an abutting two-line target is mediated by the same process as orientation discrimination was reported by Waugh et al. (1993). The rationale of their experiment was similar to that depicted in Figure 2.28A–D. They measured Vernier acuity in the presence of superimposed one-dimensional band-limited spatial noise. The effect of mask orientation on line-detection threshold and on Vernier offset threshold for the two-line target was similar to the curves in Figure 2.28D. Detection threshold for the Vernier target was most elevated when the mask was parallel to the Vernier target. But Vernier offset threshold was most elevated when the mask was inclined roughly 10 to 20 degrees to the Vernier target; Vernier offset threshold was *lowered* when the mask was parallel to the Vernier target. Explaining their finding along the same lines as the Figure 2.28D data, Waugh and her colleagues suggested that Vernier acuity is determined by the relative activity of orientation-tuned neurons, and that the two most important neurons are the pair whose orientation tuning curves differ most in slope.

However, if this is the case it is not clear why the effect of contrast on Vernier acuity is a power function whose exponent is 0.5 to 0.8 while, as indicated by Figure 2.30, orientation discrimination threshold is largely independent of contrast (Krauskopf, 1976; Foley-Fisher, 1977; Watt & Morgan, 1983a; Regan & Beverley, 1985; Bradley & Skottun, 1987; Morgan & Regan, 1987).

Noting that Vernier threshold is usually expressed in spatial units such as seconds of arc (even for the Figure 2.18 target, where threshold was assessed as a just-noticeable displacement of the centroid), Morgan and Aiba (1985a) revisited an alternative line of thought that had been developed by Hamilton Hartridge (1947, 1950), who pointed out that, because spatial discriminations can be regarded as distinguishing between different distributions of light within the retinal image, spatial discrimination thresholds can be expressed in terms of contrast thresholds. In an attempt to apply the Hartridge approach to Vernier acuity, Morgan and Aiba used the target shown (highly magnified) in Figure 2.21A. The lines were thin and so close that they could not be resolved. The luminances of the tops (T1, T2) and bottoms (B1, B2) of the lines could be varied independently. When the luminances of all four segments were the same, the percept was as illustrated in Figure 2.21B: a vertical bar. But when the luminance of T2 was less than T1 and the luminance of B1 was less than B2, the percept was more like

Figure 2.21C: a percept of spatial displacement created by changing local contrast without any change of spatial location.

Observers could detect a spatial offset of about 5 to 20 seconds of arc between the centroids of the light distribution in upper and lower halves of the target—very similar to ordinary Vernier thresholds. But, because of their unusual procedure, Morgan and Aiba were able to express Vernier acuity as a contrast threshold. Figure 2.22 illustrates their basic idea. Adjacent foveal photoreceptors (circles) detect the luminance boundary between the top and bottom of the target. When they allowed for both the blurring effect of the eye's optics and the integration of light within the area of the photoreceptor, Morgan and Aiba found the value of $\Delta L/L$ at Vernier threshold to be 0.8%, in good agreement with the contrast required to detect a thin black line (see Figure 1.12).

Morgan and Aiba showed that the peak of the light distribution did not predict the data; the relevant feature was the centroid. See Kontsevich and Tyler (1998) for a differing view.

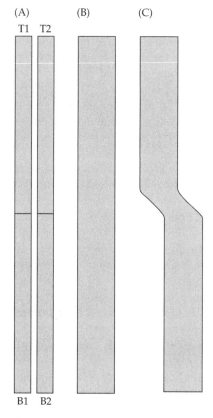

2.21 The two-line Vernier target. This target allowed M. J. Morgan and T. S. Aiba to express Vernier acuity in terms of contrast sensitivity.

Provided that the Vernier target is not moving faster than a few degrees per second, motion does not degrade Vernier acuity (Westheimer & McKee, 1975; Morgan et al., 1983; Carney et al., 1995). But as retinal image speed is increased beyond a few degrees per second, Vernier threshold starts to increase.

One proposed explanation for this effect of image motion is that motion is equivalent to the well-known effects of contrast and exposure duration. Motion spreads the stimulus energy over space and time; if the spatial spread is wider than the relevant receptive fields or the temporal spread is longer than their integration time, then stimulus visibility will be reduced and Vernier threshold will rise. (Visibility can be defined as the number of times that the target exceeds its detection threshold.) An alternative explanation is that the most important spatial

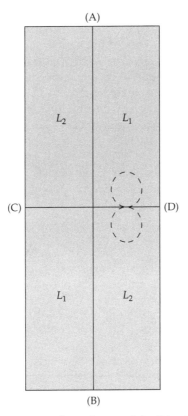

2.22 Morgan and Aiba's contrast detection model of Vernier step acuity. L_1 and L_2 are the luminances of two bars. If the bars are sufficiently thin, spatial mixture occurs and the whole target is perceived as having a Vernier offset with a magnitude proportional to the ratio L_1/L_2. The classical Vernier target is a limiting case with either L_1 or L_2 equal to the luminance of the background. In this model, adjacent foveal photoreceptors (cones) detect the luminance edge between the top and bottom of the target. After Morgan and Aiba (1985).

filters for analyzing the spatial information carried by a rapidly moving target are wide filters, while for a stationary target the most important filters are narrow. Chung et al. (1996) compared these two candidate hypotheses and came down in favor of the second one.

Bisection acuity.   Bisection threshold is an alternative measure of an individual's sensitivity to relative location. Figure 2.23A depicts a bisection target that has no overlap between the two reference lines and the test line. If, for example, we used the method of constant stimuli to measure bisection threshold, there might be eight targets organized as follows: four targets with the test line distant x, $2x$, $3x$, and $4x$, respectively, below the midline; four targets with the test line distant x, $2x$, $3x$, and $4x$, respectively, above the midline. The eight targets would be presented in random order, and the observer instructed to signal whether the test line was closer to reference line 1 than to reference line 2 or vice versa. Westheimer (1977) reported that, for the kind of target shown in Figure 2.23A, bisection threshold was between ⅟30th and ⅟50th of the separation between the reference lines over a range of reference line separations from 2 to 4 minutes of arc. Klein and Levi (1985) later reported that, to a first approximation, bisection threshold was a constant fraction of reference line separation (in their case) over a range of reference line separations from 2 to 10 minutes of arc. For their smallest reference line separation (0.8 minutes of arc), bisection threshold was close to 6 seconds of arc.

Klein and Levi (1985) also used the target depicted in Figure 2.23B. They found that the Weber fraction for bisection was approximately half that for the target shown in Figure 2.23A, and that the Weber fraction was "more-or-less constant" over a range of reference line separations from 10 minutes of arc down to 1.2 minutes of arc. The lowest threshold was approximately 1.3 seconds of arc. Klein and Levi attributed the difference in the Weber fractions for the two kinds of target to the availability of a luminance cue when the Figure 2.23B target was used that was not available when the target shown in part A was used.

Noting that "when the separation of the reference lines is small, the visibility of the dark line produced by offsetting the test line is hampered by the test line's proximity to the sharp luminance discontinuity that the pattern makes with the dark background," and that "the addition of flanking lines provides a luminance pedestal similar to the pedestal of the Westheimer effect" (Westheimer, 1967),

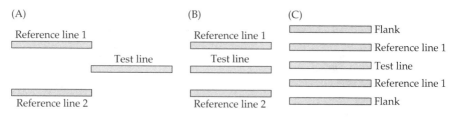

2.23 Targets for measuring bisection acuity.

Klein and Levi collected bisection using the target depicted in Figure 2.23C. The lowest bisection threshold was now reduced to 0.85 (SE = 0.04) seconds of arc.*

According to Levi and his colleagues, reports were published in the early 1860s by Fechner and by Volkman (Levi et al., 1988; Levi & Klein, 1990) that thresholds for relative position obey Weber's law, (e.g., bisection threshold approximates a constant fraction of approximately 0.03 to 0.05 of the distance to be bisected). Many authors have since confirmed the finding (Hirsch & Hylton, 1982; Levi & Klein, 1983; Klein & Levi, 1985; Toet et al., 1987; Yap et al., 1987a,b; Burbeck, 1987). Nevertheless, Levi and his colleagues proposed that bisection acuity does *not* obey Weber's law in all stimulus conditions. Previous reports that Weber's law for position is generally correct, they argued, could be attributed to a confounding of the effects of separation and eccentricity (Levi et al., 1988; Levi & Klein, 1990).

Challenging this proposal, Morgan and Watt criticized the experimental design used by Levi et al. (1988) and described a task that "we believe to be a more direct test of the eccentricity hypothesis for spatial interval acuity." (See Morgan & Watt, 1989, p. 1458.) They reported that the just-noticeable difference in the length of an arc (whose center of curvature was located on the fovea) was proportional to arc length over the range 10 to 500 minutes of arc. "Our results do not support a recent suggestion that the Weber relation is mainly due to greater positional uncertainty in the peripheral retina" (Morgan & Watt, 1989, p. 1457). "Whatever the correct explanation of the Weber relationship for length discrimination, our present results show that it cannot be considered entirely a consequence of eccentricity" (Morgan & Watt, 1989, p. 1462).

Replying to the comments of Morgan and Watt, Levi and Klein replotted some of the Morgan and Watt data as a function of the angle subtended between the endpoints of the arc and the fixation point rather than as a function of the length of the arc. They argued that the Morgan and Watt task laid more cognitive load on the observer than the Levi et al. (1988) task. They proposed that, "both the target separation and eccentricity can impose sensory limitations on the precision of positional acuity, and thus contribute to the Weber fraction for position" (Levi & Klein, 1989).

Bar width discrimination and bar separation discrimination

The task of judging which of two pairs of successively presented parallel bars or lines has the wider separation is another spatial discrimination whose threshold can be less than the shortest distance between foveal photoreceptors. The just-noticeable difference in line separation is about 5 seconds of arc for a pair of lines whose mean separation is between 1 and 4 minutes of arc, though this discrimination threshold rises considerably for smaller or greater mean separations (Westheimer & McKee,

---

* This value improved on the world record for visual discrimination as listed by the Guinness Book of Records, previously held by a German student, who, it was claimed, could identify people at a distance of 1.6 km.

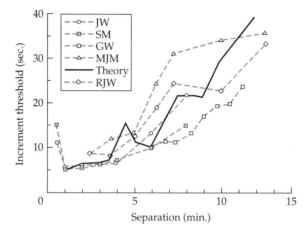

2.24 Discrimination of the separation between two lines. Data points show the effect of the separation between two lines on the just-noticeable difference in that separation. Data from four different studies: J.W. and S.M. from Westheimer & McKee, 1984; G.W. from Westheimer, 1984; M.J.M.. and R.J.W. from Watt & Morgan, 1983. The heavy line shows the prediction of Wilson and Gelb's line-element model. From Wilson (1991b).

1977; Watt & Morgan, 1983b). The data points in Figure 2.24 show how the just-noticeable difference varies with separation up to about 12 minutes of arc.

As to the effect of contrast, when line separation is below about five minutes of arc, separation discrimination threshold falls as a power function of contrast. But for larger separations (10 minutes of arc), separation discrimination threshold is independent of contrast, once contrast is more than about three times bar detection threshold (Morgan & Regan, 1987). This is similar to the effect of contrast on both orientation discrimination (Figure 2.30) and on spatial-frequency discrimination (Regan et al., 1982). As will be discussed in the section on coincident detectors later in this chapter, these two different regimes for line separation discrimination have been modeled in quite different ways.

Spatial-frequency discrimination

The just-noticeable difference between the spatial frequencies of two clearly visible gratings is far less than the range of spatial frequencies to which a spatial filter (in a psychophysical model) or a cortical cell (in neurophysiology) will respond. In addition, the just-noticeable difference in a grating's spatial frequency is little, if at all, affected by changing the grating's orientation and contrast at the same time as its spatial frequency. In the following section I review these findings in the light of the challenges they present to modelers of the discrimination process.

Labeled lines and the problem of explaining why spatial-frequency discrimination is so acute. Watson and Robson (1981) assumed that only one spatial filter is excited at grating detection threshold, so that the spatial frequencies of two gratings can be discriminated at threshold only if they are sufficiently different that the gratings excite different filters. This rationale is similar to that adopted by Thomas and Gille (1979) when estimating the orientation bandwidth of spatial filters. Watson and Robson found that the spatial frequencies of two gratings could be discriminated at contrast detection threshold, provided that the difference in spatial frequencies was sufficiently large. They came to the following conclusion:

The outputs of individual filters carry a spatial-frequency label.

Seven labeled filters span the range from 0.25 to 30 cycles/deg. at low temporal frequencies, while at high temporal frequencies only three are required.

At suprathreshold contrast levels the spatial-frequency discrimination story is quite different. Discrimination threshold falls steeply as contrast is increased until, at about three times above detection threshold, it reaches a value of about 2 to 5%, remaining approximately constant as contrast is further increased (Regan et al., 1982; Skottun et al., 1987; Bown, 1990).

At high contrasts, discrimination threshold for foveally viewed gratings is approximately independent of spatial frequency up to 20 to 30 cycles/deg. (depending on the individual observer), and can be as low as 13% at 50 cycles/deg. before discrimination fails precipitously (Campbell et al., 1970; Hirsch & Hylton, 1982; Regan et al., 1982; Smallman et al., 1996).

But when grating contrast is only just above detection threshold (Woodward et al., 1985), or the grating is viewed in peripheral vision at 10 degrees of eccentricity (Richter & Yager, 1984), then the spatial-frequency discrimination curve shows maxima and minima rather than being flat. In terms of the finding shown in Figure 2.25, these maxima and minima can be taken to indicate that only a small number of spatial filters are activated by low-contrast or peripherally viewed gratings.

The ability of human observers to discriminate as little as a 2 to 5% difference of spatial frequency between two successively presented suprathreshold gratings contrasts sharply with the comparatively broad spatial-frequency bandwidths of psychophysical channels and also of even the most selectively tuned neurons in monkey primary visual cortex. Psychophysical bandwidth estimates range from about 1.2 to 2.0 octaves (see footnote on page 78) full bandwidth at half-sensitivity (Blakemore & Campbell, 1969; Watson & Robson, 1981; Wilson, 1991b). Some cortical cells have full bandwidths at half-sensitivity as low as 0.5 octaves, but most range between 1.0 and 1.5 octaves (DeValois et al., 1982).

Thus, spatial-frequency discrimination can be regarded as a kind of hyperacuity in the same sense that wavelength discrimination is a hyperacuity and the discrimination of the direction of motion in depth is a hyperacuity. (Beverley & Regan, 1973, 1975).

A proposed explanation for the discrepancy between spatial-frequency discrimination threshold and the bandwidth of frequency-tuned neurons is that spatial-frequency discrimination is determined by the slope rather than by the band-

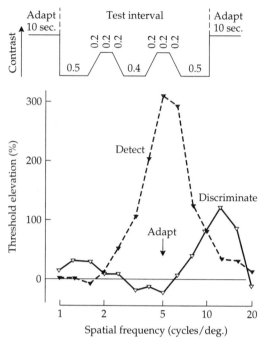

2.25 Postadaptation spatial-frequency discrimination. Changes in contrast detection thresholds (dashed line) and in spatial-frequency discrimination threshold (solid lines) caused by inspecting a sinusoidal grating of spatial frequency 5 cycles/deg. From D. Regan and Beverley (1983a).

width of the spatial-frequency tuning function. This hypothesis has been framed in both opponent-process (Campbell et al., 1970; Regan et al., 1982; Regan & Beverley, 1983a) and line-element formats (Wilson & Gelb, 1984; Wilson & Regan, 1984); see Appendix D. An opponent-process version is illustrated in Figure 2.29B. This opponent-process hypothesis is consistent with data on cue summation (Thomas & Olzak, 1990).

> One prediction of the hypothesis is that spatial-frequency discrimination depends on neurons that respond maximally to stimuli other than the ones to be discriminated.

See Regan (1982) and Regan et al. (1982) for a discussion of this idea. This theoretical prediction is consistent with single-neuron evidence in cats (Bradley et al., 1985). At the psychophysical level in humans, the hypothesis predicts that, if contrast sensitivity at spatial frequency S is reduced by adaptation or by visual dysfunction, spatial-frequency discrimination threshold will be elevated, and the elevation will not be at spatial frequency S, but at frequencies offset from S.

Elevations in spatial-frequency discrimination in patients with multiple sclerosis (discussed on p. 203) and in normal observers after adaptation (Figure 2.25) were consistent with this prediction. As well, postadaptation threshold elevations were higher at frequencies above S than below S, consistent with physiological evidence that the slope of the high-frequency segment of the neural tuning curve is steeper than that of the low-frequency segment (Tolhurst & Thompson, 1981; Bradley et al., 1985; Parker & Hawken, 1985).

Greenlee and Thomas (1992) reported that they were unable to detect the postadaptation elevation of spatial-frequency discrimination threshold at a test frequency about one octave higher than the adapting frequency shown in Figure 2.25. One possible explanation for this disagreement is that Regan and Beverley sought to produce strong adaptation by using an adapting grating of 100% contrast whose mean luminance was 4.6 times higher than that of the test gratings, while Greenlee and Thomas used an adapting grating whose mean luminance was the same as that of the test grating and whose contrast was 70% that, presumably, produced a weaker adapting effect.

The findings shown in Figure 2.25 imply that if we accept the six-mechanism model of Wilson and his colleagues (Figures 2.13 and 2.48), the spatial-frequency discrimination curve for a spatially localized foveated target should show multiple peaks and valleys even at high contrast levels. Experimental evidence is controversial (Westheimer, 1984, 1985; Hirsch, 1985; Wilson, 1991a,b; Toet & Koenderink, 1987; see Wilson & Wilkinson, 1997).

The effect on spatial-frequency discrimination threshold of superimposing a masker grating on the test grating is a severe test of frequency-discrimination models. In an experiment reported by Regan (1985a), each trial consisted of two grating presentations. The spatial frequency of one grating was $5(1 + x)$ cycles/deg. and the spatial frequency of the other was $5(1 - x)$ cycles/deg. The order of presentations was random, and there were 11 different values of x. Observers were instructed to signal whether the grating presented second had a higher or lower spatial frequency than the grating presented first. Masker gratings were optically superimposed on the test gratings.

When the masker grating had a constant spatial frequency, its major effects on discrimination could be explained trivially. By basing discrimination on beat patterns, observers were able to use the masker grating as a frequency reference; when the frequencies of the masker and test gratings were close, a small change in test frequency produced a large change in the beat pattern so that the masker produced threshold *reduction*. Discrimination threshold could be as low as 0.2% (Regan, 1985a). However, when this artifact was removed by jittering the masker's spatial frequency from trial to trial, the masker produced threshold elevations, and the chief findings were as follows.

---

1. When the masker and test gratings were parallel, a much larger elevation of discrimination threshold was produced when the frequency of the masker grating was a little higher than the frequency

of the test grating than when the frequency of the masker grating was a little lower (Figure 2.26).

2. When the masker and test gratings were orthogonal, there was little or no measurable effect.

A comparison of Figures 2.25 and 2.26 brings out the point that the elevation of discrimination threshold was greatest when the masker grating had a *higher* frequency than the test grating, but when the adapting grating had a *lower* frequency than the test grating. Nevertheless, the effect of the masker grating can be explained along the same lines as the effect of the adapting grating—in terms of the hypothesis that slope determines discrimination threshold. The three critical points are as follows: (1) the spatial frequency of the masker grating varied randomly from trial to trial; (2) the two most important neurons for discrimination respond to only a limited range of spatial frequencies; and (3) the high-frequency slope of the neural spatial-frequency tuning function is steeper than the low-frequency slope (Tolhurst & Thompson, 1981; Bradley et al., 1985).

One of the two neurons that are most important for spatial-frequency discrimination (b in Figure 2.27A) responds best to a spatial frequency a little lower than that of the test grating, and the other (c in Figure 2.27A) responds best to a spatial frequency a little higher than that of the test grating. (The most sensitive neuron (a) does not change its response when the spatial frequency of the test

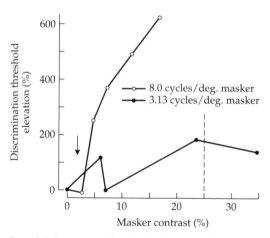

2.26 Masking of spatial-frequency discrimination. Masked spatial-frequency discrimination thresholds for a vertical 5.0 cycles/deg. luminance-defined grating are plotted versus the contrast of a vertical superimposed luminance-defined masker grating. Between successive presentations, the spatial frequency of the masker grating was randomly varied by up to ±20 % about its nominal value of 3.13 or 8.0 cycles/deg. Test grating contrast was 25 %, as indicated by the vertical dashed line. Contrast detection threshold for the masker gratings is arrowed. After D. Regan (1985a).

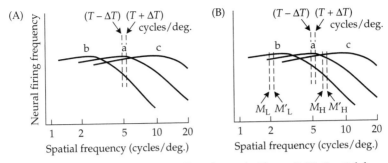

2.27 Proposed explanation for the finding shown in Figure 2.26. Spatial-frequency masking data can be explained by assuming that spatial-frequency discrimination threshold is determined by the relative activity of excited neurons. After Regan (1985).

grating changes from $(T - \Delta T)$ to $(T + \Delta T)$ or vice versa.) If the masker grating's frequency is always higher than the test frequency, it is possible to select a range of masker frequencies (M_H to M'_H in Figure 2.27B) such that relative sensitivities of the two neurons most important for discriminating the test frequency (neurons b and c) vary considerably over the range of the masker frequencies used. Thus, the random trial-to-trial variation in masker frequency will create a large random trial-to-trial variation in the relative sensitivities of the two neurons that are most important for discrimination. The consequence will be a large elevation of spatial-frequency discrimination threshold for the test grating.

The situation is quite different when the masker frequencies are always lower than the test frequency. The sensitivity curves of the two relevant neurons will both have shallow, near-identical slopes. Consequently, the random trial-to-trial variations in masker frequency (from M_L to M'_L in Figure 2.27B) will create comparatively little random variation in the relative sensitivities of the two neurons that are most important for discrimination. It follows that the elevation of discrimination threshold for the test grating will be considerably less than when the masker frequencies are always a little higher than that of the grating (D. Regan, 1985a).

On the grounds that spatial-frequency discrimination for foveally viewed gratings is not improved by increasing the number of cycles beyond 2.5, Hirsch and Hylton (1982) suggested that observers carry out the spatial-frequency discrimination task for a multi-bar grating by discriminating the separation between adjacent bright (or dark) bars, spatial pooling over cycles being negligible. From this viewpoint it is not surprising that the relative activity of multiple spatially tuned filters driven from the same location should have been proposed as an explanation for both spatial-frequency discrimination and for two-line separation discrimination. It is not clear, however, whether the failure of this model to account fully for data on two-line separation discrimination (Morgan & Ward, 1985) also compromises its plausibility as an explanation of spatial-frequency discrimination (see the section on coincidence detectors in this chapter).

Spatial-frequency discrimination between gratings of different orientations and contrasts. As already mentioned, Bradley et al. (1985) showed that some *individual* neurons have sufficiently steep spatial-frequency tuning curves and sufficiently low response variance to reliably respond to spatial differences that are just-detectable behaviorally. However, the response change of only one neuron cannot explain the following two findings.

1. Spatial-frequency discrimination threshold is the same between parallel gratings and between orthogonal gratings (Burbeck & Regan, 1983; Bradley & Skottun, 1984; Regan, 1985b; Olzack & Thomas, 1991, 1992).
2. Spatial-frequency discrimination threshold is approximately the same when spatial frequency, orientation, and contrast vary simultaneously as when spatial frequency is the only variable (Vincent & Regan, 1995).

The firing of a single neuron cannot explain these findings because identical changes of firing can be produced by a change in spatial frequency, or by a change of orientation, location, and so on.

A proposed explanation is that spatial-frequency discrimination threshold is determined by the relative activity of neurons tuned to different but overlapping ranges of spatial frequency, but that have identical tuning to orientation and other similar variables. Spatial-frequency information from orthogonal gratings is available at the discrimination stage.

(See Regan, 1982; Burbeck & Regan, 1983a; Regan & Beverley, 1983.)

The first of the findings just listed is difficult to explain in terms of the line-element model of Wilson and his colleagues (Wilson & Gelb, 1984; Wilson, 1991b), because different orientations are represented by locations that are far apart in *filter response space* (see Appendix D).

Next we consider the following two findings: spatial-frequency discrimination threshold falls steeply as contrast is progressively increased above detection threshold but remains approximately independent of contrast for contrasts more than two to three times above contrast detection threshold (Regan et al., 1982; Thomas, 1983; Skottun et al., 1987; Bown, 1990); spatial-frequency discrimination threshold is unaffected when contrast changes at the same time as spatial frequency (Regan et al., 1982; Vincent & Regan, 1995). The earlier proposal that contrast independence is achieved physiologically by second-stage opponent processing (Regan 1982; Regan & Beverley, 1983a) now seems unnecessarily complex in light of the finding that, at least in cat, contrast-independence of spatial-frequency discrimination threshold is a property of the first-stage striate cortex frequency-tuned neuron itself (Skottun et al., 1987); the connectivity between striate cortical neurons required to account for human ability to ignore simultaneous changes in, for example, orientation when discriminating spatial frequency does not seem to be necessary when the variable to be ignored is contrast.

The effect of grating orientation on spatial-frequency discrimination threshold and the oblique effect for spatial-frequency discrimination. Hirsch and Hylton (1984a) reported that a plot of spatial-frequency threshold discrimination versus orientation showed peaks and troughs and, furthermore, that there was a clear periodicity of 60 degrees. They attributed this periodicity to the hexagonal packing of central foveal cones (Color Plate 7).

Heeley and Timney (1988), however, failed to find a 60 degree periodicity in the results of any of their three observers. On the other hand, they used a stimulus field that subtended 7 degrees and, as illustrated anatomically in Color Plate 7 and Figure F.9 and demonstrated perceptually by moiré fringes (pp. 477–481), cone packing is regularly hexagonal only within the central fovea. Although they found some periodicity (at low spatial frequencies), Heeley and Timney stated that the pattern of periodicity was not consistent between observers. However, because they did not describe how they ensured accurate and reproducible alignment of the observer's head, it is difficult to evaluate this finding.*

Orientation Discrimination, Angle Discrimination, and Curvature Discrimination

In the following section I review experimental findings on the ability of humans to distinguish between the orientations of luminance-defined simple targets such as lines or gratings. I also review data on three related topics: judging the implicit orientations of complex targets, judging angles, and discriminating curvature.

Orientation discrimination for luminance-defined form

The just-noticeable difference in the orientations of two clearly visible gratings or lines is far less than the range of orientations to which a spatial filter (in a psychophysical

---

* Methodological details may be important here. For example, when collecting the data shown in Figure 2.31, Regan and Price (1986) paid close attention to ensuring that, over the many weeks of data collection, the observer's head was always aligned identically. The observer's head was firmly fixed within a heavy metal cage. And the alignment was checked frequently by reference to dents in the skull, congenital and acquired. (Author D. R. has a convenient small irregularity at the front of the skull, the result of an over-ambitious attempt to hook a fast bouncer in 1953: cricket provides even more to the vision scientist than the previously reported [Regan, 1992] academic challenges.) A second concern was that the presentation of oblique gratings would cause the observer's eye to rotate in its socket about its visual axis (torsion) and thus cause grating orientation in retinal coordinates to differ from grating orientation with respect to the head. Regan and Beverley (1985) estimated the size of this torsion by first presenting the eye with a briefly flashed vertical line so as to create a vertical afterimage and then presenting gratings whose orientations were other than vertical. Ocular torsion was evident when the presentation was long. So we reduced the presentation duration until no torsion was evident, and this presentation duration (0.6 seconds) was used by Regan and Price. The torsion effect just described can be 1 to 2 degrees when the observer views a grating inclined at 15 degrees from the vertical (Crone, 1973, p. 93). And with the aim of reducing the effective number of orientation-tuned elements, we used a small stimulus field (1.0 deg. diameter) located off the central fovea (at 1.25 deg. eccentricity).

model) or a cortical cell (in neurophysiology) will respond. In addition, the just-noticeable difference in grating or line orientation is little, if at all, affected by changing the target's spatial frequency and contrast at the same time as its orientation. In the following section I review these findings in the light of the challenges they present to modelers of the discrimination process.

Labeled lines and the problem of explaining why orientation discrimination is so acute. A heightening of interest in the psychophysics of orientation tuning of spatial contrast filters and the psychophysics of orientation discrimination can be traced back to Hubel and Wiesel's (1962) report that the stimulus feature of orientation is sufficiently important to merit the anatomical substrate of orientation columns, a substrate that can be rendered visible to naked-eye examination of the visual cortex (Hubel et al., 1978). By means of this organization the brain creates multiple maps of the visual world; these maps are displaced relative to one another, each map being for a narrow range of orientations. Mountcastle (who had, in the 1950s, discovered the columnar arrangement of the cortex while studying somatosensory cortex) noted a possible reason for this curious arrangement: that, in general, a "columnar arrangement allows the mapping of several variables simultaneously in a two-dimensional matrix with the preservation of topology" (Mountcastle, 1979).

The orientation discrimination threshold for high-contrast lines or gratings is 0.15 to 0.5 degrees (Andrews, 1965, 1967; Andrews et al., 1973; Westheimer et al., 1976; Westheimer, 1979; Burbeck & Regan, 1983a). For short lines, orientation discrimination fulfills Westheimer's (1975) definition of a hyperacuity as a spatial discrimination that transcends the 25 seconds of arc separation between cones in the central fovea, since a 0.3 degree change in the orientation of a line of length 0.5 degrees corresponds to a displacement of less than 25 seconds of arc of the line's ends (see pp. 44–48).

> Orientation discrimination for longer lines or for gratings of any extent can be regarded as a kind of hyperacuity in the same sense that wavelength discrimination in color vision can be regarded as a kind of hyperacuity.

Thomas and Gille (1979) showed that the outputs of individual spatial filters carry an orientation label, but that the half-amplitude orientation-tuning bandwidth of a filter is very broad (10 to 30 degrees). But human observers can discriminate a 0.15 to 0.5 degree difference in the orientations of two successively presented lines or gratings. This presents a challenge for theorists.

Reports that the bandwidths of the most selectively tuned cells in monkey primary visual cortex are far broader than 0.5 degrees (Hubel & Wiesel, 1968; DeValois et al., 1982) present a similar challenge to those who would explain human behavioral performance at the level of cortical neurons.

A proposed explanation for the discrepancy between orientation discrimination threshold and the bandwidth of orientation-tuned neurons is that orientation discrimination is determined by the slope rather than by the bandwidth of the orientation tuning function. This hypothesis has been framed in both opponent-process (Westheimer et al., 1976; Regan, 1982; Regan & Beverley, 1985) and line-element formats (Wilson & Gelb, 1984; Wilson & Regan, 1984), and owes its rationale to the classical theory of color vision (see Appendix D).

The opponent-process version has it that a discrimination between orientations θ_1 and θ_2 would be made by comparing the outputs of two mechanisms that are opposed in the sense that one mechanism is more sensitive to θ_1 than to θ_2, while the other is more sensitive to θ_2 than to θ_1 (see pp. 36–39). This opponent-process hypothesis is consistent with data on cue summation (Thomas & Olzak, 1990). One prediction of this hypothesis is that orientation discrimination depends on neurons that respond maximally to stimuli other than the ones to be discriminated (Regan, 1982; Regan &Beverley, 1985). The prediction is consistent with single-neuron evidence in cat (Bradley et al., 1985). At psychophysical level in human, this "discrimination is determined by slope" hypothesis predicts that, if the sensitivity of the neuron tuned to a particular orientation (θ) and spatial frequency (S) is reduced by either adaptation or visual dysfunction, discrimination thresholds for orientation and spatial frequency will be elevated at orientations and frequencies that are offset from θ and S (Regan, 1982; Regan et al., 1982). The prediction is explained in Figure 2.28A and B in the case of orientation discrimination.

Figure 2.28A shows the notional excitation pattern over many orientation-tuned neurons produced by a grating of orientation θ_1 slightly anticlockwise of vertical (continuous line) and a grating of orientation θ_2 slightly clockwise of vertical (dashed line), vertical being 0 degrees. Figure 2.28B illustrates that, because of the shape of the particular excitation curves shown, the difference between the two excitation patterns is greatest for neurons that prefer orientations considerably offset from the vertical (θ_3 and θ_4), so that information about the change of grating orientation is carried by weakly excited neurons. Since there is no difference between the two excitation patterns near the vertical, the most strongly excited neurons carry no information about the change of grating orientation. Bradley et al. (1985) have experimentally demonstrated this theoretical point in the context of individual cortical neurons.

Figure 2.28C illustrates the point just described in terms of the excitation of individual neurons whose sensitivity profiles are labeled a, b, and c. Sensitivity profiles a and c are the two whose slopes differ maximally at orientation 0 degrees. These will be the most important for orientation discrimination because the difference between their outputs changes most when grating orientation changes from θ_1 to θ_2. The output of the most excited neuron (labeled b) changes negligibly when grating orientation changes from θ_1 to θ_2. The psychophysical data of Figure 2.28D are consistent with this prediction. The dotted line confirmed previous reports (Gilinsky, 1968; Blakemore & Nachmias, 1971), that detection threshold elevations are greatest when the test and adapting gratings are parallel, and fall to half the maximum value when the test grating is at an angle of about 10 degrees to the adapting grating. The continuous line shows that discrimination thresholds behaved quite differently. These were most elevated when the test grating's orientation was offset

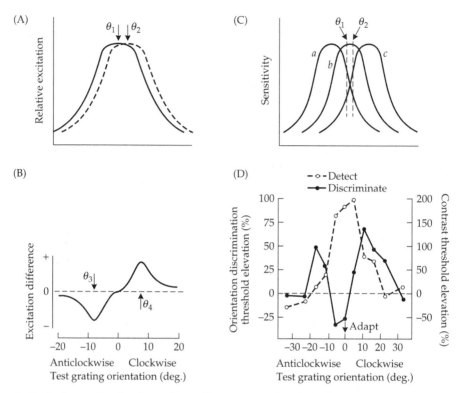

2.28 A change in stimulus orientation causes a change in the pattern of activity among a population of orientation-tuned neurons driven from the same retinal location. (A) The notional excitation patterns produced within a population of orientation-tuned filters by gratings of orientations θ_1 (continuous line) and θ_2 (dashed line). (B) The difference between the two excitation patterns shown in part A. (C) When the orientation of a stimulus grating changes from θ_1 to θ_2, the response of the most strongly excited neuron (b) changes negligibly, but there is a large change in the relative excitations of neurons a and b. (D) After adapting to a high-contrast vertical grating (zero on the abscissa) the contrast required to detect a test grating is elevated (dashed line and right ordinate). The detection threshold elevation is greatest for a vertical test grating. Orientation discrimination threshold is also elevated (continuous line and left ordinate), but the greatest elevation is for test gratings whose orientations are inclined at 10 to 20 degrees from the vertical. From Regan and Beverley (1985).

from the adapting grating's orientation. This finding is in accord with the hypothesis that orientation discrimination is determined by the slope of the neural orientation tuning function. In Figure 2.28D, the offset is from 11 to 17 degrees. Further relevant psychophysical evidence has been reported by Thomas and Olzak (1990).

So far, this discussion has been restricted to how the shape of the orientation tuning curve affects orientation discrimination threshold. Clearly, this cannot be the only determinant of orientation discrimination threshold. If the entire discrimination process were noise-free, discrimination threshold would approach zero, and this, of course, is not the case. Figure 2.29A shows three possible sources of noise (noise 1, 2, and 3) that, together with the maximum slope of the tuning of the orientation-tuned primary cortical neurons might, in principle, limit discrimination threshold (Regan & Beverley, 1985).

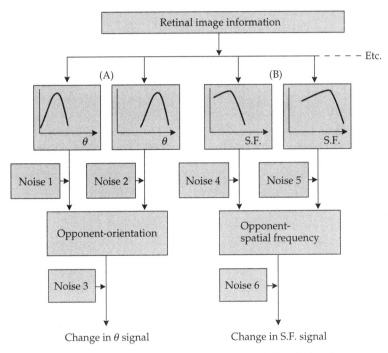

2.29 Outline of an opponent process model of spatial discrimination. Any small region of the retina on which a spatial pattern is imaged excites a population of neurons, each of which is sensitive to orientation, spatial frequency, temporal frequency, contrast, and so on. (A) A change of orientation is signaled by a change in the relative activity of a subpopulation that prefers different orientations, but that has exactly the same tuning with respect to all other visual dimensions. The most important neurons for discrimination are the two whose sensitivity curves differ most at the orientation of the stimulus. The signal for each neuron is contaminated by noise that may be correlated to some extent. The two neurons feed an opponent mechanism that may suppress all or part of the peripheral noise, but adds additional noise to the "change in orientation" signal. (B) Two neurons, different from the two in A, are most important for signaling a change in spatial frequency. For simplicity, the nonlinear contrast transducer function stage (see Figures 2.12 and 2.16) is omitted.

Depending on (1) the kind of noise at the level of the orientation-tuned filters and (2) the way in which "relative activity" is computed, the effect (if any) of peripheral noise on orientation discrimination threshold can be reduced by the opponent processing. If the two most important neurons have noise that is identical at every instant (noise 1 and 2 in Figure 2.29A), the residual noise level after subtractive opponency will be zero. This point is exploited in the design of the conventional differential amplifier for microvolt-level signals. (This extreme case is mentioned only to clarify the theoretical principle.) Nevertheless, in practical terms it is known that, although the noise is not identical in different visual neurons, it is not in general totally independent (Toyama et al., 1981).

However, as noted by Regan and Beverley (1985), even in the case that noise in first-stage orientation-tuned neurons were to be entirely suppressed, orientation discrimination threshold would not be indefinitely low because it would be limited by more central noise at the stage where relative response is encoded stage (noise 3 in Figure 2.29A, see also pp. 36–39). If the central noise were dominant and also independent of the outputs of the more peripheral neurons, then it would be easy to explain why orientation discrimination threshold is unaffected when contrast changes at the same time as orientation and that, as shown in Figure 2.30, orientation discrimination threshold is approximately independent of contrast for contrasts more than 2 to 3 times above detection threshold (Burbeck & Regan, 1983a; Regan & Beverley, 1985; Vincent & Regan, 1995).*
Unfortunately, we have little direct evidence as to the relative importance of peripheral and central noise in human vision. On the other hand, in animals the response variance of only one neuron in striate cortex needs to be considered when explaining the magnitudes of behavioral discrimination thresholds (Bradley et al., 1985). However, as already noted, a change in the firing of a single

---

* Regan and Beverley (1985, p. 153) stated: "If discrimination is limited by noise in outputs *a* and *b*" (*a* and *b* being the outputs of the orientation-tuned neurons most important for discrimination), "suppression of part of this noise allows the possibility of more acute discrimination. On the other hand, this point has little importance if discrimination is limited by noise at the opponent stage. Unfortunately, few or no physiological data are available on the three crucial points: the degree of correlation between the noise level of adjacent orientation-tuned neurons; the dependence of noise level on the firing frequency of orientation-tuned neurons; the balance between the noise levels of orientation–tuned neurons and more central orientation-opponent elements." Bown (1990) stated incorrectly that Regan and Beverley had ignored the possible role of central noise and had discussed the discrimination process entirely in terms of peripheral noise. "Many models of discrimination (Wilson, 1986; Klein & Levi, 1985; Regan & Beverley, 1985) have assumed that all suprathreshold discrimination tasks share a common noise source, neglecting the central noise shown in Fig. 1" (Bown, 1990, p. 450). On the basis of this incorrect statement (see also Heeley and Buchanan-Smith, 1994), he labeled Regan and Beverley's model an "error propagation model," stated that it should be rejected because it ignored central noise, and emphasized the importance of central noise. Heeley and Buchanan-Smith (1994) have presented suggestive evidence that discrimination threshold is limited by noise that arises after the initial filter stage.

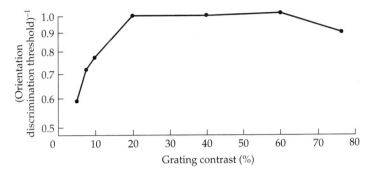

2.30 Orientation discrimination threshold is approximately independent of grating contrast. When contrast is more than about three times above grating detection threshold, threshold is approximately constant. From Regan and Beverley (1985).

neuron in striate cortex could carry many meanings. It does not signal unequivocally a change of orientation, or spatial frequency, or indeed any other variable.

The proposed explanation that contrast independence is achieved physiologically by second-stage opponent processing (Regan, 1982; Regan & Beverley, 1985) now seems unnecessarily complex in the light of the subsequent finding that—at least in cat cortex—contrast independence of orientation discrimination threshold is a property of the first-stage striate cortex orientation-tuned neuron itself (Skottun et al., 1987). The connectivity between individual striate cortical neurons required to account for human ability to ignore simultaneous changes in, for example, spatial frequency when discriminating orientation does not seem to be necessary when the variable to be ignored is contrast.

The *reduction* in postadaptation orientation discrimination threshold at the adapting orientation evident in Figure 2.28D indicates that the activity of the most excited neurons are detrimental to the discrimination process. Discrimination improves when they are rendered less active by adaptation. I suppose that the difference signal shown by the continuous line in Figure 2.28B is, in fact, not noise-free as shown, but is superimposed on noise. Consequently, the experimental observer's task can be regarded as discriminating, within the ensemble of neurons, signal-plus-noise from noise alone. The neurons that prefer orientations near the vertical will be most excited by the test gratings, and noisy fluctuations in their outputs will make an important contribution to the total noise in the difference signal. By desensitizing these neurons, the adapting grating will reduce the noise in the difference signal, and produce the small reduction in discrimination threshold evident in Figure 2.28D.

Orientation discrimination between gratings of different spatial frequencies.
Bradley et al. (1985) showed that some individual neurons have sufficiently steep tuning curves and sufficiently low response variance to allow them to respond reliably to changes of orientation and changes of spatial frequency that

are just-detectable behaviorally. They concluded that behavioral discrimination threshold can be explained without postulating statistical averaging among many neurons.

Nevertheless, they acknowledged, behavioral *performance* cannot be explained in terms of the response change of only one neuron. In particular, Burbeck and Regan (1983a) and Bradley and Skottun (1984) had reported the following: orientation discrimination threshold was the same between gratings of the same spatial frequency and between gratings of widely different spatial frequencies (2 versus 5 cycles/deg. and 1 versus 8 cycles/deg.).

These authors concluded that:

> Information about the orientations of gratings whose spatial frequencies are different is available at the discrimination stage, and orientation is processed independently of spatial frequency.

The finding has subsequently been confirmed (Olzak & Thomas, 1991, 1992, 1996; Heeley et al., 1993; Thomas & Olzak, 1996).

If spatial frequency is plotted radially and orientation is plotted as azimuth in polar coordinates, the pooling mechanism revealed by the studies just cited can be represented as an elongated area centered on the origin (Olzak & Thomas, 1996).

More recently it has been shown that orientation discrimination threshold is little, if at all higher, when orientation, spatial frequency (and contrast) vary simultaneously than when orientation is the only variable (Vincent & Regan, 1995).

These findings are difficult to explain in terms of the line-element model of Wilson and his colleagues (Wilson & Gelb, 1984; Wilson, 1991b), because gratings of very different spatial frequencies are represented by locations that are far apart in filter response space (see Appendix D).

The effect of grating orientation on orientation discrimination threshold and the oblique effect for orientation discrimination. If we follow the line of thought summarized on pages 116–121, the finding that a plot of orientation discrimination threshold versus orientation round the clock exhibits sharp peaks and troughs (Figure 2.31) can be understood if the 180 degrees of possible orientations are sampled by neurons that are sharply tuned to orientation at only a few (as few as four) fixed orientations (Regan & Price, 1986).

Although orientation discrimination sensitivity in Figure 2.31 was lower when the grating was at 45 degrees than when it was vertical or horizontal, there is a roughly threefold *increase* of sensitivity at 45 degrees compared with neighboring orientations. This suggests an alternative explanation for the well-known *oblique effect for orientation discrimination*.

> The oblique effect is a consequence of only a few orientations' being sampled by sharply tuned neurons.

In attributing the peaks and troughs in Figure 2.31 to the organization of cortical orientation-tuned mechanisms, this hypothesis is quite different from the explanation proposed by Hirsch and Hylton (1984) for their finding that a plot of

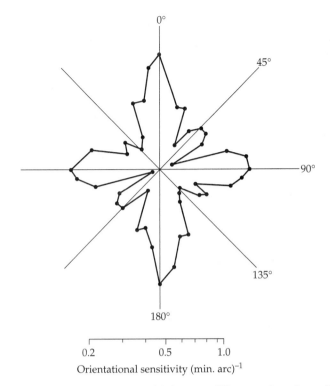

2.31 The effect of orientation on sensitivity to a difference in orientation.
In this polar plot, the reciprocal of orientation discrimination threshold is plotted as radius with mean grating orientation as azimuth. Because the maximum variation of orientation is 180 degrees, the curve has mirror symmetry. From Regan and Price (1986).

spatial-frequency discrimination threshold versus grating orientation shows peaks and troughs with a 60-degree periodicity. They attributed the periodicity to the *earliest* stage of visual processing: the hexagonal packing of foveal cones.

A subtle point here is that contrast detection thresholds do not show the peaks and troughs evident in Figure 2.31, presumably because detection can be supported by neurons that are broadly as well as sharply tuned to orientation. Also, neurons tuned to considerably fewer orientations (as few as two) may be involved when targets are temporally modulated or briefly presented (Camisa et al., 1977; Foster & Ward, 1991), possibly because the role of phasic neurons is favored with respect to the role of sustained neurons (see footnote on p. 88).

Discrimination of implicit orientation

Observers are able to discriminate small differences in the orientation of the axis of symmetry of many line figures, even when none of the lines that compare the figure are parallel to the axis of symmetry (Li & Westheimer, 1997).

Figure 2.32 shows how orientation discrimination threshold for an ellipse varied with the aspect ratio of the ellipse. Threshold was essentially constant for aspect ratios between 0 and 0.5 and then increased steeply until, at an aspect ratio of 1.0 (a circle), the task became impossible. Li and Westheimer concluded that, since the ellipses have continuously varying orientation information along their contours, what is being discriminated is not the orientation of individual segments of contour, but the implicit orientation of the figure as a whole.

The solid line in Figure 2.33 shows that orientation discrimination threshold for a cross is independent of the angle of the cross over a range of angles from zero to 90 degrees. To control for the possibility that observers might have based their discrimination responses on changes in the orientation of one or other of the individual lines that comprised the cross, Li and Westheimer removed one of the lines and measured orientation discrimination for the remaining line. Open symbols (dashed line) in Figure 2.33 should be comprised with the data for the cross (filled symbols, solid line). Although thresholds were similar when the cross

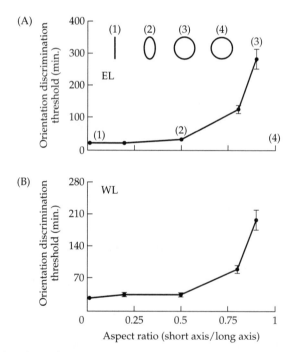

2.32 Implicit orientation I. Symbols show experimentally measured just-noticeable differences in the orientation of configurations ranging from a vertical line through vertically elongated ellipses to a circle (the just-noticeable difference is, of course, infinitely high for a perfect circle). The stimuli used to obtain various numbered points on the curve are illustrated with their corresponding numbers. Note that the orientation discrimination threshold for an ellipse with a 30 mm arc long axis and 15 min arc short axis (inset 2) is approximately as low as for a 30 mm arc line (inset 1). From Li and Westheimer (1997).

angle was near-zero (and, therefore, the individual line was near-vertical in the
control experiment), threshold for the individual line was already far higher than
for the cross when the cross angle was greater than about 10 degrees (and, therefore, the line was inclined at more than 5 degrees to the vertical). (Figure 2.31
shows evidence that there is a steep increase of orientation discrimination threshold when mean inclination departs from the vertical by only a few degrees, and
that there may be a subsequent small *reduction* of threshold as the tilt approaches
45 degrees.) The crucial points here are as follows:

1. The demonstration that orientation discrimination threshold for
   the cross as a whole is dissociated from orientation discrimination
   threshold for either of the lines that comprise the cross.
2. Additionally, and remarkably, orientation discrimination threshold for the cross as a whole showed an oblique effect when its axis
   of symmetry was inclined to the vertical by a sufficiently large
   angle. The same was true for the ellipse.

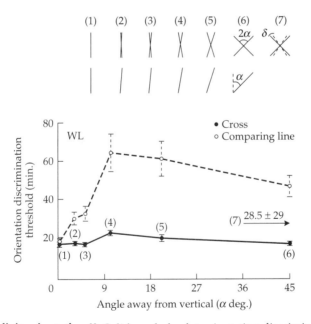

2.33 Implicit orientation II. Solid symbols plot orientation discrimination thresholds for the axis of symmetry of a cross. The mean orientation of the axis of symmetry was vertical. The angle of the cross progressively increased along the abscissa, as
indicated by the upper row of inserts. Progression was quantified in terms of the
angle (α) between either line and the vertical. The solid arrow indicates the orientation discrimination for a cross whose containing angle was randomly varied
between 70 and 90 degrees from trial to trial. Open symbols plot orientation discrimination thresholds for one of the lines that comprised the cross. From Li and
Westheimer (1997).

Li and Westheimer went on to show that performance was disrupted when the two lines were presented in succession rather than simultaneously. It seems unlikely that Li and Westheimer's data on orientation discrimination for the cross target might be explained in terms of a proposed mechanism that is sensitive to the angle between two lines, even though the angle-sensitive mechanism is distinct from the mechanism that underlies orientation discrimination (see Figure 2.37) and requires both lines to be present simultaneously. For example, angle discrimination threshold remained low when the axis of symmetry of the cross was rotated throughout a random angle from trial to trial, while orientation discrimination threshold for the axis of symmetry remained low when the angle was varied randomly from trial to trial. And angle discrimination threshold was unaffected by randomly varying the lengths of the two lines on a trial-to-trial basis (see Figure 2.37), while orientation discrimination for the axis of symmetry was disrupted by this manipulation.

Li and Westheimer pointed out that their conclusions parallel those of Wenderoth and his colleagues, who reported evidence that the visual system can extract virtual axes of symmetry from patterns and that a virtual axis acts like a weak, but real, line (Wenderoth et al., 1993; Wenderoth & van der Zwan, 1991).

Evidence for a *coincidence detector* that might account for the findings reported by Li and Westheimer is discussed on pp. 156–169.

Burbeck and Zauberman (1997) used the kind of stimulus illustrated in Figure 2.34 to test the following hypothesis of how the orientation of an object as a whole is encoded: (1) perceived orientation is based on the distribution of local edge orientations, the distribution being calculated independently of location; (2) large-sized filters that are driven from one location in the visual field and that respond to the object as a whole determine perceived orientation; (3) the orientation of the object's *core* determines perceived orientation

The concept of *core* (Burbeck & Pizer, 1995) can be understood by referring to Figure 2.35. The wavy lines in Figure 2.35A represent the boundaries of the antiphase target shown in the left half of Figure 2.34, and the wavy lines in part B represent the boundaries of the in-phase target shown in the right half of Figure 2.34. The small ellipses represent small orientation-tuned contrast-sensitive receptive fields.

The kind of untextured uniformly illuminated targets illustrated in Figure 2.34 could not provide evidence for true *coincidence detectors*. (A coincidence detector is, by definition, insensitive to targets between the two local filters that feed it; see pp. 156–169.) Nevertheless, for reasons described there, I have shown in Figure 2.35 the outputs of any given pair of local receptive feeds feeding a coincidence detector.

In Figure 2.35, the output of any given coincidence detector is labeled with the mean location of the two filters so as to identify the local core (C) of the target. Thus, as proposed by Burbeck and Zauberman (1997), the image is segmented into regions by identification of its boundaries.

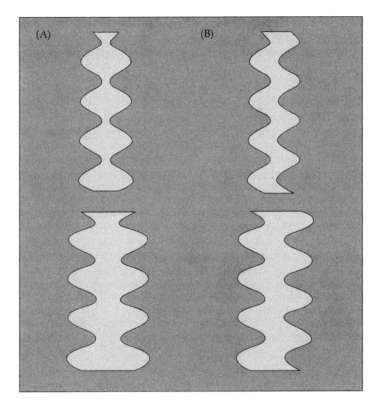

2.34 Implicit orientation III. This figure shows four targets with sinusoidally modulated edges. The upper and lower pairs differ only in their average widths. The left and right members of each pair differ in the phase difference of the edge modulators: antiphase for the left figures, in-phase for the right figures. From Burbeck et al. (1996).

The type of coincidence detector depicted in Figure 2.35 differs from the type originally proposed in that its output is labeled with the mean location rather than with the separation of the two small receptive fields (see the section in this chapter on coincidence detectors and Figure 2.53). A further distinction is that the coincidence detectors depicted in Figure 2.35 respond to lines of different orientations (part A) as well as to parallel lines rather than being sensitive to parallel lines only. Direct evidence that the human visual system contains coincidence detectors of this kind is reviewed on pp. 156–169.

As can be seen by inspecting the right half of Figure 2.34, the same amplitude of edge modulation has a greater effect on the perceived location of the local center of the target for the narrower target than for the wider target. In formal experiments carried out by Burbeck and Zauberman, observers were instructed to estimate the

(A) Axis of symmetry

(B) Axis of symmetry

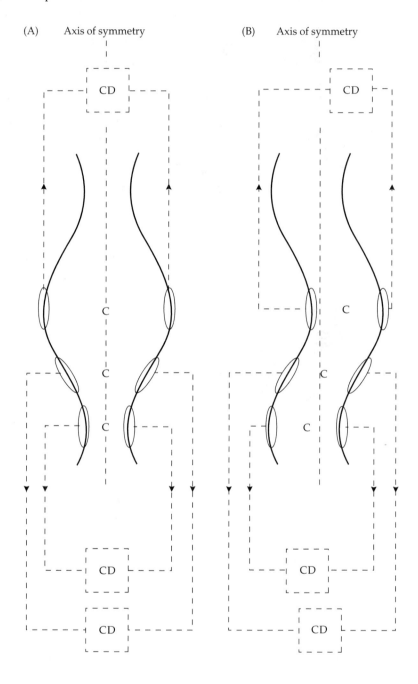

local center of the target at some given height on the target. Confirming the informal observation, the wiggliness of the perceived center reduced as the target's width was increased. Furthermore, the wiggliness of the perceived center also decreased when the spatial frequency of the edge modulation was increased.

In terms of the coincidence detector concept illustrated in Figures 2.35 and 2.53, these findings suggest that, if each of the two receptive fields that feed a coincidence detector is wide, line separation discrimination threshold will be higher than if the two receptive fields are narrow. This idea would explain why discrimination threshold for line separation is higher when the two lines are both viewed peripherally than when both are viewed foveally.

Burbeck and Zauberman (1997) stated that, for objects with a straight core (e.g., left half of Figure 2.34 and Figure 2.35A), the local orientation of the core gives the orientation of the object, but if the object does not have a straight core (e.g., right side of Figure 2.34 and Figure 2.35B), then an additional stage of processing such as averaging along the length of the object would be required to determine the object's overall orientation.

Orientation discrimination for objects with a straight core has some common ground with the discrimination of implicit orientation using crossed-line or elliptical targets (Figures 2.32 and 2.33).

According to Burbeck and Zauberman (1997, p. 180), the advantage the core concept has over the concept of large-sized filters is that it is based on the responses of smaller-scale filters, and hence could be more precise. They added, "The core is, in theory, a better source of information about object orientation than are the object's edges because the core disambiguates a change in width from a bend in the object."

The research of Burbeck and her colleagues was restricted to targets whose interiors were untextured and of uniform luminance, so that their concept of *core* would need to be extended to account for data on judging the implicit orientation of textured targets. In an experimental study of this kind Lánský, Yakimoff, and Radil (1988) used the targets depicted in Figure 2.36A–E. Figure 2.36A shows an irregular pattern of dots whose implicit orientation (indicated by the straight line) was defined as the axis for which the sum of the squared distances from each dot was a minimum. Short lines replaced the dots in parts B–E, the lines being centered on the locations previously occupied by the dots. The difference between the implicit orientation of the pattern and the orientation of the short

◀ **2.35 Extension of the *coincidence detector* concept.** This hypothetical coincidence detector (CD) differs from the one illustrated in Figure 2.53 in that it is activated by simultaneous stimulation of two narrow receptive fields that are some distance apart *and that may or may not prefer the same orientation*. By definition, a coincidence detector is not affected by stimuli in the region between the two narrow receptive fields. The output of the coincidence detector is labeled with the location (C), the point midway between the two receptive fields.

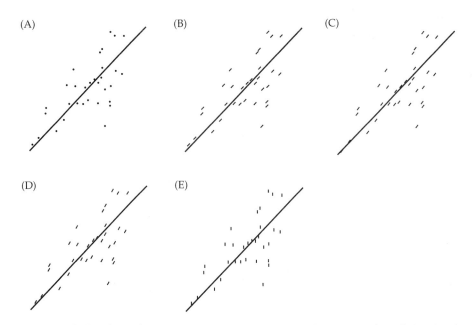

2.36 Implicit orientation IV. Targets used to find how the perceived implicit orientation of an *irregular pattern of lines as a whole* are affected by the orientation of the individual lines. The continuous lines indicate the least-squares axis of the pattern. The angle between this axis and the lines is 5.7 degrees in part (B), 11.5 degrees in (C), 22.9 degrees in (D), and 45.8 degrees in (E). In part (A), the lines were replaced by dots. After Lánský, Yakimoff, and Radil (1988).

lines was 5.7 degrees in part B, 11.5 degrees in part C, 22.9 degrees in part D, and 45.8 degrees in part E.

A straight line whose orientation was controlled by the observer was super-imposed on the dot pattern in Figure 2.36A. Observers were instructed to adjust the line until its orientation matched the perceived orientation of the dot pattern. Lánský et al. found that settings did not differ significantly from the implicit orientation of the dot pattern in Figure 2.36A. This was also the case for patterns labeled (C) and (E) in that figure.

Patterns B and D gave quite different results. For pattern B, implicit orientation was perceived as rotated about 1.3 degrees towards the orientation of the short lines, while for pattern E the implicit orientation was perceived as being rotated about 1.5 degrees away from the orientation of the short lines. Lánský et al. proposed that there is an interaction between local and global orientation, and that the interaction has a periodicity of about 45 degrees.

It does not necessarily follow that orientation *discrimination* threshold should parallel this effect on perceived *absolute* orientation. For example, orientation discrimination threshold for a vertical bar composed of short lines was the same whether the mean location of the short lines was vertical or horizontal (Regan, 1995).

Angles

The irritation felt when it becomes clear that the corners of a carefully constructed picture frame are not right angles speaks to our exquisitely acute ability to discriminate angles. Regan and Hamstra (1992a) reported that the just-noticeable difference between angles formed by two intersecting lines ranged from 0.7 to 1.6 degrees over eight observers. A weakness of this study was that the two lines were orientated symmetrically about the vertical, so that observers might have used the orientation of one or the other line as a cue to their angle of intersection. In a later study, observers were required to discriminate trial-to-trial changes in the angle of the Vee formed by two lines (θ_1 and θ_2 in Figure 2.37), while the Vee was rotated bodily through a random angle on a trial-to-trial basis. This random variation ensured that the orientation of neither individual line (e.g., β) provided a reliable cue to the Vee angle. The length of each arm of the Vee also varied randomly on a trial-to-trial basis so as to eliminate any consistent relationship between the Vee angle and the distance between the ends of the line (*ab* in Figure 2.37).

The just-noticeable difference in angle was 1.0 degrees and 1.8 degrees for two observers in the situation that no reliable cue to the task was provided by the orientation of either of the two straight lines that comprised the Vee.*

On the basis of this finding Regan, Gray, and Hamstra (1996a) proposed that:

> The human visual pathway contains a mechanism that encodes the difference between the orientations of two lines; this mechanism is quite distinct from the opponent-process orientation mechanism proposed by Westheimer et al. (1976) and Regan and Beverley (1985).

When the Vee angle was changed by equal and opposite rotations of the two arms of the Vee, the just-noticeable difference in the Vee angle was the same with and without the trial-to-trial random bodily rotations of the Vee. The reason for this finding was that, in the "equal but opposite" rotation condition, angle discrimination threshold was reached before orientation discrimination threshold was reached for either arm of the Vee. This finding suggests that the data reported by Regan and Hamstra (1992a) were true angle discrimination thresholds.

In an independent study, Snippe and Koenderink (1994) reported on human visual discrimination of 2D fronto-parallel angles. Although their angles were defined by bright dots at the ends of invisible lines rather than by continuous bright lines, their main results and conclusions were essentially the same as those reported by Regan and Hamstra (1992a) and Regan et al. (1996a). On the basis of

---

* Some years after this study was published I discovered with chagrin that what I had thought to be something that might interest vision researchers was a triviality to the dental profession. The examination book of perception tests faced by students wishing to enter dental school at the University of Toronto had long included a test that required the candidate to order according to angle a set of Vees that were bodily rotated as in Figure 2.37. The smallest increment of angle was 1 degree. And this was one of the easier tests!

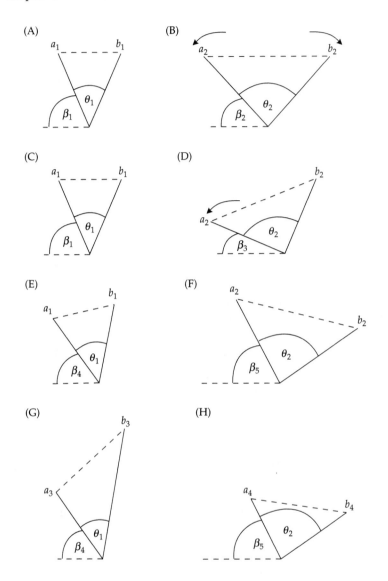

2.37 Discrimination of Vee angle. Vee angle was changed either by rotating each arm in opposite directions through the same angle (A and B) or by rotating only one arm of the Vee (C and D). (A–D) When the angle of the Vee increases from θ_1 to θ_2, the orientation (β) of the left arm of the Vee decreases, and the distance (ab) between the ends of the Vee increases. (E,F) The Vee rotates bodily either clockwise or anti-clockwise so as to remove line orientation (β) as a reliable cue to Vee angle. (G,H) The length of each line varies so as to remove distance ab as a reliable cue to Vee angle. From Regan, Gray, and Hamstra (1996a).

similar experiments, Chen and Levi (1996) also concluded that the human visual system contains a mechanism sensitive to angle that is distinct from the orientation-sensitive mechanism.

We offered an explanation for the "with random bodily rotation" discrimination threshold for Vee angle [$(\Delta\theta)_{\text{Th.WR}}$], that was framed in terms of the following sequence of visual processing.

1. The orientations of each arm of the Vee are simultaneously encoded within the visual pathway.
2. The difference between these two orientations is encoded at a second stage of processing.

To estimate the amount of information that is lost at the second stage of processing, we proceeded as follows. We measured a "without random bodily rotation" discrimination threshold for Vee angle [$(\Delta\theta)_{\text{Th.NR}}$] in the situation that the orientation of only one arm of the Vee was changed. This threshold can be regarded as the just-noticeable difference in the orientation of one arm of the Vee in the presence of the second arm of the Vee. If the visual system loses no information in encoding the difference between the orientations of the two arms of the Vee at the second processing stage, then we can assume that the discrimination threshold for the Vee angle would approximate $\sqrt{2(\Delta\theta)^2}_{\text{Th.NR}}$.

We concluded that, although the "with random bodily rotation" thresholds were not greatly higher than the thresholds predicted on this basis (0.92 versus 1.1, 0.82 versus 1.26, and 1.40 versus 1.82 degrees for mean Vee angles of 53 degrees, 108 degrees, and 72 degrees, respectively), the differences were statistically significant, indicating that some information is lost at stage two of the simple sequential processing model described above (Regan et al., 1996a).

Nevertheless, when viewed in the context of the from 12 to 26 degree bandwidths of the most sharply selective neurons in primary visual cortex of nonhuman primates, the 1.0 to 1.4 degree discrimination threshold for angle is scarcely less remarkable than the much-discussed 0.15 to 0.8 degree orientation discrimination threshold for an isolated single line. As mentioned on pages 108–115, I proposed that the original meaning of hyperacuity might be extended to sensory coding mechanisms that use broadly tuned filters in cases where discrimination threshold is found to be considerably smaller than the bandwidths of the filters as, for example, in the case of discrimination threshold for the direction of motion in depth (Beverley & Regan, 1973, 1975). Angle discrimination threshold also fits this definition. In addition to that point, angle discrimination threshold was 1.5 degrees for a Vee whose arms were 0.23 degree long. This corresponded to a 10.5 arc second movement of the end of either arm of the Vee, so that angle discrimination for short lines also falls within Westheimer's (1975) original definition of a hyperacuity.

To return to our original theme, many people feel that they can judge with high accuracy that an angle such as the corner of a picture frame is a perfect right angle. With the possible exception of 45 degrees (halfway between vertical and horizontal), one does not have similar confidence in recognizing arbitrary angles such as, for example, 145 degrees. Although (by making many repeat measurements) we showed that discrimination threshold was significantly lower for a Vee angle of 90 degrees than for other angles, the differences were quite small (e.g., 1:1.35), and by no means in accord with one's subjective impressions.

> The reason why these differences were so small might have been a result of the psychophysical method used to measure discrimination threshold.

Turning from discrimination threshold for angle I next discuss the perception and reproduction of angles. Early work on this topic focused on the claim, first put forward by Helmholtz (1962/1866), that acute angles are overestimated whereas obtuse angles are underestimated (Jastrow, 1892; Beery, 1968; Fisher, 1969; MacLean & Stacey, 1971; Ross, 1976; Wenderoth & White, 1979; MacRae & Loh, 1981). Experimental support for Helmholtz's claim was first reported by Jastrow (1892), but this and similar later studies have been criticized on several grounds. One was the possibility that observers could have used the orientation of one or other of the lines that formed the angle to judge the angle (Beery 1968; Robinson, 1972). According to Wenderoth and White (1979), the technique of naming absolute angle used by Fisher (1969) is suspect because "it is impossible to ascertain the degree to which errors merely reflect the use of verbal labels." A further criticism of research stemming from Helmholtz's claim is that earlier researchers failed to exclude the possibility that the effect might be a consequence of asymmetric errors caused by ceiling effects near angles of 0 degrees and 180 degrees (MacRae & Loh, 1981).

The finding that in some (but not all) conditions, orientation discrimination threshold for a line can be lower than angle discrimination threshold (Regan et al., 1996a) renders the interpretation of these early studies even more difficult.

We returned to the question "Is a right angle special?" by instructing observers to make 30 successive settings of a verbally specified Vee angle (Gray & Regan, 1996). It was not surprising that the accuracy of setting was considerably better when the angle was 90 degrees than when it was an arbitrary angle (e.g., 0.4 degrees for 90 degrees compared with 5.9 degrees for 145 degrees) because, as illustrated in Figure 2.38, a visual cue for judging a perfect right angle is available that is not available for any other angle. More surprisingly, differences between the accuracy of setting for 90 degrees and for angles other than 90 degrees were reduced to insignificance when observers were provided with only one initial demonstration of the angle to be set. Differences in accuracy were reduced even further when observers were provided with feedback that signaled both the direction and magnitude of the error of the setting (on a four-class scale)—though the standard deviation of settings was always significantly lower for 90 degrees than for angles other than 90 degrees (this standard deviation is a measure of angle discrimination threshold).

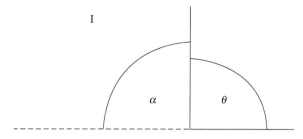

2.38 A method for judging that an angle is exactly 90 degrees. When the angle θ of the Vee formed by the two continuous lines is 90 degrees, $\theta = \alpha$. From Gray and Regan (1996).

Curvature

It was Fred Attneave's cat who, though asleep at the time, most memorably demonstrated the importance of contour curvature extrema for shape specification (Figure 2.39). More recently, computational models of shape segmentation and encoding have been based on the sequence of curvature extrema that is encountered while traversing a closed contour (Hoffman & Richards, 1984; Richards et al., 1986).

The curvature aftereffect (Gibson, 1933) provided a strong hint that the human visual system may contain a specialized mechanism for processing curvature. Given the well-established evidence that many cortical neurons are selective for line orientation, the suggestion that curvature sensitivity is based on the analysis of local orientations (Blakemore & Over, 1974) was physiologically plausible. But it was left to Watt and Andrews (1982) to provide psychophysical evidence for this idea.

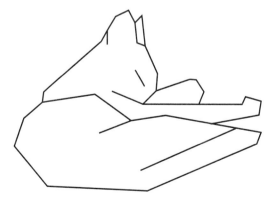

2.39 Attneave's cat. A drawing made by abstracting 38 points of maximum curvature from the contours of a sleeping cat, and connecting these points appropriately with a straight edge. From Attneave (1954).

They used the kind of target depicted in Figure 2.40A to measure the just-discriminable difference in line curvature. The lower (reference) lines had a fixed curvature, while the curvature of the upper (test) line was varied from trial to trial. Observers were required to signal which line had the greater curvature. Watt and Andrews found that curvature discrimination was a new kind of hyperacuity. Threshold corresponded to maximum differences in retinal position of less than 5 seconds of arc.

They then addressed the following question: How does curvature analysis work, and what are its limitations? But before going further we should step aside to discuss what is meant by *curvature*.

In Figure 2.40B, angle θ is, by definition, equal to S/R radians, where S is the length of the segment of the circle shown bold and R is the radius of the circle. The relation between radians and degrees can be understood as follows. The circumference of a circle is $2\pi R$, so that there are $2\pi R/R = 2\pi$ radians in a circle. Therefore, 2π radians are equivalent to 360 degrees, so that one radian is approximately 57 degrees.

The tangent of angle θ is defined as O/A (i.e., the ratio between the opposite and adjacent sides of the right angled triangle shown; you play SOHCAH with your TOA). As θ grows smaller, tan θ approximates more and more closely the value of θ in radians. (The difference is about 1% for $\theta = 10$ degrees, 4% for $\theta = 20$ degrees, 9% for $\theta = 30$ degrees, and 20% for $\theta = 45$ degrees.)

Now to curvature. The concept of the *curvature* of a line can be understood as follows. As we move from point x_1 to point $(x_1+\Delta x)$ along the curved line in Figure 2.40C, the value of y increases from y_1 to $(y_1 + \Delta y)$. The mean slope of the line (i.e., tan θ) over that small segment of the curve is equal to $\Delta y/\Delta x$. As we allow the value of Δx to approach zero, the value of the ratio $\Delta y/\Delta x$ approaches a finite value written as $\lim_{\Delta x \to 0} (\Delta y/\Delta x)$ *that is not zero*. This limiting ratio is more succinctly written dy/dx, and is equal to the slope of the tangent to the line at the point (x_1, y_1). Next, we see that curvature is the spatial rate of change of slope.

In Figure 2.40D I have drawn in the tangents to the curve at $x = x_1$, and $x = (x_1 + \Delta x)$. The two tangents differ in orientation by angle $\Delta \theta$. The length of the curved segment between the two points is ΔS. The mean *curvature* over that segment is defined as $\Delta \theta/\Delta S$. The curvature at point (x_1, y_1) is defined as $\lim_{\Delta x \to 0} (\Delta \theta/\Delta S)$, i.e., *the rate of change of orientation of the tangent with respect to distance along the line*.

In Figure 2.40E I have drawn the tangents to the circle at points P_1 and P_2. The *orientation range* $(\theta_1 - \theta_2)$ is equal to $\Delta \theta$, and $\Delta S = R\Delta \theta$ (the angles being expressed in radians). The mean curvature (i.e., rate of change of slope) over segment ΔS is equal to $\Delta \theta/\Delta S$ and this is equal to $\Delta \theta/R\Delta \theta$. By allowing point P_2 to approach point P_1 so that ΔS tends to zero, we see that the curvature at point P_1 is equal to $(1/R)$, i.e., *the reciprocal of the radius of curvature*.

I now return to the experimental work of Watt and Andrews. They faced no easy task in attempting to disentangle the effects exerted on curvature discrimination threshold by both line length and orientation range from the effect of curvature itself. For example, they found that, when they used lines whose length was 10

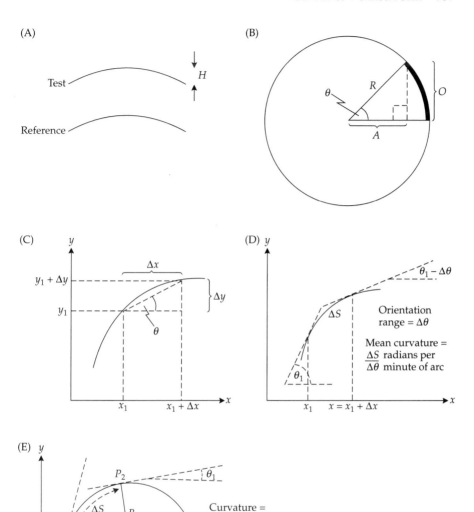

2.40 Curvature. (A) Stimulus configuration used by Watt and Andrews to measure the just-noticeable difference in curvature for different reference curvatures. (B) Relation between the *radian* and the degree. (C) Definition of slope at any given point on a line. (D) Definition of *orientation range* and a definition of *curvature* framed in terms of the spatial rate of change of slope. (E) Curvature expressed as the reciprocal of radius of curvature. Part A after Watt and Andrews (1982).

minutes of arc, curvature discrimination threshold *fell* as the reference curvature was increased; but threshold *increased* as the reference curvature was increased when they used lines three times longer.

They decided to approach this tricky problem by quantifying the observer's *efficiency* at the task of curvature discrimination (efficiency being defined as the ratio between ideal performance and human performance, where response error variance is the measure of performance; see pp. 142–143).

The effect of orientation range on efficiency for a line of fixed length (10 minutes of arc) is shown in Figure 2.41. Efficiency peaks at an orientation range of about 40 degrees; then falls steeply as the orientation is increased above 40 degrees; then rises to a second peak. By showing that the first peak remained at an orientation range of 40 degrees when line length was increased from 10 to 20 minutes of arc, Watt (1984b) proved that the 40 degree efficiency peak was determined by orientation range rather than by curvature.

Watt and Andrews addressed the possibility that their observers might have based their discriminations on trial-to-trial variations of distance H in Figure 2.40A rather than on trial-to-trial variations of curvature.

> The test line was a different length and therefore a different height from the standard in many, but not all of the versions of the experiment that I ran. The standard therefore didn't provide a direct comparison for H . . . [and] when thresholds are plotted as ΔH vs. H, then the data from different line length conditions do not overlap, whereas they do when performance is expressed as curvature . . . using relative efficiency rather than thresholds gets rid of one half of the geometric problem. Plotting efficiency as a function of the right measure of the independent variable should result in a single plot for various different stimulus conditions. This is what I found: efficiency as a function of H didn't work, but efficiency as a function of C did. (R. J. Watt, personal communication, January 1999)

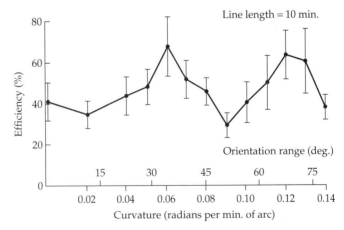

2.41 Efficiency of curvature discrimination. Relative efficiency for curvature discrimination as a function of stimulus curvature (and, consequently, orientation range) for stimuli of fixed length 10 minutes of arc. From Watt and Morgan (1982).

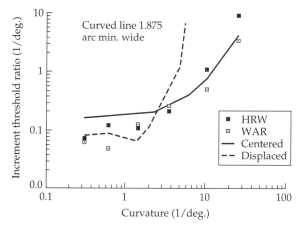

2.42 The effect of curvature on the just-noticeable difference in that curvature.
Data shown for two observers (the authors). The solid curve shows the predictions of
Wilson and Gelb's line-element theory. It takes into account filter responses from only
the curvature maximum as illustrated in Figure 2.57A. The broken line shows the predictions of a model framed in terms of a comparison between the outputs of orientation-tuned filters fed from one small region of the visual field and the outputs of orientation-tuned filters fed from a second small region of the visual field some distance
away from the first region, as illustrated in Figure 2.57C. Overall visual performance
is given by the lower envelope of these two curves. From Wilson and Richards (1989).

The second peak of efficiency reveals the presence of a second mechanism for
processing curvature, whose activity is restricted to highly curved short lines
(Watt & Andrews, 1982).

Line length also affects the efficiency with which observers perform the curvature discrimination task. Efficiency falls for lines longer than about 0.5 degrees
(as is also the case for several other hyperacuity tasks). On this point, Watt and
Andrews (1982, p. 459) reported some interesting informal observations on the
appearance of bigger targets:

> . . . all subjects reported that the larger stimuli appeared distorted. The distor-
> tions were such that the ends of the larger curves appeared to be "droopy" or
> were "bent downwards." These distortions were intermittent in occurrence, and
> not necessarily apparent in both test and comparison curves. They appeared to
> take about one second to build up. If a heavy outline of a circle is carefully fixat-
> ed, after a short time the circle appears to take on the shape of a smoothed poly-
> gon with about 10 edges. In each case this distortion could be due to interactions
> between adjacent curvature analyzers, for example, if there were no overlap
> between adjacent analyzers the "joints" might become perceptually apparent.

Filled and open symbols in Figure 2.42 plot curvature discrimination thresholds for the two observers in a study by Wilson and Richards (1989). The
researchers measured curvature discrimination thresholds using, as stimuli, a
parabola grafted to a pair of straight lines orientated at ±45 degrees, so that the

first derivative (i.e., slope) would be mathematically continuous.* (Curvature was quantified as the reciprocal of the radius of curvature.) The continuous and broken lines plot the predictions of two models (see p. 170).

Psychophysical Models of the Processing of Luminance-Defined Form along One Dimension

Although we pretend to worship **facts**, the real life of science lies in these free-floating **ideas**: . . . new facts make no sense without fitting them together with old facts, and then what matters is whether they change people's ideas.

H. Barlow in *Vision*, C. Blakemore (Ed.) (1990), p. XV

Till their own dreams at length deceive 'em
And oft repeating, they believe 'em

Matthew Prior (1664–1721)

It must be considered that nothing is more difficult to carry out, nor more doubtful of success, nor more dangerous to handle, than to initiate a new order of things.

Niccolò Machiavelli (1649–1527), *The Prince* (1981)

Overview: Local signals and comparisons of signals from distant locations

In this section I outline the endeavors of several authors to create a model that can account for the detection and spatial discrimination of luminance-defined form. A candidate model must explain how the visual system extracts the boundaries of objects from the pattern of luminance variation within the retinal image. A candidate model should also parallel the failures of human spatial vision, and thus account for optical illusions.

The aim of several of the authors cited in this section has been to provide a single model that can account for the entirety of psychophysical data on contrast detection and spatial discriminations. Although this aim may well be achievable—and, indeed, considerable progress has been made towards its achievement—there remains a suspicion that the human visual system may use different stratagems for different tasks. For example, there are at least five possible stratagems for the Vernier acuity task. In a particular target configuration, one stratagem may be more effective than all others, while in a second target config-

---

* A continuous function is a function for which a small change in the independent variable causes only a small change, and not a sudden jump, in the dependent variable. For a mathematical expression of this definition, see Daintith & Nelson (1989), p. 72.

uration a different stratagem may be the most effective (see also Watt et al. 1983; Watt 1984a; Morgan, 1986a). And it is quite possible that, in any given Vernier target configuration, the brain uses whichever of the several possible stratagems is the most effective. More generally the brain may use whichever of several possible stratagems is most suitable for the organism's immediate goal, even to the extent of modifying the connectivity of the visual pathway by means of task-dependent descending signals.

What if the organization of the visual pathway depends on the organism's immediate goal? If this suspicion is correct it might not be possible to bring the entirety of psychophysical data on spatial vision within the grasp of one model. Caveats about the analysis of biological systems vis a vis the analysis of human-designed systems are discussed on pp. 400–402.

Most formal models start with the assumption that the retinal image passes through a parallel array of local spatial filters, each of which is sensitive to only a limited range of spatial frequencies and orientations. This initial stage of processing is often assumed to be linear (linearity is defined on pp. 389–391), and nonlinearities are placed at stages subsequent to the initial stage. Most modelers also assume that every local area in the retinal image is served by several filters, each of which is most sensitive to a different spatial frequency or to a different orientation.

A complication is that nonlinear interactions between visual responses to suprathreshold gratings of different spatial frequencies have been observed psychophysically (Pantle, 1973b; Tolhurst & Barfield, 1978; DeValois & Switkes, 1982; Sagi & Hochstein, 1985; Platt & Sagi, 1993; Foley, 1994). And on pages 85–91 I described nonlinear suppression (up to 20-fold) that has been observed (by recording electrical signals from the human brain) between gratings whose spatial frequencies differ by up to more than three octaves (i.e., eightfold). Such interactions are not surprising in view of the reported interactions between single cortical cells that prefer widely different spatial frequencies (e.g., Albrecht & DeValois, 1981; DeValois & Tootell, 1983). The implication of strong nonlinear interactions between visual responses to gratings of widely differing spatial frequencies is that it would not be possible to predict fully the visual response to a complex spatial pattern from a knowledge of visual response to sinusoidal gratings presented one by one.

Several models are framed entirely in terms of the signals from *a small individual area* of the retina (see pp. 144–155 and 170). In contrast, other modelers invoke the concept of *coincidence detectors* that compare signals from two remote, small retinal areas and *ignore signals from the region between these two small areas.*

The coincidence detector concept was introduced to explain data on only one kind of spatial discrimination, but was later extended to other kinds of spatial discrimination. In its original form, the coincidence detector receives input from two narrow filters, each of which is activated by thin line. When the two narrow filters are activated simultaneously, the output of the coincidence detector is much larger than the sum of the outputs produced by activating the filters in temporal sequence. The output of the kind of hypothetical coincidence detector shown in Figure 2.53 is labeled with the *separation between the two narrow filters* (see pp. 156–169). In an extension of this idea designed to account for curvature discrimination, the coincidence detector again receives input from two distant locations, but this time responds, not only to a pair of parallel lines, but also to pairs of lines whose orientation differ. The output of this kind of coincidence detector carries a label that represents the *orientation difference between the two lines as well as the separation between the two lines* (see p. 170). The crossed-line and Vee stimuli, described in the sections on implicit orientation and angles in this chapter, would stimulate this proposed coincidence detector. In a third application of the concept, the coincidence detector again receives input from two distant locations and responds to pairs of parallel lines and to pairs of lines whose orientation differ, but the output of this kind of coincidence detector is labeled with the *mean location of the two lines*, thus signaling the location of the *core* (see pp. 123–130).

As a first step, most authors have restricted their attention to one-dimensional variations of luminance. But even with this restriction the task has proved to be formidable.

The ideal observer

How can an observer's performance in different tasks be compared? For example, is a particular individual better at the Vernier acuity task than at the line separation task? At first sight this might seem to be one of those questions that, being impossible to answer, seem a little silly to pose. But not so. It was Dennis Andrews who conceived a way of addressing this kind of question.

He introduced the following concept: the *efficiency* with which an observer performs a task is equal to the ratio (ideal performance)/(actual performance), where response error variance is the measure of performance (Andrews, 1967; Andrews et al., 1973). His proposal was to compare human performance "with the statistical precision of an ideal machine which has the same retinal transducer as the human subject. This ideal device loses stimulus spatial information only in its 'optics' and 'retinal' sampling, all subsequent processing follows the statistical methods of maximum likelihood." (Watt & Andrews, 1982, p. 451.)

Andrews' "ideal device" is often called an *ideal observer*, i.e., an imaginary observer who uses all the relevant information in the retinal image.

Comparing efficiencies rather than thresholds (expressed, for example, in seconds of arc) has the advantage that one is comparing the observer's use of the available information rather than confounding this with the different amounts of information available in different tasks. Using this approach, Andrews et al. (1973) found that the variation of threshold with line length for the tasks of orientation discrimination, curvature discrimination, and Vernier step discrimination involved two mechanisms (see, for example, Figure 2.41). Watt (1984b) used ideal observer analysis to reveal four kinds of visual cue that could be used to achieve hyperacuity performance. And Geisler (1984) also analyzed hyperacuity performance in terms of the ideal observer. All found that hyperacuity thresholds fall considerably short of ideal observer predictions. And on pp. 245–250, I describe how Sekiguchi, Williams, and Brainard used the ideal observer approach to provide remarkable insights into the processing of color-defined form.

Early filters

The attention of most modelers is focused, not on the real spatial distribution of *luminance* within the retinal image, but rather on the spatial distribution of *the outputs of hypothetical filters*. To these modelers, the problem presents itself as a challenge to explain how the spatial distribution of filter outputs represents the boundaries of objects.

In many models the hypothetical spatial filters have the "Mexican-hat" property of being insensitive to a uniform luminance.

Such filters replace a spatial variation of (all-positive) values of luminance with a (related but different) spatial variation of filter output that can assume negative as well as positive values.

The Fourier analysis model

Misunderstanding can arise if the solid validity of the physics and mathematics of Fourier methods in optical engineering is confused with the psychophysical or physiological hypothesis that the human visual system analyzes the retinal image in terms of its spatial-frequency content.

The physical stimulus can be described validly in spatial-frequency terms whether or not the brain performs spatial-frequency analysis.

In its most extreme form, the Fourier analysis model of spatial vision asserts that "the striate cortex transforms the topographic representation of visual space . . . into a Fourier transform or spatial representation" (Pollen et al., 1971) (see also Glazier et al., 1973; Pollen & Taylor, 1974). Note that Pollen et al. are talking about the striate cortex as a whole rather than any individual neuron.

Putting aside the question of how this procedure might be carried out, this linear transformation of the retinal image would do no more than redescribe the spatial pattern of luminance in terms of spatial frequency—a complementary *though totally equivalent* description (see Appendix B). The visual pathway would be required to make sense of a Fourier transform (in which all spatial positional information was, by definition, absent) rather than of a spatial pattern. The basic question "How do we see things?" is not addressed. As discussed on p. 399, linear processing does no real "work" towards interpreting the retinal image. A linear process, as it were, repeats all or part of what it has been told in a boneheaded manner (though, perhaps, more loudly or more quietly) without comment and without editing. "It is as though one were to claim that speech perception was explained by the auditory system performing a perfect translation from, for example, French to English. Nothing would be gained, but many neural resources would be wasted" (Wilson & Wilkinson, 1997, p. 941).

And as noted forcefully by Reichardt and Poggio (1981, p. 187), "every nontrivial computation has to be essentially nonlinear, that is, not representable (even approximately), by linear operations."

It is the nonlinearities in visual processing that are of interest. They operate in a "lock and key" manner and code the important features of the retinal image (see, for example, the MIRAGE model described next). And as to the practical realization of a Fourier transform, the phase spectrum would have to be obtained as well as the power spectrum. For example, the sound of a sharp crack, and the sound of continuous white noise (e.g., escaping steam) have the same power spectra. They differ only in their phase spectra (see pp. 415–416). Figure 1.20 speaks to the importance of information carried by the phase spectrum of a pattern. Recall that on pp. 53–60 I reviewed evidence that the human visual system does not encode explicitly the phase spectrum of a complex pattern as a whole. Rather, it seems that the visual system encodes the spatial distribution of local contrast within the pattern.

Taking a more conservative attitude to the Fourier analysis model, Robson stated that "the visual system does perform some rudimentary piecewise (patch by patch) spatial analysis of the visual image and the activity levels of at least some of the neurons in the visual cortex can usefully be thought of as local spectral coefficients . . ." (Robson, 1975, p. 109), but that, "if the visual cortex is a spatial analyzer, it is certainly an analyzer of very modest capabilities, able to do no more than analyze patches of the visual image into their first three harmonic components" (Robson, 1975, p. 112).

Note that in Robson's formulation of the Fourier analysis model, positional information (though coarse) is retained; that cells with different receptive field sizes are present in even–symmetric and odd–symmetric pairs in every small area of the visual field (so as to extract local spatial phase); and that the three spectral components are extracted by virtue of three receptive field sizes.

Centroids, spatial derivatives, and zero-crossings

The Watt and Morgan (1985) model was developed from the theory of local signs via the centroid analysis of Westheimer and McKee (see pp. 98–106). Bearing in mind the fact that the boundaries of any object's retinal image are blurred, Watt and Morgan (1983a) investigated the accuracy with which observers can locate a blurred edge. As illustrated in Figure 2.43, they used three kinds of edge *blurring function*: Gaussian, rectangle, and half-cosine. They defined the blurring function as the differential (with respect to distance) of the luminance distribution across the blurred edge. Thus, for example, in Figure 2.43 the differential of a ramp luminance distribution is a rectangle. For any given kind of blur, the amount of blur can be quantified in terms of the standard deviation of the blurring function.

Watt and Morgan (1983a) reported that:

Blurring function   Blurred edge   Modeled response

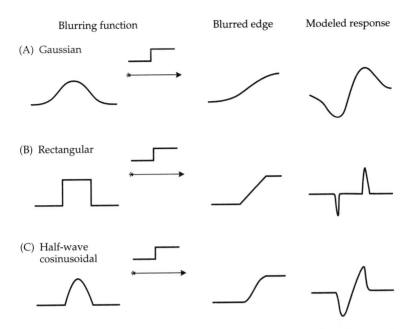

2.43 Blurring functions. The leftmost column shows three kinds of blurring function. The second column shows a step edge, and the third column shows the result of convolving the step edge with the blurring function. This is the physical stimulus. The rightmost column shows the second spatial derivative of the retinal light distribution (after allowing for the line-spread function of the human eye). From Watt and Morgan (1983a).

> Thresholds for discriminating the relative location of a blurred edge were approximately 10 times less than the standard deviation of the blurring function, even in the case of Gaussian blur.

This finding challenged Watt and Morgan with this question: "What feature of the stimulus is being extracted to allow this precise judgment?" Watt and Morgan (1983a) initially formulated their approach in terms of the first (i.e., dL/dx) and second (i.e., d^2L/dx^2) spatial derivatives of the luminance distribution in the retinal image. The meaning of these terms is explained in Figure 2.44 and Figure 2.45A–I.

Figure 2.44 explains what is meant by a *spatial derivative*. The curve represents part of a luminance distribution. At distance $x = x_1$ along the abscissa the luminance is L_1, and at distance $x = (x_1 + \Delta x)$ the luminance is $(L_1 + \Delta L)$. The increment of distance Δx, though finite, is small. The mean rate of change of luminance (i.e., the mean slope of the curve) over distance increment Δx is $\Delta L/\Delta x$. As we allow Δx to grow smaller and smaller, the ratio $\Delta L/\Delta x$ becomes a better and better approximation of the slope of the curve at point x_1. As Δx approaches zero the ratio

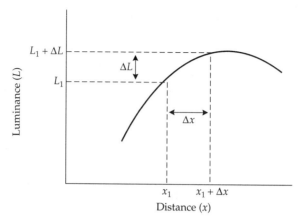

2.44 Definition of the term "spatial derivative." The first derivative of L with respect to x is $\displaystyle\lim_{\Delta x \to 0} (\Delta L / \Delta x)$.

$\Delta L / \Delta x$ does not approach zero. Provided that the curve is smooth, it asymptotically approaches a finite ratio called the derivative of L with respect to x at $x = x_1$, and written dL/dx. A formal discussion will be found in any book on elementary calculus.

For purposes of illustration we consider a Gaussian variation of luminance in Figure 2.45A–F, but the same account applies to any physically realizable luminance distribution. The first derivative of luminance (L) with respect to distance (x) is the local slope of the curves in parts A and D. As shown in parts B and E, the slope dL/dx is zero at the maximum or minimum of the Gaussian, and rises to local positive or negative peaks (called *extrema*) partway along the left and right flanks of the Gaussian. Similarly, parts C and F, respectively, plot the local slope in parts B and E. Although the luminance maximum in part A and the luminance minimum in part D are both represented by a zero-crossing in the first derivative (see parts B and E), they are distinguished by opposite sequences of maxima and minima in the second derivative (parts C and F). And the luminance maximum is represented by a negative peak in the second derivative (part C), while the luminance minimum is represented by a positive peak in the second derivative (part F). Note also that the maximum rates of luminance change in parts A and D are represented by positive and negative extrema in the first derivative (see parts B and E), and by zero-crossings in the second derivative.

The uppermost row in Figure 2.43 shows a similar analysis for blurred edge whose *blurring function* (see below) is a Gaussian. The first spatial derivative of the blurred edge is a Gaussian and the zero-crossing in the second derivative (modeled response) locates to the maximum spatial rate of change of luminance in the blurred edge.

Following the approach of Marr and Hildreth (1980), Watt and Morgan assumed that zero-bounded regions in the second spatial derivative were *indivis-*

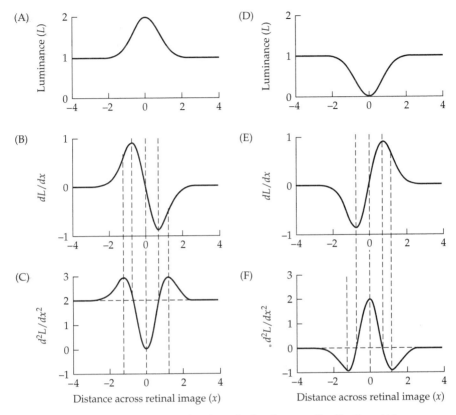

2.45 First and second spatial derivative of a luminance distribution. (A)
Gaussian variation of luminance added to constant luminance. (B) First spatial
derivative of (A). (C) Second spatial derivative of (A). (D) A Gaussian variation of
luminance subtracted from a constant luminance. (E) First spatial derivative of (D).
(F) Second spatial derivative of (D).

ible spatial primitives akin to the ancient Greek (but not the modern) concept of the
indivisible *atom*.

The Watt and Morgan model is, perhaps, more easily understood when
expressed in terms of filter outputs rather than in terms of spatial derivatives,
and indeed this is how they expressed the more formal development of their
model (Watt & Morgan, 1985).

Before going on, we should step aside to understand why it is that a Mexican-
hat spatial filters extracts from the distribution of luminance in the retinal image
a tolerable approximation to the second spatial derivative. For ease of explanation, suppose that the filter's center and surround have rectangular profiles and
that, when stimulated by a uniform luminance of one unit (Figure 2.46A) the
response of the inhibitory center is −2 units and the response of each excitatory
lobe is +1 unit, so that the output is zero (Figure 2.46B). When stimulated by a

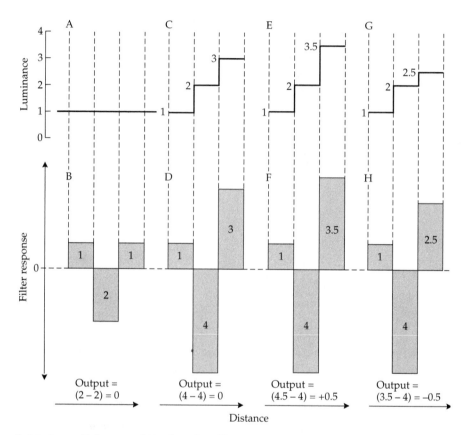

2.46 A parallel array of Mexican-hat filters converts a spatial variation of luminance into an approximation of the second spatial derivative of that variation.

stepped luminance distribution the output is zero when the steps are of equal height (Figure 2.46C,D). When the third step is higher than the first two, the output is positive (Figure 2.46E,F). When the third step is lower than the first two, the output is negative (Figure 2.46G,H).

Thus, an inhibitory-center Mexican-hat filter with a width considerably less than the luminance distribution in Figure 2.45A will give a zero output for the zone of uniform luminance, a positive output for the left segment of the curve where the slope is increasing, a zero output at the point of inflection at the center, and a negative output for the right segment of the curve where the slope is decreasing. In short, the output of the array of narrow-width Mexican-hat filters will resemble the second derivative shown in Figure 2.45C.*

---

* This equivalence is not exact because dL/dx in Figure 2.45B,E is the slope of the luminance distribution at an indefinitely small point along the luminance distribution in Figure 2.45A,D, while the output of any given filter approximates the average over some finite area.

Column four in Figure 2.43 can be regarded as the response of a parallel array of narrow-width Mexican-hat filters when stimulated with the blurred edges shown in the third column.* The uppermost and lowest "modeled responses" in Figure 2.43 have a sharply located zero-crossing where the response transitions from negative to positive. Marr and Hildreth (1980) proposed that these zero-crossings carry, in a compressed form, the spatial information provided by luminance variations across the retinal image, and that the zero-crossings provide a scale-invariant representation of object boundaries.

Taking issue with the generality of this proposal, Morgan (1991) stated that the proposal is incorrect when several bars and edges are near neighbors, or when retinal image information exists at several spatial scales. He went on to make three further criticisms of the Marr and Hildreth (1980) theory of edge detection:

1. Zero-crossing cannot be the only form of information extracted from edges, since observers can discriminate different amounts of edge blur as well as different kinds of blurring function (Watt & Morgan, 1983a).
2. Observers can locate a sharply defined edge more precisely than a blurred edge.
3. The location of zero-crossings in the filtered retinal image is very sensitive to luminance noise in the retinal image (Watt & Morgan, 1985).

Watt and Morgan (1983a) proposed that edges are represented and located in terms of the positive and negative peaks in the fourth column of Figure 2.43 rather than by the zero-crossings. In particular, they proposed that:

The perceived location of the edge is midway between the centroids of these peaks.

---

* Some students may be puzzled by Morgan and Watt's choice to explain column four in terms of "convolving the physical stimulus with the second derivative of the line-spread function of the human eye." (Convolution is a mathematic procedure discussed on pp. 427–430.) Presumably they generated their "modeled responses" by using the common kind of digital computer. Standard computers have only one central processor (or, at most, two). Consequently they perform mathematical operations in temporal sequence rather than in parallel. Therefore, Morgan and Watt were forced to use convolution to simulate the quite different way—i.e., by very many simultaneous operations performed in parallel—in which the visual system performs spatial filtering. Some programmable electronic devices have been constructed that are equivalent to a large number of parallel computers. Morgan and Watt would have obtained essentially the same results had they used such a device to compute their "modeled responses" by passing the luminance distribution in the retinal image through a very large array of parallel, identical, DOG filters whose width was matched to the eye's line-spread function. But very few other laboratories could have checked their findings. And their model would not, as it is, be available to anyone with a PC. (Further to this point, a hardware integrated circuit that emulates the information processing carried out by retinal photoreceptors, horizontal cells, and bipolar cells was described by Mahowald and Mead in the *Scientific American* issue of May 1991. This analog computer is equivalent to very many parallel processors.)

They noted that the locations of the two peaks are much more resistant to luminance noise in the retinal image than is the location of the zero-crossing. Watt and Morgan (1983a) also showed that the distance between the positive and negative peaks corresponds closely to the perceived extent of blur. Morgan (1991) notes that the established merit of zero-crossings in modeling psychophysical data is due to the fact that they nearly always lie halfway between the positive and negative peaks.

So far as failures of human spatial vision are concerned, Watt and Morgan (1983a) offer explanations for the Chevreul illusion as well as for Mach bands.

In a formal development of their model called MIRAGE (**M**ultiple **I**ndependent filters, half-wave **R**ectified, **A**veraged and **G**ated for **E**xtraction of the primitive code), Watt and Morgan (1985) proposed that, at any location in the visual field, the responses of different-sized filters are summed. This reduces the effect of noise. Importantly, the positive responses of all filters and the negative responses of all filters are summed separately. As illustrated in Figure 2.47, this

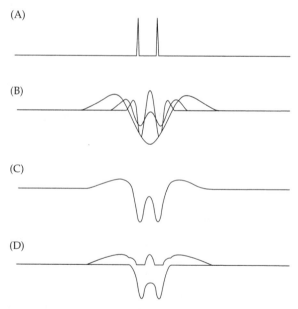

2.47 The mechanism for visual resolution according to the MIRAGE model.
(A) Two bars separated by the minimum angle of resolution. (B) The responses of filters of several widths shown superimposed. Note that only the narrowest filter resolves the two lines by producing a central region of positive response. (C) The sum of all filter responses. The central bump does not cross zero, and would be difficult to detect in noise. (D) The sum of the positive components of filter responses is shown separately from the sum of negative components. The resolution of the smallest filter is preserved, indicating the importance of the rectification stage in MIRAGE. From Watt and Morgan (1985).

prevents the resolution of the smallest filter from being lost (see Morgan & Watt, 1997). The effect is to create two types of spatial primitive: large, coarse-scale ones and small, fine-scale ones. Watt and Morgan (1985) showed that the effect of separately summing the positive and negative components of filter responses was to preserve the spatial pattern at the two extremes of spatial scale. (Morgan and Watt [1997] proposed that the rectification stage corresponds to the operation of on-center and off-center retinal ganglion cells; see Appendix E).

MIRAGE contains four filters, each of 1.7 octave bandwidth, spaced at one octave intervals from 3.4 to 27.2 cycles/deg. As already mentioned, these filters are even–symmetric (i.e., mirror–symmetric about their midlines like the DOG in Figure 1.21 or the Gabor function in Figure 2.49A).

> In MIRAGE, the physical retinal image can be transformed into a list of discrete (and symbolic) primitives, and the primitives can be interpreted to allow inferences about important spatial features in the visual scene.

For example, the code for an edge is a region of on-activity in the output of the filter array, bounded on one side by a zero region and on the other by a region of off-activity.

It is this transformation that distinguishes the MIRAGE model from models in which retinal image information is subjected to some linear transformation that merely re-expresses the same information. It is at this stage where we see real action: the "lock and key" stage, the "nontrivial" stage of Reichardt and Poggio (1981, p. 187).

According to Watt and Morgan (1985) the chief distinctions between, on the one hand, the MIRAGE model and on the other hand, the Fourier analysis model and the zero-crossing model (Marr & Poggio, 1979; Marr & Hildreth, 1980; Marr, 1982) are as follows:

- In MIRAGE, note is not taken of the center frequency of each filter.
- In MIRAGE, a symbolic code is not generated until the signals from all filter sizes have been combined.

The MIDAAS model proposed by Kingdom and Moulden (1992) differs from MIRAGE in that the interpolation rules are applied to the outputs of different-sized filters before rather than after they are combined. According to Morgan and Watt (1997, p. 1074), this implies that "if each channel finds an edge, in different places, then there will be two edges in the final combination."

Line-element models

In contrast with MIRAGE, the line-element model of Wilson and Gelb (1984) does not pool the signals from filters of different sizes. Rather, the response of differently sized filters (six sizes of even–symmetric filter at each retinal location) are kept separate and, after passing through a compressive nonlinearity, are used to provide a representation in a multidimensional filter output space). Figure 2.48 illustrates how—according to Wilson and Gelb—the spatial-frequency information in any

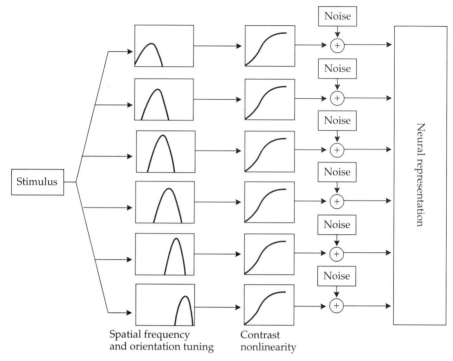

2.48 Schematic of the Wilson and Gelb line-element model of spatial pattern discrimination. A spatial pattern is processed in parallel by linear filters that are selectively sensitive to both orientation and spatial frequency. Each filter is followed by a stage of nonlinear transduction. The result is a representation of the pattern as a point in a multidimensional filter response space. Each small area of the pattern feeds six filters at each of about six orientations (about 12 at high spatial frequencies). The spatial profile of any given filter is the sixth spatial derivative of a Gaussian function. From Wilson (1991b).

given small area of the retinal image is analyzed. They suppose that similar analyses take place simultaneously at several orientations.

A spatial target is represented as a point in the multidimensional filter output space. The discriminability of any pair of targets is given by the distance between their point representations within this space. Appendix D provides a further discussion of line-element models.

The model of Nielson et al. (1985) and Watson (1983) is qualitatively similar to the Wilson and Gelb model. The main differences are as follows: eight rather than six filter widths; there is an even–symmetric and odd–symmetric pair of Gabor functions for each filter width rather than a single even–symmetric filter profile (Figure 2.49 illustrates Gabor functions); the filter outputs are not subjected to a

(A) Even   (B) Odd

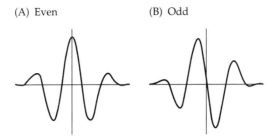

2.49 Even and odd Gabor functions. The functions shown have spatial-frequency full bandwidths of about one octave. From Klein and Levi (1985).

compressive nonlinearity. As well, pattern discrimination is based on the activity of all filters in the model rather than just spatial nearest neighbors; perhaps this explains why some predicted thresholds are lower than experimentally measured thresholds.

Viewprint

To account for their findings on bisection acuity (see pp. 115–123), Klein and Levi (1985) proposed a model that combines space analysis and size analysis. They labeled this model "viewprint," by analogy with the voiceprint (sonogram) used to analyze continuous speech or birdsong. A viewprint of a spatial pattern is equivalent to viewing the pattern through an array of bandpass spatial filters of different sizes and positions, as illustrated in Figure 2.50.

Klein and Levi noted that viewprint analysis differs from the spatial filtering approach (Figure 2.48) in which a visual pattern is analyzed by a small number of spatial filter sizes that prefer well-separated spatial frequencies. In contrast, "viewpoint analysis stresses the *continuous* nature of size sampling." In Figure 2.50 the local spatial filters are Cauchy functions. The filters are always present as pairs, one even–symmetric and one odd–symmetric, so that spatial phase (for the image patch analyzed by the pair) is recovered.

Rather than following Nielson et al. (1985) in using the balance between the outputs of the even– and odd–symmetric filters in any given pair to determine phase, Klein and Levi used the sum of the squares of these outputs (*Pythagorean sum*) to extract local response magnitude independently of phase (the *energy model*), though they retained the sign (+ or –) of the response. They stated that, "there are features that appear in the viewprint that do not stand out either in the original spatial profile of the stimulus or in its Fourier transform" and that, "viewprints of our bisection stimuli are in good agreement with the subtle nuances of our bisection data."

Because the Pythagorean sum is phase-independent, one of the merits of the viewprint model is that, by encoding the size of any object, i.e., by locating the

Space

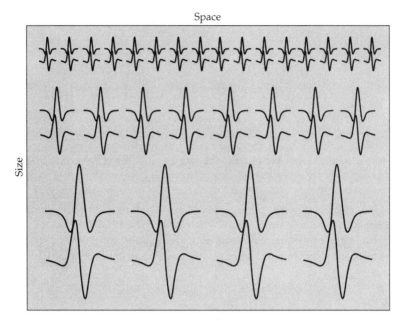

Size

2.50 Viewprint. Schematic representation of dual space-size analysis. Shown here are pairs of symmetric and antisymmetric receptive fields of different sizes (increasing downwards) at a variety of locations. After Klein and Levi (1985); figure kindly provided by S. Klein.

difference between the object's boundaries rather than their absolute locations, object perception would be rendered resistant to retinal image motion caused by the incessant movement of our eyes (Klein & Levi, 1985; Klein, 1992).

Multipoles

Klein and his colleagues have also explored a radically different approach to Vernier and other hyperacuities. Rather than discussing hyperacuity tasks strictly in terms of a spatial discrimination, they modeled a hyperacuity task in terms of detecting a difference signal in the context of the multipole concept. Multipoles are illustrated and defined in Figure 2.51. For example, adding a thin line (the test) to one-half of an edge (the pedestal) produces an edge with a Vernier step, and adding a dipole (the test) to a line (the pedestal) produces a line Vernier target (Figure 2.52).

This approach to Vernier acuity is similar to that adopted by Hartridge and by Morgan and Aiba (1985a)—see Figure 2.22—except that it required no assumptions (S. Klein, personal communication, January 1999). Basing predictions on sensitivity to a difference signal resembles an *ideal observer* approach but, "we differ from previous ideal observer calculations in that we avoid assumptions made by Andrews, Geisler, and others. We replace assumptions by making a direct

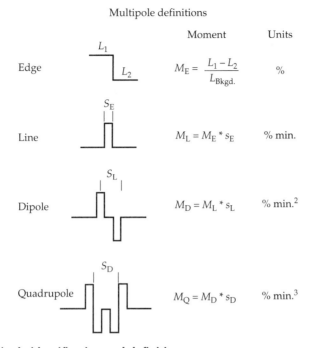

Multipole definitions

2.51 Multipole identification and definition.

The first column names each multipole in increasing order and depicts its luminance profile (where L is luminance and S is the separation, in minutes of visual angle, of the two preceding multipoles of which it is composed). The next column defines each multipole moment or strength, where M is the moment and S is the separation in minutes, L_{Bkgd} refers to the average of the L_1 and L_2 luminance (for the edge) and to the surrounding luminance (for the higher-order multipoles). The moment of each multipole is the moment of the lower-order constituent multipoles multiplied by their separation in minutes. The last column indicates the units for each multipole. After Carney and Klein (1997).

measurement of the difference signal in a detection task" (S. Klein, personal communication, 1999).

   According to Klein, Casson, and Carney (1990), edge Vernier acuity can be predicted from an observer's own line detection threshold (provided that edge contrast is low).

   This approach has been applied to several hyperacuity tasks including the line and edge Vernier tasks (Carney & Klein, 1997) and three-line bisection (Carney & Klein, 1989). According to Carney and Klein (1997), when analyzed in terms of multipoles, Vernier step threshold is up to four times *higher* than resolution.*

---

* But, in hindsight, "our task of judging one vs. two lines could be based on line blur rather than the actual seeing of two lines that would be needed for true resolution" (S. Klein, personal communication, January 1999).

2.52 Vernier acuity targets analyzed into dipoles.
The upper row shows how the Vernier step for an edge can be produced by adding a line to one half of an edge. The lower row shows how the Vernier step for a line can be produced by adding a dipole to one half of an edge. After Carney and Klein (1997).

Coincidence detectors

All the models I have reviewed so far are framed in terms of the signals from a small individual retinal area. In the following section I discuss a quite different approach to modeling spatial vision, which is based on the concept of *coincidence detectors*. Coincidence detectors compare signals from two small areas of the retina that are some distance apart and ignore signals from the region between these two small areas. In the following section I propose a hybrid class of model. In particular, I suggest that spatial vision can be more generally described in terms of models in which information from coincidence detectors and information from small individual areas of the retina are taken into account before the stage at which the spatial attributes of retinal images are processed.

Introduction. It might seem reasonable to suppose that line separation discrimination would be based on a comparison of the absolute locations of the two lines.

However, although that cannot always be ruled out, several models are framed in quite different terms.

It has been proposed that the separation between two lines (or the width of a bar) can be signaled by the relative activity of filters with center-surround receptive fields similar to the one illustrated in Figure 2.1 that are all *driven from the same retinal location*, but have different spatial extents (Regan & Beverley, 1983a; Wilson & Gelb, 1984; Klein & Levi, 1985; Nielson et al. 1985; Wilson, 1991a,b). The heavy line in Figure 2.24 plots line separation discrimination thresholds predicted by the line-element theory of Wilson and Gelb (1984).

Clearly, this model requires filters whose spatial extents are larger than the separation between the two lines (or the bar width), and so there are problems with widely separated lines. But even apart from that caveat, the proposal does not fully account for all the data on separation discrimination, even for closely separated lines. For example, Morgan and Ward (1985) measured the just-noticeable difference in separation for lines whose mean separation was 3, 6, or 12 minutes of arc. In all three cases, the just-noticeable difference in separation was little affected by the presence of nearby flanking lines that were sufficiently close to the target lines to corrupt the signals from local filters.

The coincidence detector hypothesis. A proposed explanation for the findings reported by Morgan and Ward was framed in quite different terms than the relative activity of multiple filters driven from the same retinal location. This proposal, illustrated in Figure 2.53, is that a pair of narrow-width spatial filters driven from different locations provide input to a *coincidence detector** whose output is maximal when the two filters simultaneously receive optimal stimulation, e.g., from a two-line stimulus that falls on their receptive field centers (Regan & Beverley, 1985, footnote 42; Morgan & Regan, 1987). The output of the coincidence detector is *labeled with the distance between the two filters that feed it.*

> Because the two filters that provide its input are narrow, the coincidence detector is not sensitive to stimuli located within the space between the two filters.

Consider three pairs of receptive fields, (A, A′), (B, B′), and (C, C′) in Figure 2.53. The outputs of each pair are coupled together nonlinearly so that, for example, signal *a* is much stronger when both receptive fields are simultaneously stimulated than is the sum of their responses when stimulated in temporal

---

* During the first-year undergraduate lecture course on nuclear physics given by P. M. S. Blackett in 1954, he described a vacuum tube coincidence detector that, with his colleague Occhialini, he had used to ensure that photographic cameras were triggered only when an ionizing particle had just passed through his Wilson cloud chamber. With this device they discovered the positive electron, the first discovered particle of antimatter. That is the conceptual source of Figure 2.53. (See pp. 36–39 for a more pointed illustration of the values of cross-fertilization across departmental boundaries.)

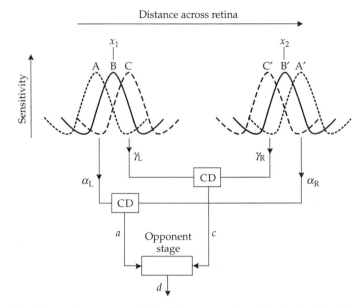

2.53 Coincidence detector model of line separation discrimination. Narrow spatial filters are connected in pairs to hypothetical coincidence detectors (CD). By definition, a coincidence detector does not respond to stimulation within the region between the two narrow filters that feed it. The output of this kind of a coincidence detector is labeled with the separation between its two input filters. The coincidence detectors feed an opponent-process stage whose output (d) signals line interval independently of line contrast and translation. From Morgan and Regan (1987).

succession.* Functionally, this hypothetical form of coupling is equivalent to a coincidence detector. Such coupling can be achieved in several ways. For example, the product $a = \alpha_L \alpha_R$ can fulfill this requirement. I suppose that several such coincidence detectors can be driven from any given region in the visual field, and that each of these coincidence detectors has a different separation between its pair of receptive fields.

I next discuss how the coincidence detector concept can explain the findings of Morgan and Regan (1987). They found that line separation discrimination threshold is approximately independent of contrast for contrasts above about 10% and is unaffected by variations in the contrast of one line, or of translations of the lines.

In order to understand the point clearly, first consider the extreme case. Suppose that two lines are initially positioned at the centers of the B and B' recep-

---

* Another illustration of Reichardt and Poggio's (1981, p. 187) point that "every nontrivial computation has to be essentially nonlinear."

tive fields, and that the separation of the lines is S_1. Symmetrically located pairs of receptive fields such as AA' and CC' will give equal coincidence detector outputs; for example, $a = c$. Suppose now that the lines increase their separation slightly to S_2 while line contrast is held constant. Signals β_L and β_R from B and B' will not change appreciably, because the lines are still located on the locally horizontal tops of the B and B' receptive field profiles. On the other hand, signals α_L and α_R will increase so that a will increase, and at the same time, signals β_L and β_R will fall, so that c will decrease. Consequently, the output of the opponent stage will change from zero, and the polarity of the change will encode increase versus decrease of line interval. This process is rather robust; the initially silent opponent elements will respond to a change of line separation with a polarity of output that is somewhat independent of the relation between line contrast and the output of a receptive field. Thus, an opponent process can ensure that a change of line interval is not confounded with a change of line contrast, even though the receptive field outputs α_L, α_R, and so on in Figure 2.53 depend both on line position and on line contrast. Line separation is not confounded with contrast, whether the opponency is ratio or subtractive.

The exact form of opponency does become important, however, if we make the further demand that interval discrimination threshold is *not quantitatively affected by contrast* and we assume that the lower limit of discrimination threshold is not set by noise at the opponent stage. (If it is noise at the opponent stage that limits discrimination threshold, the problem does not arise; see footnote on page 120.) The form of opponency required is determined by the way in which stimulus contrast affects the receptive field outputs α_L, α_R, and so on. At first sight one might suppose that if α_L, α_R, and so forth, depended on log contrast, then ratio opponency would be required, while if α_L, α_R, and so forth, were linearly dependent on contrast, then subtractive opponency would be required. This is incorrect. The crucial factor requiring ratio opponency is that amplitude versus contrast plots *differ in slope, but all have the same intercept* as illustrated in Figure 2.54A. It is irrelevant whether the contrast dependence is linear, logarithmic, or indeed any other monotonic function. The crucial factor requiring subtractive opponency is that the amplitude-contrast plots *have the same slopes but have different intercepts*, as illustrated in Figure 2.54B. Again, whether the contrast dependence is linear, logarithmic, or some other monotonic function is immaterial (Regan & Beverley, 1983a, 1985).

Next we discuss the situation that the contrast of both lines changes simultaneously. Consider the case that the opponent process in Figure 2.53 is equivalent to taking a ratio (rather than, for example, simple subtraction). We have, then, $d = a/c$.

Suppose that, when both lines have the same contrast C_1, the initial line positions x_1, x_2 elicit signals α_L, α_R, γ_L, and γ_R, so that the opponent output is

$$d = \alpha_L \alpha_R / \gamma_L \gamma_R \tag{2.1}$$

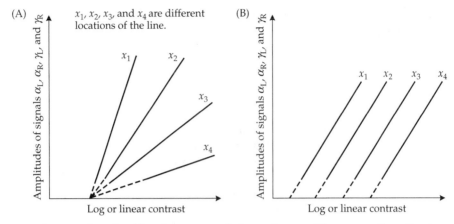

(A) $x_1, x_2, x_3,$ and x_4 are different locations of the line.

2.54 Proposed explanation for contrast independence of line separation discrimination threshold: I. Two possible relationships between line contrast and the signals α_L, α_R, γ_L and γ_R in Figure 2.53. In order to account for the observed contrast independence of line separation discrimination threshold in terms of an opponent-process hypothesis, ratio opponency would be required in case A, but subtractive opponency would be required in case B. Note that it is irrelevant whether the dependency on contrast is log or linear. From Morgan and Regan (1987).

Suppose that, without any change in contrast, the lines are moved further apart. Let e be the fractional rise in magnitude of the signals from one pair of receptive fields ($e > 1.0$), and g be the fractional fall in magnitude of the signals from the other pair ($g < 1.0$). Therefore, the two coincidence detectors' outputs are now given by

$$a' = e^2\alpha_L\alpha_R \text{ and } c' = g^2\gamma_L\gamma_R \qquad (2.2)$$

so that the output of the opponent stage is now

$$d' = e^2\alpha_L\alpha_R/g^2\gamma_L\gamma_R \qquad (2.3)$$

The change in opponent output ($d' - d$) caused by the increase in line separation is equal to

$$\alpha_L\alpha_R/\gamma_L\gamma_R[(e^2/g^2) - 1] \qquad (2.4)$$

Of the many pairs of active receptive fields, the pair that gives the largest opponent signal will be the pair whose sensitivity curves have the greatest difference of slope. Now suppose that the above calculation is repeated with the lines at a constant contrast C_2 where $C_1 \neq C_2$. We assume that the effect of line contrast is the same for signals α_L, α_R, γ_L, and γ_R, and takes the form illustrated in Figure 2.54A. Then if, at contrast C_1, the amplitudes of these signals are α_L, α_R, γ_L, and γ_R, then at contrast C_2 these amplitudes will be $S\alpha_L$, $S\alpha_R$, $S\gamma_L$, and $S\gamma_R$, where S is a scaling factor obtained from Figure 2.54A. Thus, for the smaller line interval, the opponent output at contrast C_2 will be

$$d = (S^2\alpha_L\alpha_R)/(S^2\gamma_L\gamma_R) = (\alpha_L\alpha_R)/(\gamma_L\gamma_R) \tag{2.5}$$

the same as at contrast C_1 (Equation 2.1 above), and at contrast C_2 the opponent output for the wider line interval will be

$$d' = (e^2S\alpha_L\alpha_R)/(g^2S\gamma_L\gamma_R) = (e^2\alpha_L\alpha_R)/(g^2\gamma_L\gamma_R) \tag{2.6}$$

which is also the same as at contrast C_1 (Equation 2.3 above).

Next we consider the situation that the lines have unequal contrasts. Following a similar argument, it is straightforward to show that the opponent element's output will not change if the contrast of one line is increased (or decreased) while the contrast of the other line is held constant, though contrast independence will fail at very low contrasts (see below). Therefore, the output of a ratio-opponent element will depend on the separation between the stimulus lines but not on line contrast, provided that: (a) the effect of contrast on receptive field output is as illustrated in Figure 2.54A and is the same for all receptive fields, and (b) line contrast is sufficiently high to excite multiple receptive field pairs with a sufficiently wide range of separations to support opponency. Failure of contrast independence will presumably occur when contrast is less than about two or three times contrast threshold for receptive field B or for receptive field B′ in Figure 2.53 (Regan et al., 1982; Regan & Beverley, 1985).

Note that if the excitation function differs from that shown in Figure 2.54A, a different form of opponent computation might be required to ensure that line separation discrimination threshold is quantitatively independent of contrast. For example, if the excitation plots were parallel, but displaced by different distances along the contrast axis as in Figure 2.54B, then subtractive rather than ratio opponency would be required to explain contrast independency (Regan & Beverley, 1985).

Next we turn to the effect of flanking lines. It is clear that if flanking lines are always located sufficiently far outside the receptive fields A, B, C and A′, B′, C′ of Figure 2.53 then they will have a negligible effect on the receptive field outputs α_L, α_R, and so on. If we assume that relevant receptive field diameters were several times narrower than the standard interval of 6 minutes of arc used in the flanking line experiment (i.e., roughly as illustrated in Figure 2.53) then, since a flanking line was never closer to a test line than 5.25 minutes of arc, we can understand why the flanking lines did not have any appreciable effect on separation discrimination (Morgan & Ward, 1985).

Now we discuss the effect of translating both lines with no change of line separation. Suppose that two lines are initially positioned at the centers of the B, B′ receptive fields, and then both move slightly leftwards due, for example, to an eye movement. Signals β_L and β_R will not change appreciably because the two lines are still sited on the locally horizontal tops of the B, B′ receptive field profiles.

Signal α_L will rise to $(1 + x)\,\alpha_L$ and signal α_R will fall to approximately $\alpha_R/(1 + x)$. Therefore, the output of stage CD in Figure 2.53 will be given by

$$a = (1 + x)\alpha_L[\alpha_R/(1 + x)] = \alpha_L\alpha_R \qquad (2.7)$$

after the translation. Before the translation, the output of stage CD was given by $a = \alpha_L\alpha_R$, so that the signal a is the same after as before the translation and, by a similar argument, signal c is the same after as before translation. Therefore, the opponent signal d is the same after as before translation. Thus, the opponent arrangement of Figure 2.53 unconfounds a change in line separation from a translation. (This argument does not necessarily apply to continuous motion because differences in the dynamics of individual elements might then be involved.)

Although it seems more plausible that only a few coincidence detectors can be driven from any given retinal location, for completeness we finally consider the case that any given retinal location accesses coincidence detectors with an effectively continuous distribution of receptive field separations. The continuous line in Figure 2.55A shows the notional distribution of excitation in such an ensemble of coincidence detectors when the eye is stimulated by two lines separated by the standard interval (S_1), and the dashed line shows the distribution when the lines are separated by a different line separation (S_2). The change of separation shifts the peak of the distribution along the abscissa. Figure 2.55B illustrates that a quite different situation obtains when the line separation (S_1) does not change, but instead the contrast of the two lines rises or falls by the same amount; the peak of the distribution does not shift along the abscissa, though the whole curve may be displaced along the ordinate with or without some change in shape. This is also the case when the contrast of one line rises or falls relative to the other line. We require that a contrast change is not confounded with an interval change. The key idea is as follows:

A change in line separation produces a two-lobed difference curve that is positive on one side of the standard interval S_1 and negative on the other side; an increase of separation gives the mirror image of a decrease. On the other hand, a change in line contrast produces a difference curve that is symmetrical about point S_1 on the abscissa, and is either wholly positive or wholly negative.

The shift in the peak of the excitation distribution curve distinguishes between line separation increment and contrast change; in effect, the coincidence-opponent element described above (Figure 2.53) senses the shift by responding to the consequent two-lobed shape change.

It has been suggested that the coincidence detector model of separation discrimination might not apply to the case of two widely separated targets, each of which consists of a high-frequency carrier modulated by an envelope such as DOG or Gabor waveform. The spatial-frequency spectrum of the target does not contain information about the modulating waveform (see pp. 423–426). Certainly, it is known that separation discrimination threshold for such targets is low

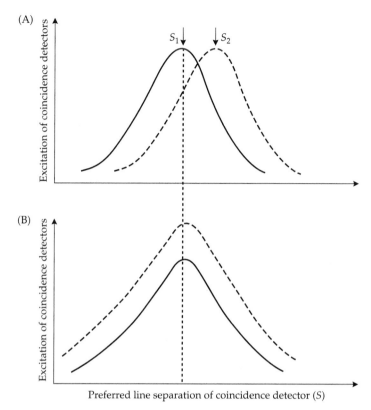

2.55 Proposed explanation for contrast independence of line separation discrimination threshold: II. (A) The distribution of excitation within an ensemble of coincidence detectors for line pairs of the same contrast but different separation. (B) The distribution of excitation for line pairs with the same separations but different contrasts. From Morgan and Regan (1987).

(Burbeck, 1987). However, as discussed on pp. 93–98 and 426–427, and in Appendix E, although there is no power in the *stimulus display* at the low spatial frequencies that correspond to the modulating envelope, known nonlinearities of visual neurons would recover this information by demodulating the pattern.

The hypothetical coincidence detectors may share common ground with the nonlinear lateral interactions between orientation-tuned cortical neurons that feature in many models of texture segregation (e.g., NLI box in Figure 4.12). In particular, the long-distance lateral connections between orientation-tuned neurons in primary visual cortex described by Gilbert and his colleagues might provide a physiological basis, not only for the coincidence detectors, but also for the lateral interactions invoked in models of texture segregation (Gilbert & Wiesel, 1985, 1990; Gilbert et al., 1990).

It has been stated by Wilson (1991b) that, if coincidence detectors for every pair of spatial filters were hard-wired, their number would be implausibly large. In this context it would be interesting to quantify limitations in the density and length of the long-distance lateral connections within primary visual cortex and to search for corresponding variations in psychophysical line-interval discrimination threshold. But, as discussed on pp. 30–33 and 402, it may be that coincidence detectors are either not hard-wired (see arrowed dashed lines in Figure 1.10), or they exist only for close separations.

If we assume that line separation discrimination threshold depends on the maximum slope of the two receptive field profiles, then we can understand why line separation discrimination threshold rises steeply with retinal eccentricity (Wilson, 1991a).

As mentioned earlier, Morgan and Regan found that discrimination threshold for line separation was not affected by random variations in the contrast of one of the lines. This finding tells us that discrimination performance was not based on analysis of the phase spectrum of the target. The basis for this conclusion is that changing the contrast of one of the lines while not changing the location of either line changes the phase spectrum of the pair of lines as a whole. Therefore, if observers had based their discriminations of line separation on the phase spectrum of the two lines, information about line separation would have been corrupted by the noisy variations in line contrast.

> The coincidence detector proposed by Morgan and Regan analyzes the retinal image in the spatial domain rather than the spatial-frequency domain. The coincidence detector is not linear; not approximately linear, not even piecewise linear. It does not transform the retinal image linearly. It does "real work" on the retinal image in the Reichardt and Poggio (1981, p. 187) sense.

Evidence for several kinds of coincidence detectors. The output of the hypothetical coincidence detector depicted in Figure 2.53 carries a *separation label.* Kohly and Regan (1999b,c) recently found direct evidence for the existence of coincidence detectors that carry labels other than the separation label.

I will first discuss experiments on orientation. Figure 2.56A explains the definitions of α_T and β_T. (Note that these two angles are much exaggerated in the figure.) Angle $2\alpha_T$ is the difference between the orientation of the two test lines ("pigeon toed" versus "splay footed") and angle β_T is their mean orientation. The mean value of S_T was 1.0 degrees of visual angle. In a temporal method of constant stimuli "reminder" design (pp. 8–17), the observer's task was to signal whether the test lines in the second of two presentations was more "pigeon toed" than in the first presentation, and whether the mean orientation of the two lines was clockwise with respect to the mean orientation of the first presentation.

To ensure that no receptive field that was sufficiently wide to "see" both test lines could contribute reliable information about the task, a pair of "noise" lines

(Figure 2.56B) was placed between the test lines, and their mean orientation was varied from presentation to presentation quite independently of the trial-to-trial variations of α_T and β_T. A report by Morgan and Ward (1985) is the basis for this idea, though their noise lines were located outside the test lines.

Because we varied α_T and β_T orthogonally, the observer could not have based responses on the orientation of one line alone. It was necessary to compare both lines. To prevent the observer's foveating the two lines in succession or from shifting focal attention from one line to the other, presentation duration was restricted to 20 msec. Phosphor afterglow was rendered invisible by optically superimposing the lines pattern on a uniformly illuminated field that had the same color as the stimulus lines. And to prevent the observer's using any after-image of the test lines, a 20-line masker pattern was presented immediately after each 20 msec. presentation. The masker lines were randomly located within an area 1.5 times wider that the 4-line test pattern, and the orientation of any given masker line was randomly selected from the range of possible orientations of the test lines. The masker pattern was selected randomly from 10 stored patterns. A fresh selection of masker was made for every individual presentation.

There were eight values of α_T, eight of β_T, and eight of β_N, all symmetrically placed about zero. The values of α_T, β_T, and β_N were orthogonal within the set of 512 different trials. The observer was required to discriminate both α_T and β_T after each trial. Thus, as described in Chapter 1, in the section on psychophysical methods, three psychometric functions could be plotted for each task (see Figure 1.7).

We found that observers could discriminate trial-to-trial variations in α_T while ignoring trial-to-trial variations in both β_T and β_N. They could also discriminate trial-to-trial variations in β_T while ignoring trial-to-trial variations in both α_T and β_N. Discrimination thresholds were 2.0 ± 0.1 degrees for α_T and 2.4 ± 0.1 degrees for β_T.

Because the trial-to-trial variations in β_N would have corrupted the signals from any spatial filters that responded to both test lines, it follows that the observers' responses were based on a comparison of signals from orientation-tuned filters that were excited by the two test lines, and whose receptive fields were sufficiently narrow that were not affected by variations in the orientation of the noise lines shown in Figure 2.56B. We concluded that:

> The human visual system contains coincidence detectors whose outputs carry a $2\alpha_T$ (orientation difference) label and coincidence detectors whose outputs carry a β_T (mean orientation) label. Whether a single coincidence detector's output carries more than one label remains an open question.

The type of coincidence detector just described could account for the finding that the just-noticeable difference in orientation between two simultaneously presented lines separated by up to several degrees is little different from the larger of the just-noticeable differences in the orientation of either line presented individually (Regan,

(A)

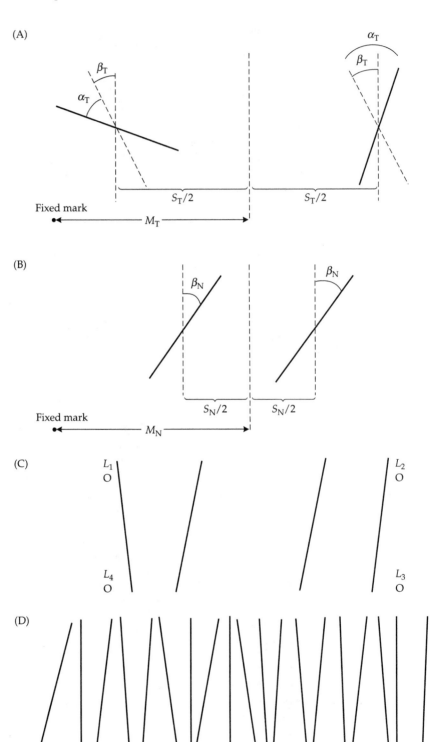

Fixed mark

(B)

(C)

(D)

1984, unpublished data). (The two-line target was stabilized by means of a double-Purkinje eye tracker to ensure that observers could not compare the orientations of the two lines by successive inspection.)

We measured discrimination thresholds for the location (M_T) and the separation (S_T) of the two test lines by assigning separation (S_T)$_{REF}$ and location (M_T)$_{REF}$ to the reference pair of test lines. We used four test values of S_T and four test values of M_T such that the values of S_T and M_T were orthogonal within the stimulus set. This design ensured that the location of one or other individual test line provided no reliable cue to either task. To ensure that observers could not base their responses on the output of wide spatial filters that "saw" both test lines, we varied S_N and M_N orthogonally with respect to the variations of S_T and M_T. This would corrupt both the M_T and S_T signals from any filter that saw both test lines.

We found that observers could discriminate trial-to-trial variations in M_T while ignoring simultaneous trial-to-trial variations in M_N and S_T. They could also discriminate S_T while ignoring simultaneous trial-to-trial variations in S_N and M_T. We concluded that:

The human visual system contains coincidence detectors whose outputs carry a label for M_T (mean location of the two test lines) in addition to the previously proposed coincidence detectors whose outputs carry a label for S_T (separation of the two test lines) (Figure 2.53). Whether a single coincidence detector's output carries more than one label remains an open question.

In subsequent experiments we found that observers could dissociate and discriminate all four variables after each trial.

Coincidence detectors whose outputs carry an orientation difference label would be capable of signaling the angle between to lines independently of the orientation of either line (Figure 2.37). Coincidence detectors whose outputs carry orientation difference and separation labels would be capable of signaling curvature (Figure 2.57C). Coincidence detectors whose outputs carry a mean orientation label would

---

◀ **2.56 Does the human visual system contain coincidence detectors whose outputs carry orientation difference, mean orientation, and mean location labels?**
(A) The mean orientation of the two test lines was β_T degrees, the difference between their orientations was $2\alpha_T$ degrees, the separation between their midpoints was S_T degrees of visual angle, and their midpoint was located M_T degrees of visual angle from a fixed mark. (B) The mean orientation of the two "noise" lines was β_N degrees, the separation between their midpoints was S_N degrees of visual angle, and their midpoint was located M_N degrees of visual angle from a fixed mark. The two pairs of lines were combined to create the stimulus illustrated in part C. Note that the values of α_T, β_T, and β_N are considerably exaggerated in parts A and B. Part C gives a better impression of the values used in the experiment. $L_1 - L_4$ in part C were fixation marks. Following each 20 (or 100) msec. presentation, a 20-line masker pattern centered on the location of the 4-line stimulus was presented for 100 msec. A typical masker pattern is illustrated in part D.

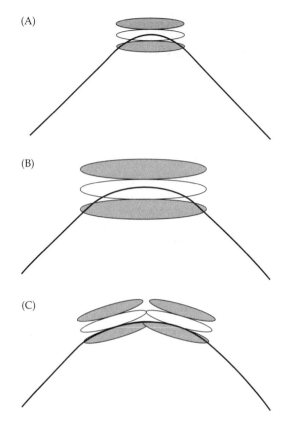

2.57 Schematic of curvature processing by orientation-selective spatial filters.
Receptive fields are shown with an excitatory center (white) and inhibitory flanks
(gray). Although not shown, filters centered on the same locations but with other orientations are also involved in processing curvature. (A) A filter with a small receptive
field tuned to high spatial frequencies would give a differential response to sharp
curvature. (B) Filters with larger receptive fields would be required to cover the same
extent of a more gradual curve. (C) An alternative scheme is to compare the orientations of two distant segments of the contour. From Wilson and Richards (1989).

be capable of signaling the implicit orientation of shapes such as ellipses or crosses (see Figures 2.32 and 2.33). Coincidence detectors whose outputs carry M_T
(mean location) label would be capable of signaling the midpoint of an object's
outer boundaries independently of the object's internal texture (see Figures 2.34
and 2.35).

  If we assume that, like the discrimination of line separation, opponent processes support the discriminations of orientation difference ($2\alpha_T$), mean orientation
(β_T), and mean position (M_T), then, according to the algebra set out earlier in this

section, the discrimination will be substantially independent of the contrast of either line, and thus independent of the phase spectrum of the target as a whole. In other words:

> The family of nonlinear coincidence detectors just described analyzes the luminance distribution across the retinal image in the spatial domain rather than the spatial-frequency domain.

A last point: discriminations based on the relative activity of the coincidence detectors can be modeled in terms of an opponent process, as depicted in Figure 2.53, or by a line element within the multidimensional response space of the coincidence detectors. They cannot, however, be modeled by a line element within the multidimensional response space of the spatial filters, as in the Wilson and Gelb (1984) line-element model (Figure 2.48).

Models of bisection acuity

As mentioned on pp. 106–107, many authors have reported that an observer who has been instructed to bisect the distance between two contours performs the task with a trial-to-trial error that is a constant fraction of the distance between the two contours. It was thought for many years that bisection threshold obeys Weber's law. One candidate explanation is framed in terms of the pattern of response within a population of filters that are all driven from the same retinal location (Klein & Levi, 1985; Wilson, 1986). For large separations, however, this explanation becomes less likely because the local filter would have to be very large (Weber's law holds up to at least 10 degrees) and maintain high sensitivity (Levi et al., 1988).

A second candidate explanation is framed in terms of the spatial grain of the visual system (Hering, 1899; Matin, 1972; Burbeck, 1987; Klein & Levi, 1985). The basic idea is that the spatial grain of the cortex varies linearly with eccentricity so that the positions of the two outer lines become increasingly uncertain as their eccentricity increases. Levi, Klein, and Yap offered the following explanation to account for their finding that when eccentricity was held constant, bisection threshold was independent of line separation over a range of separations from 2 to 10 degrees. In other words, this was a failure of Weber's law, but see pp. 106–107.

Levi et al. (1998, p. 603) stated: "When we attempt to gauge the distance between widely separated objects it is unlikely that we do so on the basis of the outputs of large spatial filters: rather it appears that we make such judgements by estimating the cortical distance which separates the two targets of interest. Our results suggest that the judgement of the separation of widely separated objects is similar to distance measurement using a ruler on the cortex, in that the error of measurement is independent of the separation between objects." This proposal shares common ground with the coincidence detector concept described and illustrated in Figure 2.53.

Models of curvature discrimination

The solid line in Figure 2.42 plots curvature discrimination thresholds predicted by the line-element theory of Wilson and Gelb (1984). Recollect that the line-element theory assumes that the discrimination is based on local mechanisms as illustrated in Figure 2.57A,B. According to this line of thought, small orientation-tuned receptive fields support the discrimination of sharp curvature (part A of Figure 2.57), while progressively larger receptive fields support the discrimination of progressively gentler curvatures (part B). Comparisons between the activations of receptive fields of the same size but that prefer different orientations would yield a measure of curvature (Wilson, 1985).

The line-element theory successfully predicts curvature discrimination thresholds for mean curvatures above about 2 degrees^{-1}, but not for lower values (continuous line in Figure 2.42). To account for these data, Wilson and Richards (1989) proposed a two-mechanism theory of curvature discrimination. Evidence for two distinct mechanisms had been reported previously by Watt and Andrews (1982)—see Figure 2.41—and also by Ferraro and Foster (1986), who reported that a plot of discrimination threshold versus curvature showed a notch at about 5.4 degrees^{-1}. The second process proposed by Wilson and Richards was, in distinction to the first process, not local. They proposed that the outputs of two distant narrow filters are compared as illustrated in Figure 2.57C. Here there is a preferred response to two narrow receptive fields that are situated some specific distance apart and whose orientations differ by some specific angle that is nonzero. Wilson and Richards excluded the possibility that a local process using broad filters could account for discrimination at low curvatures by using bandpass-filtered stimuli that contained no low-frequency information.

The dashed line in Figure 2.42 shows that this "remote comparison" hypothesis predicted the low-curvature threshold data. This hypothesis was framed in the spirit of earlier proposals that curvature detection is performed by comparing the responses of orientation-tuned cells stimulated by different regions along the curved line (Blakemore & Over, 1974; Watt & Andrews, 1982; Koenderink & Richards, 1988; Koenderink & van Doorn, 1986).

The result of Wilson and Richards' control experiment with bandpass-filtered targets indicates that their hypothetical second mechanism fits the formal definition of a *coincidence detector*. Direct evidence that the visual system contains coincidence detectors whose outputs are labeled, not only with the separation between two lines, but also with the difference between their orientations is reviewed on pp. 156–169.

Shortcomings

All the models of spatial discrimination discussed so far conflict with, or fail to explain, some of the available data. One reason for this failure is, perhaps, the neglect of possible roles, not only for memory, but also for cognitive factors such as selective attention (e.g., Sagi & Julesz, 1985; Adini & Sagi, 1992; O'Regan,

1999). Although the neural mechanism that underlies the willful direction of selective attention is not understood, it is well established that a task-dependent change in selective attention can cause short-term physiological changes such as, for example, a change in the visual tuning properties of single neurons in monkey (Maunsell, 1995). And, as to the short-term storage of precise sensory information, it may be relevant that, in human, regions of *visual sensory cortex* are involved in the conscious storage and retrieval of visual information, and that these regions bring into play structures involved in the active maintenance of stored information (Ungerleider, 1995). I will return to this issue on pp. 184–191.

From One to Two Dimensions

All of the research I have discussed so far has been restricted to investigations of the visual processing of spatial information along only one dimension. But the retinal image of an object is two-dimensional. In the following section I discuss the extent to which models based on experimentally measured responses to gratings, lines, bars, and so on, can account for experimental findings on the detection and spatial discrimination of two-dimensional targets.

Bessel function targets

The question whether the visual processing of two-dimensional targets can be completely understood in terms of responses to gratings was addressed by Kelly and Magnuski (1975). They compared detection thresholds for Bessel function targets with detection thresholds for gratings, including among their observers J. G. Robson, whose grating contrast sensitivity curve is plotted as open circles in Figure 1.19 (pp. 386–389 discuss Bessel functions.) The Bessel function of order zero used by Kelly and Magnuski looked like a series of concentric bright and dark rings whose local contrast fell with distance from the center of the pattern, as illustrated in Figure 2.58A. Kelly and Magnuski found that plots of detection thresholds versus spatial frequency for the Bessel function target could not be predicted from a knowledge of the corresponding data for the grating target. In particular, the two sensitivity curves crossed at a spatial frequency below 1 cycle/deg., and then diverged; the difference between the two sensitivities was approximately proportional to spatial frequency (Figure 2.59).

They concluded that the visual processing of a two-dimensional spatial pattern is not a linear, isotropic, homogeneous process. So that:

> In going from one to two dimensions, grating psychophysics does not provide sufficient data to understand fully the early processing of two-dimensional form.

In attempting to explain their finding, Kelly and Magnuski noted that the amplitude of the largest component in the two-dimensional Fourier transform of their Bessel function target varied inversely with the target's nominal spatial frequency,

(A)   (B)

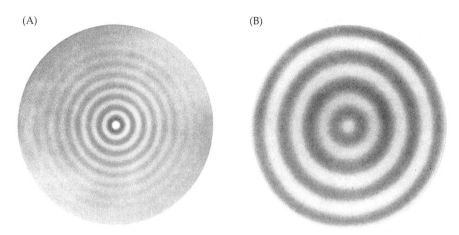

2.58 Two-dimensional targets. (A) The kind of Bessel function target used to obtain the data shown in Figure 2.59. (B) Circular sinusoidal target (cosine phase). From Kelly and Magnuski (1975).

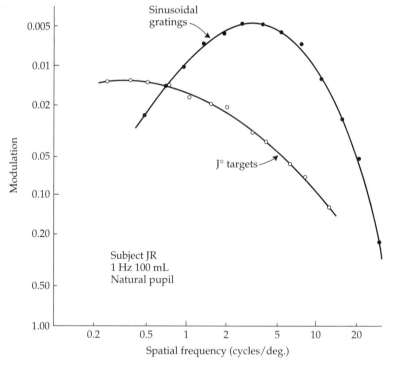

2.59 Contrast sensitivity as a function of spatial frequency for a sinusoidal grating and a Bessel function target of order zero. Both patterns were counterphase-modulated at a temporal frequency of 1 Hz. Observer was J. G. Robson (see Figure 1.19). From Kelly and Magnuski (1975).

while the amplitude of the corresponding component for the grating target did not depend on spatial frequency. On this basis they proposed that detection thresholds for the circularly symmetric patterns that they used—the Bessel function and a circularly symmetric pattern whose luminance varied radially according to a cosine waveform, as illustrated in Figure 2.58B—and the detection threshold for sinusoidal grating targets could be explained by assuming that threshold was, "governed, not by local contrast or any other feature in the stimulus domain, but rather by the component of maximum amplitude in the two-dimensional Fourier transforms of those stimulus patterns" (Kelly & Magnusky, 1975, p. 911). The two-dimensional Fourier transform is discussed briefly on p. 422. Bracewell (1965) and Brigham (1974) provide a formal treatment.

Orthogonal gratings: Discrimination and masking

As mentioned earlier, Burbeck and Regan (1983a) found that the spatial-frequency discrimination threshold was the same between parallel gratings and orthogonal gratings. They concluded that the spatial-frequency discrimination stage can access and compare spatial-frequency information across orthogonal orientations. Bradley and Skottun (1984) independently reported similar results and came to similar conclusions. This finding, subsequently confirmed by Olzak and Thomas (1991, 1992), indicates that:

> Even though a grating's characteristic spatial frequency exists only along one dimension, at some level in the visual system the neural representation of spatial frequency is generalized over two dimensions.

This level cannot be the firing of an individual simple (orientation-tuned) cell in primary visual cortex—if we assume that information conveyed by a neuron is encoded entirely in terms of the number of spikes or by firing frequency (see footnote on p. 33). The finding just described cannot be explained by the two-stage model depicted in Figure 2.29B. Nor is it explained by the line-element model of Wilson and Gelb (Figure 2.48), because orthogonal gratings are represented by widely separated locations in multidimensional filter–output space (Appendix D). A simple explanation for the findings just cited would be that the visual system contains a third-stage mechanism that sums across all orientations the outputs of filters that prefer any given spatial frequency. If spatial frequency is plotted radially in polar coordinates with orientation as azimuth, the sensitivity of such a mechanism can be represented as an annular area centered on the origin. Olzak and Thomas (1996) proposed that such a mechanism exists, and estimated the thickness of the annular area to be less than one octave.

However, the proposal that a hard-wired summation mechanism intervenes between the spatial filters and the discrimination stage is not consistent with the finding that, although a parallel jittered-frequency masker could produce a large elevation of spatial-frequency discrimination threshold (open circles in Figure 2.26), no elevation was produced by an orthogonal jittered-frequency masker (Regan, 1985a). Although Olzack and Thomas (1991) reported elevations for an orthogonal *constant-frequency* masker, they were far smaller than the maximum elevation shown in Figure 2.26. In retrospect, the finding reported in Regan (1985a) is crucial to the rejection of the summation hypothesis, and for that reason merits independent investigation.

Before returning to this problem, I will review research on aspect-ratio discrimination.

Aspect-ratio discrimination and the aspect-ratio aftereffect

In the following section I review experimental research on human visual ability to discriminate simple two-dimensional shapes such as rectangles and ellipses, and discuss evidence that the human visual system contains a specialized mechanism that is sensitive to a target's aspect ratio while being relatively insensitive to the target's area.

Aspect-ratio discrimination. The most elementary kind of two-dimensional shape is one that can be specified by the ratio of two distances along fixed perpendicular meridians within a fronto-parallel plane (e.g., a rectangle or an ellipse). For example, the shape of any given rectangle or any ellipse can be completely specified by its aspect ratio a/b, where a is its height and b its width. Two rectangles (or two ellipses) would be said to differ in shape if their aspect ratios could not be equated by a relative rotation within a front-parallel plane.*

We measured both the absolute accuracy and the precision (i.e., the discrimination threshold) with which observers could judge the aspect ratio of a (solid) sharp-edged perfect square or (outlined) perfect circle of height a and width b (Regan & Hamstra, 1992a). In order to remove either height or width as a reliable cue to aspect ratio we varied the area of the target randomly on a trial-to-trial basis.

The *accuracy* of judging aspect ratio was remarkably good: errors in a/b ranged from 0.7% to 0.4% for squareness judgments, and from 1.4% to below 0.5% for judgments of circularity. The *precision* of judging aspect ratio (i.e., the discrimination threshold or just-noticeable difference of aspect ratio) was as low as 1.6%, even when area was randomly varied from trial to trial so as to remove the linear dimensions a and b as a reliable cue. We concluded that:

> The human visual pathway contains a mechanism that is sensitive to some relation between a target's height and width, a mechanism that is rather insensitive to the target's height, width, or area.

---

* For our present purpose we define two areas within the fronto-parallel plane as having different shapes if their relative dimensions along N different azimuths within the fronto-parallel plane cannot be equated by rotating one area with respect to the other about an axis normal to the fronto-parallel plane. We suppose the N azimuths to be drawn in fixed coordinates within the fronto-parallel plane at equal angular intervals so as to cover uniformly the

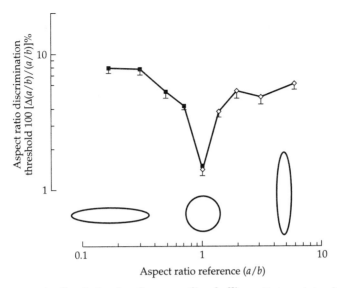

2.60 Aspect-ratio discrimination for an outlined ellipse. Data points plot the just-detectable percentage change in aspect ratio for outlined ellipses of different aspect ratios. The area of the test ellipse was randomly varied from trial to trial. The mean area was the same as that of a circle of diameter 1.0 degrees. From Regan and Hamstra (1992a).

Figure 2.60 shows that discrimination threshold* was a U-shaped function of aspect ratio, with a sharp minimum at an aspect ratio of 1.0. Suppose that aspect ratio is encoded as follows:

1. Encode height (a) and width (b).
2. Combine a and b by, for example, encoding a/b.

For a square of side length 0.5 degrees, an aspect-ratio discrimination threshold of 1.6% implies that a and b are both encoded with a precision of better than 20 seconds of arc.

The aspect-ratio aftereffect. We found that adapting to a bright solid rectangle produced a briefly lived change in the perceived aspect ratio of a subsequently presented test rectangle. After an observer adapted to a vertically elongated rectangle,

---

available 360 degrees of angle. For arbitrary shapes, the precision with which two shapes can be discriminated will be higher, the higher the value of N (Regan & Hamstra, 1992a).

* Although discrimination was clearly based on some relation between a and b, it was not clear whether this relation was a/b, or $(a − b)$, or some other function of a and b.

a square test target appeared to be elongated horizontally, and after an observer adapted to a horizontally elongated rectangle, a square test target appeared to be elongated vertically (Regan & Hamstra, 1992a).

Next I describe quantitative measurements of this *aspect-ratio aftereffect*. Following an initial adaptation period of 10 minutes, one of 10 test rectangles was presented for 0.5 seconds, then the adaptation was refreshed for 7 seconds, then another test rectangle was presented for 0.5 seconds, and so on. The test rectangles had different aspect ratios that were symmetrically placed about 1.0 (square).

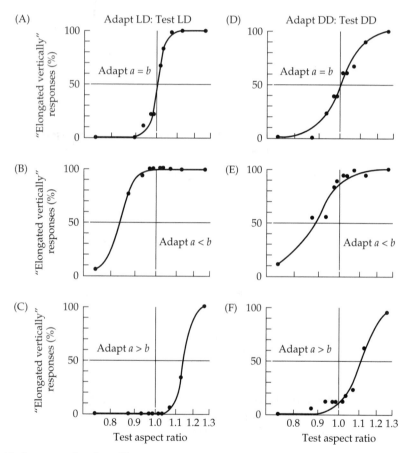

2.61 Aspect-ratio aftereffect. (A) The probability of judging that a luminance-defined test rectangle composed of random dots was elongated vertically rather than horizontally is plotted (as ordinate) versus the aspect ratio a/b of a test rectangle of height a and width b. On the abscissa, 1.0 corresponds to a perfect square. (B) After adapting to a rectangle of aspect ratio 1/1.5, but using the same test stimuli as in A. (C) After adapting to a rectangle of aspect ratio 1.5, but using the same test stimuli as in A. (D–F) Same as for A–C, but for a cyclopean rectangle. After Hamstra (1994).

An important point is that the same test aspect ratios were used in all three adaptation conditions. Observers were instructed to signal whether the test rectangle was elongated vertically or horizontally.

The data shown in Figure 2.61A are similar to the data we collected after adapting to a solid sharp-edged square (aspect ratio $a/b = 1.0$). The point of subjective equality (i.e., the 50% point on the psychometric function) was very close to 1.0. In other words, after the observer adapted to a square, a test square—unsurprisingly—looked square. On the other hand, Figure 2.61B shows that after an observer adapted to a horizontally elongated rectangle of aspect ratio 1/1.5, the point of subjective equality shifted to the left, and Figure 2.61C shows that after adapting to a vertically elongated rectangle of aspect ratio 1.5, the point of subjective equality shifted to the right.

In the first experiment we used test rectangles that all had the same area as that of the adapting rectangle. The post-adaptation data were very similar to those shown in Figure 2.61A–C. Figure 2.62A–F shows why these data could be explained in terms of Köhler & Wallach's "contour repulsion" idea (see pp. 48–53 and Figure 1.15). In Figure 2.62, adapting rectangles of aspect ratios (a/b) equal to 1/1.5, 1.5, and 1.0 are depicted by continuous lines, while test rectangles of aspect ratios 1/1.3 and 1/3 are depicted by dashed lines. The arrows indicate how contour repulsion could produce a spurious aspect-ratio aftereffect.

In a control experiment the test rectangles were still all equal in area, but now the area was half that of the adapting rectangle. Consequently, the relationship between the boundaries of the test and adapt rectangles was as depicted in Figure 2.62G–L, so that the contour repulsion hypothesis predicted quite different aftereffects than those observed. These observed effects were very similar to those shown in Figure 2.61A–B. This control experiment rejected the contour repulsion explanation for the aspect-ratio aftereffect. In point of fact, we collected the data shown in Figure 2.61A–C using test rectangles whose areas varied randomly between an area equal to that of the adapting rectangle and 0.2 of that area. We concluded that:

The human visual system contains a mechanism that is sensitive to the aspect ratio of a target while being, to a first approximation, insensitive to the target's height, width, or area.*

---

* An alternative explanation is that adaptation distorts the representation (or perception) of the frontal plane (J. D. Victor, personal communication, June 1996). And, "Could the aspect ratio data be understood in terms of a recalibration of the vertical and horizontal metrics, such as what happens after wearing an astigmatic telescope that only magnifies in one direction?" (S. Klein, personal communication, January 1999).

A similar two-dimensional aspect-ratio aftereffect that is substantially interdependent of the area of the test target (and also its location) and transfers from luminance to color (Rivest et al., 1997) was subsequently reported by Suzuki and Cavanagh (1998); see also Rivest et al. (1998) and Suzuki & Rivest (1998).

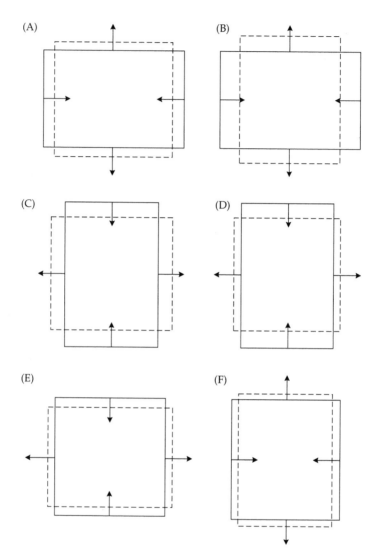

2.62 The aspect-ratio aftereffect is not caused by Köhler and Wallach's contour repulsion. Adapting rectangles of aspect ratios (a/b) equal to (1/1.5), 1.5, and 1.0 are depicted by continuous lines. Test rectangles of aspect ratios (1/1.3) and 1.3 are depicted by dashed lines. The arrows indicate a hypothetical repulsion of the test rectangle's boundaries (see Figure 1.15). In A–F the adapt and test rectangles all have the same area. In G–L (facing page) the area of the test rectangle is the same as in A–F, but the test rectangles all have an area that is sufficiently smaller than the adapt rectangles that all four boundaries of the test rectangle always fall within the boundaries of the adapt rectangle. From Regan and Hamstra (1992a).

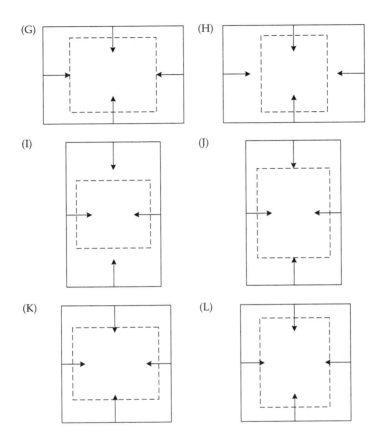

The schematic in Figure 2.63A outlines an attempt to account for aspect-ratio discrimination for a solid rectangle whose area is randomly varied from trial to trial. The signal v from a vertically tuned LD filter is inhibited by the signal h from a horizontally tuned LD filter fed from the same retinal location. One way of achieving cross-orientation inhibition is as follows. Suppose that $v = A \ln (C_V + n)$ and $h = A \ln (C_H + m)$, where C_V and C_H are, respectively, the contrasts of the stimuli for the vertically and horizontally tuned filters, A is a constant, and n and m are RMS levels of noise referred to the input and expressed in terms of contrast. I assume that the output V is given by

$$V = v - kh = A \ln(C_V + n) - Ak \ln(C_H + m) \tag{2.8}$$

where k is a constant < 1.0. For a rectangle of moderate to high contrast (i.e., $C_V \gg n$, $C_H \gg m$), Equation (2.8) reduces to

$$V \approx [A \ln (C_V / C_H^k) \tag{2.9}$$

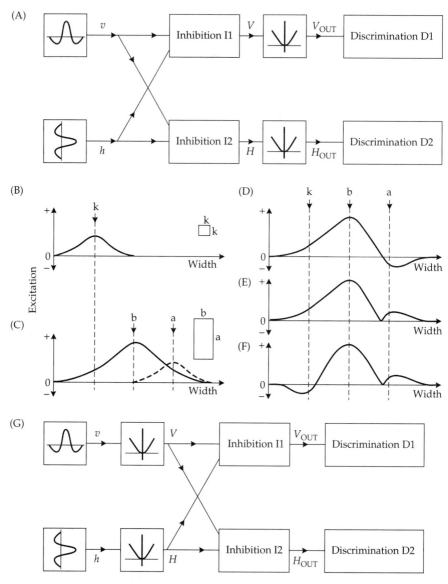

2.63 Schematic of the processing of aspect ratio. (A) The summed signal v from a population of spatial filters that prefer different widths is inhibited by the signal h from spatial filters and CDs tuned to vertical widths before passing through a rectifier stage. Signal h is similarly inhibited by signal v. (B) Signal V_{OUT} produced from stimulating the eye with a square of area k^2. (C) The continuous and dashed lines show, respectively, the inputs v and h to stage I1 that result from stimulating the eye with a rectangle of aspect ratio a/b, where $ab >> k^2$. (D) The resulting signal V. (E) The resulting signal V_{OUT}. (F) The difference between the responses to the large rectangle and the small square. (G) Alternative version of part A in which rectification precedes cross-orientation inhibition.

In Figure 2.64 I assumed that $C_H = C_V$, the noise level $m = n = 1.0$, k = 0.5, and expressed contrast as a multiple of the noise level. The dashed line in Figure 2.64 (left-hand ordinates) illustrates that V is a compressive function of contrast.

An alternative to Equation (2.8) can be written as

$$V = A \ln (C_V + n) - A \ln (kC_H + m) \qquad (2.10)$$

which, for a rectangle of moderate to high contrast, reduces to

$$V \approx A \ln (C_V / kC_H) \qquad (2.11)$$

The continuous line in Figure 2.64 (right-hand ordinate) shows that V is again a compressive function of contrast, but differs in that saturation is more complete and its onset is at a considerably lower contrast. This is because the inhibition is very weak for a rectangle of low contrast, but it rapidly becomes strong as the rectangle's contrast is progressively increased. Equation (2.10) is consistent with the following findings. Aspect-ratio discrimination threshold is independent of contrast over a wide range of contrasts; observers can discriminate trial-to-trial variations of aspect ratio while ignoring trial-to-trial variations of contrast. Equation (2.9), on the other hand, predicts some small effect of contrast.

Before reaching the discrimination stage, signal V is subject to full-wave rectification. The threshold/rectifier characteristic illustrated in Figure 2.63A is linear over most of its range, but has either a hard threshold (i.e., the slope of the characteristic

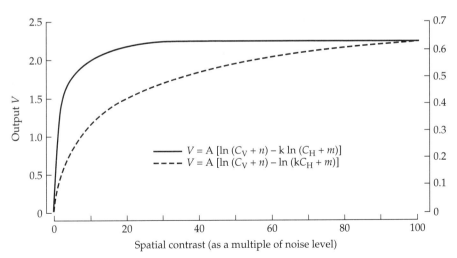

2.64 Effect of stimulus contrast on the signal labeled V in Figure 2.63A. Plots of $A \ln (C_V + n) - Ak \ln (C_H + m)$ (continuous line, left ordinate) and $A \ln (C_V + n) - A \ln (kC_H + m)$ (dashed line, right ordinate) versus contrast, in the case that $C_H = C_V$, $m = n = 1$, and k = 0.5. Key: C_V and C_H are, respectively, the contrasts of vertical and horizontal contours; m and n are RMS noise levels referred to the input. Contrast is expressed as a multiple of noise level.

is mathematically discontinuous at the threshold point), or has an accelerating slope near the origin.*

Objective evidence relevant to the hypothesis illustrated in Figure 2.63A has been obtained by recording electrical brain responses from humans. As mentioned in the section on adaptation and masking in this chapter, there is a strong nonlinear interaction between orthogonal gratings, an interaction that can be revealed by contrast-modulating one grating at frequency F_1 and the other at frequency F_2 (Morrone & Burr, 1986; D. Regan & M. P. Regan, 1986, 1987, 1988). The interaction shows aspects of divisive inhibition (Morrone & Burr, 1986), but cannot be purely multiplicative, because components other than $(F_1 \pm F_2)$ are prominent (D. Regan & M. P. Regan, 1986, 1987, 1988). The generation of these multiple *cross-modulation* frequency components can be modeled in terms of a rectifier stage (M. P. Regan & D. Regan, 1988).

A superthreshold solid rectangle will excite many vertically and horizontally tuned filters to greater or lesser extents, depending on their preferred heights and widths, so that any given rectangle will create a pattern of excitation over many filters. Following Watson and Robson (1981) I assume that the output of each filter carries a width label. Suppose that the eye is stimulated by a solid square of area k^2. Figure 2.63B depicts the pattern of excitation (V_{OUT}) arriving at the discrimination stage D1 in Figure 2.63A. The amplitude of this signal is low, because the cross-interactions are strong between vertical and horizontal filters tuned to the same width (D. Regan & M. P. Regan, 1987). Suppose now that the square is replaced by a rectangle of aspect ratio a/b, whose area is considerably larger that the area of the square. The continuous line in Figure 2.63C shows the excitation pattern (v) within the vertically tuned filters. The dashed line shows the signal arriving at inhibitory stage I1 from the horizontally tuned filters. The output (V) of I1 is depicted in part D. Part E shows the rectified signal V_{OUT} at the input to discrimination stage D1. Part F shows the difference between the inputs to discrimination stage D1 produced by the square and the rectangle. This difference pattern encodes the change in aspect ratio. By attending to the relative heights of the two positive peaks in the difference pattern, observers could dissociate the direction of the change of the rectangle's aspect ratio from its change in area.

For clarity of explanation, the rectangle's aspect ratio in Figure 2.63C–F is very different from the square's in Figure 2.63B. Consequently, the maxima in the difference pattern would correspond to filters that prefer widths little different from b and a. However, when measuring aspect-ratio discrimination threshold experimentally, the rectangle's aspect ratio would be close to 1.0, and in this situation the maxima in the difference pattern would correspond to filters that prefer widths other than b and a. (See earlier discussions on spatial frequency and orientation discrimination for gratings and Figure 2.25.)

---

* As pointed out by Spekreijse and van der Tweel (1965), it is difficult to distinguish between the two possibilities in systems where a noise source is located before the rectifier (see also Spekreijse, 1969; Spekreijse & Oosting, 1970; Spekreijse & Reits, 1982).

The hypothesis illustrated in Figure 2.63A also explains why aspect-ratio discrimination threshold is a U-shaped function centered on an aspect ratio of 1.0. Because the inhibitory cross-connections are strongest between filters that prefer the same width (Regan & Regan, 1987), the amplitude of the signal V_{OUT} will be lower for a square stimulus than for a rectangular stimulus. Thus, as illustrated in parts B–F, when only one of the two targets to be compared has an aspect ratio of 1.0, the excitation pattern V_{OUT} will change, not only in shape, but also in the area under the curve; but when both targets have aspect ratios considerably different from 1.0, the excitation pattern V_{OUT} will still change in shape, but the change in area will be proportionally less.

The schematic shown in Figure 2.63A also accounts for the processing of information carried by grating stimuli. It can account for the finding that spatial-frequency discrimination thresholds are similar for two successively presented orthogonal gratings and for two successively presented parallel gratings. And the accelerating shape of the rectifier's effective characteristic at points close to the origin combined with the compressive transformation of stimulus contrast provide an explanation for the "dipper" shape in Figure 2.15.

In Figure 2.63A the compressive and the accelerating segments of the transducer function are modeled sequentially, and in that order. A proposal that the two segments should be modeled sequentially, but with the accelerating segment first is discussed on pp. 250–253; see also Figure 2.16D. Figure 2.63G sets out this alternative organization. We must now write:

$$v = A \ln (C_V + n), \quad (C_V + n) > T_V \tag{2.12}$$

$$v = 0, (C_V + n) < T_V$$

and

$$h = A \ln (C_H + m), \quad (C_H + m) > T_H \tag{2.13}$$

$$h = 0, (C_H + m) < T_H$$

where T_V and T_H, respectively, are the hard thresholds for the upper and lower threshold/rectifier stages in Figure 2.63G. Provided that $(C_V + n) > T_V$ and $(C_H + m) > T_H$, the signal (V) reading the discrimination stage D1 is now given by equation (2.14):

$$V = v - kh = A \ln (C_V + n) - Ak \ln (C_H + m) \tag{2.14}$$

or, alternatively,

$$V = A \ln (C_V + n) - A \ln (kC_H + m) \tag{2.15}$$

As was the case for Equation (2.8), for a rectangle of moderate to high contrast, Equation (2.14) reduces to Equation (2.9), and Equation (2.15) reduces to Equation (2.11).

The patterns of excitation for the functional model shown in Figure 2.63G differ from those shown in parts B–D in that the rightmost lobe in part F is inverted as shown in part D. But just as was the case for the schematic shown in part A, by attending to the relative heights of the peaks in the difference pattern, observers could dissociate the direction of change of the rectangle's aspect ratio from its change in area.

As they stand, however, the hypotheses illustrated in Figure 2.63A and G are not compatible with the finding that a masker whose spatial frequency is jittered on a trial-to-trial basis about a mean of 8.0 cycles/deg. produced a much larger elevation of discrimination threshold for 5 cycles/deg. test gratings when the gratings were parallel (open symbols in Figure 2.26) than when the gratings were orthogonal.

So far we have focused on the role of the broadly selective LD filters in the first stage of the Figure 2.63A schematic, and the operation of the model in its "regional binding" mode (see pp. 39–40). This mode of operation does not, however, account for the finding that aspect-ratio discrimination threshold for an outlined target is at least as low as for a solid target (Regan & Hamstra, 1992a, and Figure 2.60). A bright solid rectangle with a dim surround will strongly excite filters tuned to its width (b) and height (a), but an outlined rectangle of aspect ratio a/b will excite these filters only weakly. A model of aspect-ratio discrimination for outlined targets can be framed in terms of the coincidence detector concept (CD boxes in Figure 2.53). A high-contrast outlined shape will create a pattern of excitation over many coincidence detectors, any given one of which signals a different vertical or horizontal separation. I propose that the outputs of coincidence detectors feed an aspect-ratio analyzer similar to that shown in stages 2–4 in Figure 2.63A or G.

The coincidence detector contribution to the inputs of subsequent stages accounts for aspect-ratio discrimination for outline targets, and it explains why we can, with equal facility, discriminate the aspect ratios of solid and outlined shapes (see first footnote on p. 40).

The coincidence detector signal also allows the model to encode with especially high precision a change in the aspect ratio of a solid target that has high contrast and sharp edges. When the coincidence detectors determine the functioning of the model, the model is operating in its "boundary detection" mode rather than its "regional binding" mode (see pp. 39–40). The idea just described can explain why the aspect-ratio aftereffect transfers from a solid sharp-edged rectangle to an outlined ellipse (Regan & Hamstra, 1992a).

For a more elegant approach to the analysis of two-dimensional patterns in general I refer the reader to Koenderink and van Doorn (1979).

Short-term memory and attention: What roles do they play in visual discriminations?

As mentioned earlier in this chapter, one reason why none of the models I have reviewed so far can explain all the experimental data on human spatial vision may be that they all neglect the roles of memory and selective attention in the collection of psychophysical data. In principle, if memory and selective attention play important roles in the collection of psychophysical data, it might be impossible to understand fully these data if the roles of memory and selective attention are ignored.* More generally, before framing a psychophysical model of the early processing of spatial information, it may be necessary to specify a model of how observers carry out the psychophysical task (such as temporal 2AFC) that produced the data on which the model is to be based.

In the following sections, I first review a popular view of how observers perform the temporal 2AFC task, a view that is based on the concept of *short-term visual memory*. Next I discuss the possible role of selective attention in the generation of psychophysical data. In the last part of this section I provide an introductory outline of Michel Treisman's *criterion-setting theory* (CST). I thank Professor Treisman for providing, in an exchange of letters, an introductory overview of CST, and for allowing me to quote excerpts of his letters to me.

The effect of interpenetration interval on various discrimination thresholds: The concept of visual short-term memory. Donald MacKay pointed out that in everyday life we use our eyes in an active exploratory manner when gathering visual information much as, when in a pitch-dark room, we identify an object by running our hands over it. One possible reason why we gather visual information in this manner is that, although our visual field covers about 160 degrees of visual angle horizontally and about 135 degrees vertically (Scott, 1957), high acuity is restricted to a region (the fovea) only about two degrees in diameter. So we explore an object by successively fixating different locations on it with the 3 degree^2 fovea, using the roughly 10,000 degree^2 remainder of the visual field to alert us to the presence of objects that merit foveal inspection.

According to Gouras (1991b, p.187), the fovea

> is essentially a diurnal organ, lacking in nocturnal photoreceptors. . . . Animals without foveas have a type of vision where oculomotor control of the eye is much more limited than in foveate animals. In foveate animals both saccadic and tracking eye movements appear in order to bring the fovea to targets of interest and to hold the fovea on these targets. This is a major change in visual function. With a fovea stationary objects are sought out, followed and analyzed in great detail. This leads to continuous microsaccades and microdrifts that restore and maintain vision of objects which would otherwise remain stationary on the retina (Ditchburn & Ginsburg, 1952; Foley-Fisher & Ditchburn, 1986). . . . Color vision and high spatial resolution are, in fact, major attributes of foveal vision.

---

* It may not be fanciful to draw an analogy between this line of argument and Heisenberg's realization, expressed in the Heisenberg uncertainty principle, that the results of a physical measurement can only be understood in the context of how the physical measurement was made.

But our immediate concern is that the process of inspecting an object by successive fixations clearly demands some way of integrating visual information over successive fixations.

In 1960 George Sperling reported evidence for a short-term store of visual information (see also Averbach & Sperling, 1961). But the storage time of this *iconic memory* is only a few hundred milliseconds, and storage can be disrupted by a subsequently presented mask. Furthermore, the store is tied to retinal position, and so it is not suitable for integrating information over successive fixations.

Phillips distinguished Sperling's iconic memory from a more schematic *short-term visual memory* that has a decay period of 10 to 20 seconds and is not tied to retinal location, and whose contents are not disrupted by masking (Phillips, 1983). Subsequently, Irwin proposed that *short-term visual memory* is responsible for integrating visual information across the successive fixations that comprise our inspection of an object (Irwin, 1991).

The *short-term visual memory* hypothesis should be distinguished from the concept of visual long-term memory (Klatzky, 1980; Humphreys & Bruce, 1989). Visual long-term memory stores an abstract representation of the object as a whole, while *short-term visual memory* retains at least some of the detailed features of a spatial pattern, in other words, something akin to the "viewer-centered surface description" of Marr (1982).

In an attempt to measure the dynamics of *short-term visual memory*, we measured *orientation discrimination threshold* using a temporal two-alternative forced choice procedure (see Figure 1.5B and pp. 8–17), and varied the interval between the two presentations that constituted a *trial* (Regan & Beverley, 1985). For one observer, thresholds were not significantly different (4% difference) for interpresentation intervals of 1 second and 10 seconds. For a second observer, thresholds were significantly but not greatly (37%) different for the 1- and 10-second interpresentation intervals. In a subsequent study on *spatial-frequency discrimination threshold* I varied the interpresentation interval from 0.4 to 20 seconds. The results are shown in Figure 2.65. For one observer, thresholds were exactly the same for interstimulus intervals of 0.4 and 10 seconds (5.5 ± 0.9% and 5.5 ± 0.6%). I claimed that there was no significant difference between thresholds at 0.4 and 20 second intervals (Regan, 1985b).*

Because of my ignorance of the literature on memory I failed to cite previous discussion of the short-term visual memory hypothesis when proposing that an observer's response following any given *trial* could be explained within the following conceptual framework:

---

* After re-analyzing my data, Lages and Treisman (1998) stated that I had erred in using a two-tailed *t*-test instead of a one-tailed *t*-test and went on to show that, when the data for each subject were combined and analyzed properly, there was a significant difference between thresholds for the 0.4- and 20-second intervals. So I should have better said that threshold increased by 0.0% for observer B, by 28% for observer A, and 11% for observers A and B combined as interpresentation duration increased from 0.4 to 10 seconds, and by 36% for observer B, 48% for observer A, and 41% for observers A and B combined as interpresentation duration increased from 0.4 to 20 seconds.

1. Neurally encode the orientation or spatial frequency of the grating presented first during the particular trial (alternative possibilities are a running average of the last few presentations or a long-term average of all previous presentations).
2. Store that neural representation.*
3. Neurally encode the orientation or spatial frequency of the grating presented second.
4. Compare the two neural representations (Regan, 1985b; Regan & Beverley, 1985).

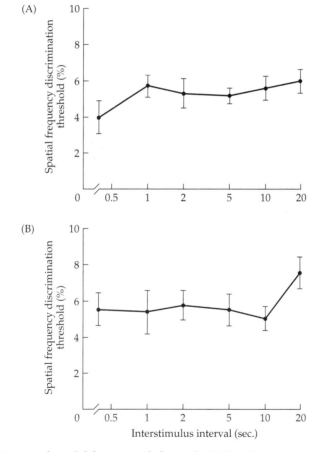

2.65 Storage of spatial-frequency information? Plots for two observers of the effect of interpresentation interval on spatial-frequency discrimination threshold measured using a temporal 2AFC procedure. From Regan (1985b).

* According to Sachtler and Zaidi (1992), when a psychophysical task requires memory storage ("even the barest amount of memory"), color information is considerably more useful than luminance information.

In terms of this way of looking at the spatial-frequency data, visual storage of information was near-perfect up to about 10 seconds.* This finding was confirmed by Magnussen et al. (1990). I also found that, even when the two gratings were orthogonal, spatial-frequency discrimination threshold remained constant while the interpresentation interval was increased from 0.4 to 10 seconds, thus extending the conclusion of Burbeck and Regan (1983a) that a single spatial-frequency discrimination mechanism accepts spatial-frequency information independently of whether the reference and test gratings are parallel or orthogonal. Lages and Treisman (1998) strengthened this conclusion with data obtained using a quite different approach: sequential dependencies of the observer responses. I concluded that spatial-frequency information is stored in a way that is independent of orientation (Regan, 1985b). Not only the spatial frequency but also the velocity of a grating seems to be stored near-perfectly in short-term visual memory (Obergfell et al., 1989).

As to how many parameters can be stored at the same time without greatly degrading discrimination threshold, the answer seems to be at least three (Vincent & Regan, 1995); see Figure 1.7.

On the other hand, the storage of other simple stimulus attributes is far from perfect: short-term visual memory for these attributes appear to be "leaky." These features include the separation between two bars, and the contrast of a grating (Vogels & Orban, 1986; Greenlee, 1990; Fahle & Harris, 1992).†

Lee and Harris (1996) investigated the decay through time of the representation of grating contrast. The intent of their experimental design was to prevent their observers from performing the discrimination task by building up an internal representation of the central value in the range of stimuli presented. They noted previous reports that, when discriminating the separation between two lines, observers performed almost as well when the reference stimulus was present on every trial as when the reference stimulus was never presented, i.e., each trial consisted of a single presentation of a test stimulus (Westheimer & McKee, 1977; Morgan, 1992). To counter the possibility of an observer's learning the stimulus set, Lee and Harris interleaved many different reference contrasts in random order. There were three groups of reference contrasts. The reference contrast could assume any value between $(5 - 2x)\%$ and $(5 + 2x)\%$ or between $(15 - 2x)\%$ and $(15 + 2x)\%$ or between $(60 - 2x)\%$ and $(60 + 2x)\%$, where x was (approximately) contrast discrimination threshold. In any given trial, the test contrast differed from

---

* Using a different experimental approach, Tanaka and Sagi (1998) found evidence that spatial filters in early vision retain an input trace up to 16 seconds, far beyond the perceptual integration range.

† The findings of Magnussen et al. (1995) conflicted with our report that orientation discrimination is little, if at all, elevated by increasing the interpresentation interval from one to 10 seconds (Regan & Beverley, 1985).

the particular reference value by one of several possible increments (positive or negative). Three psychometric functions were obtained in any given run.

Lee and Harris attempted to distinguish between the following three possible ways in which short-term memory for contrast might decay:

1. Memory literally fades (i.e., the stored representation of contrast decreases progressively with time).
2. All contrasts converge to a central or average value.
3. The stored representation of contrast remains constant in magnitude, but becomes increasingly noisy as time progresses.

Lee and Harris reported that, as they increased the interval between test and reference presentations from 1 through 3 to 10 seconds, contrast discrimination threshold rose progressively, following a power law. The rate at which threshold increased was the same for all spatial frequencies. It was not the case that the representation of contrast for a grating of high spatial frequency faded more quickly than the representation of contrast for a grating of low spatial frequency. In particular, Lee and Harris found that discrimination threshold for interstimulus interval t seconds was equal to kt^n. The value of k decreased from 0.8 for the reference grating of 5% contrast to 0.1 for the reference grating of 60% contrast. The exponent n was 0.38 for all stimulus frequencies at all three reference contrasts used. This compares with an exponent of 0.6 for the power-law relationship between contrast discrimination threshold and reference contrast for a fixed inter-presentation interval (Legge, 1980).

Does selective attention play a role in visual discrimination? We can rescue the idea illustrated in Figure 2.63A or G from its failure to explain the effects of a jittered masker on sensitivity to a grating (Regan, 1985a) if we assume that observers can attend selectively to the pattern of activity among vertically tuned spatial filters or to the pattern of activity among horizontally tuned spatial filters or to the output of the aspect-ratio encoder depicted in Figure 2.63A,G and, furthermore, can switch attention rapidly from one to another. This hypothesis would account for the observation that spatial-frequency discrimination between orthogonal gratings can be acute. Relevant here is evidence that, when an observer is instructed to attend to the width of a rectangle, width discrimination threshold is not elevated by trial-to-trial variations of height that remove aspect ratio as a reliable cue. The converse is the case for height discrimination (Regan & Hamstra, 1992a; Regan et al., 1986b). And, as mentioned earlier, when instructed to attend to a rectangle's aspect ratio, observers can make acute discriminations, even when the rectangle's area is varied from trial to trial so as to remove both height alone and width alone as reliable cues (Regan & Hamstra, 1992a).

An alternative view of the discrimination process. Lages and Treisman (1998, p. 571) stated that "findings which show an effect of an earlier stimulus on the judgment of a later one should not automatically be taken as evidence for a sensory memory of the first stimulus." M. Treisman (personal communication, June 1998) noted that the "neural representation" conceptualization of the discrimination process, described on pp. 185–189, "assumes that some isolated and unique set of information is stored that relates to the characteristics of the stimulus first presented on each trial and that could presumably be used for various purposes, one of which is that it is referred to for comparison when a second stimulus is presented on that trial and a discrimination decision must be made."

Treisman and his colleagues have developed a conceptualization of the discrimination process that is fundamentally different from the conceptualization reviewed on pages 185–189 (Treisman & Falkner, 1984, 1985; Treisman & Williams, 1984; Lages & Treisman, 1998). According to their "criterion-setting" theory (CST), the information that is used when making a discriminative response is not a neural representation (memory) of one or more past stimuli (but see first footnote on p. 188). Rather, "on each trial during the experiment the subject is presented with a stimulus. This stimulus produces a central sensory effect on the decision axis. What the subject records is the relative displacement of the input on each trial from the criterion at that moment. This measure (the sensory indicator trace) will be used on later trials to adjust the criterion. If the indicator trace is positive (the input was above the criterion), it will be used to shift the criterion upwards on later trials. These traces are stored individually, they decay, and their net effect is encapsulated in the criterion value" (M. Treisman, personal communication, March 1998). In other words, "the CST view is that the information necessary to make a decision is stored by altering a parameter of the decision mechanism (the value of the criterion). A crude analogy would be with firing a gun. If you always hit too far to the right of a briefly glimpsed target you might try to remember better where the target was each time (improving the individual neural representations), or you might alter the setting of the gun-sight (adjust the criterion in relation to past errors" (M. Treisman, personal communication, June 1998).

"Both sensory memory theory and CST rely on the concept of memory, but they differ in what they envisage is retained in memory, a representation of the stimulus, or specification for the response criterion. Sensory memory theory implicitly assumes that retention is limited by unavoidable damage to stimulus traces, by decay or interference. CST assumes that the value of the stabilization decay parameter is set to optimize performance. Thus, stabilization may extend over a few trials or over many" (Lages & Treisman, 1998, p. 570).

The CST conceptualization of the discrimination process renders the model outlined in Figure 2.63A,G compatible with the data reviewed earlier. As was the case for the "neural representation" conceptualization, it accounts for spatial-frequency discrimination between successively presented orthogonal grating. And in elegant style it accounts for the findings reported by Regan (1985a) using an orthogonal jittered masker. Recollect that there was no standard stimulus: on each trial there were two test gratings presented in random order, one of which departed from a base frequency by $+x$, the other by $-x$, and there were 11 values of x. The observer was asked to judge the second in relation to the first. "In this case CST says that the subject is not comparing neural representations of the two test gratings on each trial in isolation from other trials." He or she "is comparing the second input with a criterion which has been established over time by the deviations above and below it of the preceding inputs from the succession of (first and second) test stimuli previously presented. (Data were collected when performance had stabilized). Thus the criterion will be at or near the mean of the stimuli presented (the base frequency)" (M. Treisman, personal communication, June 1998). The observer responds on the basis of trial-to-trial variations in the spatial frequency of the *test* gratings only, so only the test gratings contribute to the location of the response criterion. And Lages and Treisman (1998) showed that the criterion setting theory can account for the finding (Regan & Beverley, 1985; Regan, 1985b) that discrimination threshold is independent of interstimulus interval up to at least 10 seconds, not in terms of a persisting neural representation of spatial frequency or orientation, but rather in terms of a persisting neural representation of the criterion value.

On the other hand, it is not self-evident how the CST approach would account for the finding that discrimination threshold for some simple stimulus attributes such as spatial frequency, velocity, and (possibly) orientation should be independent of interpresentation interval for intervals up to 10 seconds, while discrimination thresholds for other attributes such as line separation and contrast—that seem to be as simple as spatial frequency and velocity—increase as interpresentation interval is increased.

Disordered Processing of Luminance-Defined Form in Patients

As noted in the section on disordered vision in Chapter 1, studies of disordered vision might help to identify the submodalities and abstract features that, according to the *sets of filters* hypothesis, are processed independently and in parallel (*A, B, C,* and so on, in Figure 1.10). In the remaining sections of this chapter, I provide some illustrations of this approach to analyzing the visual processing of luminance-defined form.

Contrast sensitivity loss that is selective for spatial frequency and orientation, and is caused by a neurological disorder

To the extent that the pathology responsible for an observed disorder of visual function is documented, it may be instructive to compare the characteristics of the functional loss with the putative site and nature of the pathology.

Pathology central to the retina.   The ability to see and recognize objects has traditionally been assessed entirely in terms of high-contrast visual acuity for luminance-defined optotypes, and the Snellen letter reading chart has been the most favored of the acuity tests. Figure 2.66A shows a Snellen-type chart.* It is instructive to spell out the rationale of the Snellen test. The rationale is that the smaller the high-con-

(A)

ZRDOVCN5	
HRVCOSKZ	2
NDCOHRVS	3
KVRZCOHS	4
ZNVKDSOR	5
DCRVHNZK	6
OSKCVRZN	7
SNHKCDVO	8
NRDCOKSZ	9
VHCRZDH	10
....	11

(B)

NRVCDSOH	
ZKSCODRN	2
VHNKZCSO	3
KRDHVZNC	4
HVOZSDRK	5
SKCDVHOR	6
ZNKOSDCR	7
NHSVKZCR	8
ZVNDHKOS	9
....	10
......	11

2.66 Regan high- and low-contrast visual acuity charts. Letter size increases by a constant fraction (1.26:1) in successive ascending rows, so that letter size doubles every third line. Thus, a fall in acuity of (say) one line means the same thing, whatever the observer's initial visual acuity. The third line from the bottom has letters that subtend 5 minutes of arc when viewed from 20 feet (approximately 6 meters). An observer who can read this line from 20 ft (or 6 m) is said to have 20/20 (or 6/6 in metric measure, or 1.0 decimal) visual acuity. If the smallest letters that can be read from a distance of 20 ft (or 6 m) by a particular observer are twice the size of those on the 20/20 line, and could be read from 40 ft by a second observer with 20/20 acuity, then the first observer is said to have 20/40 acuity.

---

* The reason I provided three lines below the 20/20 line is that a sudden loss of acuity from 20/10 to 20/20 may be as significant clinically as a sudden loss of acuity from 20/20 to 20/40. For example, the development of an interocular difference of 6/3 in one eye versus 6/6 in the other may be the first indicator of macular degeneration. The context here is that the acuity tests used in many hospitals (especially when the test device is a poorly adjust ed projector) do not display sufficiently sharp letters to test acuity better than 20/20. So there is a ceiling at 20/20.

The convention of regarding "normal" acuity as 20/20 (6/6) is quite arbitrary. In point of fact, the 20/20 visual norm sets a below-average standard (Frisén & Frisén, 1981). According to Tayler (1981), in normally sighted European males, binocular acuity can be as high as 6/1.9, 32% of the population being 6/2.4 or better, and 93% being 6/6 or better. And the binocular acuity of Australian nonurban aboriginal males (measured at long viewing distances under a bright Australian sun) can be as high as 6/1.5—better than in European males at the 0.001 level, and four times more acute than the 20/20 norm.

trast luminance-defined letters that can be read correctly, the better is spatial form vision. This, by and large,* is an adequate rationale for prescribing spectacles for correcting refractive errors that cause the retinal image to be blurred (e.g., short sight, long sight, astigmatism). But the rationale is flawed when a patient's visual loss has a retinal or visual pathway component.

Bodis-Wollner (1972) showed that brain injuries can result in a loss of contrast sensitivity at low spatial frequencies that spares visual acuity (see also Bodis-Wollner & Diamond, 1976). On the face of it, this kind of visual loss seems to confound common sense, so that it is easy to understand why—until quite recently when simple tests for detecting low-contrast visual loss became widely available—some patents had difficulty in convincing physicians that their complaints had an organic basis (in neurology, nonorganic symptoms are called "hysterical"; see Brain and Walton [1969], pp. 994–1006.†) This designation can be especially distressing for a patient who feels sure that he or she has a physical problem. A simple test is to compare a patient's visual acuity using a high-contrast letter chart such as that shown in Figure 2.66A with visual acuity measured with a low-contrast letter chart such as that shown in Figure 2.66B. Some patients who can read the 6/6 or even the 6/3 line on the high-contrast chart are unable to read low-contrast letters that are quite clear to the normally sighted eye (Regan & Neima, 1983, 1984b; Regan, 1988).‡

It is now well established that a substantial proportion of patients with multiple sclerosis and optic neuritis§ who have normal Snellen acuity and normal acuity for high-contrast gratings show loss of contrast sensitivity over a broad range

---

* In addition to refractive error and to dysfunction of the central visual pathway, failure to read the small letters on a Snellen chart (e.g., Figure 2.66A) can be caused by defective control of direction of gaze. A problem of this kind can sometimes be recognized when the patients' errors are in fact correct identifications of the letter to the left or right of the designated letter. A gaze error of as little as 5 minutes of arc can be detected by comparing the patient's visual acuity measured with a Snellen chart such as those shown in Figure 2.66A and with visual acuity measured with a repeat-letter chart such as that shown in Figure 2.20. If the score on the repeat-letter chart is significantly higher than that on the Snellen chart, a gaze defect is indicated. The opposite finding is consistent with the poor Snellen score's being caused by abnormal lateral interactions between adjacent contours (Kothe & Regan, 1990; Regan et al., 1992b).

† Criteria for distinguishing between organic and hysterical origins of the symptoms presented by patients with suspected multiple sclerosis are discussed in Brain and Walton (1969), pp. 503–504.

‡ An alternative to measuring low-contrast acuity using a chart composed of letters of the same contrast but different sizes (as in Figure 2.66) is to measure contrast sensitivity using a letter chart comprised of letters of the same size but different contrasts. (Pelli et al., 1988). However, according to Elliot and Bullimore (1993), low-contrast acuity charts are preferred for measuring an eye's susceptibility to glare, for example, in screening professional highway drivers or in evaluating the disabling effect of early cataract (see Regan, 1991c; Regan, Giaschi, & Fresco, 1993a,b).

§ A sudden loss of visual acuity that is usually unilateral and that usually recovers within a few weeks and is associated with edema (swelling) and temporal pallor of the optic disc

of intermediate or low and intermediate spatial frequencies when tested with sinusoidal gratings (Regan et al., 1977; Bodis-Wollner et al., 1978; Zimmern et al., 1979). Visual loss is often greater at temporal frequencies of 4 to 8 Hz than for static gratings; visual loss can be quite different between corresponding points in left and right eyes and can vary greatly within the visual field of one eye (Kupersmith et al., 1983, 1984; Hess & Plant, 1983, 1986; Medjbeur & Tulunay-Keesey, 1985; Regan & Maxner, 1986; Plant, 1991).

Figure 2.67A,B shows control data: the mean contrast sensitivity curve for 19 control eyes with well-corrected sharp vision (dashed curve in part A), and corresponding data when their vision was blurred by a one diopter positive lens (continuous line in part A). Figure 2.67B shows the difference between the two curves in part A, bringing out the point that the effect of blur is to reduce sensitivity to fine detail (high spatial frequencies), and hence to reduce high-contrast visual acuity as measured on a Snellen-type chart such as the one illustrated in Figure 2.66A, while sparing sensitivity to coarse detail (low spatial frequencies).

Figure 2.67C compares contrast sensitivity curves for the right and left eyes of a patient with multiple sclerosis. It is evident that the pattern of visual loss for this patient is the mirror image of the pattern of loss caused by blurring the retinal image—selective loss of sensitivity at low spatial frequencies that spares sensitivity to high frequencies in Figure 2.67D versus the opposite pattern in part B. For this patient, high-contrast visual acuity (see part C) was the same in both eyes.

The pattern of loss revealed in Figure 2.67D could not have been caused by front-of-the-eye (refractive media) problems. Therefore, it must have been caused by dysfunction of the retinal or central visual pathway.

> In such cases a patient might have 20/20 visual acuity yet be insensitive to low-contrast targets and thus, for example, be unable to see an approaching truck in foggy conditions.

The pattern of loss shown in Figure 2.67C,D is less common than the pattern of loss shown in Figure 2.67E,F. Part E compares contrast sensitivity curves for the right and left eyes of a second patient with multiple sclerosis. It can be seen that, although the left eye's sensitivity is the same as that of the right eye at the lowest and highest spatial frequencies, it is lower at intermediate spatial frequencies. Part F brings out the spatial-frequency selectivity of this bandpass loss of contrast sensitivity.

Patients with this kind of visual loss can experience something that, at first sight, seems to run counter to common sense. In an investigation of the effect of

---

(i.e., optic neuritis) is often experienced by patients later diagnosed as having multiple sclerosis. Multiple sclerosis is associated with demyelination of nerve axons in the central nervous system. Demyelination occurs at multiple local sites that seem to be distributed more or less randomly. Visual problems are assumed to be caused by demyelination of optic nerve axons, demyelination of axons in white matter underlying visual cortex, and possibly demyelination of myelinated fibers within striate visual cortex (McAlpine et al., 1965; Lumsden, 1970; McDonald, 1974).

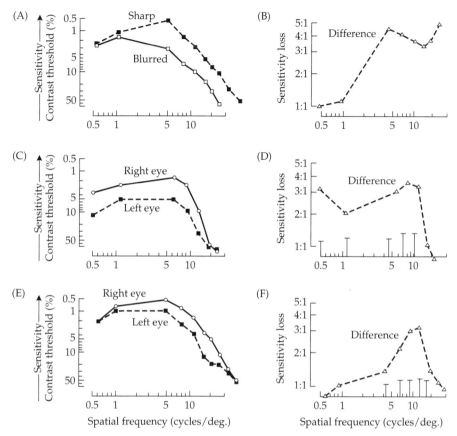

2.67 Spatial-frequency selectivity of contrast-sensitivity loss in patients with multiple sclerosis. (A) Effect of blur in control subjects. Data points plot contrast sensitivity for a sinusoidal grating (ordinate) versus the grating's spatial frequency with the grating sharply accommodated (solid symbols) and with the retinal image blurred by viewing through a +1 diopter lens (open symbols). Data are means for 19 eyes. (B) Difference between the continuous and dotted lines in part A. (C) Data points plot contrast sensitivity for the left (solid symbols) and right (open symbols) eyes of a patient with multiple sclerosis. (D) The difference curve reveals selective loss at low and intermediate spatial frequencies, the mirror image of the pattern of loss in part B. (E) Data points plot contrast sensitivity for the left (solid symbols) and right (open symbols) eyes of a patient with multiple sclerosis. (F) The difference curve reveals bandpass selective loss at intermediate spatial frequencies. The heavy T-shaped bars in parts D and F show data obtained from 29 control subjects. They indicate the standard deviations of the difference between contrast sensitivities in the left and right eye. After Regan, Silver, and Murray (1977).

letter size (expressed as angular subtense) on letter discrimination, we asked patients to discriminate between two letters at viewing distances that ranged from 1 to 10 meters. During any given trial a letter was presented for 0.2 seconds followed, one second later, by a 0.2-second presentation of the second letter. The two letters (C and O) were presented in random order and patients were instructed to signal whether letter C was presented first or second. The letters were filtered so that their power spectra were restricted to the spatial-frequency range zero to 2.5 cycles/letter width.* Figure 2.68 provides an impression of the effects of spatial frequency bandwidth on letter appearance.

Although data for one of the six patients tested were too noisy to allow any conclusions to be drawn, the remaining five patients all showed a dip at a particular distance in the plot of percent correct discriminations versus viewing distance. The viewing distance at which discrimination failed was the distance at which the letters' spatial-frequency content (expressed in cycles/degree) was in the region of the sensitivity loss (e.g., Figure 2.67F) for that particular patient.

At this distance letter discrimination could be improved by *moving further away* from the letter display.

For our normally sighted control observers, letter discrimination, of course, either remained constant at 100% correct or grew worse as viewing distance was increased. According to Parish and Sperling (1991), letter recognition is constant over a 32:1 range of viewing distances. We observed similar, though less striking, effects when we used spatially unfiltered letters.

A loss of contrast sensitivity that is selective for high spatial frequencies, that is associated with a fall in visual acuity, and that cannot be corrected by wearing

---

* The spatial-frequency content of a letter can be specified as a certain range of cycles/degree or as a certain range of cycles/letter width. The content is, of course, the same, but the expression in terms of cycles/letter width is independent of viewing distance, so that it emphasizes the spatial information carried by a particular letter, whereas a cycles/degree expression of frequency content varies with viewing distance. Ginsburg (1978, 1981) did not need to specify viewing distance in his proposal that "Snellen letter recognition can be achieved on the basis of spatial frequencies in the range of 1.5 to 2.5 cycles/letter width." (In other words, that this range contains the minimal amount of shape information for recognition.) Parish and Sperling (1991) provide a review of subsequent writings on this topic and contribute an experimental investigation in which they applied the ideal observer approach (see pp. 142–143) to finding "which spatial frequencies are most effective for letter identification, and whether this is because letters are objectively more discriminable in these frequency bands or because we can utilize the information more efficiently . . ." They confirmed that viewing distance had no effect on letter discriminability; the object spatial frequency rather than retinal spatial frequency determines discriminability. "For our two-octave wide bands . . . performance of humans and of the ideal detector improved with frequency mainly because linear bandwidth increased as a function of frequency. Relative to the ideal detector, human efficiency was 0 in the lowest frequency bands, reached a maximum at 0.42 at 1.5 cycles per object and dropped to about 0.104 in the highest band. Thus, our subjects best extract uppercase letter information from spatial frequencies of 1.5 cycles per object height, and they can extract it with equal efficiency over a 32:1 range of retinal frequencies, from 0.074 to more than 2.3 cycles per degree of visual angle" (Parish & Sperling, 1991, p. 1399).

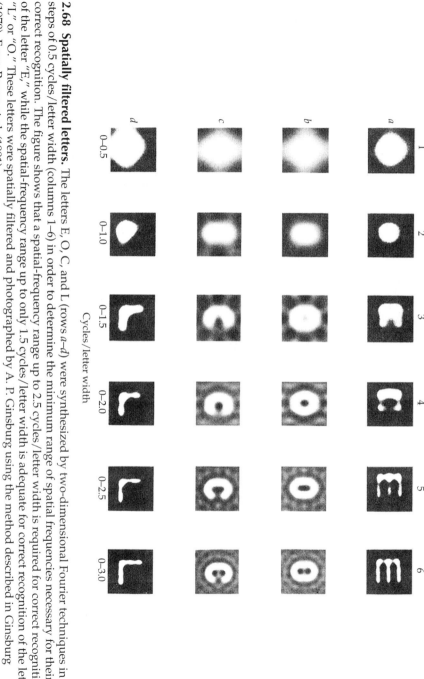

Cycles/letter width

2.68 Spatially filtered letters. The letters E, O, C, and L (rows *a–d*) were synthesized by two-dimensional Fourier techniques in steps of 0.5 cycles/letter width (columns 1–6) in order to determine the minimum range of spatial frequencies necessary for their correct recognition. The figure shows that a spatial-frequency range up to 2.5 cycles/letter width is required for correct recognition of the letter "E," while the spatial-frequency range up to only 1.5 cycles/letter width is adequate for correct recognition of the letter "L" or "O." These letters were spatially filtered and photographed by A. P. Ginsburg using the method described in Ginsburg (1978). From Regan et al. (1981).

spectacles is common in patients with multiple sclerosis and optic neuritis. But that pattern of loss is less relevant to this discussion.

Loss of contrast sensitivity in patients with multiple sclerosis can be selective for orientation as well as spatial frequency (Regan et al., 1980). At both high and low spatial frequencies, the patient whose data are shown in Figure 2.69 had similar contrast sensitivities for gratings orientated vertically, oriented horizontally, and orientated parallel to the two obliques. But near 10 cycles/deg. this patient was about 20 times less sensitive in the left eye than in the right eye for gratings with vertical and 1:30 o'clock orientation. There was no such difference in sensitivity to gratings with horizontal and 4:30 o'clock orientations. The patient's Snellen acuities for left and right eyes were not very different (20/30L, 20/20R). No astigmatism was evident when the patient was tested with a ray pattern of thin black lines.*

In subsequent studies on visual loss in patients with multiple sclerosis we confirmed that contrast threshold for grating of medium spatial frequency can depend strongly on orientation.

We also found that in some (temperature-sensitive) patients with multiple sclerosis, the plot of contrast threshold versus grating orientation changed markedly in shape over a period of weeks as the ambient temperature changed from summer to winter levels. Furthermore, the orientation dependencies of the flicker/motion threshold and the pattern threshold for a counterphase-modulated grating followed dissociated time courses through those weeks (Regan & Maxner, 1986).

On the basis of the orientation tuning of the contrast sensitivity loss shown in Figure 2.69, taken with the similarly between, on the one hand, the pattern of contrast sensitivity loss shown in Figure 2.69F, and on the other hand the curves depicted in Figures 2.8B, 2.12A–F, and 2.9, we suggested that some patients with multiple sclerosis experience selective dysfunction of cortical mechanisms that are selective for both orientation and spatial frequency (Regan et al., 1977, 1980). The reason for implicating cortical mechanisms is that sharp selectivity for orientation has not been found in neurons located peripheral to striate cortex in monkeys.

Contrast sensitivity loss that is greatest for gratings that combine low spatial frequency with fairly high temporal frequency is not uncommon in patients with multiple sclerosis. We suggested that this kind of loss is due to selective dys-

---

* The orientation-selective visual loss experienced by this patient was quite different from meridional amblyopia (neural astigmatism), a functional disorder that, it has been proposed, can be caused by prolonged retinal image blur (caused by uncorrected refractive astigmatism) experienced in early life at a time when the neural organization of the visual system is still plastic (Freeman et al., 1972; Mitchell et al., 1973; Freeman & Thibos, 1973). Although meridional amblyopia can be observed at spatial frequencies as low as 1 cycle/deg., the contrast sensitivity loss becomes progressively larger as spatial frequency is progressively increased (Mitchell & Wilkinson, 1974).

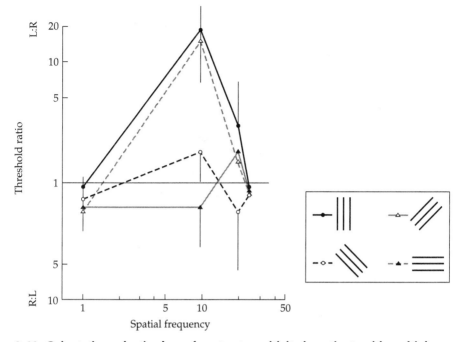

2.69 Orientation-selective loss of contrast sensitivity in patients with multiple sclerosis. Data points plot the ratio between the contrast sensitivities in the left and right eyes of a patient (ordinate) versus the test grating's spatial frequency for four orientations of the test grating. This patient's Snellen acuity was 20/30 in the left eye, 20/20 in the right. After Regan et al. (1980).

function of phasic (Y-type) neurons in the magnocellular stream (Regan & Maxner, 1986). The basis for this suggestion was as follows. Although this kind of visual loss is commonly classified as a loss of sensitivity to gratings of low and/or intermediate spatial frequencies, it can also be described as a failure to process low contrasts; visual loss can be greater at temporal frequencies of 4 to 8 Hz than for static gratings; neurons in the magnocellular stream are more sensitive to low contrasts than are neurons in the parvocellular stream, and tend to be phasic rather than sustained in their temporal properties and also to have larger receptive fields (Shapley et al., 1981).

It is generally accepted that the symptoms characteristic of multiple sclerosis are caused by focal demyelinating plaques within the central nervous system. But how can a focal demyelinating plaque produce the very specific pattern of spatial vision loss just described? In particular, where in the visual pathway are the axons of neurons that serve a narrow range of orientations and low and/or intermediate spatial frequencies spatially segregated from the axons of neurons that serve other orientations and spatial frequencies? What is the basis of their selective vulnerability to demyelination?

A basis for speculation is offered by the following findings. Some patients with Parkinson's disease experience contrast sensitivity loss at low spatial frequencies (Kupersmith et al., 1982; Regan & Neima, 1984b; Bulens et al., 1986; Bodis-Wollner et al., 1987; Regan & Maxner, 1987); the sensitivity loss can depend on orientation (Regan & Maxner, 1987; Bulens et al., 1988), spatial frequency, and temporal frequency (Bodis-Wollner et al., 1987; Regan & Maxner, 1987); the sensitivity loss can be lessened by dopaminergic precursors (Bulens et al., 1987; Bodis-Wollner & Regan, 1991); this improvement can be produced within one to two hours of *oral* administration of medication (Giaschi, Lang, & Regan, 1997). And in healthy human volunteers, the administration of dopaminergic agonists shifted the peak of the contrast sensitivity curve towards higher spatial frequencies, thus *improving contrast sensitivity*, while the peak shifted towards lower spatial frequencies during dopaminergic blockade (Domenici et al., 1985).

Is it possible that an occult neurochemical abnormality might accompany the evident demyelination in at least some patients with multiple sclerosis and that this, rather than the clearly evident demyelinating plaques, contribute to the contrast sensitivity loss whose dependence on orientation, spatial frequency, and temporal frequency is so reminiscent of the kind of loss observed in some patients with Parkinson's disease? This speculation was offered some decades ago as a possible explanation that patients with multiple sclerosis can experience delayed perception of light onset but not light offset, or delayed perception of light offset but not of light onset (Regan et al., 1976). Here, it may be relevant that the ON and OFF pathways are neurochemically distinct at retinal and LGN level (Schiller, 1986).

From the patient's point of view, the significance of the finding that many patients who have normal Snellen acuity have, nevertheless, clear losses of contrast sensitivity or some other visual function is as follows:

1. The diagnosis of multiple sclerosis is a diagnosis of exclusion. One criterion is the presence of more than one unrelated lesion of the central nervous system. (The central nervous system is the brain plus spinal cord.) Suppose that a patient presents with clear symptoms of spinal cord dysfunction, has no other neurological symptoms, and has 20/20 Snellen acuity. If the patient shows contrast sensitivity loss that is not caused by monocular diplopia (see pp. 203–205) or shows reduced visual acuity for low-contrast letters (Figure 2.66B), then the second lesion is demonstrated.

2. To compare the effectiveness of experimental therapies it is necessary to have some measure of the severity of the disease. On the face of it, changes in the severity of the patient's symptoms might seem to be the obvious way of assessing the effectiveness of therapy. The problem with this idea is that the symptoms of untreated multiple sclerosis vary notoriously from month to month—indeed, the relapsing/remitting time course is a diagnostic criterion. It is known that, in some patients, the effects of increasing and decreasing body tem-

perature mimic relapse and remission, respectively. Bearing this in mind, some authors have compared the effects of varying the body temperature of patients and nonpatients on such measures as visual acuity, contrast sensitivity, delay of the visual perception of light onset or offset, double-flash resolution, and the delay of brain responses to flicker (e.g., Galvin et al., 1976; Regan et al., 1977).

Retinal pathology. In the years following the introduction of effective therapy for glaucoma, continuing efforts have been made to improve the effectiveness of clinical perimetry. The motivation for these efforts is that current therapy can arrest the expansion of the regions of total blindness in the visual fields that are detected by standard methods. So it would be better to start treatment before rather than after the patient has suffered irreversible visual loss. With this in mind, during a routine consultation, many optometrists offer older members of society the option of having their intraocular pressure checked.

It is known that a proportion of individuals with elevated intraocular pressure go on to develop glaucoma (with its associated areas of irreversible blindness), but it is not possible to say *which* individuals with elevated pressure will develop glaucoma. And some individuals with normal intraocular pressure develop glaucoma. The dilemma is that current therapies have undesirable side effects, so cannot ethically be used before glaucoma is diagnosed—and the diagnosis currently requires areas of irreversible blindness to have developed.

Contrast sensitivity testing is one of the many approaches that have been taken in attempts to develop a means for predicting which individual patients with elevated interocular pressure will go on to develop glaucoma. If such a prediction could be made with confidence, there would be a possibility of preventing the development of blind areas.

Following up on the finding of Atkin et al. (1980) that glaucoma patients show elevated detection thresholds for foveally viewed grating, and bearing in mind that the clinical field defects characteristic of glaucoma are first seen in peripheral vision (Rock et al., 1972), we used a test grating that subtended 3.5 degrees to measure, over a 48×48 degree visual field, contrast sensitivity for counterphase-modulated (8 Hz) grating of spatial frequency 2 and 5 cycles/deg. We also measured visual fields for grating acuity and carried out standard clinical perimetry using Octopus and Goldmann perimeters. (Clinical perimetry assesses the ability to detect a small test spot, i.e., the ability to detect a highly localized light rather than the ability to detect spatial contrast.)

Results in 15 control eyes confirmed the finding (reviewed on pp. 67–71) that log contrast sensitivity and log cutoff spatial frequency fell off linearly with eccentricity (for a target of constant diameter and temporal frequency). Of the 15 patients with elevated intraocular pressure (but with no diagnosis of glaucoma) eight had localized elevations of contrast detection threshold for the 5 cycles/deg. grating and four also for the 2 cycles/deg. grating.

> Although these localized losses of contrast sensitivity could be gross—in some cases total—no field defect was detectable for grating acuity or by means of clinical perimetry.

Less interesting, in four of the 10 patients with glaucoma we detected field defects that were not evident on clinical perimetry or by testing with gratings. In a separate study we based our approach on the work of Kulikowsky and Tolhurst, described on pp. 71–74 (Regan & Neima, 1984). Figure 2.6 shows that two putative mechanisms can be uncovered by asking observers to set thresholds for just-detectable flicker/motion and for just-detectable spatial pattern while viewing a temporally modulated grating. Figure 2.7 shows how the ratio between these two thresholds varied with eccentricity for 10 normally sighted control subjects.

We replicated the measurements shown in Figure 2.7 for six patients with glaucoma, 10 patients with elevated intraocular pressure (and 10 patients with multiple sclerosis). The balance between pattern-detection threshold and flicker/motion-detection threshold was markedly abnormal in part or all of the visual field for many patients. There were examples in all patient groups. In some patients, flicker threshold was elevated with respect to pattern threshold, while others showed the converse abnormality.

Of 10 patients with elevated intraocular pressure and no visual field defect evident on clinical perimetry, eight had a significantly abnormal ratio between pattern and flicker/motion thresholds at some location in the visual field.

We concluded that the ratio between pattern and flicker/motion thresholds is more sensitive to visual field damage than is conventional perimetry or visual acuity perimetry. Regan and Neima (1984a, p. 314) offered the following explanation for the finding just described:

> It is known on morphological grounds that ganglion cells' dendritic trees have a wide range of sizes even within a single class of ganglion cells (Boycott & Wässle, 1974). Suppose that the dendritic sites most distant from the cell body are more vulnerable to functional loss in ocular hypertension and glaucoma than are the dendritic sites less distant from the cell body, perhaps because of the greater distance that a signal must travel from the outer boundary of the tree before reaching the cell body. Then, for any given dendritic tree, the most distant dendritic processes would be the first to lose their ability to transmit neural signals. The biggest dendritic trees would be most vulnerable, and these presumably belong to the ganglion cells with large receptive fields that govern visual sensitivity to our low spatial-frequency test gratings. Less vulnerable would be the ganglion cells with smaller dendritic trees that presumably govern visual acuity.*

---

* From 1940 to the end of World War II, English schoolchildren were strongly encouraged to attend the "Saturday morning pictures" where their riotous tendencies could be, more or less, kept in check by feeding them a diet of cowboy movies, whose pseudo-lethal violence seemed to bear no relation to the real thing that, shatteringly, entered their lives from time to time. (More serious stuff like *Bambi* could upset children who knew about killing and

This psychophysically based hypothesis is consistent with the subsequent physiological finding that the thickest ganglion cell axons are preferentially dysfunctional in glaucoma (Quigley et al., 1987, 1988; Glovinsky et al., 1991; Quigley, 1999).

Degraded spatial-frequency discrimination caused by a neurological disorder

On pp. 108–115 and 115–123 I discussed evidence for the hypothesis that spatial-frequency discrimination and orientation discrimination are determined by the relative activity of spatial filters. A prediction of this hypothesis is that insensitivity of a filter that prefers spatial frequency S cycles/deg. and orientation θ degrees would elevate spatial-frequency discrimination threshold at test frequencies offset from S, and it would elevate orientation discrimination threshold at test orientation offset from θ (Regan, 1982). Figures 2.25 and 2.28 show evidence consistent with these predictions in the case of short-lived insensitivity caused by adaptation.

We found that patients with contrast sensitivity loss caused by multiple sclerosis showed the predicted elevation of spatial-frequency discrimination threshold (Regan et al., 1982). For example, a patient whose pattern of contrast sensitivity loss resembled that shown in Figure 2.67D had high contrast detection thresholds from 1 to 8 cycles/deg. Her spatial-frequency discrimination thresholds were normal from 1 to 8 cycles/deg. (at about 6 to 7%), but were much higher at frequencies above 8 cycles/deg.; at 12 cycles/deg., two gratings had to differ in spatial frequency by 25% before she could tell them apart.

How would the visual world look to this woman? Fine detail would be clearly visible, so the visual problem would be quite different from the familiar problem experienced by people with disorders such as short sight, amblyopia, or macular degeneration. *She would see a distorted world as distinct from a blurred world.*

Contrast sensitivity loss that is selective for spatial frequency and orientation, and is caused by refractive error

Some caution is called for when interpreting contrast sensitivity loss that is selective for orientation and spatial frequency. A sharp "notch" in the contrast sensitivity

---

who were themselves orphaned. Also, there were 3.5 million British children who were evacuated to safer locations, many spending years away from their parents in the care of randomly selected strangers. Some of these strangers provided loving care, some treated their evacuees as near-slaves [Wicks, 1989], and some evacuees endured years of physical abuse.) The idea of the Saturday morning pictures was, presumably, to allow our mothers more time to do useful things like filling shells with high explosives, helping to make bombers, parachutes, and so on. Johnny Mack Brown was dear to our hearts, because he was continuously in action; less highly regarded figures such as Gene Autry and Roy Rogers wasted time singing and talking to women—activities greeted with loud boos and catcalls. In at least one of his movies, Johnny Mack Brown conveyed to me a clear message: When the Pony Express rider crosses hostile Indian country, the further the journey, the less likely is the rider to arrive at his destination. This is the conceptual basis for our large dendritic field hypothesis of contrast sensitivity loss in ocular hypertension and glaucoma. So I called it "the Pony Express hypothesis."

Diplopic view of one grating

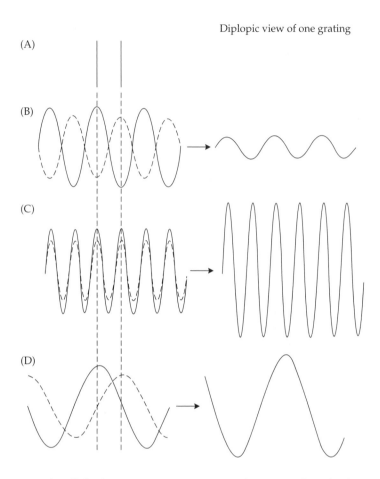

2.70 Monocular diplopia can cause one or more sharp "notches" in the contrast sensitivity curve. (A) In monocular diplopia, a single bright line is seen as double. (B) For a sinusoidal grating, the two images partially or completely cancel when the grating's period is exactly twice (or exactly two-thirds, and so on) of the diplopic separation between the two lines. Cancelation grows rapidly less as the grating's spatial frequency is increased (C) or decreased (D). From Regan (1989).

curve can result from small-angle monocular diplopia (double vision) of either optical or neural etiology—a not uncommon condition that can be either chronic or temporary (Fincham, 1963; Stampfer & Tredici, 1975; Records, 1980; Carney et al., 1981).

Chronic "notches" of optical origin are shown in Apkarian et al. (1987). In some normally sighted individuals it is possible to produce transient diplopia or neural original by occluding one eye while visually stimulating the fellow eye by, for example, a counterphase-modulated pattern of sharp-edged checks (Regan &

Maxner, 1986). And transient optical diplopia can be produced by deforming the eye mechanically with a tightly fitting eye patch (Regan & Maxner, 1986).

As its name implies, monocular diplopia manifests itself as a double image when a single target (e.g., a line or a letter) is viewed monocularly. When a spatially repetitive target such as a grating is viewed, the dysfunction shows as one or more orientation-selective "notches" in the contrast sensitivity curve. It has been suggested that these dips are produced by destructive interference between the two images (Regan & Maxner, 1986; Apkarian et al., 1987; Woods et al., 1996). Figure 2.70 illustrates this explanation. For example, if the angular deviation between the two images of a single small dot is about 2 minutes of arc, the contrast sensitivity curve would be expected to show its first notch at a spatial frequency of about 15 cycles/deg. This kind of sharp notch differs from the kind of contrast sensitivity loss observed in many patients with multiple sclerosis, Parkinson's disease, and amblyopia that extends either over a broad range of intermediate spatial frequencies or over a broad range of low and intermediate spatial frequencies, has a patchy distribution over the visual field, and is tuned to temporal frequency. Monocular double vision is readily detected by testing vision with a single narrow line.

CHAPTER 3

Color-Defined Form

Visual pigments of vertebrates and invertebrates are similar and ancient.
T. H. Goldsmith, *The Perception of Colour*, 1991

In the country of the blind, the one-eyed man is king.
Erasmus, *Adagia*, 1500

Preamble

Though they, as a species, must have come close to despair during their 7,000 year wait, dogs faithfully maintained their friendship with *Homo sapiens*, somehow passing on from generation to generation the belief, so evident in the dog of today, that humans were put on this earth to invent the motor car and drive them around in it. This may or may not be true. But for humans to believe that we have been given color vision to provide us with greater pleasure from sunsets, flowers, butterflies and so on,* is a kind of hubris that can, and historically has, led to nasty consequences. Very many animal classes, including many species of primate and

---

* An English television critic with leftist views who had heralded the future introduction of color TV with comments such as "unnecessary," and "money that could be better spent" changed his mind after seeing the first programs transmitted by the BBC. "Color TV will warm my old age," he wrote. "Women look much more attractive than in black and white." This comment sold many color TV sets.

other mammals, reptiles, birds, insects, and shallow-water fish possess color vision (or at least, multiple visual pigments),* although many species of nocturnal animals probably have very poor color vision. (For example, rats and cats do not learn to make color discriminations easily, and possess few cells that could support color vision [Goldsmith, 1991].)

> A predator with color vision can more easily break the camouflage of its food source, an advantage enjoyed also by herbivores (see Color Plate 5).

A second advantage offered by color vision is that characteristic patterns of coloring can help animals to recognize members of their own species—a point much exploited by birds and by the Englishmen who sport subtly striped ties to signal their membership in some cricket or gentleman's club of particularly exalted tone, or their having attended a public school.†

And an interesting idea. Having found that color information was more useful than luminance information in tasks that required memory ("even the barest amount of memory"), Sachtler and Zaidi (1992, p. 893) offered the following speculation: " . . . [T]he chromatic component of the light signal from an object is of considerably more use than the brightness component in identifying the object over viewings separated in time. The color temperature of ambient sunlight can vary over seasons and even during a day . . . but this variation is a minute fraction of the change in illuminance during a day. The light incident from an object over separate viewing would therefore be expected to exhibit a smaller variation in spectral composition than in brightness. The greater visual capability to remember chromaticities than brightnesses seems to be matched to this physical phenomenon."

The use of color in paintings (since c. 10,000 B.C.) and the historical development of color theory are related in fascinating style by Gouras (1991a).

However, in view of the formidable neural circuitry required to create visual sensitivity to color-defined (CD) form, present-day humans with defective color vision experience surprisingly little handicap. (Approximately 8% of the male population and 0.5% of the female population have congenitally defective color vision [Ruddock, 1991].) This raises the question: If color vision is (or was) so

---

* Three pigments is not the norm. Many species have two or four pigments. And pigments with maximum absorption in the near-ultraviolet part of the spectrum (at wavelengths that cannot be seen by humans) have been found in species of fish, turtles, and birds (Goldsmith, 1991).

† The British public school is very different from its namesake in the core of an American city. A British public school is not only a fee-paying private school, but a very special kind of private school. A 13-year-old who has passed the entrance examination and whose parents are willing to foot the bill is by no means necessarily acceptable at one these exalted institutions.

important, why do so many men have defective color vision? An intriguing hint is that dichromats can see color-camouflaged objects that cannot be seen by those with normal color vision (Morgan, Adam, & Mollon, 1992). Faced with a situation where the (fruit or animal) food supply was perfectly camouflaged, dichromats would eat while the normally sighted starved. In view of the very large imbalance (about 16:1) in the incidence of defective color vision in male and female humans, it would be interesting to know whether lions change their family habits when food is scarce.*

Recent reviews of color vision include *The Perception of Color* (edited by P. Gouras), *Human Color Vision* by P. K. Kaiser and R. M. Boynton, and a special edition of *Vision Research* (1998, vol. 38, no. 21). Mollon (1989) has discussed the origins and possible purposes of primate color vision.

The Concept of Equiluminance—and Caveats

Generally, threshold measurements of the pattern sensitivity of putative color pathways begins with two assumptions. First, experimenters often assume that the color sensitivities of the mechanisms are known before the experiment or that these properties can be measured with procedures such as flicker photometry. Second, the experimenter assumes that the pattern and color sensitivities are separable. This assumption is implicit in the act of measurement since, if separability fails, then the pattern and color-sensitivity curves are intertwined and we learn very little from an individual tuning curve. (Poirson and Wandell, 1993, p. 2468)

Can we see spatial form that is rendered visible by chromatic contrast alone?

Few readers who have worked through Chapter 2 will doubt that humans can detect spatial form on the basis of *achromatic spatial contrast*. Indeed, the basis for the concept of achromatic spatial contrast is given immediately by sensory experience: we can see a white object against a white ground when figure and ground have different perceived brightnesses but differ in no other way. Color-defined (CD) form, on the other hand, is a deceptively difficult topic. So we should start at the beginning by defining *color*. According to Wyszecki and Stiles (1967, p. 229): "Color is that aspect of visual perception by which an observer may distinguish differences between two structure-free fields of view of the same size and shape, such as may be caused by differences in the spectral composition of the radiant energy concerned in the observation."

Some readers may be left with the uneasy feeling that this definition, authoritative though it is, lacks substance. And indeed it is a definition of exclusion.

---

* Female lions do most if not all of the hunting as well as the feeding, educating, and rearing of cubs while the male lions rest. Other than passing on their genes (at which they are famously adept), the only role of the male lion seems to be seeing off hyenas.

When you exclude texture contrast and (by implication) achromatic contrast, motion contrast, and disparity contrast, what you are left with, if anything, is chromatic contrast.

"If anything?" The common form of congenital color blindness provides indirect evidence that something is left. For, example the structure of a sinusoidal grating composed of alternate red and green bars cannot be seen by a deuteranope when the relative intensities of the red and green bars are adjusted appropriately. A deuteranope reports an unpatterned area of uniform brightness and uniform color—even though, as is usually the case, the deuteranope has normal sensitivity to the monochromatic contrast of a red or a green grating (Birch, 1991, 1993). Yet the red–green grating is clearly visible to a normally sighted observer. We conclude that the normally sighted observer has something that the dichromat does not have. That something we call visual sensitivity to chromatic contrast. (For an objective demonstration of this point, see Figure 3.15.) For the present I will suppose that the spatial difference that renders the grating visible to us is "whatever it is in the stimulus that creates the difference in our irreducibly basic perceptual experiences of redness and greenness"—and will discuss some caveats later on.

Less compelling is a finding first reported by Liebman in 1927. She observed that, if a form and its surrounding differ sufficiently in color, the eye can segregate the form from its surrounding whatever the luminance difference between the form and its surrounding, even when the form is of sufficiently small angular size that it stimulates a retinal area that is approximately homogeneous in its color properties. She also noted that the boundaries of a sharp-edged target appear blurred close to the equiluminant point. This *Liebman effect* is even more striking when both lateral and longitudinal ocular chromatic aberrations are canceled simultaneously (Regan, 1973b).

The Liebman effect shows that *something* happens when the relative intensities of the differently colored figure and ground are set to some unique ratio. The perception of the figure's sharp edges is lost, that is, information about the high spatial frequency content of the figure is lost. But lacking here is a demonstration that the achromatic contrast system has been "silenced" to the point that figure–ground segregation is demonstrably not being supported by the achromatic contrast system, i.e.,

---

Visibility of the figure as a whole is not created by the spatial filters for achromatic contrast discussed in Chapter 2.

From the fact that the figure and ground look different subjectively (e.g., a red hue versus a green hue) it does not necessarily follow that this red–green difference is the entire or even partial cause of the figure–ground segregation. For example, it might be the case (and often is the case, see the next section) that ocular chromatic aberrations create sufficient achromatic contrast to support figure–ground segregation, and this would be just as much the case for a person with no color vision whatsoever as for a person with normal color vision.

Now we are at the crux of the problem: if our aim is to silence the achromatic system—assuming that this is possible*—it is necessary to establish the appropriate measure of achromatic contrast.

The distinction between the processing of achromatic contrast, monochromatic contrast, and chromatic contrast: Some hypotheses

I will follow the usage of Switkes and several (but not all) color vision researchers who regard *achromatic contrast* as a property of stimuli that appear white, and thus, in the three-channel standard model, would activate neither the red–green (R–G) nor the blue–yellow (B–Y) opponent systems. A white grating is isochromatic, as is, for example, a red, green, yellow, or blue monochromatic grating. But these monochromatic gratings could activate, depending on their chromaticity, both a putative luminance mechanism and one or both of the color mechanisms (E. Switkes, personal communication, December 1998). The importance of making a clear distinction between achromatic contrast, monochromatic contrast and chromatic contrast will become evident in later sections. In everyday (naked-eye) vision, the longitudinal (axial) chromatic aberration of the eye plays an important role in the perception of colored objects. The objective data shown in Figure 3.1 document this point—the difference in lens power required to sharply accommodate monochromatic targets of wavelengths 645 nm and 436 nm differ by approximately two diopters. The data shown were obtained by recording signals from the human brain, but they agree well with data obtained behaviorally. See Helmholtz (1962/1866); Ivanoff (1947); Hartridge (1947, 1950); Campbell (1957); Bradley et al. (1992); and Zhang et al. (1991).

As Marimont and Wandell (1994, p. 3113) said,

> ... it is apparent that high-spatial frequency components of the image can play little role in contrast and color appearance and that in the spatial frequency range from 5 to 20 cycles/deg. the visual system is dichromatic, because there is no contrast in the short-wavelength receptor signal.
>
> Color-matching experiments are the key behavioural experiments that define the relationship between the initial encoding of light by photopigments and the physiological response of the photoreceptors . . . . The color-matching experiments used to define the properties of the encoding of light in the CIE's 1931

---

* In discussing the idea that the magnocellular stream is the physiological substrate of the achromatic system of psychophysics, Lee et al. (1988) noted that the phasic retinal ganglion cells of the magnocellular stream that sum the outputs of medium- and long-wavelength cones could, by virtue of an early nonlinearity, respond to equiluminant red–green gratings. In other words, they suggested that it might not be possible to silence the achromatic contrast system by adjusting the luminances of the red and green components of a red–green grating. Schiller and Colby (1983) had earlier noted that individual magnocellular neurons are not silenced for any red–green luminance ratio when stimulated by red–green alternation.

As to the possibility of silencing of the parvocellular neurons of the lateral geniculate body, Schiller and Colby (1983) pointed out that each cell has a different "equiluminant point," so that all the cells within the population cannot be silenced simultaneously.

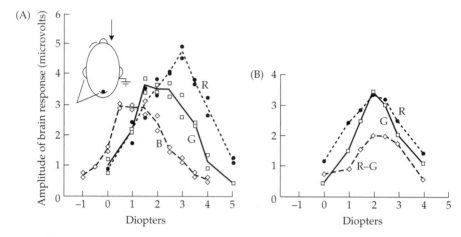

3.1 The longitudinal (axial) chromatic aberration of the human eye. I paralyzed the accommodation of one eye by applying a drug to my eyeball. This also dilated my pupil so that I viewed the stimulus (a pattern of sharp-edged monochromatic checks of side length 0.2 degrees that subtended 2.2 degrees) through an artificial pupil of diameter 2 min. The data points plot the amplitude of the 7 Hz component of brain responses produced by counterphase modulating the checks at 3.5 Hz (ordinate) versus the power of a lens placed in front of the eye. (A) Relative to the red (645 nm), the chromatic aberrations for the green (550 nm) and blue (436 nm) lights were, respectively, 0.7 and 2.0 diopters. (B) Brain responses to a monochromatic red (R), a monochromatic green (G), and an equiluminant red–green (R–G) grating recorded after canceling the eye's chromatic aberrations. Noise levels were between 0.2 and 0.3 microvolts (horizontal arrows). From Regan (1973b).

and 1964 standards are based on relatively large uniform fields. When we restrict our analysis of the photoreceptor absorptions to large uniform fields, we can avoid the effects of axial chromatic aberration for color matching.

In this section I address the following question: How can we create a spatial form (e.g., a grating) that is rendered visible by virtue of its chromatic spatial contrast only? Before addressing this practical question we must back up a little because, as discussed in the previous section, to ask the question is to assume implicitly that it is possible to see spatial form in the absence of achromatic contrast.

One of the several hypotheses that more clearly state this somewhat loosely framed assumption is depicted graphically in Figure 3.2: a *zone hypothesis* of color vision. According to such hypotheses, signals from long-wavelength (L) cones, medium-wavelength (M) cones, and short-wavelength (S) cones are summed directly to give the luminance signal.* (Though the S-cone contribution is very

---

* The discussion of psychophysical models framed in terms of two or more parallel spatial filters on pp. 262–266 sets out a radically different hypothesis.

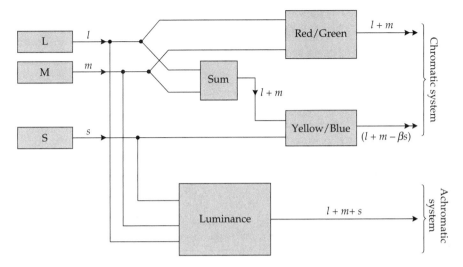

3.2 Walraven's version of the zone theory of color vision. Long-wavelength (L), medium-wavelength (M), and short-wavelength (S) cones feed red–green opponent and yellow–blue opponent color stages. The luminance signal is the sum of the three cone outputs (the S-cone contribution to luminance is very small). β is a scaling factor. From Walraven (1962).

weak, see Stockman et al. [1993]; Drum [1983]; Grinberg & Williams [1985]; and Wilson et al. [1988]). Red versus green is signaled by the difference between the L- and M-cone outputs. Blue versus yellow is signaled by first combining the L- and M-cone outputs and then subtracting the S-cone output. In this particular zone model (Walraven's), the S-cone output is first multiplied by a constant (to allow for its very small contribution to luminance and large [i.e., high *saturation*] contribution to hue perception).

In Figure 3.2 the first stage of visual processing is the absorption of light by photoreceptor cells. The long-wavelength, medium-wavelength, and short-wavelength cones operate at high intensities of light. They support color vision and high visual acuity. The rods enable us to see in very dimly illuminated environments, though with poor visual acuity and no color vision. All photoreceptors obey the *principle of univariance.* Although the light falling on, for example, a cone can vary in wavelength, the cone's electrical polarization increases with the rate at which light energy is absorbed independently of the wavelength of the light. The only effect of a change in wavelength is to change the probability that any given photon will be absorbed.* Although the output of any given cone is color-blind (it does not

---

* At the turn of the century, classical physics faced a problem that would have attracted hilarity and scorn from the general public and some wonderful articles in satirical magazines, had the general public heard of it. According to classical physics, the power radiated

distinguish between a change of wavelength and a change of intensity), the visual system achieves color vision by comparing the rates of absorption in the three classes of cone.

The kind of spectral sensitivity curves shown in Color Plate 6 are based on data obtained from individual photoreceptors by researchers exercising the highest levels of technical and scientific ingenuity (Liebman & Entine, 1964; Marks, Dobelle, & MacNichol, 1964; Brown & Wald, 1964; Dartnall, Bowmaker, & Baylor, 1983; Schnapf, Kraft, & Baylor, 1987).

But the fact is that color information, at some stage, restricted to three channels (the *trichromatic theory of vision*) had long been known. The realization can be traced back through Helmholtz (in 1866), Young (in 1802), and Palmer (1777), to Lomonosov in 1757 (Weale, 1957).* According to Wright (1970), the first set of color mixture curves was published by Maxwell in 1860—the same Maxwell who, through Maxwell's equations, gave us the basis for understanding electromagnetic radiation and who, among many other major contributions, introduced *Maxwell's demon* to the new science of thermodynamics.

The contrast sensitivity curves for isolated M cones and L cones are much as shown by the filled circles in Figure 1.19. But the isolated S-cone system is a *low-vision* system. Contrast sensitivity peaks near 1 cycle/deg., and grating acuity is 2.5 to 10 cycles/deg. (Mollon, 1982). This low acuity is a consequence of the sparse distribution of S cones (Marc & Sperling, 1977; Sperling, 1980). The frac-

---

by a red-hot poker should be infinite. The magnitude of Max Planck's achievement is brought out by the fact that this embarrassing prediction had been known by physicists worldwide for many years before he proposed that the red-hot poker radiates energy in packets. The amount of energy in a packet (called a *quantum*) depends on the wavelength of the radiation. Its value (E) is equal to hc/λ, where h is *Planck's constant* (h = 6.6×10^{-27} erg–sec.), and c is the speed of light (3.0×10^8 m/sec.). It is not possible to emit a fraction of a quantum.

Planck's hypothesis did not require that energy should be radiated in *localized* packets. The idea that quanta are localized was introduced by Einstein. Early in the twentieth century it was found that light can cause atoms to emit electrons (the *photoelectric effect*) and that the energy carried by any given electron was very much greater than that which, according to the classical electromagnetic wave theory, could have been absorbed by the atom. Some years after Planck had put forward his quantum hypothesis, Einstein proposed that light is absorbed in such a way that the energy of the light beam appears to be concentrated in localized packets (called *photons*) rather than being spread evenly over the beam and that the energy in a photon is equal to hc/λ. Einstein was awarded the Nobel Prize for this theory of the photoelectric effect.

* Because there are only three parallel color channels, many combinations of wavelengths can produce the same color sensation (metamerism). This is a general property of multi-channel systems.

The trivariance of color vision allows the colors of paints, wallpapers, car bodies, and so on to be specified in terms of three numbers. The basis for this CIE system (Appendix G) is the experimental data on color matching collected by Wright and Guild in the late 1920s. David Wright's obituary, published by the *Daily Telegraph* on 3 July 1997, and entitled "Professor David Wright: Scientist who laid the foundations for colour television in 1930," stated that, "In the late 1920s, Wright measured, for 10 observers, the way in which

tion of S cones relative to all cones is zero or near-zero in the foveola (Williams et al., 1981), rises to a peak of approximately 0.16 at an eccentricity of 1.0 deg., and falls to 8 to 10% in the parafovea (Mollon, 1983). (The foveola is an area of diameter 20 minutes of arc located at the exact center of the fovea; see Color Plate 9.) The distance between S cones in the human fovea has been estimated at about 10 minutes of arc by psychophysical means, and about 11 minutes of arc by physiological means (Williams et al., 1981; Ahnelt et al., 1987). When corrected for hexagonal packing, intercone spacings of 8 to 11 minutes of arc correspond to a Nyquist limit of about 4 cycles/deg. (Hirsch & Miller, 1987). These figures for the isolated S cones are far inferior to the 25 seconds of arc intercone separation and corresponding 56 cycles/deg. Nyquist frequency for the foveal M and L cones (see pp. 477–481).

In sharp contrast with their spatial properties, the dynamic characteristics of the three cone types are closely similar. For all three types, sensitivity falls off for frequencies above about 10 Hz, but responses can be recorded up to about 40 Hz (Stockman et al., 1993).

The hypothesis of opponent-color processing was originally proposed to account for subjective observations of color appearance. In particular, if one superimposes a green light on a red light and progressively increases from zero the luminance of the green light, there comes a point where the red hue is annihilated. Similarly, by increasing the luminance of a red light that is superimposed

---

the colours of the spectrum are matched by beams of red, green and blue light added together. . . . Wright carried out his work on colour in the Physics Department of Imperial College and, except for a short break from 1929 to 1930, he spent the whole of his career there. . . . In that interlude he was a research engineer at Westinghouse Electric and Manufacturing Company, in Pittsburgh, where he worked on color television. . . . This was long before even black-and-white television had been properly developed: but the colour television systems in use today depend on Wright's work as the basis of their reproduction of colour by the addition of areas of red, green, and blue light."

It was W. D. Wright who sparked my interest in vision research. Among the many things that he taught me, by example, and in his low-key manner, was that meticulously careful and honest experimental work is the first priority in research. Also, that you must understand how any piece of equipment works before you use it. Better still—design and make it yourself. Always use the simplest equipment that will allow you to carry out your experiment. I learned that I must remain at all times alert to the artifactual effects (which can seduce you into making a public fool of yourself) that even simple equipment can produce. To use more complex equipment than is necessary is to take unnecessary risks of being fooled by occult artifactual effects that are beyond one's wit to recognize for the rubbish they are. And Professor Wright made it clear that a deliberate failure to cite relevant previous research is dishonorable.

I once asked him which, of all the things he had done in science, most pleased him. He told me that it was his having produced, at very short notice, deep-red goggles that offered some distraction to the young men waiting to be summoned to their waiting Spitfires or Hurricanes and ordered to fly over blacked-out England in an attempt to defend the cities against the night bombers. Instead of sitting around in the dark, waiting, thinking, and trying to hold down their fear, these goggles allowed the young men to play billiards or other games while maintaining their eyes in a state of dark adaptation.

on a green light, the green hue can be annihilated. The same is true of perceived yellowness versus perceived blueness, but not of redness versus blueness, redness versus yellowness, greenness versus blueness or greenness versus yellowness. So there is something special about the red–green and blue-yellow pairings that is not a property of the other four pairings. It was Hering who, in 1870, first proposed that, following the photoreceptor stage of processing retinal image information, there is a stage at which cone outputs are combined by taking their sums and differences (Hering, 1920). The characteristics of this second, color-opponent, stage of processing have been estimated by the method of canceling perceived hues. *Chromatic valence* curves are shown in Figure 3.3.

Hurvich and Jameson used unique blue, unique green, unique yellow, and unique red lights as their cancelation stimuli, their rationale being that unique blue or unique yellow is perceived when the red–green opponent system is in equilibrium (i.e., *silent*), and unique green or unique red is perceived when the blue–yellow opponent system is in equilibrium (Hurvich & Jameson, 1955, 1957; Jameson & Hurvich, 1955). And indeed, there is an equivalence between chromatic valence data and independent data on unique hues (Bruns et al., 1984; Ayama et al., 1987).

Qualitatively similar sensitivity curves were obtained by Poirson and Wandell (1993) using a quite different approach based on their observation that the color appearance of a monochromatic squarewave grating depends markedly on its spatial frequency. The hue cancelation technique presupposes opponency. But Poirson and Wandell's approach does not.

In more recently proposed zone models, the inputs to the red–green opponent mechanism are weighted cone outputs $(k_1l + k_2m + k_3s)$, as are the inputs to the yellow–blue opponent mechanism $(k_4l + k_5m + k_6s)$ and to the luminance mechanism $(k_7l + k_8m + k_9s)$ (Sperling & Harwerth, 1971; Eisner & MacLeod, 1980; Noorlander et al., 1981; Noorlander & Koenderink, 1983; Thornton & Pugh, 1983a,b; Stromeyer et al., 1985; Cavanagh et al., 1987; Stromeyer et al., 1987; Lee & Stromeyer, 1989; Cole et al., 1993; Chaparro et al., 1994). There is general agreement that the L-cone and M-cone inputs to the red–green mechanism have similar weightings and that the S-cone input to the luminance mechanism is weak. It seems, however, that the cone weightings depend on temporal frequency (Figure 3.9) and spatial frequency (Gordon & Shapley, 1989; Marimont & Wandell, 1994). A recent tabulation of the weightings (at particular values of temporal and spatial frequency, means of three observers) is as follows: $k_1 = 0.74$; $k_2 = -0.67$; $k_3 = -0.01$; $k_4 = 0.39$; $k_5 = 0.39$; $k_6 = -0.83$; $k_7 = 0.96$; $k_8 = 0.89$; $k_9 = 0.05$ (Sankeralli & Mullen, 1996). (On pp. 262–266 I discuss a different kind of model in which an intermediate stage of processing is placed after the cones and before the opponent stage that determines color appearance).

Kranz (1975) drew attention to a caveat by asking whether different chromatic valence functions would be obtained if different canceling hues were used (noting that, if that were so, the chromatic valence functions would not mean very much). Kranz showed that a chromatic valence function would be independent of

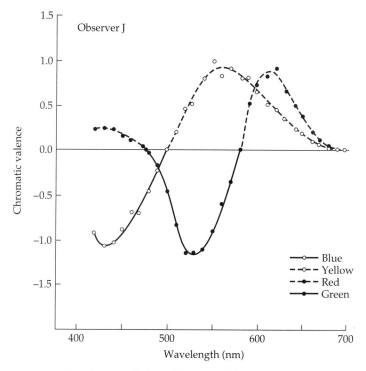

3.3 Opponent-color characteristics of human vision. The chromatic response or "valence" curves of human color vision. The red–green opponent process is indicated by filled symbols, and the blue–yellow opponent process by open symbols. From Jameson and Hurvich (1955).

the choice of canceling hues, if and only if it is a linear function of tristimulus values. (*Tristimulus values* are explained in Wright, 1991.) With this caveat in mind, Ayama and Ikeda (1989) remeasured the chromatic valence functions using three of four different cancelation hues for each of the four segments of the valence curves. They found that the shapes of the red, green, and yellow segments depended on the choice of canceling hue, though the shape of the blue segment did not. In an attempt to make quantitative sense of these findings, they proposed candidate nonlinear equations to relate the cone spatial sensitivities to the measured chromatic valence functions.

Van Dijk and Spekreijse (1983) provide a quantitative discussion of nonlinear opponency at the physiological level. Seizing onto the finding that Ethambutol (a drug used to treat patients with tuberculosis) does not affect the cone sensitivities but can cause color vision defects (Zrenner & Krüger, 1981), they investigated the effect of Ethambutol in carp, a fish with trichromatic color vision. They confirmed the Ethambutol did not affect the sensitivities of the cones, nor did it affect the horizontal cells (Figure 1.9). At this level, processing is linear for small signals, as expressed in the notation of receptive field coding with plusses and minuses (Tomita et al., 1967; Spekreijse & Norton, 1970). Nor did the drug affect simple algebraic opponency of the kind discussed earlier in this section and investigated by Sankeralli and Mullen (1996). The drug exerted a selective effect on nonlinear color-opponent properties of the responses of ganglion cells. Since Ethambutol did not influence the maintained activity of ganglion cells, and did not affect the center and surround sensitivities, vanDijk and Spekreijse concluded that it was the bipolar or the amacrine cells that were affected by the drug and that those cells were, therefore, the source of the nonlinear processing. The nonlinear process was *inhibition*.

Let Reichardt and Poggio (1981, p. 187) have the last word on this: ". . . every nontrivial computation has to be essentially nonlinear, that is, not representable (even approximately) by linear operations."

Summarizing thus far:

> Zone theories of color vision, such as the version depicted in Figure 3.2, account for the facts of color matching (i.e., the trivariance of color vision; see Wright, 1991) in terms of the first stage of processing, while the second stage explains subjective observations on the appearance of colors and data such as those shown in Figure 3.3.

Reviews of color appearance and color appearance systems are provided by Pokorny et al. (1991) and by Derenfeldt (1991).

Figure 3.4A shows a modified version of Figure 3.2 that will be more suitable for our present purpose. Figure 3.4A illustrates one of several candidate hypotheses of how spatial contrast is processed. An important difference from the hypoth-

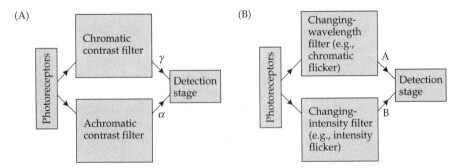

3.4 Working hypotheses. (A) The processing of chromatic and achromatic spatial contrast. (B) Temporal characteristics of chromatic and achromatic processing.
Signals γ and α carry a spatial contrast label, whereas signals A and B carry a temporal change label. Although depicted separately for convenience, the spatial characteristics in part (A) and the temporal characteristics in part (B) are the spatial and temporal characteristics of the same achromatic and chromatic systems. Part A from Regan, Kaiser, and Nakano (1993); B from Regan (1991b).

esis illustrated in Figure 3.2 is that I do not assume that the spectral sensitivity of the achromatic system is described by the CIE V_λ curve (see pp. 219–220, and Appendix G), nor even by the individual observer's spectral sensitivity curve obtained by any of the methods reviewed later in the chapter. Note also that this hypothesis specifies that achromatic system is a unity (though other hypotheses specify two or more parallel subsystems for achromatic spatial contrast, see pp. 262–266), but does allow for the possibility that its spectral sensitivity curve may vary with spatial frequency. I will return to this point later.

Achromatic contrast in Figure 3.4A is the kind of spatial contrast that renders a white grating visible, and that, throughout Chapter 2, I have referred to, somewhat loosely, as *luminance contrast* on the (so far, unjustified) assumption that the response of the achromatic contrast mechanism is a response to the luminance contrast of the stimulus. In the next section I will define the term *luminance*.

CIE luminance and "sensation luminance"

The mandate of the International Commission on Illumination (Commission Internationale de l'Éclairage, CIE) includes the task of defining the units and procedures for measuring the effect of light power on the human visual system (see Appendix G). For our immediate purpose it is only necessary to note that luminance, measured in *candelas per square meter* (cd/m^2), is the CIE-defined variable nearest to what is in everyday language called "the brightness of a surface" (though they are by no means the same thing) and, in particular, the following: Luminance is defined in terms of candelas per unit area; candelas are defined in terms of *lumens*; the lumen is, in effect, defined as follows, "one-watt power of monochromatic radiation of wavelength 555 nm provides 683 lumens"; that the watt is a unit of physically measurable *power*. In short:

> The CIE has defined the intensive effect exerted by light of wavelength 555 nm upon the human visual system (a subjective effect) in terms of a quantity that can be measured physically.

At *photopic* levels the CIE defined the intensive effect of light of wavelengths other than 555 nm by reference to the so-called V_λ curve (see Appendix G). For our present purpose, the crucial point of all this is that the concept of CIE luminance takes no account of interindividual variations of sensitivity, and that these variations can be substantial even within a particular age group.* Consequently, authors who define equiluminance in terms of the CIE standard observer—perhaps by using a photoelectric photometer whose spectral sensitivity is calibrated to match the CIE (theoretical standard observer) V_λ curve—may find that their equiluminant lights do not produce the same intensive effect on the visual systems of many if not all of their real observers.

---

* As to the effect of age on vision, Weale (1963) has documented the progressive deterioration of visual sensitivity in near-Shakespearean terms.

An alternative and more satisfactory procedure is to equate the intensive effect of the differently colored lights relative to each individual observer's spectral sensitivity curve. Three alternative procedures designated to achieve this equalization of intensive effect are described in the next section. Kaiser (1988) has called this procedure *"equating sensation luminance."*

The concept of equiluminance

The concept of equiluminance is commonly encountered in one of two contexts: (1) experiments in which the eye is stimulated by a variation of color across space and (2) experiments in which the eye is stimulated by a variation of color across time. In both cases, the aim of adjusting the two (or more) colors to equiluminance is to eliminate any stimulation of the *achromatic system*, i.e., to "silence" the achromatic system.

In our present context, the relevance of time-domain data is to allow spatial patterns of colors across space to be presented with a time course that allows the achromatic spatial system depicted in Figure 3.4A to be most effectively silenced.

Figure 3.4B illustrates one hypothesis of the distinction between the achromatic and chromatic systems for processing temporal changes. Note that the hypothesis illustrated in Figure 3.4B does not assume that the spectral sensitivity of the achromatic system is described by the CIE V_λ curve nor even by the individual observer's spectral sensitivity curve obtained by any of the methods reviewed in this chapter (though other hypotheses specify that the spectral sensitivity of the achromatic system is one of these four possibilities).

> Note also that this hypothesis allows for the possibility that temporal selectivity of the chromatic system may depend on spectral location.

"Heterochromatic flicker photometry": A candidate procedure for silencing the achromatic system

The purpose of *heterochromatic flicker photometry* (HFP) is to equate the intensive effects on a particular individual's visual system of two differently colored lights. At least two different procedures can be listed under the HFP heading. Both procedures pit the visual effects of a flickering colored light against a flickering standard light (commonly a standard white light; see Appendix G).

In the classical HFP procedure, the flicker modulation waveform may be squarewave or sinusoidal, and the modulation depth is usually 100%. The stimulus field is a homogeneous patch of light, usually of about 1 to 5 degrees subtense (so as to restrict it to a relatively homogeneous foveal region), and a white surround field is advantageous (Walsh, 1953, p. 304). When the two superimposed lights are modulated in antiphase and the modulation rate is not too high, an observer will see the light flickering in both color and brightness. If the modulation frequency is increased in small steps, a point can be reached when the color flicker just disappears and the observer sees a light of constant color whose brightness is flickering.

With the mean luminance of the standard held constant, the mean luminance of the colored light is then adjusted to give minimal flicker. At this point the luminance of the colored light is defined to be equal to the luminance of the standard white light.

The classical procedure just described has the disadvantage that the mean luminance and also the spectral distribution of the stimulus vary during the adjustment procedure, thus varying the eye's state of adaptation to both luminance and color. I introduced an alternative procedure that does not have these disadvantages (Regan, 1970). The basic idea is to increase the modulation depth of one of the two lights while decreasing the modulation depth of the other in a yoked manner, keeping the mean luminance and the chromaticity of the stimulus constant throughout. An intuitive grasp of this procedure can be obtained by inspecting Figure 3.5. Using a 24 Hz modulation frequency, I carried out modulation HFP while recording the 48 Hz brain responses generated within the observer's visual cortex. The point of minimum (near-zero) subjective flicker, shown by the arrow, was very close to the sharp minimum in the amplitude of the brain response. As would be expected, the phase of the brain response (filled triangles and dotted line in Figure 3.5) shifted through 360 degrees near the point of minimum amplitude. The relative modulations of the two lights at minimum flicker quantified the relative mean luminances of the two lights.

I repeated the procedure just discussed for several monochromatic lights whose wavelengths ranged from 440 nm (blue) to 630 nm (red), flickering each in turn against the same reference white light. Each measurement gave a curve like the one in Figure 3.5. From the minima in the curves I derived a relative luminosity curve. The relative luminosities agreed closely (to within 0.07 log units) with corresponding data obtained using psychophysical modulation heterochromatic flicker photometry.*

Pokorny et al. (1989) developed a variant of the *modulation HFP* procedure just described in which the two modulation depths are decreased in tandem (rather

---

* Regan and Lee (1993) proposed that the contributions to cortical activity in humans of the magnocellular and parvocellular streams, respectively, are reflected in the properties of the high-frequency and medium-frequency systems in the brain's response to flicker.

Human brain responses to flicker reveal three parallel systems: the low-frequency system with a peak near 10 Hz, the high-frequency system with a peak near 40 Hz (Regan, 1964; van der Tweel & Lunel, 1965; Spekreijse, 1966; Regan, 1966, 1968), and the medium-frequency system with a peak near 16 Hz (Regan, 1968, 1975a). Regan and Lee (1993) compared the following properties of magnocellular and parvocellular neurons in the macaque monkey with the properties of the high-frequency and medium-frequency responses in humans: (a) spectral sensitivity as measured by variable-modulation HFP; (b) the effects of the relative phase of the two lights in variable-modulation HFP; (c) the effects of flicker modulation depth. In all three respects, the properties of magnocellular neurons corresponded closely to the properties of the human high-frequency brain response but were quite different from the properties of the human medium-frequency response. The properties of parvocellular neurons corresponded closely to the properties of the human medium-frequency response, but were quite different from those of the human high-frequency response.

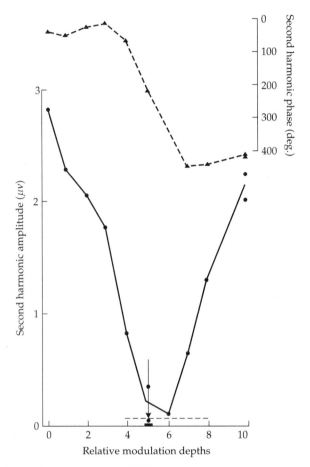

3.5 Modulation heterochromatic flicker photometry procedure for equating the luminance of two lights of different colors. An unpatterned patch of monochromatic red (630 nm) light was superimposed in an unpatterned patch of green (544 nm) light and both were sinusoidally modulated in antiphase at a frequency of 24 Hz. The modulation depth of the red and green lights were, respectively, 0% and 30% at zero on the abscissa, and 30% and 0% at 10 on the abscissa. Data points plot the amplitude and phase of a 48 Hz electrical signal recorded from the brain. The point of minimum (near-zero) subjective flicker is arrowed, with the range of six settings indicated by the bar. Zero of phase is arbitrary. The dotted line shows the noise level recorded with both lights unmodulated. From Regan (1970).

than increasing one while decreasing the other) so as to give a flicker/no-flicker endpoint rather than requiring the observer to judge the point of minimum flicker.

The HFP method is, perhaps, the most commonly used psychophysical procedure by authors attempting to silence the achromatic system.

The "minimally distinct border": A candidate procedure for silencing the achromatic system

The *minimally distinct border* technique of heterochromatic photometry developed by Boynton and Kaiser is based on the Liebmann effect described earlier in this chapter. The procedure is as follows. The stimulus is similar to the classic bipartite field of colorimetry: two untextured patches of light that are separated by a sharp border. When the colors of the two patches are the same and their luminances are matched, the sharp border disappears totally. When the two patches have different colors the border is always visible. But when the ratio between the luminances of the two patches of light is set to some unique value, the perceived sharpness of the border falls to a minimum. This unique ratio is close to the equiluminant point measured using heterochromatic flicker photometry (Kaiser, 1971; Boynton, 1973, 1978).

According to Kaiser and Boynton (1996), minimally distinct border matches have the properties of additivity, proportionality, and transitivity required of a photometric technique.*

The contribution of the short-wavelength cones to edge perception seems to be small compared with the contribution of medium- (M) and long- (L) wavelength cones. When the (M cone – L cone) difference signal across the border is zero, as in the case of a pair of tritanopic lights that differ only in the degree to which they excite the short-wavelength cones, the border is very indistinct (Kaiser & Boynton, 1996).

"Minimal motion": A candidate procedure for silencing the achromatic system

When a grating composed of two different colors is in continuous motion, the perceived speed of motion falls to a minimum when the ratio between the luminances of the two color components is adjusted to some unique value (Gregory, 1974; Cavanagh et al., 1984). And the apparent motion that is commonly evident when a pattern of differently colored checks is counterphase-modulated (individual checks appear to dart around although they are in fact stationary) is abolished for some unique luminance ratio (Regan, 1973b; Anstis & Cavanagh, 1983). The unique ratio for which continuous or apparent motion is reduced to a minimum (or abolished) is close to the equiluminant point measured by heterochromatic flicker photometry (Regan, 1973b; Gregory, 1974; Moreland, 1982; Anstis &

---

* According to Kaiser and Boynton (1996, pp. 139–371), additivity means that if stimulus A is indistinguishable from stimulus B, and C is indistinguishable from D, then A + C will be indistinguishable from B + D. "Transitivity occurs when radiances of wavelengths A and B are adjusted for equal luminance by conventional flicker photometry, and when B and C are similarly equated, after which A and C produce minimum flicker when directly exchanged (LeGrand, 1968). . . . The proportionality corollary states that when the luminances of two different colors are set to produce minimum flicker they will continue to yield minimum flicker when both colors are increased or decreased by identical factors."

Cavanagh, 1983; Cavanagh et al., 1984, 1987; Mullen & Boulton, 1992; Teller & Lindsey, 1993).

The minimal motion technique of heterochromatic photometry has been used by several authors aiming to silence the achromatic system (e.g., Mullen & Losada, 1994).

Do all methods of measuring luminance give the same result?

Lennie et al. (1993) stated that:

> All techniques for measuring spectral sensitivity require the comparison of lights of different spectral composition presented either jointly or in nulling procedures such as HFP, minimally distinct border (MDB), and brightness matching or sequentially in threshold procedures such as critical flicker fusion (CFF) and increment threshold procedures. Hence all photometric procedures that involve presentation of suprathreshold lights have the potential to adapt the three classes of cone differently. . . . The effect of this on the spectral sensitivity function will depend substantially on the method of measurement. . . . Spectral sensitivities measured by a CFF technique (Marks & Bornstein, 1974) at moderate and high luminances are narrower than those obtained with the use of conventional HFP at comparable light levels, presumably representing more extreme wavelength-dependent adaptation . . . we should not be surprised that techniques that provide different opportunities for light adaptation in the three classes of cone yield different spectral-sensitivity curves. However, we also need to consider additional factors that might explain why the different methods give rise to different spectral-sensitivity functions. An obvious possibility is that the different techniques tap different underlying mechanisms that have different spectral sensitivities. (p. 1286)

And Webster and Mollon (1993, p. 1332) concluded, "These results suggest that different measures of equiluminance tap neural pathways that can have different spectral sensitivities. At low temporal frequencies both perceived lightness and minimum-motion setting appear to depend on channels that do not represent luminance and color independently." We will return to this point on pp. 262–266 (see Figure 3.26).

"The titration method": A candidate procedure for silencing the achromatic system

The titration procedure for silencing the achromatic system has the advantage that it can provide a clear indicator that the achromatic system has indeed been silenced—a feature that is lacking in the methods described in detail on pp. 220–224. (However, this indicator may not be present in some cases where the achromatic system is, in fact, silenced.)

Because the temporal version of the titration method is more readily understood than the spatial version, I will first describe the temporal version. The temporal version was implemented with a *wavelength modulator* that I designed in 1965. This device was a double-pass monochromator that gave as output high-purity monochromatic spectral light (15 nm full bandwidth at half-power) when it was fed white light. The special feature was its unusual dynamic response characteristic: the output wavelength could be varied as a continuous function of time with a ± 3 dB small signal bandwidth of 0 to 70 Hz. A plan of the device is given in Regan and Tyler (1971a).

As illustrated in Figure 3.6A, the light fed to the wavelength modulator had already passed through a luminance modulator (a device that could vary the luminance of the light independently of the wavelength modulator) so that the light entering the observer's eye could be modulated simultaneously in wavelength

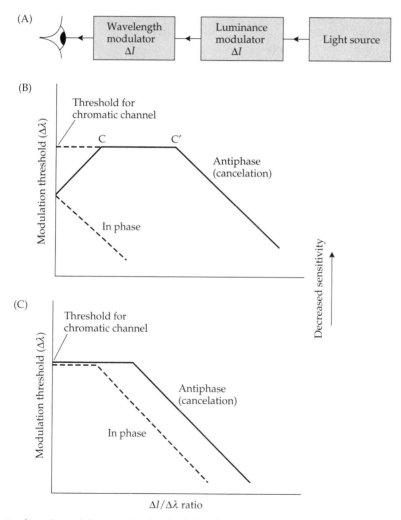

3.6 Explanation of the psychophysical titration procedure. See text for details. From Regan (1991).

and luminance by any desired waveform. The two modulations could differ in phase or frequency. The observer's eye was stimulated in Maxwellian view. The unpatterned stimulus field subtended 2 degrees.

The titration procedure, an ingenious method for silencing the achromatic system, was invented by Christopher Tyler. The principle is explained in the idealized Figure 3.6B,C. Suppose that the wavelength and the intensity of the 2 degree field are simultaneously modulated by sinusoidal waveforms with the same frequency and that the peak-to-peak amplitudes of these modulations are $\Delta\lambda$ and ΔI, respectively (Figure 3.6A). The observer is provided with a knob that reduces $\Delta\lambda$ and ΔI by the same fraction for each degree of rotation.

In the first experiment we arrange that the two modulations differ in temporal phase by 180 degrees. We start with $\Delta I = 0$ (i.e., zero added intensity modulation) and instruct the observer to adjust the knob until flicker is just detectable. Now with a small amount of added intensity modulation (a small value of the ratio $\Delta I/\Delta\lambda$) the observer again sets flicker threshold. The procedure is repeated for many values of the ratio $\Delta I/\Delta\lambda$. The continuous line in Figure 3.6B shows the following:

> Small amounts of added intensity modulation have a counterintuitive effect. Flicker threshold is elevated, that is, the observer appears to be less sensitive to flicker.

Further increases in the amount of added intensity flicker have no effect between point C and C' in Figure 3.6B. Beyond point C' further additions of intensity flicker progressively reduce flicker threshold; in other words, the observer seems to grow progressively more sensitive to flicker.

Figure 3.7 shows empirical data that correspond to the idealization shown as a solid line in Figure 3.6B. To allow for the possibility that, due to some nonlinear process (as described on pp. 93–98 and in Appendix E), the appropriate canceling waveform might be nonsinusoidal, we also used as a canceling waveform a fundamental plus a second harmonic component. Results were essentially unchanged.

The interpretation that we offered for the kind of data shown in Figure 3.7 was as follows (Regan & Tyler, 1971a). Suppose that, as depicted in Figure 3.4B, the visual pathway contains two parallel and independent systems, one sensitive to temporal changes in stimulus wavelength, the other (achromatic system) being sensitive to temporal changes of the intensive effect of light energy. In general, a change of stimulus wavelength will excite both systems. Only if the change is exactly balanced with respect to the achromatic system's spectral sensitivity will the achromatic system be silent. With zero added luminance modulation in Figures 3.6B and 3.7, we suppose that flicker threshold is determined by the achromatic system rather than by the chromatic system. We also suppose that adding small amounts of antiphase luminance modulation progressively cancels the input to the achromatic system while leaving the chromatic system unaffected.

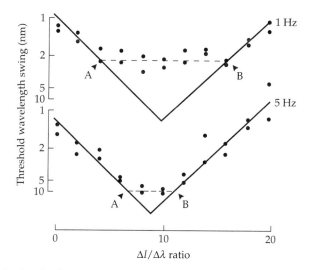

3.7 Data obtained using temporal titration. The flatness of the horizontal dotted lines indicates that the changing-intensity filter in Figure 3.4B has been silenced, so that threshold is determined by the changing-wavelength filter. After Regan and Tyler (1971a).

The flat region between C and C′ in Figure 3.6B indicates that adding different amounts of luminance modulation has no effect on flicker threshold. It follows that, between C and C′, flicker threshold is determined by something other than the achromatic system.

According to the hypothesis depicted in Figure 3.4B, that "something other" is the chromatic system. The response pattern shown in Figure 3.7 is typically obtained when the achromatic system is favored over the chromatic system by selecting a modulation frequency higher than 2 to 3 Hz and a spectral location other than the yellow and blue–green.

Figure 3.6C shows an alternative outcome to the experiment that can be observed when the flicker rate is 2 to 3 Hz or less and the spectral location is yellow or blue–green. Rather than the flat-topped inverted V of Figure 3.6B, the plot is flat initially (i.e., small amounts of added luminance modulation have no effect). Our proposed interpretation was that a change in stimulus wavelength excites the chromatic system more strongly than the achromatic system—so much more so that signal A in Figure 3.4B is considerably stronger than signal B. Consequently, flicker threshold is determined entirely by the chromatic system, and not until a moderately large peak-to-peak amplitude of luminance modulation has been added does signal B grow stronger than signal A, allowing the achromatic system to determine flicker threshold.

The flatness of the solid lines in Figure 3.6B,C indicates that the achromatic system is silent so that the chromatic system can be studied in isolation. To the extent that the corners at C and C' are sharp, and the section between is flat rather than rounded, we can conclude that threshold is determined by the chromatic or achromatic systems on an either/or (winner take all) basis, rather than by a weighted sum of the two contributions.

The effect of temporal frequency on the sensitivities of the chromatic and achromatic systems

By repeating the procedure explained in Figures 3.6 and 3.7 over a range of temporal frequencies at each of many spectral locations, we determined the effect of temporal frequency for the chromatic and achromatic systems for a spectral location in the blue–green (Regan & Tyler, 1971b). As illustrated in Figure 3.8, the chromatic system has a lowpass temporal characteristic while, as first noted by DeLange (1952, 1954, 1957, 1958), the luminance-flicker system is bandpass.* We found that this distinction holds for locations throughout the spectrum. Chromatic information is restricted to a frequency from DC to between 3 and 5 Hz, while luminance information is contained within a frequency band centered on about 10 Hz (depending on the luminance) that extends to considerably higher frequencies.†

The classical method of measuring the ability to discriminate between two different wavelengths is to present two uniform patches of light in a foveally viewed display. The two patches are continuous, and separated by a sharp boundary (Wright, 1946, 1991). The wavelength of one-half of the bipartite field is held constant. The wavelength of the other half is adjusted until both halves of the field have the same hue, then its luminance is adjusted so that the boundary disappears and both halves of the field look identical. Then a very small difference in wavelength is introduced, and luminance is adjusted until the boundary disappears. This procedure is repeated until it is impossible to make the boundary disappear by adjusting luminance. At this point, the difference in wavelength between the two halves of the field is the *wavelength discrimination threshold*.

---

* Hendrick de Lange, an electrical engineer employed by the Philips Company in the Netherlands, exerted a pivotal effect on vision research by applying methods of linear systems analysis to the study of flicker perception. His work influenced the later application of linear systems analysis to the study of spatial vision carried out by Fergus Campbell and his colleagues at Cambridge University. DeLange was also an inspiration personally. Starting in 1951 he carried out his work in his spare time with home-made equipment in a wooden shed by his house that also served to store his bicycle.

† Kelly and van Norren's (1977) "two band" model of heterochromatic flicker is a variant on the same idea. Their proposal, restricted to red–green flicker, was that at frequencies below about 5 Hz, flicker thresholds are determined by the red–green variations in the stimulus, while at flicker frequencies above about 5 Hz, thresholds are determined by the luminance variations in the stimulus.

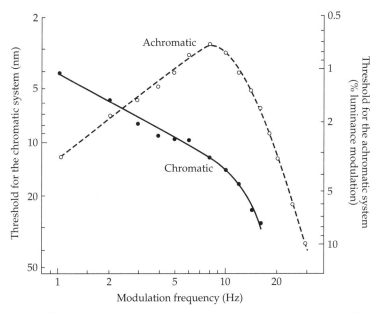

3.8 Temporal frequency characteristics of the chromatic and achromatic systems. Filled symbols represent the changing-wavelength filter in Figure 3.4B. Open symbols represent the changing-intensity filter in Figure 3.4B. The light was monochromatic with a mean wavelength of 527 nanometers and mean retinal illumination 100 trolands. After Regan and Tyler (1971b).

Figure 3.9C shows a *wavelength–discrimination curve* for one observer (C. W. Tyler) obtained by repeating the procedure just described at many locations throughout the spectrum. Two minima are evident, one in the blue–green centered on about 490 nm and one in the yellow centered on about 580 nm, in agreement with the classical data of Wright and Pitt (1934a,b); see also Wright (1946).

At first sight it might seem that temporal factors are irrelevant when the bipartite-field method is used. But this is not so. McCree (1960) showed that wavelength discrimination threshold becomes very high indeed when the observer gazes fixedly at the target so as to achieve some rudimentary level of retinal image stabilization (see also Beeler et al., 1964).* With this in mind, Christopher Tyler and I investigated the dynamic properties of the wavelength discrimination curve.

The field was a uniformly illuminated patch of light (2.0 degrees in subtense) rather than being bipartite. Using the wavelength modulator, we caused the wavelength of the stimulus to oscillate sinusoidally about some selected spectral

---

* So far as color appearance is concerned, the subjective attribute of hue fades quickly when a homogenous colored patch of light with a dark surround is viewed through a retinal image stabilizer (Clowes, 1962), but it can be restored by moving the stimulus (Gerrits, 1967).

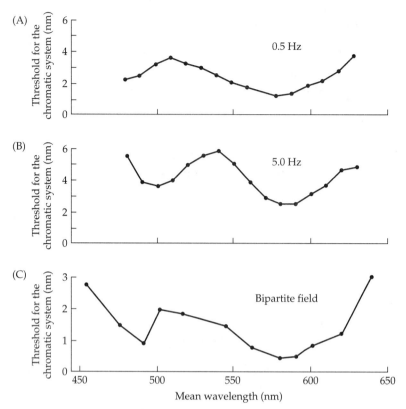

3.9 The shape of the wavelength discrimination curve depends on temporal frequency. (A, B) The wavelength discrimination curve measured by means of the titration method at frequencies of 0.5 Hz (part A) and 5 Hz (part B). (C) The wavelength discrimination curve measured by means of the classical bipartite-field method. All three curves are for the same observer (C. W. Tyler). After Regan and Tyler (1971b).

location. Then we used the titration procedure (Figure 3.6) to measure threshold for the chromatic filter shown in Figure 3.4B. We reported this procedure for many spectral locations.

Figure 3.9A shows the resulting wavelength–discrimination curve for an oscillation frequency of 0.5 Hz. The minimum in the yellow is in approximately the same location as the minimum obtained using the bipartite field procedure (Figure 3.9C). But the other minimum is at some wavelength below 480 nm. Figure 3.9B shows the wavelength–discrimination curve at a frequency of 5 Hz. The minimum in the yellow has not moved, but the other minimum has shifted considerably—it is now centered on about 500 nm. The just-noticeable oscillation of *luminance* behaved quite differently. It did not depend on spectral location for any temporal frequency between 0.5 and 10 Hz (Regan & Tyler, 1971b).

In terms of Walraven's version of the zone theory of color vision, this shift of the short-wavelength minimum shown in Figure 3.9A,B implies that β depends on temporal frequency. I will return to this issue on pp. 262–266.

Taking a more direct approach to the dynamic properties of the bipartite-field wavelength discrimination curve, I illuminated the left halves of a foveally viewed bipartite field with light from a double grating–monochromater, and the right half with light from a second double monochromator (half-power full bandwidth 3.3 nm). Field diameter was 1.5 degrees. Using heterochromatic flicker photometry, I equated the luminance of the reference half-field across the spectrum. Then I set the wavelength of the reference half-field to some value between 420 and 650 nm. While viewing the bipartite field through an SRI double-Purkinjé retinal image stabilizer, I adjusted the wavelength and the luminance of the variable half-field, following the classical bipartite-field procedure for measuring the wavelength discrimination curve.

Open circles in Figure 3.10 show an unstabilized wavelength–discrimination curve that was measured by viewing the bipartite field through the stabilizer, but with the eye movement signals disconnected from the input to the stabilizer. The discrimination thresholds followed the usual pattern. Then I repeated the measurements under stabilized retinal image conditions. Filled circles in Figure 3.10 show that thresholds were considerably elevated in the blue–green and extreme red regions of the spectrum, but were comparatively little affected in the yellow. The effect of stabilization was to transform a normal wavelength–discrimination curve into a curve that, over the range of wavelengths studied, resembles that of a tritanope.* (The tritanopic data reported by several authors is shown in Figure 10.14 of Kaiser and Boynton [1996] and Figure 10.9 of Boynton [1979].) The dotted line in Figure 3.10 is the wavelength–discrimination curve of a color-normal observer measured using a small (14 minutes of arc diameter) stimulus field that was viewed with the central fovea (Weale, 1960). This effect of reduced field size is called *small-field tritanopia*; it is caused by the sparse distribution of S cones (or their total absence within a small area surrounding the exact center of the fovea).

> All this suggests that the main effect of retinal image stabilization is to reduce or totally remove the S-cone input to the blue-yellow opponent mechanism.

When the luminance of the bipartite field was flickered at 5 Hz (25% modulation depth) while maintaining stabilization, thresholds returned to approximately

---

* For most researchers, finding a sufficient number of suitable observers is a chore. But consider the problem faced by those who would study the rare color vision defect *tritanopia* in its congenital (rather than acquired) form. In 1950 it was well known that tritan color deficiency (blue confused with green, yellow confused with violet) can be caused late in life by a variety of common visual disorders, but congenital tritanopia was thought by some to be exceeding rare (an estimate made in 1950 was one person in a million) while others thought it did not exist. Searching for tritanopes (assuming that they existed) by the usual procedure of using skilled examiners to screen a group of individuals was out of the

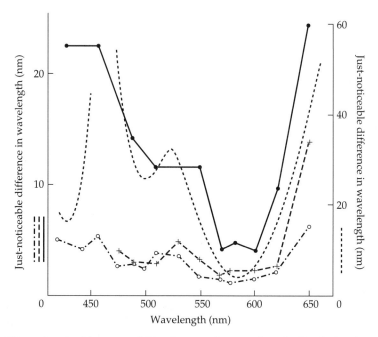

3.10 Effect of retinal image stabilization on the wavelength discrimination curves. Open circles plot wavelength discrimination thresholds measured by the classical bipartite field method in normal viewing condition. Stimulus field diameter was 1.5 degrees. Filled circles plot thresholds measured using the same procedure, but with the retinal image stabilized. Crosses plot thresholds measured with a stabilized image whose luminance was modulated at 5 Hz. For comparison, the dotted line shows a wavelength discrimination curve obtained with a field subtending 14 minutes of arc for a color-normal observer. The dotted line is based on data from Forshaw, reported in Weale (1960).

---

question. Then one day, W. D. Wright was approached by Mr. D. Wragge Morley for advice on how to print some of the Ishihara color vision test plates in an article on color blindness intended for the general reader. (The commercially available Ishihara test screens for the common red–green color vision deficiencies.) Recollecting that his friend and colleague Lt. Commander Dean Farnsworth of the U.S. Navy Medical Research Laboratory had put together a test plate for detecting blue–green and yellow–violet confusions, Wright "made his own luck" and asked that this additional test plate be included in the forthcoming article. The article was published on May 12, 1951, in the *Picture Post*, an illustrated English weekly magazine. Anyone who could read the concealed figure (perfectly camouflaged to anyone but a tritanope) was asked to write to the *Picture Post* or to Professor Wright. After sifting through the 900 letters received, Wright found 29 "almost certain" tritanopes, of whom 17 agreed to visit Imperial College for testing, of whom 7 agreed to extended testing. From the readership statistics of *Picture Post*, Wright estimated the incidence of tritanopia to be somewhere between one person in 13,000 and one in 65,000, and the ratio of men to women to be 1.6:1 (Wright, 1952; Thomson & Wright, 1953). A subsequent estimate (Kalmus, 1965) put the incidence at one in 10,000.

their unstabilized values (crosses in Figure 3.10). Reducing flicker frequency to 0.5 Hz had no further effect on wavelength discrimination thresholds except in the blue region of the spectrum, where they were further reduced in accord with the findings shown in Figure 3.9. These findings were confirmed for a second observer (Burbeck & Regan, 1983b).

In a further experiment, I first stabilized the retinal image with respect to eye movements, then introduced a controlled retinal image movement by moving the stimulus. In particular, while keeping the circular outer boundary of the bipartite field fixed on the retina, I caused the location of the boundary between the reference and test half-field to oscillate sinusoidally from side to side. The oscillation frequency that was most effective at restoring the perception that the two half-fields differed in hue was 0.5 Hz. With a peak-to-peak amplitude of 0.5 degree, each half-field looked fairly uniform, though less saturated than when unstabilized. Oscillation frequencies of 0.2 Hz, 1.0 Hz, and 5.0 Hz were considerably less effective.

Temporal summation characteristics for the chromatic and achromatic systems: Bloch's law for color and for luminance

We determined the temporal integration characteristics for the chromatic system by using the titration technique with pulsed changes of wavelength and intensity (Regan & Tyler, 1971c). Filled symbols in Figure 3.11 approximately follow

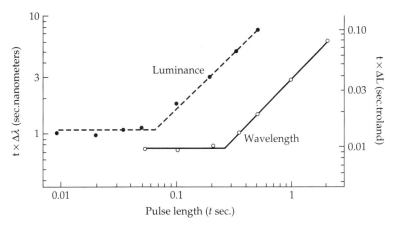

3.11 Temporal integration characteristics of the chromatic and achromatic systems. The just-detectable amplitude of a pulsed luminance change (ΔL) is inversely proportional to pulse length up to a pulse length of about 50 milliseconds (Bloch's law). This *critical duration* is marked by the abrupt change of the slope of the dashed line. The just-detectable amplitude of a pulsed wavelength change ($\Delta\lambda$) is, to a first approximation, inversely proportional to pulse length up to a considerably longer duration than 50 msec. (100 to more than 200 milliseconds, depending on spectral location). After Regan and Tyler (1971c).

Bloch's law: the horizontal segment of the curve indicates that, up to some *critical duration*, threshold is determined by the total energy in the pulse (total energy is proportional to pulse duration times pulse luminance); the segment of the curve with 45 degree slope indicates that, at longer presentation durations, threshold was reached at a particular rate of delivery of energy to the eye (i.e., by luminance).

Open symbols in Figure 3.11 show that temporal integration continues over a far longer duration for the chromatic system than for the achromatic system.* King-Smith and Carden (1976) came to similar conclusions. Schwartz and Loop (1982) found that reaction times were considerably longer when stimulation was restricted to the opponent-color system than when stimulation was restricted to the achromatic system.

The titration method used to determine
the contrast sensitivity of the chromatic contrast system

The findings shown in Figures 3.9 and 3.11 suggest that, if the 2AFC procedure were used (see Chapter 1, pp. 8–23), the chromatic contrast system would be favored with respect to the achromatic contrast system by presenting the stimuli for longer than 250 msec. with gradual onset and offset. And if the method of adjustments were used, the maximum allowed rate of adjustment should be low.

It has been found that equiluminant settings depend on the spatial frequency of the target. For example, Gordon and Shapley (1989) found that the detection of sinusoidal grating whose spatial frequency is less than 10 cycles/deg. follows the V_λ curve, while for higher spatial frequencies the relevant spectral sensitivity curve deviates from the V_λ curve.† And Marimont and Wandell (1994, pp. 3117 & 3121) stated that: "Chromatic aberration obliterates the short-wavelength cone response beyond a few cycles per degree. It also changes the shape and the peak value of the other two cone classes. When measured through the optics, the cone photopigment spectral responsivity depends strongly on the spatial frequency of the stimulus. . . . Hence contrast and color comparisons are meaningful only within relatively small spatial frequency ranges." In the light of these findings it might be that the spatial titration technique could usefully be used in studies of the early processing of CD form.

---

* The hue substitution technique (Piéron, 1931; Weingarten, 1972), a method for investigating visual system properties at equiluminance (i.e., when either CIE luminances or sensation luminances have been equated before the experiment is carried out) has been used mainly with spatially unpatterned stimuli. Post-hoc evidence exists that the achromatic system in Figure 3.4B has been at least partially isolated by means of this technique; this evidence included increased temporal integration time for pulses, elevated double-pulse resolution threshold, and increased reaction time (Bowen, 1977; Bowen et al., 1977; Pokorny et al., 1979; Smith et al., 1984).

† At single-cell level, the red–green "equivalent" point for neurons in the lateral geniculate nucleus of monkeys depends on spatial frequency (Shapley & Kaplan, 1989).

The design of a grating used in an attempt to silence the achromatic contrast system by means of titration is explained in Figure 3.12. Observers set their grating detection thresholds by varying the luminance and chromatic modulation in

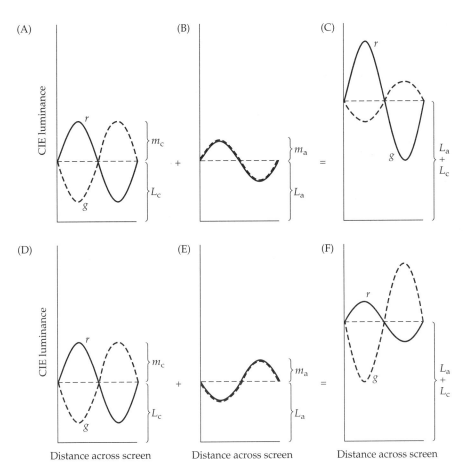

3.12 Stimulus for spatial titration. The stimulus grating comprised the linear sum of a chromatic-contrast component of fixed mean luminance (Lc) and a luminance-contrast component of fixed mean luminance (La). In our experiment Lc = La. In some cases the red modulations of the chromatic (A) and the luminance (B) components were in phase, so that in the stimulus grating (C) the red modulation was stronger than the green modulation. In other cases the red modulations of the chromatic (D) and luminance (E) components were in antiphase, so that in the stimulus grating (F) the red modulation was weaker than the green modulation. The luminance modulation/chromatic modulation ratio was equal to ma/mc. Grating detection threshold for any given ma/mb ratio was set by adjusting the values of ma and mc in a yoked manner, keeping ma/mb constant. From Regan, Kaiser, and Nakano (1993).

a yoked manner that did not change their ratio (m_a/m_c). Note that m_a/m_c is the ratio between two *modulations* rather than between two contrasts.

Figure 3.13 shows the effect of the m_a/m_c ratio on the contrast (i.e., m_c/L_c) of the chromatic contrast component of the grating (Figure 3.12A,D) at grating detection threshold. Data are shown for red–green gratings of spatial frequencies 2, 6, and 8 cycles/deg. The continuous line showing 2 cycles/deg. is approximately flat, indicating that additions of luminance modulation had essentially no effect on grating detection threshold. We concluded that, in terms of the hypothesis illustrated in Figure 3.4A, threshold was determined entirely by the chromatic contrast system. The titration data for the 6 and 8 cycles/deg. were consistent with the presence of a locally flat region near zero on the abscissa (though the flat regions are not so clear as for the temporal titration data shown in Figure 3.7). Other observers gave rounded tops in several experimental conditions, or even sharp inverted Vees instead of the locally flat areas. (If threshold were determined by a weighted sum of the contributions of the achromatic and chromatic systems rather than by a "winner takes all" rule, we would expect a rounded

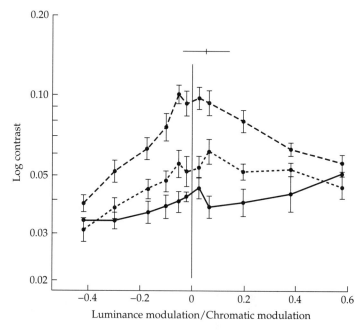

3.13 Spatial titration results. Spatial titration results for gratings of spatial frequencies 2 cycles/deg., 6 cycles/deg., and 8 cycles/deg., respectively. Grating contrast threshold is plotted as the ordinate. Luminance modulation/chromatic modulation is plotted as abscissa. An achromatizing lens was used. Vertical bars indicate ± 1 standard error. Horizontal bars indicate ±1 standard error for HFP. From Regan, Kaiser, and Nakano (1993).

rather than a flat top. And a sharp inverted Vee is what one obtains when the chromatic system is inactive—as, for example, when the experiment is repeated using two lights of the same rather than different colors.)

The horizontal bar in Figure 3.13 shows ± 1 standard error for the heterochromatic flicker photometry setting. Given that the CIE definition of luminance makes no provision for variability between observers, it is not surprising that the HFP setting departed from CIE equiluminance (zero on the abscissa) for two of the four observers, although not for the observer whose data are shown in Figure 3.13. As would be expected, the HFP settings coincided with the peak in the 16 Hz temporal titration data obtained with a spatially unpatterned field (not shown). More significantly, the "silencing" points in the 8 cycles/deg. spatial titration curves (mean of four observers) were displaced somewhat to the left of both the HFP settings and the temporal titration peaks obtained with targets whose power was restricted to low spatial frequencies. This finding accords with the theoretical predictions of Marimont and Wandell (1994) cited earlier.

But what if our model is wrong?

Switkes et al. (1988) noted that many aspects of their data could be explained in terms of a hypothesis that is quite different from the hypothesis depicted in Figure 3.4A. This alternative hypothesis is that an isoluminant chromatic grating excites a plurality of filters sensitive to achromatic contrast that have a broad distribution of chromatic balances.

A similar proposal had been made previously, but was based on a quite different kind of evidence. The relevant experimental data were electrical signals recorded from the human brain. These signals were responses to stimulation of the fovea by patterns of red and green checks (Regan & Sperling, 1971; Regan, 1973b; Regan & Spekreijse, 1974).

In the first of two experiments, the pattern of about 140 checks, each 0.18 degrees wide, subtended 3.0 degrees. Before recording started, I rendered the red and green checks equiluminant (1.0 on the lower abscissa in Figure 3.15) according to psychophysical heterochromatic flicker photometry (see pp. 220–222), and noted that they were also approximately equiluminant according to the zero apparent-motion criterion (see pp. 223–224) as well as the minimally distinct border criterion (see p. 223). The red and green checks abruptly exchanged places at intervals of 166 msec., i.e., at a frequency of 6Hz. Figure 3.14 shows how this stimulus was created. All checks were illuminated at all times with a mixture of monochromatic red and green lights. For the uppermost and lowermost of the three checks shown, the red light initially had a higher luminance than the green light so that those checks looked red. Then the luminances of the red and green lights abruptly exchanged, so that the uppermost and lowermost checks looked green. The red and green luminances followed the converse time course for the middle check of the three shown in Figure 3.14 so that it was initially green, and then turned red. The vertical arrows indicate the instants at which chromatic contrast reversed. Note that, in the situation depicted, luminance contrast did not change

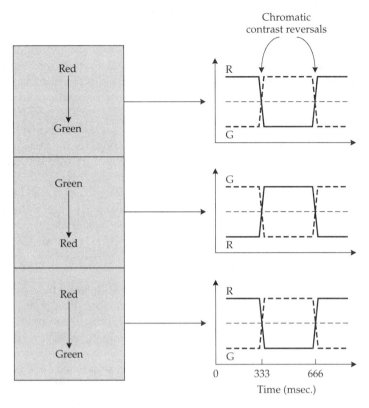

3.14 The stimulus that produced the electrical brain responses shown in Figure 3.15. The pattern consisted of alternating red and green checks. Red and green checks abruptly exchanged places 6 times per second.

at any time because the sum of the red and green luminances within any given check was constant.

The repetitive reversals of contrast produced a strong brain response at a frequency of 6Hz. The data points above 1.0 on the lower abscissa in Figure 3.15 plot the amplitude of this brain response recorded from a deuteranope (Spekreijse) and a color-normal subject (Regan). In accord with his statement that the stimulus appeared to be totally without patterning (the exchanges between red and green checks were invisible to him), the deuteranope gave no brain response. This finding suggested the following:

> The large brain response recorded from the color-normal subject was not an artifact of spurious retinal image luminance contrast caused by ocular chromatic aberration. This point was confirmed by recording brain responses to the pattern of red and green checks after canceling

simultaneously, by means of an optical technique,* longitudinal chromatic aberration, chromatic difference of magnification, and chromatic variation of deviation of the principal ray.

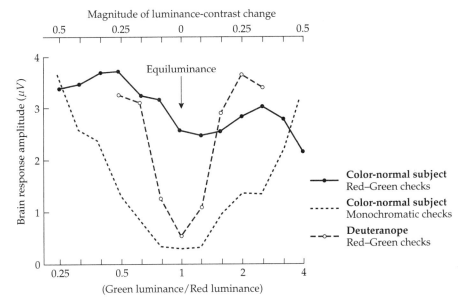

3.15 Electrical responses of the human brain produced by stimulating the central fovea with patterns of red–green checks. Subjects viewed a circular region of diameter 3.0 degrees that contained about 140 checks, each of which was 0.18 degrees wide. As illustrated in Figure 3.14, chromatic spatial contrast across the boundaries of the checks reversed 6 times per second. This stimulus produced a repetitive electrical signal in the subject's brain that consisted almost entirely of a 6 Hz frequency component. The continuous and dashed lines, respectively, show how the amplitude of this 6 Hz component depended on the Green/Red luminance ratio for a color-normal and a deuteranopic subject. (Red luminance was fixed and green luminance varied.) The dotted line indicates the results for the color-normal subject of replacing the red light with a green light of equal mean luminance. Contrast was 0.4 for the red and the green components of the pattern. The green light was of wavelength 547 nm (10 nm full bandwidth at half power) and the red light was of wavelength 640 nm (56 nm full bandwidth at half power). The overlap of spectral power was essentially zero. After Regan (1973).

---

* Achromatizing lenses that correct for chromatic difference of focus either leave the chromatic difference of magnification unaffected or make it *worse*. In any case only a small (1 to 2 degree) field can be used. On the other hand, both kinds of chromatic aberration can be canceled simultaneously over a wide field by generating gratings of different colors on

See R–G in Figure 3.1B. The longitudinal aberration to be canceled was estimated from the data shown in Figure 3.1A.

Next, we varied the luminance of the green component of the checks while holding the luminance of the red component constant. This meant that, as indicated on the upper abscissa in Figure 3.15, an abrupt change in luminance contrast now accompanied each of the abrupt changes of chromatic contrast. The deuteranopic subject gave strong responses to luminance-contrast reversals, indicating that his failure to respond at equiluminance was not caused by insensitivity to spatial contrast per se.

The brain signal from the color-normal subject remained strong for all green/red luminance ratios, indicating that his response to red/green ratios near equiluminance was not an artifact of inaccurate photometry. Finally, the dotted line shows data recorded from the color-normal subject after the red light had been replaced by a green light of the same luminance so as to remove entirely the chromatic contrast component of the stimulus, leaving only the monochromatic-contrast component.

> Although it might seem somewhat counterintuitive, it is not necessarily the case that the color-normal's brain response at equiluminance was a response to chromatic contrast rather than a response to monochromatic contrast.

The basis for this statement will become clear when I have reviewed the results of the second experiment.

In the second experiment we manipulated the red and green components of the checkerboard quite differently. In this experiment, red checks remained red at all times, and green checks remained green at all times. Figure 3.16A explains how this was done. The uppermost and lowermost of the three checks shown in Figure 3.16A were always red, but their luminances abruptly rose or fell (in synchrony) repetitively. The central check was always green. At the instant that the luminances of the red checks increased by luminance increment ΔL cd/m^2, the luminance of the green checks decreased by ΔL cd/m^2. Since the mean luminances of the red and green checks were equal, this meant that the *luminance contrast* across each edge reversed every 270 msec. (Figure 3.16B).

The traces labeled "Equiluminant Red–Green" in Figure 3.17 show that, although the deuteranopic subject gave a clear response to this stimulus, *no brain responses were recorded from the color-normal subject.* This is the mirror image of the finding in the first experiment.

That the deuteranopic subject's brain gave an electrical response is not difficult to explain. In the absence within the central fovea of the medium-wavelength

---

different monitors and optically superimposing them by means of a beam splitter. The two monitors are placed at different distances from the eye (to compensate for chromatic difference in focus) and the spatial frequencies of the grating are set to different values (to compensate for chromatic difference in magnification). See Regan, 1973b.

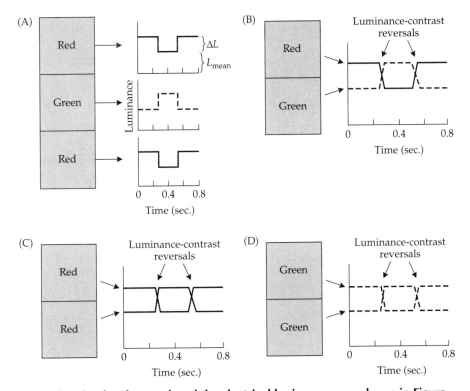

3.16 The stimulus that produced the electrical brain responses shown in Figure 3.17. (A) A pattern of alternate red and green checks (about 95 checks in total) whose sensation luminances were equal, and that subtended 2.2 degrees, was viewed with the central fovea. The luminances of the red and green checks were squarewave-modulated in antiphase. (B) The luminance difference across each edge reversed polarity every 270 msec. (C) The green light was replaced by a red light of the same luminance so that all checks were red. The luminance difference across each edge reversed polarity every 270 msec. (D) The red light in part A was replaced by a green light of the same luminance so that all checks were green. The luminance contrast across each edge reversed polarity every 270 msec.

cone and with a sparse population of short-wavelength cones (Color Plate 9), the luminance differences between checks must be signaled almost exclusively by red cones so that, viewed through the deuteranopic eye, the "Equiluminant Red–Green" condition in Figure 3.16B is approximately similar to the "Red" condition in part C and the "Green" condition in part D.

Results from the color-normal subject were more puzzling. The dotted line in Figure 3.15 shows that the color-normal subject gave strong brain responses when he viewed a contrast-reversing monochromatic checkerboard (Figure 3.16C). But, as indicated by the arrows in Figure 3.16B, luminance contrast reversals occurred in the isoluminant condition shown in part A. Why did these reversals of lumi-

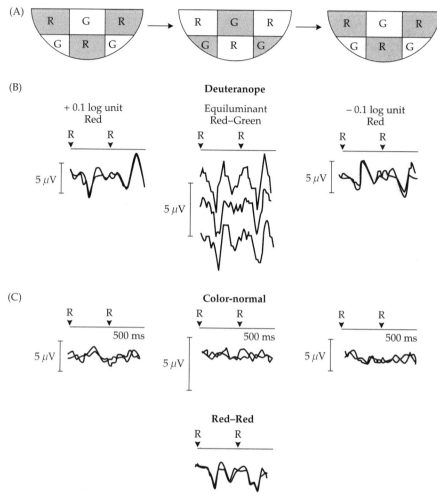

3.17 Electrical responses of the human brain produced by stimulating the central fovea with patterns of red–green checks. (A) The stimulus. Red checks remained red and green checks remained green, but their luminances alternated between a lower (shaded) and a higher (not shaded) level. The stimulus pattern contained approximately 47 checks rather than the five shown here. Maximum contrast was 11% for both the red and green components of the pattern. The horizontal diameter of the field was 2.2 degrees. Mean luminance was 8.3 cd/m². The red and green lights had the same specifications as those used in Figure 3.15. (B) Brain responses from a deuteranope. The traces labeled "Equiluminant Red–Green:" are responses to the stimulus described by Figure 3.16A,B. Traces labeled "+0.1 Log unit Red" and "–0.1 Log unit Red," respectively, were obtained by brightening and dimming the red component of the light by 18%. (C) Brain responses from a color-normal subject. Details as for part B. The traces marked "Red–Red" were obtained by stimulating with reversals of monochromatic contrast as illustrated in Figure 3.16C. Reversals of luminance contrast across the edges of the squares are marked by the arrowed R's.

nance contrast produce no brain signal, while reversals in the luminance contrast of an all-green (or all-red) checkerboard gave strong responses? It is difficult to avoid the following conclusion:

> In the *achromatic* contrast system, there is something very different about the physiological effect produced when two adjacent locations are illuminated by lights of different luminances (L_1 and L_2 cd/m^2) that have the same wavelength and the physiological effect produced when two adjacent locations are illuminated by lights of the same two luminances (L_1 and L_2 cd/m^2) that have different wavelengths.

Nevertheless, in 1974 and also still today, both these spatial patterns are said to have identical "luminance contrasts." In an attempt to account for our findings, we offered the following hypothesis:

1. At the earliest contrast-processing stage, the color-normal subject has no spatial contrast mechanism whose spectral sensitivity matches— even approximately—the equiluminant curve defined by the CIE V_λ curve or by any of the three measures of sensation luminance. This hypothesis accounts for the color-normal subjects' absence of response to the stimulus illustrated in Figure 3.16A,B.
2. The color-normal subject has a mechanism that responds to mono-chromatic spatial contrast. It consists of two (or more) parallel sub-mechanisms that have different spectral sensitivities, all of which differ considerably from the V_λ curve. This hypothesis accounts for the finding that the color-normal subject gave symmetrical contrast-reversal responses to the monochromatic stimuli depicted in Figure 3.16C,D, but gave similar responses to the pattern of alternate red and green checks depicted in Figure 3.16A,B only when the red luminance was considerably higher than the green luminance, and vice versa.

With the aim of isolating monochromatic contrast mechanisms that were most sensitive to red light I stimulated a subject's fovea with a 2×2 degree pattern of monochromatic deep red (676 nm) checks, each of which was 0.15 degrees wide (Regan, 1974, 1975a, 1979). Superimposed on the pattern was a uniform unpat-terned monochromatic patch of desensitizing light that subtended 6 degrees. The basic idea was to vary both the wavelength and the intensity of the desensitizing light so as to hold the response to the checkerboard stimulus at a constant ampli-tude and thus establish the spectral sensitivity curve of the mechanism that was responding to the red checkerboard.*

---

* One of the two ways in which this was done was to place the subject's brain within a feedback loop so that the amplitude of the brain responses directly controlled the lumi-nance of the desensitizing light (Regan, 1975b, 1979).

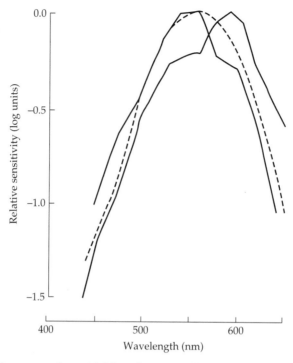

3.18 Relative spectral sensitivities of two parallel foveal mechanisms sensitive to achromatic contrast. The bold curves were obtained by measuring electrical responses recorded from the brain of a human subject. The fine dashed line shows the same subject's relative luminosity curve obtained by psychophysical heterochromatic flicker photometry. Modified from Regan (1974).

The rightmost heavy curve in Figure 3.18 was the result. The leftmost heavy curve in Figure 3.18 shows a spectral sensitivity curve obtained by replacing the red checkerboard probe with a monochromatic green (544 nm) checkerboard probe.

Figure 3.1 shows that, although a monochromatic blue (436 nm) checkerboard with 0.2 degree-wide checks gave easily recordable brain responses, they were considerably weaker than the response to all-red or to all-green checkerboards. Presumably that, coupled with the slightly smaller checks used (0.15 degree width), resulted in failure to obtain data on a putative spectral sensitivity curve of shorter wavelength than the leftmost curve in Figure 3.18.

A psychophysical equivalent of the experiment just described might be carried out as follows. Take two monochromatic checkerboard patterns, one of wavelength 590 nm, the other of wavelength 545 nm, both having the same luminance. On the basis of the findings shown in Figure 3.18, one would envisage that contrast detection threshold for the red checkerboard would be elevated about 0.4 log units more by adapting to a 100% contrast version of the red checkerboard than by adapting to a 100% contrast version of the green checkerboard. And that contrast detection threshold for the green checkerboard would be elevated about 0.4 log units more by adapting to a 100% contrast version of the green checkerboard than by adapting to a 100% contrast version of the red checkerboard. (In the design of such an experiment it would be preferable to create the monochromatic checkerboards using narrow-band interference filters or light-emitting diodes rather than by using a computer monitor, because a green of dominant wavelength 545 nm and a red of dominant wavelength 590 nm generated on a monitor would have very considerable spectral overlap, while the monochromatic lights used to obtain our brain response data had essentially zero overlap.)

An abstract by Yamamoto and DeValois (1996) reports an experiment whose design is not greatly different from that just described. They concluded that: "These results are not readily explained by the standard two chromatic opponent mechanisms and one color-blind luminance mechanism. . . . [T]he data suggest the existence of color-selective detectors that respond to effective intensity differences—i.e., non color-blind 'luminance' mechanisms." Similar conslusions were reached by Ellis et al. (1975).What would be the implications for research on the visual processing of CD form if the human achromatic contrast mechanism is indeed organized along the lines just proposed?

The implication is that it would be impossible to totally "silence" the entire achromatic spatial contrast system. But this by no means denies the possibility that stimuli could be designated to stimulate the chromatic contrast system considerably more strongly than the achromatic contrast system.

Detection of Color-Defined Form:
Contrast Sensitivity Functions for Color-Defined Form

At low spatial and temporal frequencies the contrast sensitivity function for a chromatic sinewave grating is considerably flatter than for a luminance-defined grating (compare open circles with open triangles in Figure 1.19) (Schade, 1948, 1956, 1958; van der Horst, 1969; van der Horst & Bouman, 1969; van der Horst et al., 1967; Granger & Heurtley, 1973; Kelly, 1983; Mullen, 1985). There is general agreement on this point.

The shape of the contrast sensitivity function at high spatial frequencies is more controversial than the shape of the low-frequency segment; estimates of grating acuity for chromatic gratings vary widely, probably because incompletely canceled ocular chromatic aberration(s) allowed luminance artifacts to dominate grating visibility at high spatial frequencies in some studies, even when an achromatizing lens was used (Bradley et al., 1992). A case in point is Granger and Heurtley's (1973) report that visual sensitivity to their red–green chromatic gratings was based largely on artifactual luminance contrast even at the moderate spatial frequency of 20 cycles/deg. Instead of an achromatizing lens, Mullen (1985) used a variant of the optical superimposition technique described by Regan (1973b) to simultaneously cancel longitudinal aberration, lateral aberration, and deviation of the principal ray, thus eliminating the artifactual luminance contrast cues to grating detection that had plagued earlier studies; see footnote on p. 239. (Ocular chromatic aberrations are discussed by Zhang et al., 1991, 1993.) The optical technique also allowed the large field size necessary for measurement at low spatial frequencies. (It is important to have at least five complete cycles visible in the stimulus field; see pp. 416–420.) Open triangles in Figure 1.19 plot Mullen's data for a red–green equiluminant grating that was counterphase-modulated at 0.4 Hz. She estimated visual acuity for a red–green grating to be 11 to 12 cycles/deg. compared with 34 to 36 cycles/deg. for a luminance grating of the same mean luminance and spectral content.

Sekiguchi et al. (1993a) pointed out that the spatially broadband phosphors in CRT displays restrict the chromatic contrast of isoluminant gratings and, furthermore, such CRT displays cannot produce the high luminance levels required to measure contrast thresholds at high spatial frequencies. They avoided these restrictions by using red (632.8 nm) and green (514.5 nm) laser light to generate isoluminant red–green interference fringes on the foveal retina (see pp. 436–439 and 477–481). They found that grating acuities were at least 23 cycles/deg. for all five observers tested. The highest acuity was 27 cycles/deg. compared with an acuity of approximately 48 cycles/deg. for a comparable LD grating.

Before going further we should step aside to review, stage by stage, the *ideal observer* model by means of which Sekiguchi et al. insightfully interpreted their empirical data. (The concept of the ideal observer was introduced on p. 142.) The "photon noise" stage in Figure 3.19 is the only source of noise that degrades the stimulus information, i.e., the model *does not incorporate neural noise*. Ocular transmittance data were obtained from Wyszecki and Stiles (1967). The aperture size of any given cone (the full width at half-height) was taken to be 34% of the cone spacing. The trichromatic cone sampling was calculated from photomicrographs of the long- and medium-wavelength cones in the central fovea (see Color Plate 9 and Figure 9, Appendix F), and of parafoveal short-wavelength cones (Curcio et al., 1991). Absorption spectra for the three cone types were taken from Schnapf et al. (1987). The model computes ideal observer performance by simulating the performance of an ideal decision-maker on a series of two-interval forced choice trials. The decision-maker has access to the output of the model visual system depicted in Figure 3.19. And the ideal discriminator chosen was the maximum-likelihood rule (Geisler, 1984, 1989).*

Figure 3.20A shows experimentally measured contrast sensitivity curves for the red–green and LD gratings. In Figure 3.20B, these same data are re-expressed in terms of efficiency, that is, when compared with the performance of the ideal

---

* The major difference between this model and the ideal observer model of Geisler (1984, 1989) is that the model of Sekiguchi et al. did not include a stage of ocular blurring, since this stage is not required when interference fringes are formed on the retina.

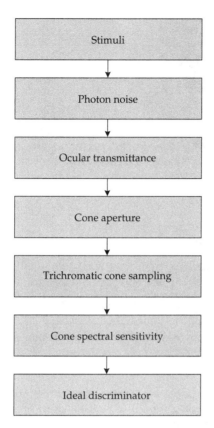

3.19 Schematic of the ideal observer model used to interpret the data shown in Figure 3.20. The output of the model visual system is computed by passing the grating stimulus, degraded by photon noise, through a series of stages. Each stage represents one factor known to affect the performance of real observers. From Sekiguchi, Williams, and Brainard (1993).

observer. This way of looking at the response data confirmed a previous report (Banks et al., 1987) that the real observer is much less sensitive than the ideal observer (10 to 30 times less sensitive) but, more to the point, it also indicated that the difference between the responses to CD and LD gratings was caused by neural rather than optical factors. If the shape of the CSFs had been determined by optical factors only, then the two curves in Figure 3.20B would have been identical (Sekiguchi et al., 1993b).

Sekiguchi et al. (1993b) also measured contrast sensitivity in the situation that short-wavelength cones were isolated. They created violet (441.6 nm) laser light interference fringes on the retina and superimposed them on a very bright (84,000 troland) uniform 6-degree diameter background of yellow (580 nm) incoherent

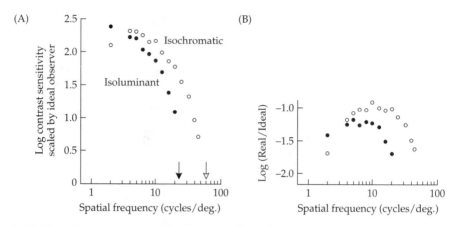

3.20 Foveal contrast sensitivity functions for color-defined and luminance-defined gratings. The eye's optics were bypassed by forming isoluminant red–green laser interference fringes on the retina. (A) Contrast threshold of a real observer. The open and filled arrows indicate the resolution limit (i.e., grating acuity) for the color-defined and luminance-defined gratings, respectively. (B) Data in part A replotted in terms of the ratio of the real observer's contrast sensitivity to the ideal observer's contrast sensitivity. Filled circles: Color-defined gratings. Open circles: Yellow luminance-defined grating. From Sekiguchi, Williams, and Brainard (1993).

light. This very bright yellow background desensitized the medium- and long-wavelength cones, but had comparatively little effect on the short-wavelength cones. As well, the violet fringes were centered on the retinal location with the highest density of S cones (at 1.0 degrees of eccentricity).

Sekiguchi et al. confirmed previous reports that the resolution limit for gratings that stimulate S cones only is considerably lower than the resolution limit for red–green isoluminant gratings, that is, 10 to 14 cycles/deg. compared with 20 to 29 cycles/deg. (Williams & Collier, 1983; Williams et al., 1983; Sekiguchi et al., 1993a). They also added the following observation.

> There is no difference between the two contrast sensitivity functions when they are replotted in terms of the ratio of real observer performance to ideal observer performance.

They concluded that: "The difference seen between the red–green isoluminant and S-cone-isolated gratings when contrast sensitivity is plotted in a conventional manner can be explained primarily by the low photon catch of the sparse S-cone submosaic. This effect is tempered by the spectral overlap of the L- and the M-cone responsivities that affect red–green isoluminant contrast sensitivity" (Sekiguchi et al., 1993b, p. 2129).

In modeling their findings Sekiguchi et al. (1993b) assumed that the differences in real observer efficiency they had found (and that, as already mentioned, must have been caused by neural rather than optical factors) could be described in terms of a spatial filter followed by additive noise that was independent of spatial frequency. They restricted their discussion to high spatial frequencies. Figure 3.21 summarizes the results of their calculations. The bottom row shows the eye's optical point spread function (see Figure 1.13). The next row up depicts the cone spacing (0.54 minutes of arc in the fovea and 0.95 minutes of arc in the parafovea). The Gaussian functions in the row above represent the profiles of cone apertures, the full widths at half-height being 0.23 minutes of arc in the fovea and 0.40 minutes of arc in the parafovea. The three Gaussians in the top row represent the profiles of the estimated neural point spread functions for the three kinds of grating:

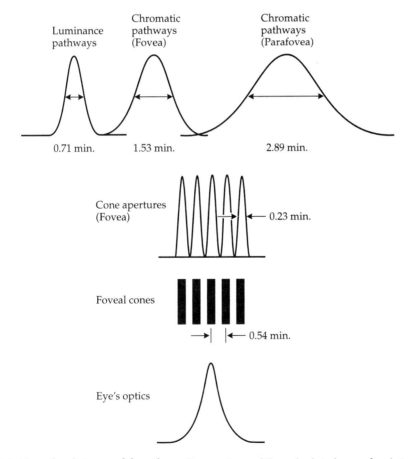

3.21 Neural point spread functions. Comparison of the calculated neural point spread functions for the processing of chromatic and luminance information with the point spread functions for the eye's optics, for the cone aperture, and for cone spacing at the fovea. From Sekiguchi, Williams, and Brainard (1993).

the luminance-defined grating; the red–green isoluminant grating; and the S-cone-isolated grating. In the fovea, the full width at half-height of the point spread function was 0.71 minutes of arc for the LD grating and 1.53 minutes of arc for the CD grating. These widths are, respectively, 3.1 and 6.8 times larger than the cone aperture at the foveal center. At an eccentricity of 1.0 degrees in the parafovea, the width of the neural point spread function was 2.89 minutes of arc for both the CD and the S-cone-isolated gratings, 7.2 times larger than the parafoveal cone aperture.

Channels for Color-Defined Form

Figure 2.10B shows the effect of test grating orientation on sensitivity to chromatic contrast after adapting to an homogenous field (filled circles) and after adapting to a high-contrast horizontal (open circles) or vertical (open triangles) red–green equiluminant grating. Orientation-dependent sensitivity loss is evident, just as in the corresponding experiment using LD gratings (Figure 2.10A), though the sharpness of selectivity is somewhat less. While post- and pre-adaptation sensitivities were approximately the same when the test and adapting gratings differed by 45 degrees, as in Figure 2.10A, in Figure 2.10B, this was not the case until test and adapting gratings differed by from 75 to 90 degrees.

Figure 2.9B shows the effect of test grating spatial frequency on sensitivity to chromatic contrast after adapting to a high-contrast equiluminant red–green grating. At each of the four adapting frequencies there was frequency-selective sensitivity loss whose peak coincided with the adapting frequency, just as for the LD gratings in Figure 2.9A (see also DeValois, 1978, and Yujiri et al., 1980).

According to Bradley, Switkes, and DeValois (1988), when grating contrasts were normalized with respect to detection thresholds for the two kinds of grating, the magnitudes of the adaptation effects were similar for luminance and chromatic gratings, and the selectivities of the effects were more similar than shown in Figure 2.9 and 2.10.

Cross-adaptation effects between chromatic and luminance gratings were comparatively small, indicating that the spatial filters for luminance and chromatic gratings are separate, an idea that is also consistent with the finding that the apparent spatial frequency of an isoluminant red-green grating can be shifted by adapting to a similar grating of a different spatial frequency, while at the same time a shift in the opposite direction is generated by adapting to a luminance grating (Favreau & Cavanagh, 1981). Furthermore, oppositely directed orientation aftereffects for CD and LD form can also exist simultaneously (Cavanagh, 1989). The separation between the processing of color and luminance breaks down, however, at a stage subsequent to spatial filtering. The evidence for this point, described next, is that masking interactions occur between chromatic and luminance gratings.

Masking functions for all four combinations of isoluminant chromatic C and achromatic (L) masker and test gratings were reported by DeValois and Switkes

(1983) and by Switkes, Bradley, and DeValois (1988), and subsequently by Mullen and Losada (1994), and by Losada and Mullen (1994). Switkes and his colleagues used the *psychophysical heterochromatic flicker photometry* criterion of sensation equiluminance, whereas Mullen and Losada used the *minimal motion* criterion.

Figure 2.15 shows the transition from facilitation to attenuation in the two same-on-same cases. Data for $L_{\text{mask}}/L_{\text{test}}$ are shown by filled triangles and for $C_{\text{mask}}/C_{\text{test}}$ by open circles. Because the specification of absolute chromatic contrast is rather arbitrary, Switkes et al. (1988) expressed test grating thresholds as multiples of the test grating detection threshold, and they expressed masker grating thresholds as multiples of the masker grating detection threshold. It is interesting that, when normalized in this way, the relation between achromatic and chromatic data was simplified and became more lawful.

Switkes et al. (1988) reported that the $L_{\text{mask}}/C_{\text{test}}$ and $C_{\text{mask}}/L_{\text{test}}$ conditions gave different functions, i.e., that cross-masking was asymmetric. Mullen and Losada (1994) found that cross-masking effects were less asymmetric than reported by Switkes et al. (1988), though some asymmetry remained. Mullen and Losada attributed the significant $L_{\text{mask}}/C_{\text{test}}$ facilitation reported at suprathreshold mask contrasts by Switkes et al. to their use of constant-phase grating.* Mullen and Losada's data for the $C_{\text{mask}}/L_{\text{test}}$ and $L_{\text{mask}}/C_{\text{test}}$ conditions, respectively, are shown in Figure 3.22A and B.

All three observers showed suprathreshold facilitation in the $L_{\text{mask}}/C_{\text{test}}$ condition (Figure 3.22B). Mullen and Losada (1994) noted that this suprathreshold facilitation was still evident even when as many as 16 phases of test and masker grating were randomized. Switkes et al. (1988) had previously found this facilitation to be very broadly tuned to spatial frequency (Figure 3.23; filled diamonds); Mullen and Losada reported the tuning curve to be not only very broad, but essentially flat.

Figure 3.23 brings out the point that the spatial frequency tuning of the attenuation effect for same-on-same masking was similarly broad for the $L_{\text{mask}}/L_{\text{test}}$

---

* Whereas in any given set of masking trials, Switkes and his colleagues used test and masker gratings of constant spatial phase, Mullen & Losada (1994) emphasized that they investigated the effect of varying the phase difference between the test and masker gratings on a trial-to-trial basis. Mullen and Losada (1994, p. 3141) explained one effect of relative phase as follows: "For example, for the detection of luminance contrast in the presence of color, adding the luminance test in a fixed phase of 180 deg causes the red to darken (appear browner) and the green to brighten. Thus, comparing one color between the two intervals, for example, to find the browner red, may be used to indicate the luminance test interval. In the random phase condition, however" (i.e., 180 degrees or 0 degrees chosen randomly), "the luminance test may cause the red to either brighten or darken and so no local color cues to the presence of the test stimulus exist." DeValois and Switkes (1983) and Switkes et al. (1988) showed their cross-masking results to be independent of the test masker's relative phase (0, 90, 180 degrees). Each phase, however, was used in a separate experiment. These authors as well as Mullen and Losada note that phase variation is a control for the presence of spurious luminance contrast caused either by chromatic aberration or by an error in estimating the isoluminant point.

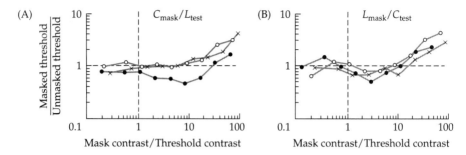

3.22 The dipper effect for cross-masking between color and luminance gratings. (A) Detection threshold elevation for a yellow luminance grating is plotted as ordinate versus the contrast of the red–green masker grating (expressed as a multiple of detection threshold for the masker grating). Data are shown for three observers. (B) Detection threshold elevation for a red–green color grating is plotted as ordinate versus the contrast of the yellow luminance masker grating (expressed as a multiple of detection threshold for the masker grating). After Mullen and Losada (1994).

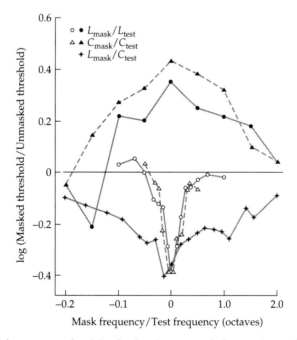

3.23 Spatial-frequency selectivity for luminance and chromatic masking. Log (normalized) threshold is plotted as a function of the ratio between the spatial frequencies of the masker and test gratings. From Switkes, Bradley, and DeValois (1998).

(filled circles) and C_{mask}/C_{test} (filled triangles) cases. (To reiterate, attenuation occurred only for high-contrast maskers.) Low-contrast maskers produced a facilitation effect whose spatial frequency tuning was similarly narrow in the two same-on-same cases (L_{mask}/L_{test} shown by open circles and C_{mask}/C_{test} shown by open triangles in Figure 3.23—see also Fig. 2.15.)

Although one of the three observers in Figure 3.22A shows suprathreshold facilitation, Switkes et al. (1988) found no suprathreshold facilitation in the C_{mask}/L_{test} condition. At suprathreshold mask contrasts, all interactions elevated detection threshold. Indeed, Switkes et al. stated that visual sensitivity to a 2 cycles/deg. luminance grating can be depressed as strongly by a chromatic grating masker as by a luminance-grating masker when the masker strengths are normalized relative to their respective thresholds (though they did not find this degree of masking at lower spatial frequencies).

Orientation Discrimination for Color-Defined Form

Webster, DeValois, and Switkes (1990) compared orientation discrimination thresholds for equiluminant sinusoidal CD gratings and monochromatic sinusoidal LD gratings. They used two types of CD gratings. One kind was designed so that contrast variations were achieved without any change in the excitation of short-wavelength (S) cones; in other words, they achieved the variations entirely by changes in the balance between excitations of long-wavelength (L) and medium-wavelength (M) cones. The second kind was designed so that contrast variations were achieved without any change in the excitation of either L or M cones, i.e., entirely by changes in the excitation of S cones.

As mentioned earlier, Webster, DeValois, and Switkes expressed grating contrast relative to the detection threshold for that particular CD or LD grating. When contrast was normalized in this way, orientation discrimination threshold for CD gratings was significantly—though not greatly—worse than for LD gratings at all contrast levels. A second finding was that orientation discrimination thresholds were similar for both kinds of CD grating. The effects of contrast were similar for the CD and LD gratings; orientation-discrimination threshold was approximately constant over a wide range of suprathreshold contrasts, but degraded sharply at low contrasts. As discussed in Chapter 2, the effect of contrast on orientation discrimination is important for models of orientation discrimination.

With the intent of finding whether the outputs of spatial filters for chromatic contrast carry an orientation label, Webster et al. measured orientation discrimination at a contrast near grating-detection threshold, adopting the rationale of Thomas and Gille (1979) described on pp. 75–83. On each trial, a single grating with one of two possible orientations was presented in one of two time intervals marked by tones. Webster et al. instructed their observers to signal whether the grating was in the first or second interval (detection) and which of the two orientations was present (discrimination). They then collected their observers' responses over a range of contrasts for each of many orientation differences. Figure 3.24A–C shows how the contrast required to detect gratings (open symbols) and to discriminate their orientations (filled symbols) varied with the difference between the two possible orientations. When the two possible orientations were only moderately different (4 to 8 degrees), the contrast required to discriminate grating orientation was considerably higher than the contrast required to detect the grating (left side of each plot), but when the difference between the two possible orientations was large, the two orientations could be discriminated at detection threshold (right side of each plot). Figure 3.24A confirms the earlier conclusion of Thomas and Gille (1979) that the orientations of two just-detectable LD gratings can be discriminated, provided that they differ by roughly 30 degrees. Webster et al. added the finding that the orientations of two just-detectable equiluminant constant-S gratings (Figure 3.24B) or constant-LM gratings (Figure 3.24C) can also be discriminated, though the difference between the two possible orientations needs to be considerably greater than for LD gratings.

Webster et al. noted that, although orientation discrimination threshold for the two types of CD gratings did not differ at high contrasts, orientation discrimination at near-threshold contrasts was poorer for constant-LM gratings than for constant-S gratings. For one subject, a difference of 35 to 45 degrees was required to discriminate constant-S gratings at threshold, while similar performance with constant-LM gratings was not achieved until the orientation difference was from 60 to 90 degrees. (Note that a 90 degree difference is the maximum possible.)

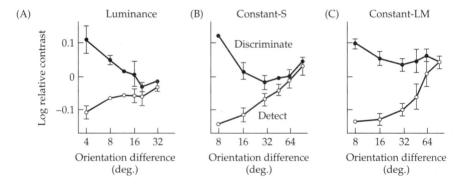

3.24 The contrast required to detect a grating and to discriminate a particular difference in orientation. Contrast threshold for detecting a grating and for discriminating its orientation are plotted as ordinate. In any given trial, grating orientation had one of two possible values. The difference between these two possible values is plotted as abscissa. (A) Luminance gratings. (B) Constant-S chromatic gratings. (C) Constant–L-M chromatic gratings. From Webster, DeValois, and Switkes (1990).

Positional Discrimination, Width Discrimination, Separation Discrimination, and Spatial Frequency Discrimination for Color-Defined Form

Compared with the large body of laboratory research on our abilities to judge the relative directions of luminance-defined objects and to discriminate their widths (see pp. 98–115), little attention has been paid to our corresponding abilities for color-defined objects. But, as discussed next, these latter abilities are by no means negligible.

Positional discrimination

It is known that moderate amounts of blur degrade Vernier acuity for a luminance-defined edge and for abutting or near-abutting luminance-defined lines (Watt and Morgan, 1984; Williams et al., 1984). Taken together with the observation that a sharp edge looks less sharp at equiluminance, this observation suggested to Morgan and Aiba (1985b) that Vernier acuity for a chromatically defined edge or line might be lower than for a similar target defined by luminance contrast. They tested this prediction using two abutting vertical green bars (each 2.6' wide and 9.5' high) with a red surround, and found that Vernier threshold does indeed rise (by 0.5 log units) near the equiluminant point. A similar finding had also been reported by other authors (Mulligan and Krauskopf, 1983; Farell and Krauskopf, 1988).

Morgan and Aiba (1985b) carried out a control experiment to show that the loss of Vernier acuity could not be attributed to a reduction of the detectability of the bars at equiluminance. They measured the narrowest bar that could just be detected in two experimental situations: (a) a green bar with an equiluminant red surround; (b) the bar and surround were the same color, but there was a 10% luminance difference. The result was that width threshold for detecting the CD bar was *lower* than for an LD bar.

The relation between positional acuity and neural receptive-field organization was treated by Morgan and Aiba (1985b) by combining the opponent-process theory of spatial discriminations with the theoretical approach to receptive field analysis of Ingling and Martinez (1983a,b). According to Morgan and Aiba, spatial position discrimination would be degraded at equiluminance because the spatial tuning of the receptive field profile is broadened and its maximum slopes reduced. The finding that Vernier offset threshold was higher for a CD bar than for an LD bar is consistent with this theoretical approach. To explain the apparently conflicting finding that detection threshold was *lower* for the CD bar than for the LD bar, they suggested that bar detection is primarily a low spatial frequency task, while high spatial frequencies are important for the Vernier acuity task.

Bar width and bar separation discrimination

I have been unable to find any reports on width and separation discrimination for CD bars.

Spatial frequency discrimination

Webster et al. (1990) measured spatial frequency discrimination as a function of grating contrast for constant-S, constant-LM, and LD gratings. The luminance data confirmed previous findings that spatial frequency discrimination is poor at low contrasts, rapidly improves as contrast is raised, becomes approximately independent of contrast at high to medium contrasts and asymptotes to a value of from 4 to 7% (Regan et al., 1982; Skottun et al., 1987). The high-frequency asymptote for CD gratings was a little higher than for LD gratings (about 1.4:1 threshold ratio), and this difference was maintained over a spatial frequency range of from 0.5 to 4 cycles/deg. (Vimal, 1988; Webster et al., 1990).

To find whether the outputs of filters for CD form carry a spatial frequency label, Webster et al. (1990) measured spatial frequency discrimination at near-threshold contrasts. Data for luminance gratings confirmed previous findings (Watson and Robson, 1981; Thomas et al., 1982). A frequency difference of between 0.75 and 1.5 octaves (i.e., a frequency ratio between 1:1.7 and 1:2.8) was required for discrimination at contrast detection threshold compared with about 1:1.05 at high contrasts. Discrimination at contrast threshold was slightly poorer for chromatic gratings, a frequency difference of between 1.5 and 2.0 octaves (i.e., a frequency ratio between 1:2.8 and 1:4) being required.

Aspect Ratio Discrimination for Two-Dimensional Color-Defined Form

I have been unable to find any information as to whether observers can ignore trial-to-trial variations in the area of a CD rectangle while discriminating trial-to-trial variations in its aspect ratio, as they can for LD, OTD, MD, and DD rectangles.

Disordered Processing of Color-Defined Form in Patients

When carrying out the Farnsworth-Munsell 100-hue test (and several variants of the Farnsworth D15 test), the observer compares the hues of small circular colored caps. These tests fall into the "successive inspection" class (see pp. 42–44). Tests of the "spatial contrast detection" class assess an observer's ability to detect the spatial boundary between equiluminant regions of different colors that are presented simultaneously to contiguous retinal areas. This class includes the several kinds of anomaloscopes (e.g., Nagel, Pickford-Nicolson) that require observers to match the two halves of a bipartite 2- to 3-degree field so that the entire field appears to be uniform in both hue and luminance. Spatial contrast detection tests also include the task of detecting equiluminant CD gratings. The several kinds of pseudo-isochromatic plates (such as the Ishihara plates and the HRR plates) test shape recognition and shape discrimination as well as contrast sensitivity (see pp. 53–60). In one kind of plate, a color-normal observer sees a figure (e.g., a number) that cannot be seen by observers with a particular type of color deficiency. In another kind of plate, one number is seen by observers with normal color vision and a different number is seen by observers with a particular type of color deficiency. Color vision tests are reviewed by Birch (1991, 1993).

The congenital deuteranopic and protanopic types of color vision defect are associated with a failure of hue discrimination over the red–yellow–green part of the spectrum. It is generally supposed that the deuteranopic defect is caused by a loss of the M- (medium-wavelength) cone type, and that the protanopic defect is caused by a loss of the L- (long-wavelength) cone type. In terms of this hypothesis it is easy to understand why the patterning of an equiluminant red–green CD checkerboard was invisible to a deuteranope, and also why this stimulus produced no electrical brain responses (evoked potentials) in a deuteranope who gave large brain responses to a monochromatic checkerboard pattern (Figure 3.15). The necessary lateral interaction signals did not exist at any level in the visual pathway (Regan & Spekreijse, 1974). It seems, however, that the known forms of inherited defects of color vision do not provide information that allows us to distinguish the processing that underlies color appearance from the processing of chromatic spatial contrast. On the other hand, some acquired defects do allow that distinction to be made.

Zeki (1990) has reviewed the 100-year history of conflict "between data and preconceived opinions" that has characterized research on central achromatopsia (i.e., loss of color vision produced centrally). It now seems to be established that damage to a region of extrastriate cortex in the lingual and fusiform gyri can produce a loss of color perception in the sense that patients report that the visual world appears to be composed of various shades of gray. In the one patient with achromatopsia who had been tested with all the required psychophysical procedures, the long-, medium-, and short-wavelength cone mechanisms were all shown to be functioning even though color perception was essentially absent (Mollon et al., 1980). Zeki notes that one interpretation of reports on achromatopsia caused by damage to the lingual and fusiform gyri is that, even though color-coded neurons are activated in the striate cortex of such patients, this is not sufficient to support the subjective experience of color.

Several authors have suggested that the region in the lingual and fusiform gyri just discussed can be regarded as the homologue of Zeki's area V4 in the prestriate visual cortex of macaque monkey (Zeki, 1973, 1977, 1980; Green & Lessell, 1977; Pearlman et al., 1978; Damasio et al., 1980; Heywood et al., 1987). It is known that this V4 cortical area in monkey is important in the processing of both color and spatial form. It has also been proposed that long-range lateral interconnections within area V4 in monkey provide a basis for *color constancy*. That is, they provide the basis for the phenomenon that perceived color of an illuminated surface remains comparatively constant when the spectral content of the light illuminating the surface is varied (Zeki, 1980). Evidence that long-range lateral interconnections within and between the homologues of V4 in the left and right hemispheres are responsible for color constancy in man was reported by Land et al. (1983).

The results described so far do not address the question whether a central lesion can dissociate different aspects of color processing. Victor et al. (1989) addressed this question in a study of a patient with acquired central dyschromatopsia (i.e., partial loss of color vision) associated with lesions in the ventromedial occipital lobe. Their conclusion was that sensitivity to chromatic contrast was normal, although the patient's performance was severely impaired on tests of color naming; in addition, the ability to distinguish one color from another (as measured by the Farnsworth-Munsell 100-hue test) was degraded.

The crucial evidence was as follows. The luminances of a red and a green patch of light were equated by heterochromatic flicker photometry, and the balance point was found to be within the normal range. Spatial contrast detection threshold for a red–green equiluminant grating was measured for static gratings of spatial frequencies of 0.3, 2.5, and 10 cycles/deg. Both the shape of the curve and absolute values of threshold were normal, similar to the open triangles in Figure 1.19.

This finding raises the speculation, yet to be investigated, that some patients might be able to see CD form (e.g., a red H with an equiluminant green surround), even though the patient perceived no difference in the appearances of the red and green areas on successive inspection—much as the visibility of the OTD letter in Figure 4.10A can be modeled in terms of the way in which the texture contrast is translated into "intensity" values, as illustrated in Figure 4.10D. In the present hypothetical case it might be that lateral inhibition between the responses of adjacent retinal points stimulated by the same color would cause the translated "intensity" values to be low except near the chromatic border.

A relevant study on normally sighted subjects was reported by Lueck et al. (1989), who used position emission tomography (PET) to measure the increase in blood flow through active regions of the brain. When a normally sighted human viewed a multicolored pattern (a Land color-Mondrian), two regions of increased activity were observed. One was in striate cortex, and the other one was some distance away in the lingual and fusiform gyri. In a control experiment, the subject viewed a display that *had the same spatial patterning as the multicolored Mondrian*, but consisted of shades of gray. The activity in the striate cortex remained the same, but the activity in the lingual and fusiform gyri fell by about one-third. However, a confound in the Lueck et al. (1989) study was that the color-Mondrian differed from the gray Mondrian in that different color appearances were present as well as color-defined boundaries. See footnote on page 33.

Psychophysical Models of the Processing of Color-Defined Form

Almost all models of color vision are based on data collected with stimulus fields that, completely or almost completely, lack spatial patterning. These data indicate that the spectral sensitivity of the achromatic system follows the V_λ curve. In modeling the processing of color-defined form, many authors have assumed that humans have a system for *achromatic contrast* and, furthermore, that the spectral sensitivity of this hypothetical achromatic contrast system follows the V_λ curve. On pages 237–245 I discussed caveats about these assumptions. In the following section I first review what might be termed mainstream models, and then present a radically different approach.

Models based on an achromatic contrast system with a V_λ spectral sensitivity

As discussed on pp. 250–253, the hypothesis that luminance and color information feed a common spatial contrast filter (Figure 2.16A) can be rejected. In attempting to account for their cross-masking data, Switkes et al. (1988) first considered the hypothesis that interactions between luminance and color gratings are all excitatory, as illustrated in Figure 2.16B. The nonlinear stage in part B is accelerating near threshold and compressive at high input levels. In part B the suprathreshold masking of luminance by color and vice versa is represented by the bold arrowed lines, indicating strong excitatory cross inputs that drive the operating point well into the compressive region at the upper end of the nonlinear characteristic, and thus reduce sensitivity to luminance-contrast increments. Figure 3.25A explains this idea in the particular case of C_{mask}/L_{test}. The excitatory cross-signal from the color system is designated in Figure 3.25A by "C_{mask} cross-signal." This cross-signal sets the operating point (OP) high on the characteristic where the slope of the characteristic is low. Because of this low slope, a large contrast increment ΔL_1 is needed to produce a just-detectable change of output Δy.

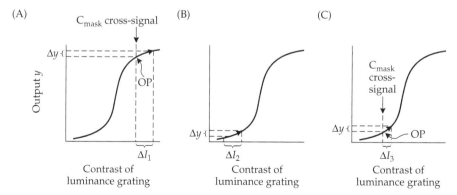

3.25 A candidate explanation for the dipper effect. The curve is the input–output characteristic of the hypothetical luminance contrast processing stage in the visual pathway. As the input level is progressively increased from zero (A,B), smaller and smaller increments of input (ΔI) are required to produce a given change of output (Δy). As the input level approaches high values (A), larger and larger increments of input are required to produce a given change of output. From Regan (1991b).

The Figure 2.16B hypothesis can be rejected because it predicts that luminance-grating detection would be facilitated by a color grating masker when the masker contrast was low, and Switkes et al. (1988) did not find this experimentally. The prediction can be understood as follows. With no masker present, the operating point is more or less near the origin, depending on the level of neural noise at the input of the nonlinearity. Figure 3.25B illustrates that this region of the characteristic has a low slope so that a comparatively large increment in the contrast of the luminance test grating (ΔL_2) would be required to produce a just-detectable change of output (Δy). Figure 3.25C shows that a weak cross-signal from the color-grating mask would shift OP, the operating point, to a steeper part of the characteristic so that a smaller luminance contrast increment (ΔL_3) would be sufficient to produce a just-detectable change of output (Δy). In other words, the Figure 2.16B model predicts incorrectly that a low-contrast chromatic masker grating would lower luminance-contrast threshold.

Although the hypothesis proposed by Mullen and Losada (1994) illustrated in Figure 2.16C accounts for the desensitizations shown in Figure 3.22A,B, it does not account for the suprathreshold facilitation observed for all three observers in Figure 3.22B.

Switkes et al. (1988) pointed out that, as illustrated in Figure 2.16D, different processing stages may be responsible for the accelerating and compressive segments of the transducer characteristic. (A more detailed account of the transducer characteristic and of contrast gain control is given on pp. 75–91.) In the spirit of their proposal I offer the all-excitation hypothesis shown in Figure 2.16D. Consider the L_{mask}/C_{test} condition. There is no subthreshold facilitation because the cross input occurs after the accelerating segment of the transducer function. At low suprathreshold values of mask contrast the solid arrowed line marked 3(+) accounts for the facilitation to the right of the vertical dashed line in Figure 3.22B. The excitatory signal marked 1(+) has little effect, because it is operating within the approximately straight central segment of the transducer function for the chromatic-contrast mechanism. As the contrast of the masker grating is progressively increased, the excitatory signal marked 1(+) shifts the operating point well into the compressive segment of the transducer function for the chromatic-contrast mechanism, thus producing a strong masking effect. This eventually overcomes the facilitation effect produced by the input marked 3(+), thus accounting for the transition from facilitation to masking shown in Figure 3.22B.

The hypothesis illustrated in Figure 2.16 D can account for the data of Switkes et al. (1988) collected in the C_{mask}/L_{test} condition and for the results of two of the three observers whose data are shown in Figure 3.22A. The suprathreshold facilitation in one of the three curves can be explained if we assume that some, but not all, observers have a cross-connection shown by the dashed line in Figure 2.16D, excitatory signal 4(+).

The hypothesis illustrated in Figure 2.16D can also account for the following findings reported by Mullen and Losada (1994). The shape of the L_{mask}/L_{test} dipper function (Figure 2.12) was unchanged by the presence of a suprathreshold luminance-contrast masker, though its overall position was shifted upward and rightward; the shape of the C_{mask}/C_{test} dipper function (Figure 2.12) was unchanged by the presence of a suprathreshold color-contrast masker. In Figure 2.12D the subthreshold facilitation observed in, for example, the L_{mask}/L_{test} condition would still be observed in the presence of a color grating, because color gratings have no access to the accelerating segment of the transducer function that receives input from luminance gratings. An overall desensitizing effect would be expected, because the excitatory signal marked 2(+) would drive the operating point even further along the compressive segment of the transducer function than would have been the case with no color grating present.

According to Ingling and Martinez (1983a,b), the observation that the contrast sensitivity function for equiluminant CD gratings is lowpass, whereas the contrast sensitivity function for monochromatic LD gratings is bandpass, does not in itself indicate that CD gratings and LD gratings are processed by different filters. They have suggested that the lowpass/bandpass distinction between chromatic and achromatic contrast sensitivity functions can be explained in terms of the color-opponent, circularly symmetrical receptive-field organization characteristic of a large proportion of the retinal ganglion cell population in monkeys (DeMonastrario & Gouras, 1975; Gouras, 1991b; Gouras & Zrenner, 1981). Ingling and Martinez (1983a,b) showed theoretically that the response of an (idealized) chromatically—and spatially—opponent filter is equal to the sum of two responses. One of these can be described as a bandpass spatial frequency filter with an achromatic (R + G) spectral sensitivity, and the other can be described as a lowpass spatial frequency filter with opponent-color (R − G) spectral sensitivity. Thus, according to this line of thought, it is an inherent property of the receptive-field organization of such opponent filters that they produce both summing and differencing signals (see also Rohaly & Buchsbaum, 1988, 1989; Kelly, 1989). At low spatial frequencies the filter would be sensitive to both chromatic and luminance gratings, while at high spatial frequencies it would be sensitive only to luminance gratings. Theoretical algorithms for decoding the output of chromatically opponent filters so as to separate the (R + G) and (R − G) signals are discussed by Ingling and Martinez (1983a,b).

On the other hand, this often-repeated statement that psychophysical spatial filters for CD form lack an inhibitory surround is inconsistent with the psychophysical evidence (shown in Figures 2.9B and 3.23, and in Losada & Mullen, 1994) that CD form filters have a bandpass characteristic (E. Switkes, personal communication, July 1996). Switkes noted that "the spatial tuning, along with the orientation specificity observed for chromatic grating detection" (Figure 3.24B,C) "points to a cortical site for the limiting mechanisms; there the chromatic double-opponent cells would provide the necessary spatial antagonism to create bandpass color mechanisms." He, along with others, suggests that "the overall lowpass color contrast sensitivity function reflects variations in the numerosity or peak sensitivity of mechanisms tuned to various spatial frequencies, rather than the filter characteristics of each mechanism" (E. Switkes, personal communication, July 1996 ; see also Losada & Mullen, 1994).

And Sekiguchi et al. (1993b) state that attempts to account for the lowpass–bandpass distinction between the contrast sensitivity curves for CD and LD gratings that is evident at low spatial frequencies (see Figure 1.19) in terms of the properties of center-surround units fail to explain the differences in neural bandwidth at high spatial frequencies depicted in Figure 3.21.

Models framed in terms of two or more parallel spatial filters sensitive to monochromatic contrast

Warning to readers who are not conversant with the color vision field: What follows is not mainstream color vision theory.

On the basis of the findings described on pp. 237–245, I proposed a hypothesis that is totally different from the hypotheses just discussed (Regan, 1972, 1973b, 1975a,b). Figure 3.26 illustrates an elaborated version of my hypothesis.

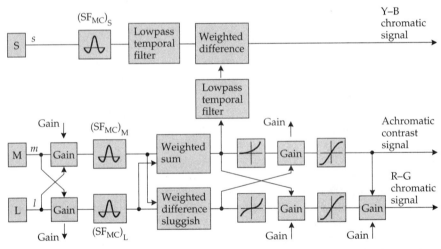

3.26 A different way of looking at the processing of chromatic and achromatic contrast. The first stage of processing any kind of spatial pattern, whether multicolored or not, is entirely in terms of monochromatic contrast. There are at three monochromatic spatial contrast filters and, at least for the long- and medium-wavelength spatial filters, nonlinear interactions between cone outputs precede spatial filtering. The outputs of these long- and medium-wavelength spatial filters are rearranged to give an achromatic-contrast signal and a red–green opponent signal. According to this hypothesis, spatial filtering precedes the color-opponent stage. Key: *l*, *m*, and *s* are the outputs of the long-wavelength (L), medium-wavelength (M), and short-wavelength (S) cones, respectively.

> The crucial feature of that hypothesis is that at the earliest stage of spatial information processing there is no spatial filter whose spectral sensitivity matches the individual's relative luminosity curve (as measured, for example, by heterochromatic flicker photometry).

Earlier I reviewed evidence that monochromatic contrast is processed by (at least) two parallel mechanisms, neither of whose relative spectral sensitivities correspond to an observer's relative luminosity curve. I proposed the pair of filters sensitive to monochromatic spatial contrast—designated $(SF_{MC})_L$ and $(SF_{MC})_M$ in Figure 3.26—to account for the findings shown in Figure 3.18 (Regan, 1972, 1973).

The shoulders visible on both the long- and medium-wavelength curves in Figure 3.18 suggest that there is an interaction between signals from L cones and M cones. An interaction would be consistent with the comment that equiluminant settings "appear to depend on channels that do not represent luminance and color independently" (Webster and Mollon, 1993, p. 1332). I assumed that this interaction reduces the gain of the achromatic-contrast and chromatic-contrast filters as illustrated in Figure 3.26.

To obtain the predictions shown in Figure 3.27A we used the Smith–Pokorny–Voss cone sensitivity functions (Kaiser & Boynton, 1996, p. 558) to compute the relative spectral sensitivities of the $(SF_{MC})_L$ and $(SF_{MC})_M$ filters (Regan & Regan, unpublished data, 2000).*

First we obtained the $(SF_{MC})_L$ curve by calculating $\log[l(1 - m/1.6m_{max})]$, where m_{max} was the maximum height of the M-cone curve. Thus, we modeled the effect of the m signal as a reduction of the contrast gain of the $(SF_{MC})_L$ filter. This reduction is of moderate strength and, being multiplicative, is nonlinear. We obtained the $(SF_{MC})_M$ curve by calculating $\log[m(1 - l/3l_{max})]$ for values of l within approximately 0.6 of l_{max} and by calculating $\log[m/(1 - l/4l_{max})]$ for lower values of l. In other words, we modeled the effect of the l signal as a moderately strong reduction of the contrast gain of the $(SF_{MC})_M$ filter at wavelengths where the L-cone signal is strong, and as a lesser reduction of the contrast gain of the $(SF_{MC})_M$ filter at wavelengths where the M-cone signal is weak. In Figure 3.27A, we have normalized the $(SF_{MC})_L$ and $(SF_{MC})_M$ curves.

In Figure 3.26 the outputs of the two monochromatic-contrast filters are summed at a stage that does not greatly degrade the dynamic characteristics of the l and m signals. The summed output, shown in Figure 3.27B, is the achromatic-contrast signal. Although its spectral sensitivity curve (measured through the eyes' optics) will vary with spatial frequency, at low spatial frequencies its spectral sensitivity curve will approximate the individual observer's relative luminosity curve as determined by heterochromatic flicker photometry. (The word "approximate" is used because of the contamination of HFP data caused by differential

---

* Computational modelling and generation of Fig. 3.27 by Marian P. Regan.

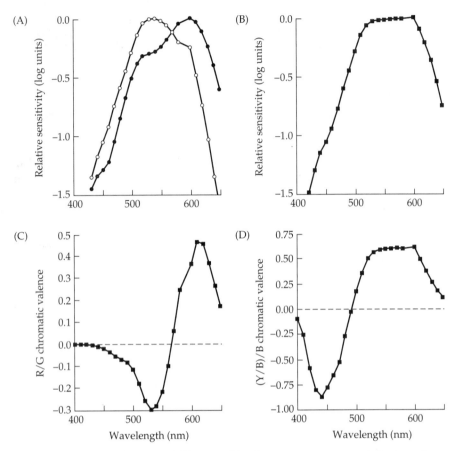

3.27 Predictions of the model illustrated in Figure 3.26. (A) Modeled spectral sensitivities for the long-wavelength and medium-wavelength monochromatic spatial filters in Figure 3.26. (B) Modeled achromatic-contrast signal. The weightings of the outputs of the (SFMC)L and (SFMC)M filters were, respectively, 0.96 and 0.89. (C) Modeled red–green opponent-process signal. The weightings of the outputs of the (SFMC)L and (SFMC)M filters were, respectively, 0.74 and 0.67. (D) Modeled yellow–blue opponent-process signal. The weightings of the outputs of the (SFMC)L and (SFMC)M filters were, respectively, 0.39 and 0.39. The weighting of the S-cone output was 0.83. The weightings were after Sankeralli and Mullen (1996).

adaptation of the three cone types; see Lennie et al., 1993.) Figure 3.27B shows the relative luminosity curve *for the spatial patterns used to obtain the data shown in Figure 3.18* predicted on the basis of the model shown in Figure 3.26.

Figure 3.26 shows that the outputs of the long-wavelength and medium-wavelength achromatic contrast filters are subtracted at a stage that attenuates high spatial frequencies with respect to low spectral frequencies (Figures 3.20 and 3.21) and is considerably more restricted in dynamic range that either of its inputs. I suppose that the resulting dynamic range is indicated by Figures 3.8 and 3.11. Figure 3.27C shows the predicted red–green chromatic contrast signal (compare with the color-appearance data shown in Figure 3.3). To explain why the location of the yellow minimum in Figure 3.9 does not depend on temporal frequency, I assume that both l and m signals experience the same lowpass filtering.

No low-wavelength shoulder is evident on the leftmost curve in Figure 3.18 that would suggest the presence of a third monochromatic-contrast filter peaking at a wavelength not greatly shorter than 545 nm. As noted earlier, I failed to pursue with sufficient vigor the question whether the brain responses shown in Figure 3.1 evoked by a monochromatic checkerboard whose wavelength (436 nm) was far into the blue end of the spectrum (its hue is sometimes called violet) was mediated via an achromatic spatial filter with peak sensitivity in the blue. So the relevant brain response data are not available. But relevant psychophysical data are. Humanski and Wilson (1992) showed that isolated short-wavelength cones feed two orientation-selective spatial filters whose sensitivities peak at 0.7 and 1.4 cycles/deg., respectively. The spatial tuning of these filters closely resembles the two filters centered on the lowest spatial frequencies that were revealed using achromatic luminance-defined targets (Figure 2.12).

In Figure 3.26 the output of the $(SF_{MC})_S$ filter is subtracted from the output of the weighted-sum stage to create the blue–yellow chromatic contrast signal. To account for the effect of temporal frequency on the spectral location of the blue–green minimum in Figure 3.9, I assume that the signals pass through different lowpass filters before being subtracted. Figure 3.27D shows the predicted yellow–blue valence curve for the spatial patterns used to obtain the data shown in Figure 3.18. In Figure 3.26 the stages that follow the weighted-sum and weighted-difference processing of the M- and L-cone signals follow Switkes et al. (1998); see Figure 2.16D.

In common with the hypothesis illustrated in Figure 3.2, the first stage in Figure 3.26 is the parallel array of independently functioning L-, M-, and S-wavelength cones, so that this alternative "nonmainstream" hypothesis is also consistent with the experimental facts of trichromacy as set out by Wright (1946, 1991).

To end this nonmainstream section, I include an excerpt from the section headed "Multiple mechanisms with $V(\lambda)$-like spectral sensitivity?" in a review entitled "Luminance." Referring to neurons in the striate cortex of macaque monkeys, Lennie, Pokorny, and Smith state:

> Although the average spectral sensitivity of neurons in the upper layers is close to V_λ, few individual neurons have the spectral sensitivity of V_λ; indeed the spectral sensitivity of many that respond well to achromatic stimuli clearly differ from V_λ, generally having narrower spectral-sensitivity functions that result from their receiving opposed (albeit weakly opposed) inputs from M cones and L cones. Cells with the weakly opponent organization are chromatically heterogeneous and form no sharply identified group, yet they are so numerous and generally have such finely tuned spatial and orientational selectivities that there

can be little doubt that they play some important role in form vision. Could this heterogeneous population of cells give rise to the $V(\lambda)$-like spectral-sensitivity functions in acuity tasks and those involving detections of punctuate light? . . . . [I]f we suppose that the visual stimulus activates several cells, linear combinations of signals from these cells might reasonably be expected to give rise to a spectral-sensitivity curve that reflects the average of the spectral sensitivities of the individual cells. (Lennie et al., 1993, p. 1289)

CHAPTER 4

Texture-Defined Form

Preamble

In the everyday visual world, shadows create bright–dark edges that could be mistakenly identified as an object's boundaries if figure–ground segregation relied entirely on luminance contrast. Differences between the surface textures of different objects can override such misleading information. Indeed, although we are seldom aware of it in everyday life, a difference in texture can, by itself, support object detection. In this section I will focus on the role of texture in supporting the segregation of objects from their surroundings, as distinct from the more-or-less related topics of texture recognition and classification, pop-out of single texture elements, rapid visual search, and spatial attention.

To carry out scientific research on the contribution of texture differences to object visibility, it is first necessary to describe different textures quantitatively, and preferably concisely. In view of the enormous number of textures we encounter in the everyday world—a brick wall, polished wood, a cat's fur, shot silk—devising a concise quantitative description that applies to all textures might seem a formidable task. On the other hand, in view of the enormous number of colors we encounter in the everyday world, a concise quantitative description of color might seem an equally formidable task, but this problem was solved more than 60 years ago (Guild, 1926, 1931; Wright, 1928–29, 1946). As discussed in Chapter 3, the basis for this achievement of color research is that all color information passes through only three *psychophysical channels* (whose physical correlates were recently shown to be the three classes of cone photopigment). The rationale for a great deal of texture research has been the hypothesis that, like color information, texture information is processed through a small number of *channels* so that, if the properties of these channels could be determined, any given texture could be specified by only a few numbers.

Recognizing the achievement of the CIE system for describing colors, many researchers in texture perception have adopted some of the approaches that have proved effective in the much older field of color research. The early laboratory researchers in color vision reduced the complexities of everyday color perception by using as their stimulus a 2 degree bipartite, foveally viewed stimulus rather than the complex combinations of spatial pattern and color we encounter in the everyday world (Wright, 1991). Following a similar line of thought, rather than using real world object textures, researchers in texture perception have used synthesized simple texture patterns that lend themselves to concise quantitative description. Borrowing further from color vision research, Whitman Richards has even attempted to apply the concept of metamerism (see the first footnote on p. 214) to research on texture perception by inventing the procedure of texture matching (Richards & Polit, 1974; Richards, 1979). The history of research on texture perception has been incisively reviewed by Bergen (1991).

Detection of Texture-Defined Form

A difference in texture between the retinal images of a spatial form and its surroundings can cause the form to segregate from its surroundings so that it can be recognized, even when the form and its surroundings are identical in luminance, color, motion, and disparity. The process is completed within 100 msec. (Beck et al., 1983; Julesz, 1981). Figure 4.1A illustrates this phenomenon that has been referred to as preattentive, instantaneous, or effortless texture discrimination by Julesz (1981), or as the formation of illusory (subjective) contours between differently textured regions (especially in the physiological literature; see Peterhans and Baumgartner, 1984), or as texture-based segmentation (especially in the computer vision literature; see Bergen, 1991). This phenomenon is the topic of this section.

> Not all pairs of textures segregate. In particular, it does not necessarily follow that, because texture elements look quite different, segregation will occur when they are placed in contiguous regions (Beck, 1966a,b; Olsen & Attneave, 1970). Figure 4.1B illustrates this point.

One way of looking at this distinction between, on the one hand, texture-based segregation and, on the other hand, differences between surface textures is that discriminating two successively inspected textures requires merely that the two textures should generate different visual signals when presented to the same retinal region at different times, whereas texture segregation requires a response when different textures are presented simultaneously to adjacent regions of the retina. In particular, certain lateral interactions are involved in the second case that are not necessarily involved in the first case.

(A)   (B)

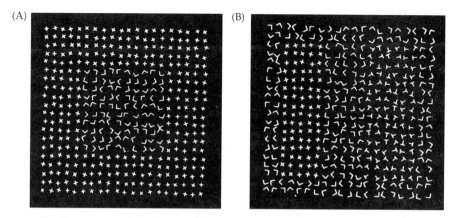

4.1 Effortless texture-based segregation. (A) The central square region has the same color and mean luminance as its surroundings. The square has clear but illusory boundaries. (B) Some pairs of textures do not segregate. Laborious element-by-element inspection reveals that the right side of the texture pattern contains a rectangular area filled with T's that is surrounded by a region filled with L's, but this region does not segregate effortlessly, as the rectangular area in the left side of the pattern does. From Bergen and Julesz (1983).

For reasons discussed later in this chapter, and because most of the research on spatial discriminations for texture-defined (TD) form has been restricted to orientation-texture-defined (OTD) form, the rest of this section focuses on orientation texture. This restriction means that a considerable amount of published work on texture perception per se, including the role of surface texture in object recognition (e.g., Joseph & Victor, 1994), is omitted.*

Nothdurft (1985b) suggested that one of the requirements for the segregation of an OTD form from its immediate surroundings is an adequately large local gradient of orientation. "Adequate," Nothdurft added, means that the orientation gradient at the boundary of the OTD form must be significantly larger than

---

* I make a sharp distinction between the retinal image of a textured object and surface texture per se. This chapter is about how we see *objects*. For example, in Figures 4.11 and 4.12, we modeled the recognition of texture-defined letters in terms of seeking the best match between internal templates and the processed retinal image of a noise-degraded letter. These internal templates were the processed retinal images of the 10 noise-free letters in the stimulus set. I do not suppose that this approach would be useful in attempting to model the recognition and classification of surface textures per se, as for example, when we very quickly classify a texture as tree bark and reject other candidate hypotheses such as a brick wall, and so on. I do not suppose that one compares the retinal image with a series of stored templates of many kinds of tree bark, many kinds of brick wall, and so on. Rather one classifies the retinal image into a general category of tree bark, rejecting a "brick wall" and other general categories. The work of Julesz and his colleagues on the statistics of textures focused on mathematically defined classes of texture rather than on the topic of this section, which is the early processing of texture-defined form in which my focus is the nature of the human visual system. In an attempt to classify surface textures Rao and Lohse (1996) have proposed a quite different approach.

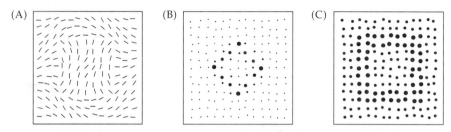

4.2 Illustration of texture segregation that cannot be explained in terms of a difference in the density of textons. (A) Texture pattern of oriented lines. The rectangular area segregates effortlessly. (B) Spatial distribution of textons, here vertical line textons. Texture segregation based on this texton distribution should generate the impression of a diamond. Response strength, indicated by spot size, is assumed to be modulated by local orientation contrast. (C) Response distribution of pools of neurons with different orientation preferences, but similar sensitivity to orientation contrast as the neurons in (B). Texture segregation borders could be determined by nonspecific summation over many orientation-selective neurons. From Nothdurft (1991).

the orientation gradient at any other location within the OTD form or its immediate surroundings, i.e., the orientation contrast gradient locally at the boundary is greater than elsewhere in the entire texture pattern. Evidence for this suggestion includes the finding that widely spaced texture elements do not segregate or pop out (Nothdurft, 1985b; Sagi & Julesz, 1987). A demonstration of this last point is given in Nothdurft (1985b). Landy and Bergen (1991) confirmed Nothdurft's suggestion by using a texture pattern for which there was no covariance between orientation gradient and spatial sampling. Figure 4.2A–C illustrates this important idea. The line orientation texture in Figure 4.2A segregates effortlessly into a rectangular area with a surround. However, the spatial distribution of a typical texton (a vertical line in this illustration) is the diamond shape shown in Figure 4.2B. (The texton concept is discussed in the section on psychophysical models). Nothdurft (1991a) noted that lines at other orientations show less regular spatial distributions and concluded that, if the perception of texture borders were based on first-order differences within maps for specific textons, we would not see a rectangle in Figure 4.2A. Figure 4.2C shows the response distribution of pools of

4.3 Texture-defined form. (A) Photograph of the texture pattern used to measure ▶ detection threshold and spatial frequency discrimination threshold for a texture-defined grating. The peak-to-peak texture contrast (β_{max}) is 90 degrees in the grating illustrated. (B) Photograph of the texture pattern used to measure aspect ratio discrimination for a texture-defined rectangle. (C) Photograph of the texture pattern used to measure Vernier acuity for texture-defined form. Part A from Gray and Regan (1998a). Part B from Regan, Hajdur, and Hong (1996b). Part C from Gray and Regan (1997).

(A)

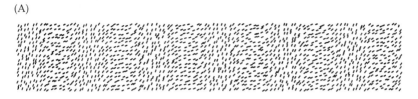

(B)

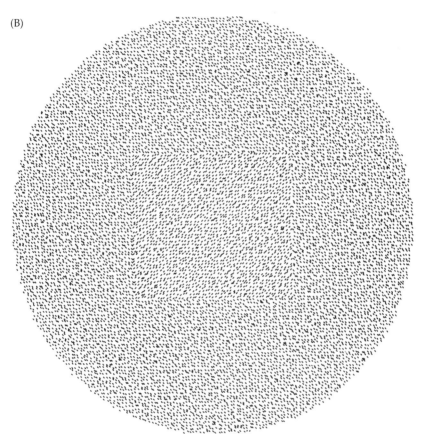

(C)

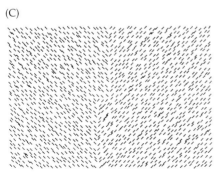

neurons with different orientation preferences but with similar sensitivity to orientation contrast as the neurons in Figure 4.2B.

Nothdurft (1985a,b; 1991b) concluded the following about the texture borders in Figure 4.2A.

> The texture borders are perceived at locations where the adjacent texture lines have large orientation differences rather than at locations where lines of a certain orientation vary in density.

The concept of orientation contrast gradient is pertinent to the interpretation of data on the detection of sinewave orientation-texture-defined (OTD) gratings such as that illustrated in Figure 4.3A. One possibility is that an OTD grating is detected when orientation contrast gradient rises above some threshold value. An alternative possibility is that a TD grating is detected when a *region-based* (Caelli, 1985) mechanism rather than an *edge-based* mechanism is sufficiently excited. In particular, we hypothesized that the TD grating is detected when the maximum difference of line orientation within the texture pattern rises above some threshold value.

To decide between these two hypotheses, we requested observers to judge which of two successive pattern presentations contained a TD grating (Gray & Regan, 1998a). As illustrated in Figure 4.3A, line orientation varied sinusoidally from left to right between extremes of $(\theta_{mean} + 0.5\beta)$ and $(\theta_{mean} - 0.5\beta)$.

Filled circles in Figure 4.4 show how the orientation contrast* required to detect an OTD grating depended on spatial frequency over the range 0.07 cycles/deg. to 7.0 cycles/deg. in the situation that the number of texture lines per grating cycle was six or more (see pp. 470–476), and the length of the texture lines was more than 1.2 minutes of arc.† (See Appendix F for a discussion of these points in the context of Nyquist's theorem.).

If orientation gradient were the only determinant of the visibility of an OTD grating, a log–log plot of detection threshold versus spatial frequency would be a straight line, threshold being halved for each doubling of spatial frequency. Filled circles in Figure 4.4 show that this was not the case.

One possible explanation for the finding that the OTD grating detection curve is not a straight line of unity slope is that bar width and orientation gradient covary for OTD sinewave gratings. In contrast, the widths of the OTD targets dis-

---

* The orientation contrast (β) between a line of orientation θ_2 and a line of orientation θ_1 is equal to $(\theta_2 - \theta_1)$ if $(\theta_2 - \theta_1) < 90$ degrees, and is equal to $[180 - (\theta_2 - \theta_1)]$ if $(\theta_2 - \theta_1) > 90$ degrees. Thus, the greatest possible orientation contrast is 90 degrees.

† For OTD gratings, there was an absolute limit to the number of spatial samples per degree of visual angle. The reason was as follows. If texture lines were not to overlap, line length had to be reduced when the number of spatial samples per degree was high; when line length became too short (less than 1.0 to 1.5 minutes of arc), the just-noticeable difference in line orientation started to rise.

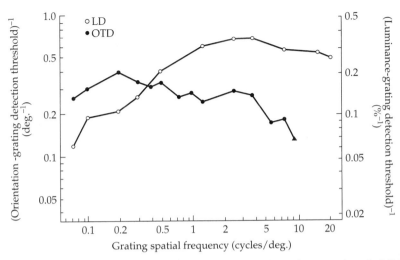

4.4 **Contrast sensitivity functions for spatially sampled gratings rendered visible by luminance contrast (open symbols) and by texture contrast (filled symbols).** The number of spatial samples per grating cycle was six or more for open and filled circles. Threshold rose when the number of samples per grating cycle fell below approximately 6. For the filled triangle there were 4 samples per grating cycle. After Gray and Regan (1998a).

cussed by Nothdurft (typically, a rectangle or an optotype) did not covary with the orientation gradient across the target's boundary.

The finding that the OTD contrast sensitivity curve is approximately flat over the 60:1 range between 0.07 cycles/deg. and about 4.0 cycles/deg. can be understood if orientation contrast information passes through an array of parallel spatial filters that prefer OTD targets of different widths and in addition, that over a range of bar widths from 7 degrees to 0.13 degrees, any given bar is detected when the total difference of orientation within the receptive field tuned to that particular grating period exceeds some fixed threshold (approximately 3.3 degrees in Figure 4.4). We arrived at the following proposal, which can be seen in the context of Nothdurft's (1985b) hypothesis that the segregation of OTD form can be based on an "adequately large" spatial rate of change of line orientation (as, very clearly, in the case of Figure 4.14).

> The segregation of OTD form can be based *either* on narrow filters that extract the boundaries of the OTD form by virtue of their sensitivity to locally steep spatial gradients of line orientation *or* (as in the case of the OTD grating data shown in Figure 4.4) on comparatively wide local spatial filters that are specialized for the detection of OTD form (see Figure 4.13) and are matched to the size of the OTD target (one grating cycle in the case of Figure 4.4A).

On the basis of a quite different kind of experimental data, Wolfson and Landy (1998) independently concluded that the human visual system contains edge-based and region-based mechanisms for texture analysis.

A spatially sampled LD grating was created by assigning the same orientation to all texture lines and imposing a sinusoidal variation of line luminance across the pattern. The contrast sensitivity function plotted as open circles in Figure 4.4 shows how the luminance contrast required to detect an LD grating depended on spatial frequency over the range 0.07 cycles/deg. to 22 degrees (see pp. 470–472 for a discussion of the effect of spatial sampling on this function).

Since the differences between the thresholds designated by filled and open circles were not affected by spatial sampling (the spatial sampling of the LD and OTD grating were the same at every point on the abscissa), we can conclude that they show a difference between the contrast sensitivity functions for OTD and LD gratings. The major differences are as follows:

1. The familiar intermediate-frequency peak in the LD grating characteristic is absent in the OTD characteristic.
2. The highest resolvable spatial frequency would be considerably less for an OTD grating (little more than 10 cycles/deg. in Figure 4.4) than the 35 to 50 cycles/deg. reported for LD gratings (Campbell & Green, 1965; Robson, 1966; Van Nes & Bouman, 1967; Smallman et al., 1996).

This second difference can be understood straightforwardly if, as discussed on pp. 288–294, receptive fields for OTD form are created by a spatial integration stage that follows the stage at which the orientations of individual texture lines are encoded.

Channels for Texture-Defined Form

We obtained evidence that the human visual system contains channels tuned to the orientation of OTD form by adopting the same rationale as that used to establish the existence of channels for LD form (Figures 2.8–2.10) (Kwan & Regan, 1998). The adapting grating was similar to the OTD grating illustrated in Figure 4.3A except that, as illustrated in Figure 4.5A, the pattern was circular rather than rectangular. Grating spatial frequency was 0.5 cycles/deg. Baselines were measured after adapting to a texture pattern that contained exactly the same texture

4.5 Examples of the stimuli used to obtain the data shown in Figure 4.6. (A) ▶
Vertical orientation-texture-defined (OTD) grating with the maximum-possible orientation contrast (90 degrees) and a vertical (0 degrees) mean line orientation. (B) Scatter pattern matched to the grating shown in part A. Each individual line in the scatter pattern corresponds to a line in the OTD grating, and vice versa, but the line orientations are ordered periodically in the grating and randomly varied in the scatter pattern. After Kwan and Regan (1998).

(A)

(B)

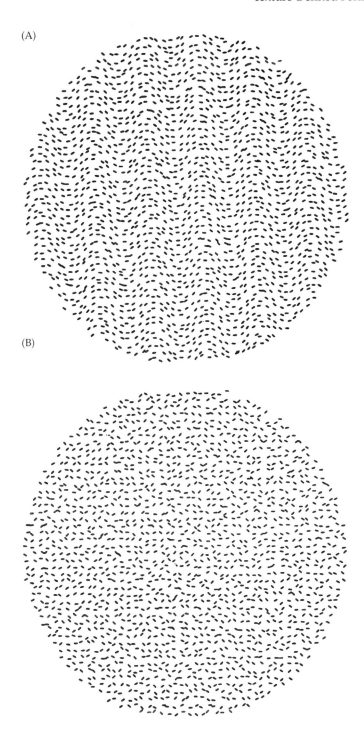

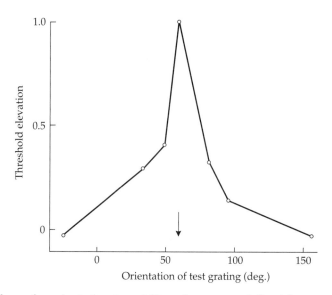

4.6 Evidence for orientation-tuned filters for texture-defined form. Ordinates plot normalized elevations of detection threshold for texture-defined test gratings caused by adapting to a texture-defined grating of high (90 degrees) orientation contrast. The adapting orientation is arrowed. Threshold elevation was given by the ratio $[(\beta_2/\beta_1) - 1]$, where β_1 and β_2 were, respectively, the orientation contrasts required to detect the grating before and after adaptation. Data points are means for two observers. After Kwan and Regan (1998).

lines as the adapting grating (Figure 4.5B). The only difference between the two patterns was that lines of different orientation were randomly scattered rather than being ordered as in Figure 4.5A.

> Thus, any difference between the adapted and baseline thresholds could be attributed to the periodicity (spatial structure) of the OTD grating rather than the adapting effect of the individual texture lines.

Figure 4.6 shows how threshold elevations produced by adapting to an OTD grating of fixed orientation varied with the orientation of the test grating. The postadaptation threshold elevation peaked at the adapting orientation and fell to zero for test gratings perpendicular to the adapting grating. When the orientation of the adapting grating was changed by 90 degrees, the threshold elevation curve shifted bodily through 90 degrees. This was the case independently of the mean orientation of the texture lines.

> These data imply that the human visual system contains orientation-tuned channels sensitive to OTD form.

Next, we asked how the sensitivity of the filter that responded most strongly to an OTD grating depended on (1) the orientation of the grating, and (2) the difference between the orientation of the grating and the mean orientation of the texture lines. We measured detection threshold for four different grating orientations (vertical, horizontal, and the two obliques) in the condition that the mean orientation of the texture lines was vertical (i.e., 0 degrees). Then we repeated the experiment with the mean orientation of the texture lines held constant at 45 degrees, 90 degrees, and 135 degrees. The result of subjecting the thresholds for all four observers in all 16 conditions to repeated measures analysis of variance (ANOVA) was that neither grating orientation nor texture line orientation had any significant effect. In particular, there was no significant difference in detection thresholds when texture lines were parallel to the grating and when they were perpendicular to the grating.

I have been unable to find any published report on spatial frequency channels for OTD form.

Orientation Discrimination for Texture-Defined Form

I measured orientation discrimination for an OTD bar using a pattern similar to that illustrated in Figure 4.3B, except that the OTD target was a bar. The diameter of the pattern was 10 degrees, and the bar subtended 5.0 degrees × 1.4 degrees (Regan, 1995). Figure 4.7A shows that orientation discrimination for the OTD bar was a U-shaped function of line orientation contrast. The minimum value of orientation-discrimination threshold occurred at about the maximum value of orientation contrast (90 degrees), and was 0.57 degrees (SE = 0.05 degrees) and 0.57 degrees (SE = 0.04 degrees) for the two observers. Orientation discrimination threshold for the OTD bar was the same whether the mean orientation of the texture lines was parallel or perpendicular to the bar.

I generated a luminance-defined (LD) bar by removing all the lines outside the OTD bar. (This procedure ensured that the OTD and LD bars had the same spatial sampling.) As I increased the luminance contrast of the LD bar above bar detection threshold, orientation discrimination threshold fell steeply, then leveled out for contrasts that were greater than detection threshold by a factor of 3 to 4 (see Figure 2.30). The lowest values of orientation discrimination threshold for the LD bar were 0.42 degrees (SE = 0.06 degrees) and 0.35 degrees (SE = 0.05 degrees) for the same two subjects. Thus, when spatial sampling was matched, the lowest orientation discrimination threshold was only slightly lower for an LD bar than for an OTD bar (between 1:1.3 and 1:1.6).

In related work on other non-Fourier targets, Westheimer and Li (1996) found that orientation discrimination threshold was "almost as good" for illusory contours and real lines, Vogels and Orban (1987) found that orientation discrimination threshold was less than twice as high for illusory contours than for LD contours, and Lin and Wilson (1996) reported that orientation discrimination threshold for a contrast-modulated LD grating was 0.5 degrees.

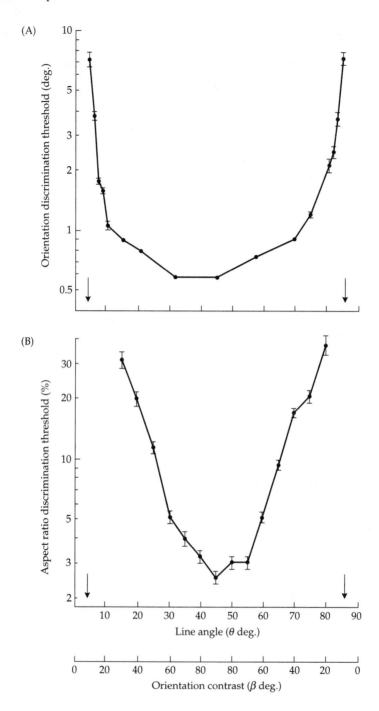

Positional Discrimination, Width Discrimination, Separation Discrimination, and Spatial Frequency Discrimination for Texture-Defined Form

Although our ability to judge the relative directions of luminance-defined objects and to discriminate their widths has attracted interest for more than a hundred years (pp. 98–115), only during the last few years have any measurements of our corresponding abilities for texture-defined objects been published. Yet, as we see below, our spatial discrimination abilities are little, if at all, inferior for texture-defined form than for luminance-defined form *provided that spacial sampling of the two kinds of target are matched.*

Positional discrimination

We estimated the precision with which position is encoded for an OTD boundary by quantifying the ability to discriminate the relative positions of local features in the Vernier step acuity and bisection acuity tasks (Gray &Regan, 1997).

Vernier acuity. We measured Vernier step acuity for the kind of pattern illustrated in Figure 4.3C. In the top half of Figure 4.3C, texture lines whose centers fall to the left of an imaginary vertical line have a different orientation from texture lines whose centers fall to the right of the imaginary line. It is the same for the lower half of Figure 4.3C, except that the imaginary vertical line is displaced horizontally. The displacement could be altered by 0.0015% of the width of the display. The Vernier task was to judge whether the displacement was to the left or to the right.

We generated a luminance-defined boundary for the Vernier task by first arranging that all the texture lines were parallel, and then replacing the orientation-defined boundary by a luminance-defined boundary. This procedure ensured that spatial sampling was matched for the OTD and LD targets.

For an OTD boundary, the effect of orientation contrast on Vernier step acuity approximated a square root law.

Open symbols in Figure 4.8A show that Vernier acuity for the OTD boundary improved as spatial sampling frequency was progressively increased up to about

◀**4.7 Orientation discrimination and aspect-ratio discrimination for texture-defined form.** (A) Orientation-discrimination thresholds (in degrees) for a texture-defined bar are plotted as ordinate on a log axis versus the orientation contrast (β degrees) and versus the orientation (θ degrees) of the texture lines. (B) Aspect-ratio discrimination thresholds (in %) for a texture-defined rectangle are plotted as ordinate on a log axis versus the orientation contrast (β degrees) and versus the orientation (θ degrees) of the texture lines. Vertical arrows show bar or rectangle detection thresholds. Part A from Regan (1995). Part B from Regan, Hajdur, and Hong (1996).

10 samples/degree. As sampling frequency increased beyond about 18 samples/degree, Vernier acuity degraded steeply. In separate experiments we showed that this degradation of Vernier acuity was not caused by the increase in the number of samples/degree. On the contrary, increasing the number of samples/degree while holding line length constant caused Vernier acuity to improve. But, in Figure 4.8A, as sampling rate increased, line length decreased. When line length fell a little below approximately 1.2 minutes of arc, the texture lines were so short that the orientations of individual lines could no longer be discriminated (in effect they were dots) and the Vernier task became impossible.

The best value of Vernier acuity in Figure 4.8A (2.5 minutes of arc) can be regarded as approaching the physiological limit for an OTD boundary. This is considerably inferior to the physiological limit of Vernier acuity (2 to 5 seconds of arc) for a high-contrast LD boundary of indefinitely high spatial sampling frequency (Westheimer, 1975, 1979; Westheimer & McKee, 1977a), presumably because a late spatial integration stage is involved in the processing of OTD boundaries. On the other hand, open symbols in Figure 4.8A show that, over a wide range of matched spatial sampling frequencies, Vernier acuity for an OTD boundary is not greatly inferior to Vernier acuity for an LD boundary (2.5:1).

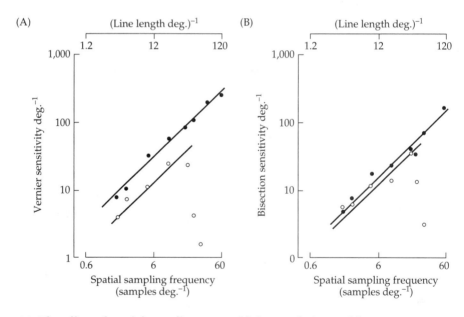

4.8 The effect of spatial sampling on sensitivity to relative position. Vernier step sensitivity (A) and bisection sensitivity (B) for texture-defined (open symbols) and luminance-defined (filled symbols) boundaries were plotted versus the number (F) of spatial samples per degree. Solid lines are best fits to the equation $S_V = a + b\,F^{1.0}$ and $S_B = c + d\,F^{1.0}$ where S_V and S_B are, respectively, the Vernier and bisection sensitivities and a, b, c, and d are constants. Vernier step sensitivity is the reciprocal of Vernier step acuity threshold expressed in degrees. After Gray and Regan (1997).

When the boundary was defined by both luminance contrast and texture contrast, Vernier step threshold was significantly lower than when the boundary was defined only by texture contrast or only by luminance contrast. The combination rule was consistent with probability summation over two independent channels (Gray and Regan, 1997).

Bisection acuity. We measured bisection acuity for an OTD boundary by occluding the lower half of the pattern shown in Figure 4.3C. The observer's task was to judge whether the texture-defined boundary was to the left or right of the center of the pattern.

Figure 4.8B shows that bisection acuity thresholds behaved similarly to the Vernier thresholds shown in Figure 4.8A, except that thresholds for OTD and LD boundaries between 2 and 18 spatial samples deg.$^{-1}$ were even more closely similar. The lowest threshold for the OTD boundary (1.7 minutes of arc) can be regarded as approaching the physiological limit for an OTD boundary. Again, this is considerably higher than the 1 to 5 seconds of arc bisection acuity threshold for high-contrast LD boundary of indefinitely high spatial sampling frequency (Klein & Levi, 1985), presumably because a late spatial integration stage is involved in the processing of OTD boundaries.

For an OTD boundary, the effect of orientation contrast on bisection acuity approximated a linear law.

Bar-width and bar-separation discrimination

We measured bar-width discrimination thresholds for the one-dimensional width or height of a TD rectangle using the display illustrated in Figure 4.3B (Regan, Hajdur, & Hong, 1996b). To remove trial-to-trial variations of aspect ratio as a reliable cue to the width discrimination, we interleaved randomly eight different values of height. Similarly, in the height discrimination task we interleaved randomly eight different values of width.

For a reference width (or height) of 13.6 degrees, discrimination thresholds for width (Th_W) and height (Th_H) were similar [Th_W = 1.8 (SE = 0.1)%, T_H = 1.4 (SE = 0.1)%, means for three observers]. These thresholds were approximately the same as corresponding thresholds for a sampled LD rectangle that was created by switching off all the lines outside the rectangle (Regan et al., 1996b).

If we assume that aspect ratio is obtained, by first independently encoding the height and width of the rectangle and then encoding the ratio a/b, we would expect that, provided no information is lost in combining a and b, aspect ratio discrimination threshold would equal $[(Th_W)^2 + (Th_H)^2]^{\frac{1}{2}}$ where Th_W is the discrimination threshold for width and Th_H is the discrimination threshold for height. The predicted values of aspect ratio discrimination threshold were 1.82 (SE = 0.1)%, 1.67 (SE = 0.15)%, and 4.6 (SE = 0.3)%, compared with the experimentally measured thresholds 2.8 (SE = 0.1)%, 2.7 (SE = 0.1)%, and 5.1 (SE = 0.3)%, respectively. We concluded that, although a significant amount of information was lost when combining information about the rectangle's width and height, the amount of information lost was small.

I was unable to find any published investigation analogous to the Morgan and Ward (1985) experiment. That experiment showed that an observer's discrimination of the separation between two LD lines could not be explained in terms of filters for LD form that are driven from the same retinal location.

Spatial-frequency discrimination

Next I discuss spatial-frequency discrimination for OTD gratings such as the one illustrated in Figure 4.3A. By inspecting Figure 4.9, readers can compare the just-noticeable difference in spatial frequency for OTD gratings (filled circles) with the just-noticeable difference in spatial frequency for sampled LD gratings (open circles).

Some procedural details are, perhaps, in order here before I get to the main points. We wanted to ensure that our observers based their responses on the task-relevant variable (i.e., spatial frequency) and ignored trial-to-trial variations both in perceived orientation contrast and in any aliasing patterns (see Appendix F). We dealt with this problem by generating a stimulus set that comprised six values of spatial frequency, six values of orientation contrast, and six values of the number of texture lines (spatial samples) per degree of angular subtense. These three variables were orthogonal within the set of 216 trial stimuli, that is, they had zero correlation. (This can be understood at intuitive level by visualizing the stimulus set as a $6 \times 6 \times 6$ cube of stimulus cells; spatial frequency varied along a direction (x) parallel to one edge of the cube, but orientation contrast and spatial sampling were constant along the x direction; orientation contrast varied along a direction (y) at right angles to direction x, but spatial frequency and spatial sampling were constant along the y direction; spatial sampling varied along a direction (z) at right angles to the x and y directions, but spatial frequency and orientation contrast were constant along the z direction.)

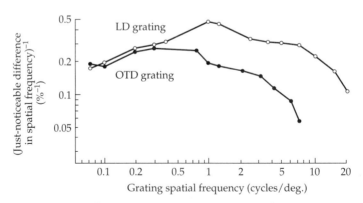

4.9 Spatial-frequency discrimination for texture-defined form. The just-noticeable difference in spatial frequency for texture-defined (filled symbols) and luminance-defined (open symbols) gratings as a function of the grating's spatial frequency. The number of spatial samples per cycle was 6 or greater for filled and open circles. Both axes are logarithmic. From Gray and Regan (1998a).

To remove any positional cue to the observer's task, the spatial phase of the grating was selected randomly from very many values between 0 and 360 degrees before every individual trial. Each trial consisted of a single presentation that was sufficiently brief (0.2 seconds) to prevent the observer's scanning the grating. The observer's task was to signal whether the spatial frequency of the grating last presented was higher or lower than the mean of the stimulus set. Before any given run, the observer could request as many presentations as desired (each of duration 0.2 seconds) of a grating whose spatial frequency, orientation contrast, and number of texture lines per degree was equal to the mean of the stimulus set.

From the averaged data recorded in several individual runs of the 216 stimulus set we constructed three psychometric functions by plotting the percentage of "spatial frequency higher than the mean" versus spatial frequency, versus orientation contrast, and versus the number of lines per degree. When spatial frequency was plotted along the abscissa the psychometric function was steep, but the other two psychometric functions were essentially flat (see Figure 1.7). We concluded that the observer based his responses on spatial frequency and ignored trial-to-trial variations both in perceived contrast and in any aliasing patterns. (Pp. 476–477 discuss how this procedure prevented the observer's using aliasing patterns as a cue to the task.)

In the LD grating, all texture lines had the same orientation. A sinusoidal variation of line contrast about a mean of 70% was impressed across the grating. (The lines could be regarded as the "carriers" of the sinusoidal grating, and the mean number of lines per degree of angular subtense is the *carrier frequency* for the comparatively low-frequency grating; see pp. 421–424 and 467–470.)

Returning to Figure 4.9, spatial sampling for the OTD and LD grating was matched at every point on the abscissa. Spatial-frequency discrimination thresholds for OTD and LD gratings were similar at low spatial frequencies. To the extent that spatial frequency discrimination threshold can be regarded as a measure of sensitivity to differences in the spatial scale of scene content, Figure 4.9 indicates that this sensitivity is the same for OTD and LD form over the range 0.07 to 0.4 cycles/deg. As spatial frequency increased beyond 0.5 cycles/deg., sensitivity to differences in spatial scale grew progressively less for OTD form relative to LD form, but the ability to discriminate different spatial frequencies for OTD form did not fail until beyond 7 cycles/deg.

Just as is the case for LD gratings, spatial-frequency discrimination threshold for OTD gratings fell steeply as the total number of grating cycles was increased from 0.5 to 2.5, but remained approximately constant as the number of cycles was increased beyond 2.5. Following the argument of Hirsch and Hylton (1982) this finding indicates that, for OTD gratings as well as LD gratings, spatial-frequency discrimination is mediated by a local process rather than being based on summation over multiple cycles of the grating. This conclusion takes us to the following question: "Is spatial-frequency discrimination based on filters whose outputs carry a *width* label, or on filters whose outputs carry a *spatial periodicity* (spatial-frequency) label, or on both?" Pages 48–53 provide a relevant discussion.

The effect of orientation contrast on spatial frequency discrimination threshold for OTD gratings was as follows. Threshold fell steeply as orientation contrast was increased up to about 15 degrees (3 to 5 times above grating detection threshold), after which, threshold remained constant up to the highest value of orientation contrast (Gray & Regan, 1998a). This saturation behavior is very similar to the effect of luminance contrast on spatial frequency discrimination threshold for LD gratings (Regan et al., 1982).

Aspect Ratio Discrimination for Two-Dimensional Texture-Defined Form

Figure 4.7B shows that aspect ratio discrimination threshold for the OTD rectangle illustrated in Figure 4.3B was a U-shaped function of line orientation contrast with the lowest threshold at or near an orientation contrast of 90 degrees. Discrimination thresholds fell considerably as orientation contrast was reduced from 30 to 90 degrees. This finding suggests that the effect of texture contrast on aspect ratio discrimination threshold cannot be predicted from its effect on the detection of OTD form, given that the detection of OTD form is improved negligibly when orientation contrast is increased from 30 to 90 degrees (Nothdurft, 1985b). The lowest values of aspect ratio discrimination threshold were 2.8% (SE = 0.2%), 2.5% (SE = 0.2%), and 5.3% (SE = 0.4%) for three observers (Regan et al., 1996b).

Observers were able to ignore simultaneous trial-to-trial variations in the area of the rectangle while discriminating changes in its aspect ratio. As discussed on pp. 174–184, this variation of area removed height alone and width alone as reliable correlates of aspect ratio so that observers were forced to base their discriminations on some *relation* between height (a) and width (b), although it was not clear whether this relation was a/b or $(a - b)$ or some other function of a and b.

To explain the findings just described, I propose that the aspect ratio of an OTD rectangle is encoded according to the schematic shown in Figure 2.63, but with the broadly tuned receptive fields sensitive to OTD form (Figure 4.13) rather than LD form, and with the *coincidence detectors* sensitive to the separation between a pair of separated, narrowly tuned receptive fields for OTD form rather than the separation between two narrowly tuned receptive fields for LD form (Figure 2.53). The processing of aspect ratio information for an OTD rectangle would be along the same lines as illustrated in Figure 2.63B–F for an LD rectangle.

Disordered Processing of Texture-Defined Form in Patients

The psychophysical procedures used to carry out intensive studies on a few experienced observers are too slow and too demanding for use in testing large numbers of patients. With this in mind we developed a simple letter reading test for assessing sensitivity to OTD form (Regan & Hong, 1994). Figure 4.10A–C illustrates a letter that is rendered visible entirely by orientation contrast. The display is divided into 80 × 80 cells, each of which contains a line. All texture lines inside the letter are horizontal and all outside the letter are vertical (as in Figure

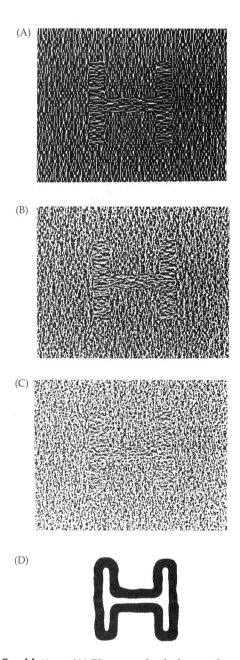

4.10 Texture-defined letters. (A) Photograph of a letter whose visibility is created entirely by orientation texture. (B) The letter's visibility is degraded by adding two randomly located noise dots per texture line. (C) Letter visibility is further degraded by adding four noise dots per texture line. (D) This image was created by passing the letter shown in part A through the model illustrated in Figure 4.12. From Regan and Hong (1995).

4.10A–C), or vice versa. One of these two options is selected randomly before any given letter is presented. The test procedure is as follows. Each trial comprises two presentations, only one of which contains a letter. In the other presentation, texture lines are randomly selected to be either all horizontal or all vertical. In half of the trials (selected randomly) the letter is presented first, and in the other half the letter is presented second. Ten different letters are presented in random order, and the observer is instructed to signal which letter was presented (recognition) and whether it was in the first or second presentation (detection). Then the procedure is repeated with letter visibility reduced by adding one randomly located noise dot per cell, then again with two noise dots per cell, and so on until a total of 100 different noise-degraded letter stimuli have been presented. In Figure 4.10A there are no noise dots, in Figure 4.10B two noise dots per cell, and in Figure 4.10C four noise dots per cell.

Figure 4.11 shows control data. Filled circles in Figure 4.11A plot the percentage of correct detections versus the number of noise dots per cell. Because there were two presentations per trial, chance level was 50% (indicated by the horizontal dotted line). Filled circles in Figure 4.11B plot the percentage of correct letter recognitions versus the number of noise dots per cell for the letter H. Because there were ten different letters, the chance level was 10% (indicated by the horizontal dotted line).

Twenty-five patients with multiple sclerosis and 25 age-matched controls carried out the following visual tests: The orientation-texture-defined (OTD) letter recognition test described above; the motion-defined (MD) letter recognition test described on pp. 324–327 (Figure 5.3); the luminance-defined (LD) low-contrast letter recognition acuity test (Regan & Neima, 1983; Regan, 1988) described on

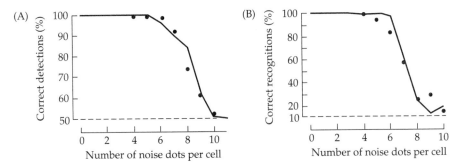

4.11 Empirical data on the detection and recognition of texture-defined letters. (A) Data points plot percent correct letter detections averaged over all 10 letters and four subjects versus the number of noise dots per cell. The continuous curve plots the theoretical predictions of the model illustrated in Figure 4.12. (B) Data points plot percent correct reading accuracy for letter H averaged over four subjects versus the number of noise dots per cell. The continuous curve plots the theoretical predictions of the model illustrated in Figure 4.12. From Regan and Hong (1995).

pp. 191–205 (Figure 2.66) for letters of 11% and 100% contrast. All patients had visual acuities within the normal range. Six patients were abnormal on TD letter recognition, of whom one was normal on all other tests. Eleven patients were abnormal on MD letter recognition, of whom four gave normal results on all other visual tests. Visual acuity for letters of 11% contrast were abnormally low in seven patients, of whom two gave normal results on all other tests.

We concluded that the neural mechanisms essential for the recognition of OTD letters, MD letters, high-contrast LD letters, and low-contrast LD letters in subjects with normal visual acuity are sufficiently different physiologically that they can be differentially damaged by multiple sclerosis (Regan & Simpson, 1995).

We offered the following explanation. Myelinated long-range horizontal fibers connect orientation-selective neurons in neighboring columns in the monkey striate cortex (Gilbert et al., 1990; Gilbert & Wiesel, 1990). If we assume that these long-range connections are the basis of sensitivity to OTD boundaries, one possible way in which multiple sclerosis could selectively disrupt the ability to recognize OTD letters might be by demyelinating these horizontal fibers. In terms of the kind of model illustrated in Figure 4.12, this damage would be at the nonlinear

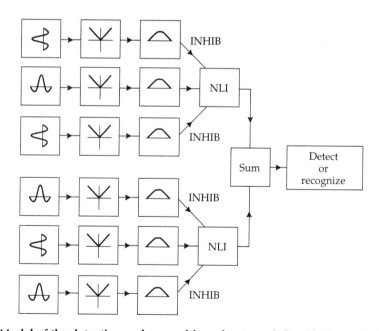

4.12 Model of the detection and recognition of texture-defined letters. Block diagram of a physiologically plausible model of the detection and recognition of texture-defined form. The sequence of processing is applied simultaneously to every pixel in the stimulus display. From Regan and Hong (1995).

lateral interaction (NLI) stage. The hypothesis that this nonlinear lateral interaction occurs in striate cortex is consistent with the report that lesions of cortical area V4 do not impair behavioral ability to detect TD form in macaque monkey (Schiller & Lee, 1991; Schiller, 1993). As mentioned on pp. 156–169, it is possible that these same long-range connections are the physiological basis for the link between the two narrowly selective receptive fields in the *coincidence detector* depicted in Figure 2.28.

Psychophysical Models of the Processing of Texture-Defined Form: Local Signals; Distant Comparisons of Global Features; Distant Comparisons of Local Features

Three broad lines of thought can be distinguished in texture perception research over the last several decades (for an incisive review, see Bergen, 1991). First, the statistically based work of Julesz and his colleagues (see footnote on p. 269). This began in 1962 with the study of texture segregation in fields of random dots with different statistical characteristics. A similar approach was also applied to texture images composed of repetitive micropatterns such as "L" and "+." Julesz (1975) proposed that texture segregation occurs between textured areas with different global statistics and, in particular, differences in second-order statistics of the luminance at different locations in the texture. Counterexamples to Julesz's conjecture were later reported (Julesz et al., 1978; Victor & Brodie, 1978).

The second approach to texture segregation research, largely associated with Beck (1966a, 1967, 1972), focused on the factors that cause textures composed of micropatterns to group together. Beck suggested that texture segmentation occurs on the basis of differences in the density of local features such as the orientation or size of texture elements (Beck, 1982). Julesz (1981, 1991) named such features *textons*, and defined textons as "conspicuous local features." As pointed out by Bergen (1991), this implies the following:

> Textons are perceptual entities and, therefore, this definition places texture segregation at a late stage of processing.

The validity of the texton hypothesis was questioned by Bergen (1991) on the grounds that, according to physiologically plausible computational models, texture segregation can occur at a processing stage earlier than the stage at which one can speak of perceptual entities. Julesz (1991, p. 757) noted that "What these textons really are is hard to define" but that the following are accepted: color, orientation, flicker motion, depth, elongated blobs, colinearity. He stated that "Some less clearly defined textons are related to ends of lines or terminators, which occur in the concepts of 'corner' and 'closure'" (Julesz, 1991, p. 757).

Nothdurft (1990) has stated that differences in the density of supposed textons are often associated with differences in either mean luminance or in the homogeneity of the luminance distribution, and that positional or luminance jitter of texture elements can strongly affect segregation, even though texton density is unaltered. He added (Nothdurft, 1990, p. 295): "From the textons reported in the literature, only differences in orientation were found to be fairly robust against such modifications" (see also Gurnsey & Browse, 1987). Going further, Nothdurft (1991b) compared the effects of a masker on the recognition of candidate textons and on the segregation of areas demarcated by a difference in texton density. Only for the line orientation texton were the masking effects similar. He concluded (p. 295) that:

> "For the other candidate textons investigated (blob size, line intersections or 'crossings' and line ends or 'terminators'), texture segregation is based on visual cues other than the candidate textons."

Like the second approach, the third approach to texture segregation research focuses on local rather than global properties of the segregating textures, but draws on our current knowledge of neural properties in monkey brain as well as on human psychophysical data. A class of physiologically plausible multiple-channel models of texture segregation have, at the first stage, local analysis by a bank of parallel linear filters, each of which is tuned to orientation and spatial frequency (Daugman, 1980, 1988; Caelli, 1985; Turner, 1986; Beck et al., 1987; Bergen & Adelson, 1988; Clark & Bovik, 1989; Fogel & Sagi, 1989; Sutter et al., 1989; Malik & Perona, 1990; Sagi, 1990; Landy & Bergen, 1991; Lee, 1991; Bravo & Blake, 1992). These are the local filters whose tuning characteristics are depicted in Figures 1.21, 1.22, 2.1, 2.8–2.11, and 2.12, the same filters that feature in models of the detection and discrimination of luminance-defined form.

A multiple-channel model that is based purely on linear mechanisms can account for segregation between many texture pairs, but several counter-demonstrations are known (Julesz & Krose, 1988; Victor, 1988; Julesz, 1991; Malik & Perona, 1990; Bergen, 1991; Chubb & Landy, 1991). For this reason, several proposed models follow the linear parallel filtering stage with one or more nonlinear stages. Different authors have variously explored rectification (Bergen & Adelson, 1988; Malik & Perona, 1990), squaring or energy computation (Adelson & Bergen, 1985; Fogel & Sagi, 1989; Sutter et al., 1989; Rubenstein & Sagi, 1990), thresholding (Rubenstein & Sagi, 1990), and nonlinear edge enhancement (Landy & Bergen, 1991). Rubenstein and Sagi (1990) included a treatment of variability across the texture pattern as a limiting factor in texture discriminating tasks.

I suggested that the low (0.57 degree) orientation discrimination thresholds for the OTD bar in Figure 4.7A could be understood by assuming that orientation discrimination threshold is determined by the relative activity within a population of orientation-tuned filters for OTD form (Regan, 1995). The data shown in Figure 4.6 are consistent with the hypothesis that the human visual pathway contains such orientation-tuned filters. By analogy with the double-opponent "convexity cell" for MD form proposed by Nakayama and Loomis (1974) that is described on pp. 324–327, we proposed that the receptive field of such a filter might be built up along the lines illustrated in Figure 4.13A–C (Gray & Regan, 1998a). (The properties of individual neurons in primary visual cortex of monkey had

previously been modeled along similar lines; see Knierem & van Essen, 1992).
When the excitatory part of the receptive field shown by the dashed circle in
Figure 4.13A is stimulated by short lines of the preferred orientation, and the
inhibitory surround is simultaneously stimulated by lines of the same orientation, the net excitation is zero. If the lines falling on the excitatory region do not
change orientation, while the lines falling on the inhibitory region are slowly
rotated, the net excitation progressively increases. Excitation reaches a maximum
in the condition shown in Figure 4.13B. Suppose, now, that we sum many receptive fields of the kind shown in Figure 4.13A and B, all of which are driven from
the same receptive field locus, but which prefer different line orientations. Such a
double-opponent receptive field will be excited by lines of any arbitrary orientation (θ_1), provided that the lines that fall on the excitatory region all have orientation θ_1 and the lines that fall outside the excitatory region all have orientation
θ_2, where $\theta_2 \neq \theta_1$. This would account for the finding, mentioned earlier, that both
orientation discrimination threshold for an OTD bar and detection threshold for
an OTD grating were the same whether the mean orientation of the lines inside
the bar was parallel or perpendicular to the bar (Regan, 1995; Kwan & Regan,
1998). If we assume that the receptive field is circular as in Figure 4.13A,B rather
than being elongated, we can build an elongated receptive field by summing the
outputs of several such double-opponent receptive fields that lie along a straight
line in retinal coordinates (dashed circles in Figure 4.13C). The resulting elongated receptive field will have the sensitivity profile for texture lines shown by the
continuous line in part C. It will be strongly excited by an OTD bar or by the bars
of the OTD grating shown in Figure 4.3A, provided that the bar's width and ori-

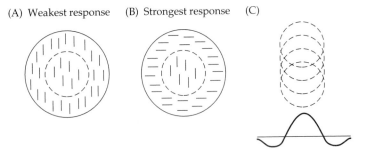

**4.13 Functional model of an orientation- and size-tuned spatial filter for orien-
tation-texture-defined form.** (A, B) The double-opponent receptive field consists of
an excitatory center (shown by the dashed circle) with an inhibitory surround.
Texture lines are shown with the preferred orientation for the excitatory region. (C)
In the case that the receptive field is not elongated, the filter is built by summing the
outputs of many such receptive fields whose centers fall along a straight line so as to
give an elongated receptive field whose profile is shown by the continuous line.
From Gray and Regan (1998).

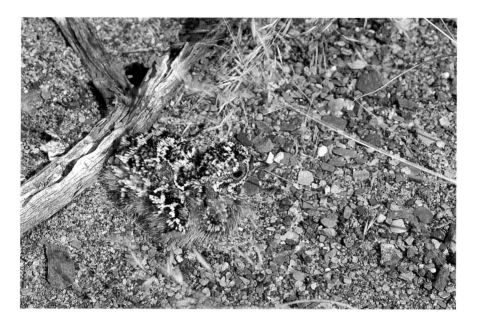

Plate 1 The possibility that this sandgrouse chick will survive to adulthood is improved by camouflage. Photograph © Michael Fogden/Animals Animals.

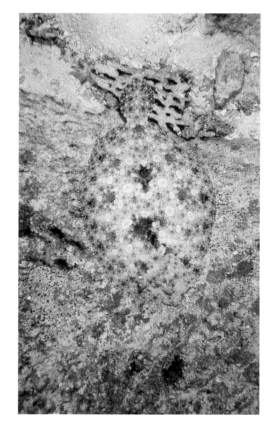

Plate 2 The flounder fish matches its surroundings in terms of mean luminance, color, and texture; furthermore, when it flattens itself against the seabed, it renders its camouflage tolerably secure against predators with binocular depth perception. Photograph © Dale Sarver/Animals Animals.

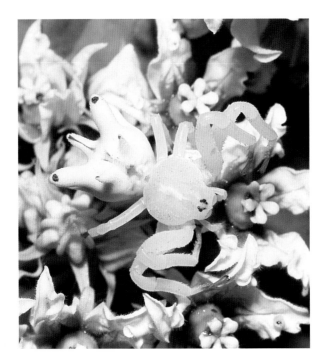

Plate 3 The crab spider merges into the three-dimensional organization of its chosen surroundings so as to defeat the camouflage-breaking capability of stereoscopic depth perception. Photograph © John Pontier/Animals Animals.

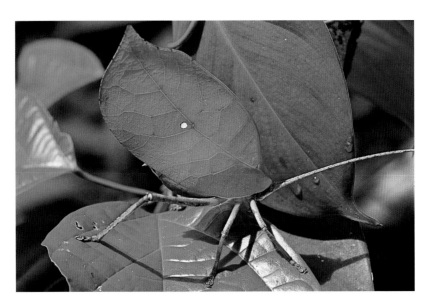

Plate 4 The leaf katydid has the misfortune to feature prominently in the diet of many birds and several species of monkey in the forests of Peru. This insect's defense is camouflage. Not only do its wings match the surrounding leaves in both color and reflectance, they are also marked so as to mimic a leaf's texturing of veins. And by crouching among leaves, it defeats the camouflage-breaking capability of binocular stereo vision. Photograph © Michael and Patricia Fogden.

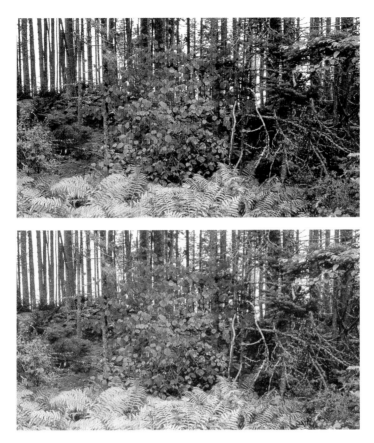

Plate 5 The red leaves are much more easily seen by an animal with color vision than by one without. Photographs © Sonja Bullaty.

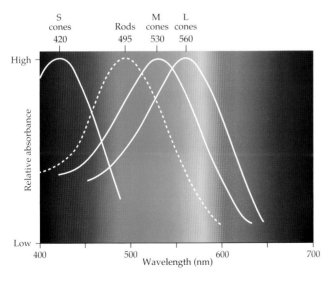

Plate 6 Absorption spectra from human S-, M-, and L-cone photoreceptors and from a human rod photoreceptor (dashed curve).

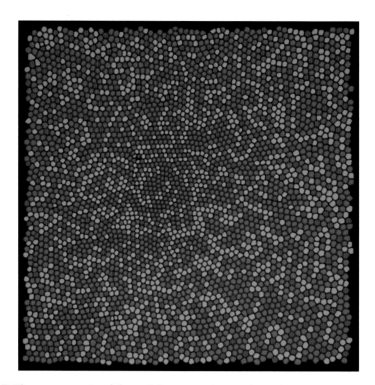

Plate 7 The cone mosaic of the rod-free inner fovea of an adult human retina at the level of the inner segment (tangential section). Superior is at the top and nasal to the left. The region is about 1 degree of visual angle in diameter (~300 μm). The center coordinates of the cone cross sections shown were obtained from the retina of a 35-year-old male (Curcio & Sloan, 1992). The outer dimensions of the cone cross sections have been defined mathematically by Voronoi regions and color-coded (L-cones, red; M-cones, green; S-cones, blue) according to the following assumptions: (1) only three cone opsin genes, those encoding the S-, M-, and L-cone pigments, are expressed; (2) the inner roughly circular area (~100 μm or 0.34 deg. in diameter), displaced slightly to the upper left quadrant of the mosaic, is free of S-cones (Curcio et al., 1991); (3) S-cone numbers in the rest of the retina do not exceed 7% and are semiregularly distributed (Curcio et al., 1991); and (4) there are approximately 1.7 times as many L- as M-cones in this region of the retina, and they are randomly distributed. The diameters of the cross sections in the center are slightly smaller than those at the outer edge to allow for close packing. From Sharpe et al. (1999), courtesy of L. T. Sharpe.

entation matches the width and orientation of the excitatory receptive field. Gorea and his colleagues have previously discussed the concept of double opponency in the context of texture segregation (Gorea & Papathomas, 1993).

The large elongated double-opponent receptive field that hypothetically detects a 5.0 × 1.4 degree bar as a whole achieves image segregation by grouping for similarity (regional binding), i.e., it is sensitive to the fact that line orientation is constant within a 5.0 × 1.4 degree area, and different outside that area. However, as pointed out by Nothdurft (1994):

> A receptive field of this kind whose width was matched to the clearly visible OTD square in Figure 4.14 would fail to detect the square.

The OTD square in Figure 4.14 is rendered visible by locally increased orientation contrast gradient across the boundaries of the square. Such a boundary would be highlighted by a class of spatially opponent receptive fields whose excitatory region was narrow. Depending on the kind of lateral interaction within the receptive field, narrow receptive fields of this kind translate the orientation gradient across a boundary into either a bright line on a dim background (as is the case for the receptive-field organization shown in Figure 4.13) or into a dark line on a bright background, as in Figure 4.10D.

It is evident that this way of representing the shape of an OTD form is analogous to an outline sketch. If we assume that receptive fields for OTD form come in a wide range of sizes, OTD targets, such as that shown in Figure 4.3B, would be represented, not only by filters matched to the width of the target, but also by narrow-width filters that highlight the OTD boundaries. On the other hand, the target shown in Figure 4.3A would be represented chiefly by filters matched to

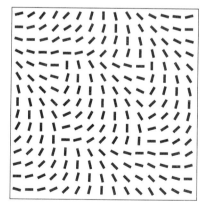

4.14 Clearly visible target that cannot be detected by filters matched to the size of the target. The segregation of the central square is not based on grouping for similarity. The boundaries of the square are rendered visible by locally increased orientation gradient. From Nothdurft (1994).

bar width, and the targets shown in Figures 4.3C and 4.14 would be represented only by narrow-width filters.

The multiple-channel model described by Regan and Hong (1995), and depicted in Figure 4.12 has a double-opponent stage, but is an example of the "boundary detector" type of model as distinct from the "regional binding" type of model (pp. 39–40). In particular, the width of the excitatory region of the double-opponent receptive field for OTD form is very small (one pixel in our model). The early stages are not greatly different from those of the earlier multiple-channel models just cited. The novel feature is that the last stage allows quantitative prediction of experimental psychophysical data, namely percent correct letter detections and recognitions.

The spatial filtering properties of visual system neurons have been modeled by several functions including difference of Gaussians and Gabor functions (Rodieck & Stone, 1965a,b; Daugman, 1980; Marceltja, 1980; Parker & Hawken, 1988). In Figure 4.12 we chose to use difference of Gaussians (DOG) filters at stage 1 on the basis of the good fit with physiological data and ease of computation (Regan & Hong, 1995). First, the stimulus illustrated in Figure 4.10A was passed through a parallel array of vertically oriented spatial filters and then passed through a parallel array of horizontally oriented filters. Stage 2 of the model was the first nonlinear stage. It follows Bergen and Adelson (1988) in that it is equivalent to summing the outputs of two half-wave linear rectifiers, one corresponding to the ON system and one to the OFF system. (Half-wave rectification models the fact that a neuron cannot fire at a negative rate; see Appendix E and p. 394.)* At stage 3 of the model, the rectified outputs of the horizontally and vertically oriented stage 1 filters are smoothed by a circularly symmetric Gaussian filter (a process equivalent to blurring). Stage 4 of the model is the second nonlinear stage. Stage 4 enhances the boundaries of the OTD target by using a nonlinear lateral interaction (NLI in Figure 4.12) to compare texture at different locations on the texture pattern. This rationale is based on Nothdurft's (1985b, 1991a, 1992) suggestion, mentioned earlier, that segregation between two orientation textures, and also the perception of the texture boundary, arise from local differences in orientation near the border rather than from global differences in the orientation statistics of the two textures. At stage 4 of the model, the signal from vertically tuned filters driven from any given pixel on the display is inhibited nonlinearly by the signals from horizontally tuned filters driven from the region surrounding that point on the display (NLI, upper half of Figure 4.10).† Likewise, the signal from horizon-

---

* In the abstract of their 1988 paper, Chubb and Sperling stated: "the results and examples from the domain of motion perception are transposable to the space-domain problem of detecting orientation in a texture pattern." Their "elaborated Reichardt detector" incorporated rectification at an early stage of processing.

† The rationale for choosing cross-orientation inhibition as a boundary-enhancing process was based on two physiological lines of evidence. First, in human subjects, brain responses evoked by superimposed orthogonal gratings reveal a strongly nonlinear mutual nonlinear inhibition (Morrone & Burr, 1986; Regan & Regan, 1986, 1987, 1988). Second, cross-orientation

tally tuned filters driven from any given pixel in the display is inhibited nonlinearly by the signal from vertically tuned filters driven from the region surrounding that point on the display (NLI, lower half of Figure 4.12). At stage 5 of the model, the processed outputs of the horizontally and vertically tuned filters of stage 1 are summed, thus pooling the processed outputs of stage 1 vertically tuned and horizontally tuned filters. Stages 4 and 5 of our model together create a spatially opponent receptive field for OTD form that is analogous to the spatially opponent receptive fields for LD form of simple cells in the primary visual cortex. Here, the excitatory region of the receptive field is very narrow (one pixel). A narrow receptive field of this kind would detect the texture-defined square in Figure 4.14.

The sequence of processing depicted in Figure 4.12 was applied to every one of the 640 × 480 pixels in the stimulus display of Figure 4.10A, giving a display in which the boundaries of the letter were dark compared with the rest of the display (Figure 4.10D). The process was repeated for the letter "H" with one noise dot per cell, two noise dots per cell (Figure 4.10B) and so on up to 11 noise dots per cell. As the number of noise dots increased, irregular dark blobs appeared over the pattern, whose effect was to reduce the salience of the letter boundaries. Then, this process was repeated for each of the other nine letters.

We modeled the observer's cognitive detection strategy as a search for any part of a letter (i.e., "to detect a part is to detect the whole") as follows. The letter-segment detector at stage 6 of the model was an outlined black bar that was cross-correlated with the output of stage 5 of the model. This gave a signal-to-noise level that, after weighting with a cumulative normal distribution (Green & Swets, 1974), was plotted as the continuous curve in Figure 4.11A. The fit between the predictions of the model and the empirical data points is close. It is not difficult to predict letter detection data if we assume that the observer's strategy was to search for a part of the whole letter. Even when we removed the second nonlinear stage (i.e., that edge-enhancement algorithm), the predictions were as close as those shown in Figure 4.11A.

In the spirit of Landy and Bergen's (1991) concept of multiple parallel cross-correlations (see also Burgess, 1985),* we modeled letter recognition as follows.

---

inhibition is well established at the single-cell level in the visual cortex of cat and monkey, and cortical cells can show orientation-selective effects from stimuli outside the classical receptive field (Nelson & Frost, 1978; Burr et al., 1981; Toyama et al., 1981; Morrone et al., 1982; DeValois & Tootel, 1983; Bonds, 1989; Gilbert et al., 1990). The alternative choice of lateral inhibition between signals from filters tuned to the same orientation would translate the texture boundary into a bright line on a dark area rather than the dark line on a bright area in Figure 4.10D but would not affect our present conclusions or the predictions of our model, although the choice might be metabolically more efficient. There is physiological evidence for lateral within-orientation inhibition (Knierim & van Essen, 1992).

* On pp. 43–59, 66–85, and 98–112 of Regan (1989), I provide a detailed discussion of how prior knowledge can be used to extract a signal from noise. I set out several caveats, including an emphasis on the fact that the method used to enhance the signal-to-noise ratio in

Starting with test letters having one noise dot per cell, one letter (e.g., Figure 4.10B) was processed up to stage 5 of the model. Then the output of stage 5 was separately cross-correlated with each of ten templates. Each template was the output of stage 5 when the input to the model was the highest-visibility version of one of the 10 letters (e.g., Figure 4.10A). This procedure was repeated for the other nine letters with one noise dot per cell. Next for each of the 10 test letters, we calculated the ratio between its cross-correlation coefficients for the other nine letters. From this ratio we obtained a predicted percent correct recognition score. This procedure was repeated for the 10 test letters with two noise dots per cell, for the 10 test letters with three noise dots per cell, and so on. (The "template matching" procedure just described is equivalent to the notion of discrete filters, one for each letter of the alphabet).* The predicted recognition scores, plotted as a continuous curve in Figure 4.11B, were a close fit to the empirical data points.

It is more difficult to predict letter recognition data than letter detection data. Predictions were inaccurate when we removed the third stage of the model. And models lacking the second nonlinear stage failed badly. We conclude that a border-enhancing algorithm is necessary to model letter recognition.

Note that, according to our model, the process underlying letter detection is *qualitatively* different from the process underlying letter recognition.

When observers were reading an appreciable percentage of letters incorrectly (right half of Figure 4.11B), the model often assigned a considerably higher cross-correlation to an incorrect letter than to any other letters including the letter actually presented. This implies that some incorrect responses would occur, not because the observer was guessing, but because the observer actually saw a letter other than the one presented. Several observers (including me) stated that this was indeed the case. On occasion I would recognize a letter with a good degree of confidence, but it was not the letter actually presented, and sometimes not even one of the 10 letters in the stimulus set.

---

effect defines the nature of the signal. Although this discussion is framed in the context of electrical signals generated by the human brain, much of the logic and mathematics has more general applicability and, in particular, relevance to psychophysical modeling.

* This template-matching scheme might be regarded as an extreme version of the more general hypothesis that the visual system analyzes visual patterns by comparing them with a fixed repertoire of internally represented components including global features, such as *symmetry, area, compactness,* and *jaggedness*; local features, such as *local orientation* and *curvature*; and spatial relations between local features, such as *above, right of,* and *joined to* (Sutherland, 1968; Gibson, 1969; Zusne, 1970; Barlow et al., 1972; Sutherland, 1973; Reed, 1973; Leuwenberg & Buffart, 1978; Foster, 1980).

CHAPTER 5

Motion-Defined Form

Preamble

Helmholtz

A strong hint that camouflage can be broken by relative motion is provided by the common observation that many carnivores are adept at remaining absolutely still and that this skill is also highly developed in their prey (Color Plate 1). However, Helmholtz seems to have been the first to point out (in 1866) that self-motion can also cause image segregation by means of motion parallax.

> Suppose, for instance, that a person is standing still in a thick woods, where it is impossible for the person to distinguish, except vaguely and roughly, in the mass of foliage and branches all around him what belongs to one tree and what to another, or how far apart the separate trees are, etc. But the moment that person begins to move forward, everything disentangles itself, and immediately he gets an appreciation of the material contents of the woods and their relations to each other in space, just as if he were looking at a good stereoscopic view of it. (Helmholtz, 1866/1962, pp. 295–296)

Helmholtz's explanation was that, because they are at different distances from the moving eye, the individual trees have different retinal image velocities, an effect he termed motion parallax. Because the different shapes of the trees are revealed as well as their individualities, Helmholtz's observation also provides an informal demonstration that the eye is capable of some degree of shape discrimination for form that is rendered visible by motion parallax.

The reader can demonstrate Helmholtz's observation on motion parallax by placing the drawing of the bird on the bookmark included with this book over the pattern in Figure 5.1 and following the directions in the figure caption.* When the bird is stationary it is almost perfectly camouflaged, but when it is moved, the eye immediately segregates the bird as a whole from its surroundings. When the bird stops moving, it merges back into its surroundings.† For our present pur-

(A)

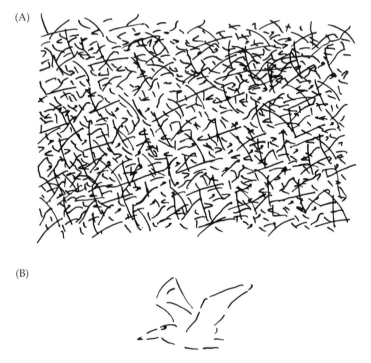

(B)

5.1 Flying bird. If a transparency of (B) is superimposed on a transparency of (A), the bird is almost perfectly camouflaged, but when (B) is moving with respect to (A), the bird is visible and its shape is recognizable. The bird is composed of 21 pen strokes in an ordered array. (Its shape was inspired by an advertisement for *Guinness*.) The background is composed of the same 21 pen strokes arranged randomly. The principle of this demonstration was described in a children's book published in the 1930s, but the basic idea dates at least from Victorian times. From Regan (1986a).

* If the bookmark is missing, try photocopying Figure 5.1A and B onto separate transparent sheets, both figures being enlarged to the same extent. Then place one sheet on top of the other on an overhead projector.

† Although the bird seems to appear as soon as it starts to fly, it does not disappear the instant that it stops moving. Its visibility fades away curiously slowly. I speculated that,

pose, the crucial point is that the bird is not only detected—its shape can also be recognized.

Two kinds of visual information caused by self-motion, each of which can be used in two ways

There are two kinds of visual information created by self-motion. Figure 5.2A illustrates the first kind in its pure form. When the moving observer fixates point F, the retinal images of objects that are closer than F and objects that are more distant than F slide across one another without changing size. This is the effect that Helmholtz called motion parallax.

> Motion parallax does two things. It can segregate the retinal images of objects that are at different depths. And it provides information about the relative distances of objects.

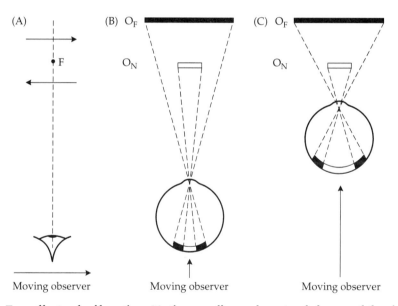

(A) F

Moving observer

(B) O_F O_N

Moving observer

(C) O_F O_N

Moving observer

5.2 Two effects of self-motion: Motion parallax and a rate of change of the size of an object's retinal image. (A) Motion parallax. (B, C) The retinal images of O_N and O_F have different relative rates of expansion.

---

in addition to the aftereffect caused by adapting the first-stage filters for unidirectional local motion (Reichardt detectors), there might be some longer-lived aftereffect caused by adapting the filters for MD form (e.g., Reichardt pool cells [Reichardt et al., 1983a,b]). This speculation would be consistent with the finding that the integration time constant of filters sensitive to MD form is considerably longer than the integration time constant of filters sensitive to local velocity (Figure 5.9). Evidence consistent with this speculation was reported by Shiori and Cavanagh (1992).

Figure 5.2B,C illustrates, in its pure form, the second result of self-motion. As the observer moves directly towards the fixed objects O_N and O_F, the retinal images of O_N and O_F expand (together with any texture elements on the surfaces of O_N and O_F).

> A differential rate of expansion of the retinal images of objects that are at different distances can do two things. It can segregate the retinal images of the different objects (Beverley & Regan, 1980). And it provides information about the relative distances of the objects.

The pattern of retinal image motion produced by looking along a line that is neither perpendicular to (as in Figure 5.2A) nor along (as in Figure 5.2B,C) the direction of motion can, mathematically, be expressed as a vector sum (the *resultant*) of the patterns of retinal image motion illustrated in Figure 5.2A,C, and D (see Appendix I). This mathematical fact does not necessarily imply that the human visual system can resolve a complex pattern of retinal image motion into these two components. But there is experimental evidence (Regan & Beverley, 1980) for the following.

> The human visual system can dissociate changes in the size of an object's retinal image from translational motion of that same retinal image.

Most of Chapter 5 focuses on the detection and spatial discrimination of form that is rendered visible by motion parallax. But, in addition, on pp. 309–310 I discuss the early processing of spatial form that is rendered visible by the kind of relative motion illustrated in Figure 5.2B,C. And later in the chapter I review how the visual system uses the information created by self-motion to recover the relative distances of objects.

What is it about motion parallax that breaks camouflage?

At first sight, Helmholtz's observation might be taken to imply that relative velocity alone is sufficient to support the detection and recognition of motion-defined (MD) form. However, this conclusion does not necessarily follow, because real-world motion parallax confounds several cues to figure–ground segregation, even when figure and ground have exactly the same luminance, color, texture, and binocular disparity. These cues include the following:

1. Retinal image velocity is different on either side of the MD boundary.
2. During any given time interval, different distances are moved by points within the figure and within the ground.
3. Texture continuously appears and disappears along the MD boundary (except for those parts of the boundary parallel to the direction of relative motion).

In order to investigate the role of relative velocity in figure–ground segregation it is necessary to dis-confound the three variables just listed. Figure 5.3A–E illustrates one way in which this can be done. Figure 5.3A is a photograph of a random pattern of dots on a computer monitor. A letter Z is perfectly camouflaged within the pattern. To demonstrate the letter, in Figure 5.3B camouflage is broken by removing all the dots outside the letter, so that the letter is rendered visible by luminance contrast. Figure 5.3C is a time exposure in which the dots inside the letter are moving rightwards, while the dots outside the letter are stationary. This abrupt change in dot speed across the boundaries of the letter is capable of rendering the letter visible to a normally sighted individual, but the photographic time exposure renders the letter clearly visible by *texture contrast* rather than by *motion contrast* (motion contrast is defined on pp. 301–304). In principle, the letter in Figure 5.3C could be seen and recognized by an individual who was totally blind to motion per se. For example, temporal integration in the well-known cortical neurons that are sensitive to the length

5.3 Motion-defined letters. Parts A–E are photographic time exposures of a computer monitor. (A) A letter is perfectly camouflaged within a pattern of random dots. (B) The letter is revealed by switching off all dots outside the letter. (C) Dots within the letter move rightwards at speed V, while dots outside the letter are stationary. (D) Dots within the letter move rightwards at speed V, while dots outside the letter move upwards at speed V. (E) Dots within the letter move rightwards at speed V, while dots outside the letter move leftwards at speed V. The letter is almost invisible to the camera, but was clearly evident when viewed by normally sighted individuals. After Regan et al. (1992b).

(A)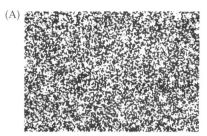

(B)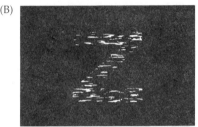

(C)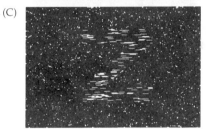

(D)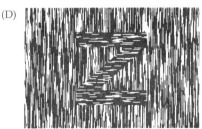

(E)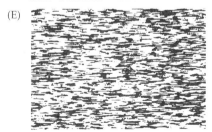

and orientation of a line might cause them to respond to a moving dot as though the moving dot were a line of some specific length and orientation, much as illustrated by the camera film's temporal integration in Figure 5.3C. Again, Figure 5.3D is a time-exposure of dots inside and outside the letter moving at right angles at the same speed; the temporal integration of the camera film reveals the letter by orientation texture contrast. In Figure 5.3E the dots inside and outside the letter move at equal speeds in opposite directions. The letter is almost perfectly camouflaged in the photographic time exposure, because the camera is insensitive to the direction of motion; yet the letter is seen clearly by a normally sighted observer.

Careful inspection shows that camouflage, though close, is not quite perfect in Figure 5.3E; the trajectories of some dots near the vertical boundaries of the letter are shorter than those in the rest of the display. This was because dots continuously appeared and disappeared along those boundaries.

Addressing this texture appearance/disappearance issue, we compared detection thresholds for a motion-defined bar in two conditions.

> Condition (1). Test stimulus: Dots within the bar and outside the bar moved at the same speed but in opposite directions. Reference stimulus: Dot speed was the same as for test stimulus, but dots within the bar and outside the bar moved in the same direction. Thus, in this first condition, relative motion was the only cue that could render the bar in the test stimulus more visible than the bar in the reference stimulus.
>
> Condition (2). Test stimulus: Same as in first condition. Reference stimulus: Dot speed was zero. Thus, in this second condition both the appearance/disappearance cue and the relative motion cue rendered the bar in the test stimulus more visible than the (perfectly camouflaged) bar in the reference stimulus.
>
> Bar detection thresholds were not significantly different in the two conditions. We concluded that detection threshold for MD was determined by the relative motion cue, and that the contribution of appearance/disappearance cue was negligible (Regan & Hamstra, 1992b).

A second control experiment for the appearance/disappearance problem was to generate a complete new dot pattern several times per second so that dots frequently appeared and disappeared all over the pattern rather than only along the vertical figure–ground boundaries so that the dot pattern looked like the "snow" of a detuned television set. Nevertheless, the motion-defined form was clearly visible (Regan, 1986a).

Figure 5.3E shows that the letter is almost perfectly hidden to a *stationary* camera. However, if the observing eye tracked one set of dots, the retinal image would differ from the display so that texture contrast could once again contribute to the letter's visibility. To control for this possibility, I stabilized a random-dot display on the retina by means of a double-Purkinje eye tracker (Regan, 1986a). In this situation, having effectively eliminated both the blur-line and the texture creation/destruction cues to image segregation, we can attribute the visibility of the form entirely to relative velocity.

Having carried out these control experiments, I noted that visual performance was little affected when I removed retinal image stabilization. This finding indicates that a camouflaged target (or at least, a camouflaged target that subtends only a few degrees) is rendered visible chiefly by motion contrast rather than by texture contrast or by accretion/deletion of texture even when the retinal image is unstabilized and the dot pattern is not recreated many times per second—provided that the dots move at equal speeds in opposite directions (Regan, 1986a).

Detection of Motion-Defined Form

Thus far we have seen that a difference in the velocities of texture elements within and outside an object's retinal image can *by itself alone* render the object visible. In the next section I distinguish between several of the different kinds of "difference in the velocities of texture elements."

Two ways in which motion parallax can render visible a spatial form

It will be useful to make a distinction between two ways in which a two-dimensional form can be rendered visible by motion alone.

- MD Form Type A: Moving figure. A perfectly camouflaged textured figure can be rendered visible by its bodily translation relative to its identically textured surrounding. This is an example of motion parallax, as illustrated in Figure 5.2A. Figure 5.1 provides a demonstration.
- MD Form Type B: Stationary figure. A perfectly camouflaged textured figure whose boundaries remain stationary relative to its identically textured surroundings can be rendered visible by motion of the texture within the form relative to the texture surrounding the form. Figures 5.3E and 5.5 explain this kind of MD form.

Physically identical spatial forms of types A and B can produce quite different percepts (see footnote on page 315.)

Two kinds of motion contrast

It will be useful to make a distinction between two kinds of motion contrast: motion contrast associated with motion parallel to the boundary and motion contrast associated with motion perpendicular to the boundary.

I have used the phrase *motion contrast* as shorthand for something along the following lines: "a quantitative measure of the relation between the velocities of two contiguous regions of homogeneously moving texture elements expressed so as to capture the basis for the visibility of the boundary between the two regions that is created entirely by their relative motion." In previous reports I adopted the following working definitions: the magnitude of spatial contrast for (shearing) motion parallel to the boundary BB' in Figure 5.4A is given by $|V_1\sin\theta_1 - V_2\sin\theta_2|/(1 + |0.5[V_1\sin\theta_1 + V_2\sin\theta_2]|)$, when the components of the velocity vectors V_1 and V_2 parallel to BB' have the same direction as illustrated in Figure 5.4A, and $|V_1\sin\theta_1 + V_2\sin\theta_2|/(1 + |0.5[V_1\sin\theta_1 - V_2\sin\theta_2]|)$, when the two components have opposite directions; the magnitude of spatial contrast for motion perpendicular to the boundary BB' (i.e., for compressive/expansive motion) is given by $|V_1\cos\theta_1 - V_2\cos\theta_2|/(1 + |0.5[V_1\cos\theta_1 + V_2\cos\theta_2]|)$, when the components of the velocity vectors V_1 and V_2 perpendicular to BB' have the same direction as illustrated in Figure 5.4A, and $|V_1\cos\theta_1 + V_2\cos\theta_2|/(1 + |0.5[V_1\cos\theta_1 - V_2\cos\theta_2]|)$ when the two components have opposite directions.

A distinction between motion-defined (MD) form and luminance-defined (LD) form is that the mean velocity in the region of the MD boundary can be zero, as illustrated in Figure 5.4B for shearing motion and in Figure 5.4C for compressive/expansive motion while, as discussed on pp. 420–422, the mean luminance in the region of an LD boundary can never be zero (see Figure 1.18B). The knotty problem of how to express the difference between the luminances across an LD boundary in a rationally based relationship with the mean luminance is discussed on pp. 53–60 and 470–476. For want of relevant experimental evidence I will not discuss the analogous problem for MD boundaries.

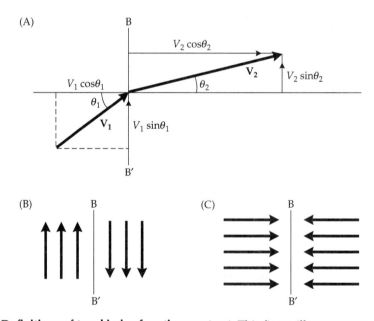

5.4 Definitions of two kinds of motion contrast. This figure illustrates pure shearing contrast (part B), pure compressive/expansive contrast (part C), and a combination of the two (part A).

Next I discuss whether the two kinds of motion contrast are processed differently by the human visual system.

It has been reported that the effect of bar width and presentation duration on detection threshold for a foveally viewed MD bar are the same for the two kinds of motion contrast (Regan & Beverley, 1984). However, the experiment described next revealed a distinction. Figure 5.5A–D illustrates a rationale that was originally developed for dissociating early and late processing in stereoscopic vision (Regan & Beverley, 1973a), but here is used to "dissect apart" the properties of first -stage motion detectors and second-stage MD contrast detectors (Regan, 1986b). I adopted the Reichardt model of sensitivity to MD form: first-stage filters sensitive to local velocity feed second-stage filters sensitive to MD form (Reichardt et al., 1983a,b). On the assumption that the effect of adaptation would depend on temporal frequency (as it does, for example, for flicker adaptation [Smith, 1970; Pantle, 1973a; Regan & Beverley, 1978a]), I attempted to separate the first-stage and second-stage filters by adapting them to different temporal frequencies.

During the adaptation period, the three vertical bars in Figure 5.5 were continuously visible; all dots executed 0.5 Hz triangular-wave oscillations. There was a

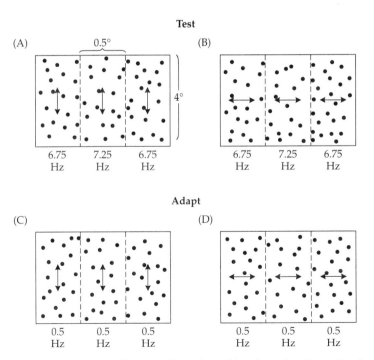

5.5 Method for unconfounding the detection of local motion from the detection of motion-defined form. See text for details. From Regan (1986b).

phase difference of 180 degrees between the central bar and the two outer bars. All dots had the same speed and hence the same peak-to-peak amplitude of oscillation. I assumed that viewing the continuously visible MD form for several minutes would adapt the observer's second-stage filters. Unavoidably, the first-stage local motion filters would also adapt. But if the adaptation were frequency-selective its effects would be small for frequencies far from 0.5 Hz.

There were two test stimuli. For both test stimuli, all dots outside the central bar oscillated sinusoidally at 6.75 Hz, and all dots within the central bar oscillated sinusoidally at 7.25 Hz. Thus, the bar's visibility oscillated at a low ("beat") frequency that served as a "signature" of the bar's presence. For one of the two test stimuli, the central bar was rendered visible by pure shearing motion (Figure 5.5A), while the other was rendered visible by compressive/expansive dot motion at right angles to the boundaries of the central bar (Figure 5.5B).

I measured baseline thresholds after adapting to a stationary dot pattern. After adapting to the pure shearing-motion stimulus illustrated in Figure 5.5C, threshold for detecting the pure shearing-motion central test bar illustrated in Figure 5.5A was elevated considerably more than threshold for detecting the compressive/expansive test bar.

A second adapting stimulus was similar to that illustrated in Figure 5.5C except that dot motion was at right angles to the boundaries of the central bar (Figure 5.5D). Adapting to this stimulus produced no threshold elevation for either of the two test bars.

This experiment indicated that different filters supported the detection of MD bars that were rendered visible by relative motion parallel to and perpendicular to the boundaries of the foveally viewed bar, a conclusion that is consistent with the report that a large difference in visual sensitivity to the two kinds of MD boundary can be produced by viewing the boundaries in peripheral vision (Richards & Liberman, 1982).

In order to assess the role of the first-stage dot-motion filters in the threshold elevations just described, I carried out the following control experiment. In the adapting stimuli all the dots oscillated in-phase at 0.5 Hz (so that no bar was ever visible, but the local-motion detectors were adapted to 0.5 Hz). For the test stimuli, all dots oscillated in-phase at 7.0 Hz (so that no bar was ever visible, but the local motion detectors were adapted to 7.0 Hz). I measured threshold elevations for detecting dot motion. There were no significant elevations. I concluded that the observed threshold elevations for detecting MD bars was entirely determined by the second-stage filters sensitive to MD form with negligible contribution from the first-stage local-motion filters.

Detection of spatial form defined by shearing motion; contrast sensitivity functions for motion-defined form

Nakayama and Tyler (1981) created sinewave gratings for MD form as illustrated in Figure 5.6. Each dot in a random pattern oscillated sinusoidally with the same frequency along a horizontal direction. The amplitude of oscillation was constant in a horizontal direction, but varied sinusoidally in a vertical direction, thus pro-

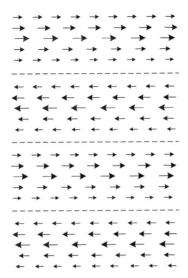

5.6 Motion-defined grating. Nakayama and Tyler's method for generating a motion-defined sinewave grating. Each dot in a pseudo-random pattern oscillated sinusoidally at the same temporal frequency in a horizontal direction. Oscillation amplitude was constant in a horizontal direction, but varied sinusoidally in a vertical direction. Each arrow represents the velocity of one dot at one instant in time. From Nakayama and Tyler (1981).

ducing shearing motion. Note that dot density remained constant at all locations within the dot pattern.

Figure 5.7 shows the contrast sensitivity function for MD form defined by shearing motion. Sensitivity does not fall off at the lowest spatial frequencies.* On the other hand, at high spatial frequencies, sensitivity falls off from about 0.7 cycles/deg., and grating acuity is 5 to 10 cycles/deg. in Figure 5.7.

Is this high-frequency rolloff a property of the visual system or might it be an artifact of spatial undersampling? (Spatial sampling is discussed in Appendix F.) There were approximately 129 dots across the 6 degree height of the display used to collect the data shown in Figure 5.7, so that the number of spatial samples per cycle did not fall to 6 until grating frequency reached 1.8 cycles/deg. So if the effect of the number of random dots per grating cycle on sensitivity to MD gratings is similar to

---

* Golomb et al. (1985) reported that sensitivity fell as spatial frequency was reduced from about 0.28 to 0.04 cycle/deg. But their display subtended only 19 degrees, so that the number of cycles on the screen would fall below 5 as spatial frequency passed 0.26 cycle/deg., and at a spatial frequency of 0.40 there would be less than one cycle on the screen (see pp. 53–60 and 416–420 and Figure B.7). Rogers and Graham (1983) reported that sensitivity to an MD grating falls off at spatial frequencies below the lowest frequency used by Nakayama and Tyler (1981). Again, however, it is not clear to what extent this low-frequency falloff was a result of using a grating that contained only 1 cycle at the largest period used (25 degrees per cycle).

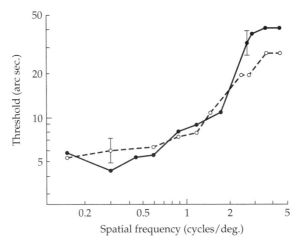

5.7 Contrast sensitivity function for a motion-defined grating. Ordinates plot the peak-to-peak amplitude of oscillation for the dots at detection threshold for the motion-defined grating. Each dot in the pattern oscillated at a temporal frequency of 2 Hz. Field size was 6 degrees (vertical) × 5 degrees. From Nakayama and Tyler (1981).

its effect on LD and OTD gratings (pp. 470–476), the considerable fall in sensitivity between 0.7 and 1.8 cycles/deg. evident in Figure 5.7 can be regarded as a property of the visual system.

A comparison of Figures 5.7 and 1.19 shows that sensitivity to an LD grating extends to much higher spatial frequencies than sensitivity to an MD grating. But this comparison is not entirely fair, because the gratings used to collect the luminance data in Figure 1.19 had a very large number of spatial samples per gratings period.

Spatial summation for motion-defined form

Nakayama and Tyler (1981) concluded that the spatial summation field size for detecting MD form is approximately 2 degrees—somewhat larger than for detecting LD form. The 2 degree estimate, however, was based on the full width of the summation field; the width at half height would have been closer to 1 degree (C. W. Tyler, personal communication, November 1996). Using a different approach, Richards (1971a) had previously arrived at a similar estimate.

In a more direct attempt to measure spatial summation, Regan and Beverley (1984) found that detection thresholds for an MD square fell as the square's area was progressively increased from 0.1 to 5 deg.². For a foveally viewed target, the curve leveled out at a threshold of approximately 0.1 degrees/sec., consistent with a circular spatial summation area (Gaussian profile) of roughly 0.4 degrees diameter for MD form. Log spatial summation area was approximately proportional to eccentricity. The (circular) spatial summation area for a solid foveally viewed LD square was approximately 0.2 degrees in diameter.

Figure 5.8 brings out the relation between target size and retinal eccentricity on detection threshold for MD form. For any given target area, the logarithm of threshold motion contrast is proportional to eccentricity. But the slope depends on the area of the target.

Temporal summation for motion-defined form

Open circles in Figure 5.9 show how the motion contrast required to detect an MD target varied with presentation duration. For points that fell on the horizontal segment of the continuous line, target detection threshold was reached at a constant value of presentation duration × (motion contrast), i.e., by a constant distance moved by the dots. For points that fell on the segment with 45 degree slope, target detection threshold corresponded to a constant value of motion contrast (Regan & Beverley, 1984).

Open circles in Figure 5.9 show that, for presentation durations up to the *critical duration* of about 0.6 seconds, the visual system integrates motion contrast.*

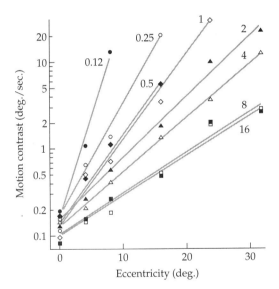

5.8 Log detection threshold for motion-defined targets is proportional to viewing eccentricity. The effect of eccentricity is less for larger targets. Motion contrast at detection threshold for motion-defined targets is plotted as ordinate. The log-linear relationship holds for targets of areas ranging from 0.12 to 6 degrees2, a 130:1 range, and holds over a 200:1 range of thresholds. After Regan and Beverley (1984).

---

* Rather than the standard method of fitting temporal integration data with lines of 45 degrees and zero slopes (Graham, 1965), we fitted our luminance data to the single-stage equation $(Th)_t = (Th)_\infty(1 - e^{-t/\tau})$, where $(Th)_t$ was the threshold for a presentation duration of t seconds, $(Th)_\infty$ was the threshold for a very long presentation duration, and τ seconds

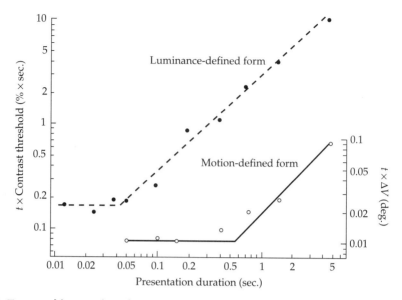

5.9 Temporal integration characteristics for motion-defined form and luminance-defined form. Motion contrast at target-detection threshold is, to a first approximation, inversely proportional to presentation duration up to a presentation duration of about 0.6 seconds. This *critical duration* is marked by the abrupt change of slope of the continuous line. Luminance contrast at target detection threshold is, to a first approximation, inversely proportional to presentation duration up to a presentation duration of about 0.06 seconds. Both targets had an area of 1.0 degrees². After Regan and Beverley (1984).

We measured the *critical duration* for a comparable LD target by switching off all the dots outside the MD target and measuring the luminance contrast at target detection threshold. Filled symbols in Figure 5.9 are in accord with the well-known finding (*Bloch's law*) that the critical duration for LD form is about 0.05 seconds. We concluded that:

> Temporal integration for MD form approximates Bloch's law. And temporal integration for MD form extends to a duration about 10 times greater than for LD form.

Figure 5.9 can be compared with Figure 3.11. The finding that temporal summation extends over a considerably longer time for detecting an MD object than

was the temporal integration time constant. The advantage of this method of estimating integration time over the method of drawing two asymptotes of 45 degrees and zero slope is that all data points are taken into account. The value of τ was 0.061 seconds. Data points for the MD target could not be modeled by a single integration stage. But they were well-described by two cascaded stages (correlation coefficient 0.98), the first stage being that used for the luminance data. The second stage had a much longer time constant (about 0.75 seonds) (Regan & Beverley, 1984).

for detecting an LD object (Regan & Beverley, 1984) is accounted for by the Reichardt "pool cell" model (W. Reichardt, personal communication, October 1984).

Different rates of retinal image expansion: A possible aid in segregating an object's retinal image from the retinal image of the object's surroundings

How are the multitude of pattern elements produced by the initial analysis of the retinal image subsequently organized or integrated into a number of groups, each of which corresponds to a separate object in the outside world? How does the visual system assign a particular retinal image contour to a particular object and a particular retinal image pattern element to the surface of that particular object? This process of organization can be regarded as the *interpretation* of the retinal image. (The same problem emerges in artificial intelligence as the problem of parsing groups of features such as lines and intersections into objects.) Since the early work of Marr and his colleagues, this problem has received increasing attention (Marr, 1976, 1982; Marr & Poggio, 1976; Marr & Nishihara, 1978; Marr et al., 1979; Marr & Hildreth, 1980).

A related problem is to explain why the visual system does not often confound the edges or boundaries of one object with the edges of a different object. The fact that, when such confounding does take place it often occurs with stationary objects, led us to suggest a way in which information provided by self-motion might aid image interpretation (Beverley & Regan, 1980a). Note that the suggestion is framed in terms of early processing rather than in terms of leisurely cognitive evaluation of what one sees. The key to our suggestion was the finding that there is a strong nonlinear interaction between responses to the values of $\theta/(d\theta/dt)$ across different meridians of the retinal image (Beverley & Regan, 1980a).*

- When the values of $\theta/(d\theta/dt)$ between boundaries of an untextured object's retinal image are equal across all meridians, the object as a whole appears to move in depth, but when the value of $\theta/(d\theta/dt)$ along one meridian is reduced, the perceived speed of motion in depth is considerably reduced, and time to collision is overestimated (Beverley & Regan, 1979a; Regan & Beverley, 1978b, 1979c; Gray & Regan, 1999a).
- If the values of $\theta/(d\theta/dt)$ are equal for all texture elements within the retinal image of a textured object and are also equal to the value of $\theta/(d\theta/dt)$ for the boundaries of the object, then the object and its surface texture appear to move in depth as a solid entity, but if the value of $\theta/(d\theta/dt)$ for texture elements is less than the value of $\theta/(d\theta/dt)$ for the boundaries of the object's retinal image, the speed of perceived motion in depth *for the object as a whole* is reduced (see Gray & Regan, 1999b, for relevant evidence and a proposed explanation for this phenomenon).

---

* This interaction causes large errors in estimating the time to collision with a tumbling nonspherical object (such as a Rugby football or an American football) that is approaching the eye at constant speed (Gray & Regan, 1999a).

We proposed that the characteristics of early visual processing just described could, in the everyday three-dimensional world of objects, guide the visual system in organizing the multitude of pattern elements and contours in the retinal image into groups, each of which corresponds to a different object by utilizing the geometrical fact that "for an object moving in depth, there is a fixed relationship between the velocities both of surface features and of boundaries, and this relationship is determined by the distance of the object from the eye. Objects at different distances have different velocity relationships. . . . It follows that our proposed system might fail to distinguish between objects at the same distance" (Beverley & Regan, 1980a, p. 158).

Channels for Motion-Defined Form

Hogervorst, Bradshaw, and Eagle (1998) reported evidence that, at least for motion-defined *corrugations in depth*, the visual system contains independent spatial-frequency channels, whose bandwidths (around 1.5 octaves) are similar to those found in the disparity domain (see also Hogervorst et al., in press).

Figure 5.10 explains their optical arrangements. The display screen was covered with a pattern of randomly scattered dots. When the observer's head was

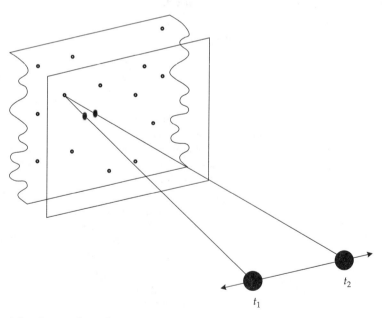

5.10. Stimulus used to obtain the data shown in Figure 5.12. The observer moved his head side to side over 13 cm in a direction parallel to a display that was viewed from 70 cm. One eye was covered. From Hogervorst, Bradshaw, and Eagle (1998). Figure kindly provided by M. A. Hogervorst.

still, the dots did not move. Then the observer moved his head from side to side at a frequency of about 1 Hz. A head-position sensor was linked to the dot display in such a way that head movements caused the dots to move relative to one another. The linkage was designed so that the retinal image in the observer's eye was exactly as though he was moving his head from side to side while viewing a surface that really was corrugated sinusoidally in depth. As was already well known, the arrangement produces the impression that the observer is viewing a corrugated surface even though the dot pattern is flat. (When the observer's head stops moving, the illusory corrugation collapses and the dot pattern appears to be flat.)

Hogervorst et al. used the *notched noise* approach (Patterson, 1976) to search for spatial-frequency channels. Figure 5.11 illustrates their rationale. They measured the detectability of corrugations of a particular spatial frequency in the presence of two noise bands placed symmetrically about the corrugation frequency. They reasoned that "spatial-frequency tuning should become apparent

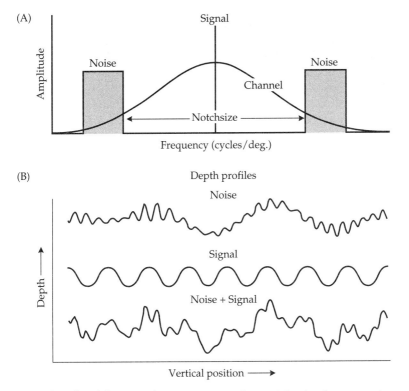

5.11 Rationale of the experiment. The waveform of the depth corrugations consisted of a sinusoid ("signal") that was flanked by noise on either side. From Hogervorst, Bradshaw, and Eagle (1998). Figure kindly provided by M. A. Hogervorst.

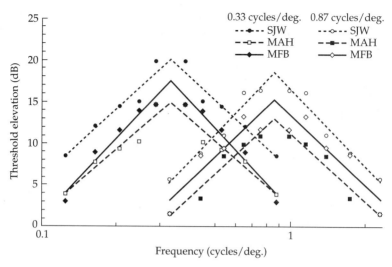

5.12 Spatial-frequency tuning curves for corrugated surfaces rendered visible by relative motion. The data shown in this figure provide evidence that the human visual system contains channels for motion-defined form. From Hogervorst, Bradshaw, and Eagle (1998). Figure kindly provided by M. A. Hogervorst.

in an increase in threshold elevation with decreasing notchsize." Figure 5.12 shows their data.

Hogervorst et al. concluded:

> "The parallax-sensitivity function is comprised of a series of independent channels with bandwidths around 1.5 octaves. These bandwidths are similar to those found in the stereo domain."

Orientation Discrimination for Motion-Defined Form

Following the line of thought illustrated in Figure 5.3, I arranged that a bar that was perfectly camouflaged within a pattern of stationary random dots was rendered visible by motion contrast. Since the dots inside and outside the rectangle moved at the same speed but in opposite directions, motion contrast was equal to twice the dot speed. Filled circles in Figure 5.13A show that, unsurprisingly, orientation discrimination threshold for a dotted MD bar of high dot contrast was high at dot speeds just above bar-detection threshold (filled circle with arrow) and fell as motion contrast was increased (Regan, 1989b). Less predictably, orientation discrimination threshold was approximately constant for motion contrasts greater than about three times bar detection threshold (compare with Figure 2.30).

The curve shown is presumably the left segment of a broad U-shaped function; at very high dot speeds each dot would look like a line, and observers would

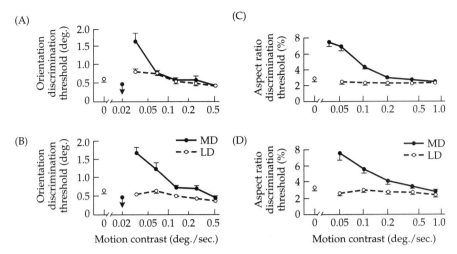

5.13 Orientation discrimination and aspect-ratio discrimination for motion-defined form. (A, B) The effect of motion contrast on orientation-discrimination threshold for a dotted bar whose visibility was created by relative motion (MD), and for the same dotted bar whose visibility was created by luminance contrast (LD). Orientation detection thresholds are arrowed. Dot contrast in part (B) was 0.7 log units lower than in part (A). (C, D) The effect of motion contrast on aspect-ratio discrimination threshold for a dotted rectangle whose visibility was created by relative motion (MD), and for the same dotted rectangle whose visibility was created by luminance contrast (LD). Dot contrast was 0.7 log units lower in part (D) than in part (C). The random pattern contained approximately 1,000 dots, each of which subtended 2 minutes of arc. The pattern subtended 2.2 deg. × 2.2 deg., and mean dot separation was 6 minutes of arc. The bar subtended 1.5 deg. × 0.22 deg. Parts A and B after Regan (1989b). Parts C and D after Regan and Hamstra, 1991.

not be able to discriminate leftwards from rightwards motion. Consequently, at high dot speeds the bar's visibility would fall to zero, and orientation discrimination threshold would rise correspondingly.

The lowest value of orientation discrimination threshold was 0.5 degrees, and this was the same as that for an LD bar (open circles) that was created by removing all the dots outside the bar.

To account for this very low orientation discrimination threshold for an MD bar, I proposed that the visual system contains orientation-tuned filters for MD form, and that orientation discrimination threshold is determined by the relative activity among a population of such filters tuned to different orientations (Regan, 1989b). A comparison of Figure 5.13A and B brings out a tradeoff between luminance contrast and motion contrast. In Figure 5.13B, the luminance contrast of the dots was 0.7 log units lower than in Figure 5.13A, and a higher dot speed was required to reduce threshold to 0.5 degrees.

Positional Discrimination, Width Discrimination, Separation Discrimination, and Spatial-frequency Discrimination for Motion-Defined Form

Although, as mentioned earlier, our ability to judge the relative directions of luminance-defined objects and to discriminate their widths has attracted interest for more than a hundred years, only during the last few years have any measurements of our corresponding abilities for motion-defined objects been published. Yet, as we see below, our spatial discrimination abilities are little, if at all, inferior for motion-defined form than for luminance-defined form, *provided that spatial sampling for the two kinds of target is matched.*

Positional discrimination: High precision for discriminating relative position co-exists with low accuracy for estimating absolute position

The edges of a suprathreshold motion-defined rectangle appear to be strikingly sharp—especially in view of the large spatial summation fields for MD form (pp. 306–307) and low grating acuity (shown in Figure 5.7) for MD form (Regan & Beverley, 1984). Whether this illusion of sharpness implies that we can discriminate the relative location of an MD edge with the high precision corresponding to its perceived sharpness is an empirical question that I addressed by measuring Vernier acuity for an MD target (Regan, 1986a).

Figure 5.14A illustrates one of three stimulus configurations used. In this configuration, the MD bar was stationary but the dots moved at equal speeds in the directions shown. The retinal image of the stimulus was stabilized to prevent the eye from tracking the dots and thus creating a texture contrast cue to the Vernier step. A new dot pattern was created every 0.125 sec. so as to minimize the dot disappearance/appearance cue to the Vernier step.

The main finding was that Vernier step threshold for the MD bar was not significantly different from Vernier step threshold for an LD bar that was created by removing all dots outside the bar (so that the two bars had the same spatial sampling frequency). Vernier step threshold was 27 seconds of arc for the best subject and 45 seconds of arc for the worst (Regan, 1986a). At first sight, Vernier step thresholds of 27 to 45 seconds of arc might seem poor compared with the best values in the literature for a narrow bright line (2 to 5 seconds of arc). To check that these high values were not a result of generally poor vision in the observers tested, it was confirmed that these values all had normal Vernier step thresholds for a solid bright bar (5 to 8 seconds of arc).

A more revealing way of evaluating the 27 to 45 seconds of arc Vernier step thresholds for the dotted MD bar is to compare them with the size of the dots (120 sec. arc diameter) and the mean interdot separation (7,200 sec. arc). Thus, the formal psychophysical measurement of Vernier acuity supported the subjective impression that the edges of the MD bar were much more sharply defined than the mean dot separation—by a factor of over 250:1. And the cognitive level of processing played no evident role in this edge sharpening. In light of these num-

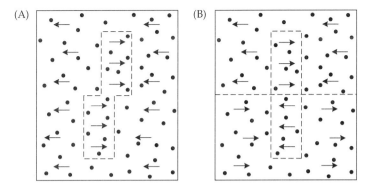

5.14 Vernier acuity target for motion-defined form. A random pattern of about 1,000 bright dots contained a perfectly camouflaged Vernier step target shown by the dashed line. The target was rendered visible in one of two ways. As illustrated, dots inside the target were moved at the same speed, but in the opposite direction from dots outside the target, the target remaining stationary. Alternatively, the target and all the dots within it moved bodily at the same speed but in the opposite direction from all the dots outside the target. (B) Mislocation of motion-defined form. When a straight bar is rendered visible by the dot motions illustrated, the bar appears to contain an illusory Vernier step similar to that illustrated in part A.

bers, we are faced with the problem of explaining why the 27 to 45 seconds of arc Vernier step thresholds for the MD bar are so *low*.

Some authors have suggested that Vernier acuity for bright-line targets can be explained in terms of sensitivity to the luminance distribution in the retinal image (see pp. 98–106), but this cannot be the case for an MD bar, because there were no luminance cues to the bar's presence. An intriguing clue is provided by observers' reports that they made Vernier discriminations, not on the basis of seeing the Vernier step, but rather on the basis of an illusory tilt of the whole bar.* On this basis, I suggested that Vernier acuity for the MD bar was determined by the relative activity of orientation-tuned neural mechanisms sensitive to the MD bars (Regan, 1986a; see Appendix D).

We reported that errors in estimating the absolute location of an MD target can be gross—as large as several degrees in peripheral vision—while discrimination threshold for relative location remains at around one minute of arc (Regan & Beverley, 1984). Although this effect is largest in peripheral vision, it can be demonstrated in foveal vision by using the Vernier target illustrated in Figure

---

* When the MD bar was stationary and the dots inside and outside the bar moved at equal speeds in opposite directions, observers reported that the bar appeared to be straight but tilted, and they could not see a Vernier step. When the dots inside the bar and the bar moved bodily in the opposite direction and at equal speed to the dots outside the bar, observers reported that the Vernier step was visible and the bar was not tilted. But the radically different percepts had no effect on psychophysical performance. Vernier acuity was the same in the two situations.

5.14B. As in Figure 5.14A, the bar is stationary and the dots move at equal speeds in the directions shown. But note how the directions of motion in Figure 5.14B differ from those in Figure 5.14A. Observers reported that the upper and lower halves of the bar appeared to have a Vernier offset similar to that illustrated in Figure 5.14A - even though they were exactly in line. If the directions of all dot motions were now reversed, the illusory Vernier offset was seen in the opposite direction. Similar observations have been reported by Anstis (1989); Ramachandran and Anstis (1990); and DeValois and DeValois (1991). However, in spite of this considerable failure in the *accuracy* of locating the MD bar, the *precision* of relative location (i.e., Vernier offset threshold) was the same for the Vernier target just described and for the Vernier target illustrated in Figure 5.14A.

Bar-width and bar-separation discrimination

I have been unable to find any study on separation discrimination threshold for MD boundaries or bars and, in particular, any analog of the Morgan and Ward (1985) experiment described on pp. 107–108 and 156–169. (Morgan and Ward [1985] showed that an observer's discriminations of the separation between two LD lines could not be explained in terms of filters for LD form that are driven from the same retinal location.)

Spatial-frequency discrimination for motion-defined form

I have been unable to find any study on spatial-frequency discrimination for MD form.

Aspect Ratio Discrimination for Two-Dimensional Motion-Defined Form: Local Signals and Distant Comparisons

We rendered a rectangular area within a random-dot pattern visible by moving the dots inside and outside the rectangle in opposite directions (along an oblique line so that the vertical and horizontal edges of the rectangle would have the same combination of compressive /expansive and shearing motion). The dot pattern was the same as was used in the orientation discrimination study just described. We interleaved randomly rectangles of three mean areas to ensure that neither the height (a) nor width (b) of the rectangle provided a reliable cue to its aspect ratio a/b (Regan & Hamstra, 1991).

Figure 5.13C shows that aspect-ratio discrimination threshold for an MD rectangle of high dot luminance contrast fell as motion contrast was progressively increased up to about three times bar-detection threshold. As was the case in Figure 5.13A, the curve was presumably the left half of a broad U-shaped function. The lowest aspect-ratio discrimination threshold was approximately 2%, and this was the same as aspect-ratio discrimination threshold for an LD rectangle created by removing all dots outside the MD rectangle. Figure 5.13D shows that, just as for orientation discrimination, aspect ratio threshold showed a tradeoff between luminance contrast and motion contrast.

And just as for LD rectangles (see Figure 2.60), aspect-ratio discrimination threshold for MD rectangles is a U-shaped function of aspect ratio, with the lowest value at an aspect ratio of 1.0 (Regan & Hamstra, 1991).

To explain the findings just described, I propose that the aspect ratio of an MD rectangle is processed according to the schematic shown in Figure 2.63A, but with broadly tuned receptive fields sensitive to MD form (Figure 5.22C) rather than LD form, and with the coincidence detectors sensitive to the separation between two narrowly tuned receptive fields for MD form (Figure 5.26) rather than the separation between two narrowly tuned receptive fields for LD form as in Figure 2.53. The processing of aspect-ratio information for an MD rectangle would be along the same lines as illustrated in Figure 2.63B–F for an LD rectangle.

Spatial Processing of Form Defined by Short-range Apparent Motion

The random-dot stereogram was devised by Bela Julesz (1960, 1971). Figure 5.15 shows one of his stereopairs. When the images are viewed in binocular fusion, a central square is seen floating above its surround in vivid depth, yet when one eye is closed, the square disappears and one sees a flat pattern of random dots.

Figure 5.16 explains the principle. "The left and right images are identical random-dot textures except for certain areas that are also identical but shifted relative to each other in the horizontal direction as though they were solid sheets. The shifted areas (denoted by A and B cells) cover certain areas of the background

5.15 A stereopair provided by Bela Julesz. Hold a pencil horizontally above the page at such a height that with the right eye closed, the point appears to fall on the center of the right picture, and with the left eye closed the point appears to fall on the center of the left picture. Look at the pencil point and wait.

(denoted by 1 and 0 cells; and owing to the shift, certain areas become uncovered (denoted by X and Y cells). If the horizontal shift is kept always an integral multiple of cell size, then no cell of the background will ever be partly covered by the shifted areas, and thus no monocular cue will be present" (Julesz, 1971, pp. 20–21).

Spekreijse and I projected slides of a stereopair kindly given to us by Bela Julesz (Figure 5.15) onto a screen, and we viewed the screen from a distance such that the individual cells subtended 10 minutes of arc. First we used a stereopair for which the central region was displaced by one cell. When we optically superimposed the two patterns on the screen and abruptly alternated between them, we found that, at the moment at which one pattern replaced the other, we saw a sudden brief appearance of the central square region of the pattern that moved either leftwards or rightwards depending on which of the two patterns was presented second.

Bela Julesz had provided us with two additional stereopairs. The central square region was displaced by two cells in the second stereopair, and by four cells in the third. When we replaced the first stereopair with either of the other two stereopairs, we saw no moving central square area. Instead, all the individual dots appeared to jump in random directions at the instant of transition.

Corresponding to these subjective observations, a clear brain response was produced when the displacement was one cell (i.e., 10 minutes of arc), but there was no brain response when the displacement was either two cells (i.e., 20 minutes of arc) or four cells (i.e., 40 minutes of arc [Regan & Spekreijse, 1970]). Thus, the illusion that the central area of the pattern moved as a coherent whole failed when the displacement was somewhere between 10 and 20 minutes of arc.*

Anstis (1970) also reported that global motion could be produced as described above, but did not use sufficiently large jumps to observe the breakdown. Braddick (1974) reported that the interval between the two pattern presentations should not exceed 100 msec. (see also Baker & Braddick, 1985), and he noted that

* This was one control experiment in a study whose purpose was to find whether it was possible to demonstrate brain responses that were specific to a change in binocular disparity. As already mentioned, we used a Julesz stereopair. The brain responses were evoked by switching abruptly between two conditions. In one condition both eyes viewed one of the two patterns. In the second condition the right eye continued to view the same pattern, while the left eye saw the second pattern. However, when the displacement of the central rectangle in the pattern viewed by the left eye was 10 minutes of arc, strong brain responses were produced by binocular stimulation. But strong responses were also recorded when the right eye was occluded. On the other hand, when the displacement was either 20 or 40 minutes of arc there was no brain response when the right eye was occluded (and, correspondingly, no percept of so-called short-range motion). But large brain responses were recorded when the occluder was removed from the right eye. We concluded that these responses were not caused by monocular stimulation of the right eye, but rather reflected binocular interactions.

Some authors (e.g., Tyler & Julesz, 1980) have discussed the concept of d_{max} for stereopairs, and it has been suggested that the values of d_{max} for short-range motion and for stereopsis are similar (Glennerster, 1998). This suggestion is difficult to reconcile with our finding that (in our experimental conditions) the short-range motion percept and its associated brain response failed somewhere between 10 and 20 minutes of arc, but the percept of a jump in depth and its associated brain response were still strong at 40 minutes of arc.

1	0	1	0	1	0	0	1	0	1
1	0	0	1	0	1	0	1	0	0
0	0	1	1	0	1	1	0	1	0
0	1	0	Y	A	A	B	B	0	1
1	1	1	X	B	A	B	A	0	1
0	0	1	X	A	A	B	A	1	0
1	1	1	Y	B	B	A	B	0	1
1	0	0	1	1	0	1	1	0	1
1	1	0	0	1	1	0	1	1	1
0	1	0	0	0	1	1	1	1	0

1	0	1	0	1	0	0	1	0	1
1	0	0	1	0	1	0	1	0	0
0	0	1	1	0	1	1	0	1	0
0	1	0	A	A	B	B	X	0	1
1	1	1	B	A	B	A	Y	0	1
0	0	1	A	A	B	A	Y	1	0
1	1	1	B	B	A	B	X	0	1
1	0	0	1	1	0	1	1	0	1
1	1	0	0	1	1	0	1	1	1
0	1	0	0	0	1	1	1	1	0

5.16 How the stereopair shown in Figure 5.15 was made. See text for details. After Julesz (1971).

this timing constraint seems not to apply to classical "long-range" apparent motion. (Long-range apparent motion can be seen with interstimulus intervals up to 350 msec. [Kolers, 1972] and even 500 msec. [Burt & Sperling, 1981].)

Braddick (1974), who has studied this effect intensively, dubbed it short-range motion, to distinguish it from the classical apparent-motion effect that operates over considerable distances (Kolers, 1972), but the validity of the distinction has been challenged (Cavanagh & Mather, 1989). Braddick (1974) gave the label d_{max} to the critical distance beyond which motion of the central rectangle as a whole is not seen (15 minutes of arc in his study, between 10 and 20 in ours) (see also Anstis, 1980; Braddick, 1980).[*]

Reichardt (personal communication, November 1969) suggested that the effect might be explained in terms of autocorrelation along the lines of his motion detector, and variants of this approach have been widely favored (see Ramachandran & Anstis, 1983; Cleary & Braddick, 1990a,b).

A great deal of attention has been paid to the conditions required to create the briefly lived visibility of the moving area of dots, but the spatial processing of the moving area has been virtually ignored.

> It is not known how spatial discrimination thresholds for this transiently visible form compare with spatial discrimination thresholds for an MD form that is created by continuous motion (as for example, in Figures 5.13 and 5.14).

[*] Subsequent studies showed that dmax scales inversely with spatial frequency (Chang & Julesz, 1985; Cleary & Braddick, 1990b). Eagle (1998, p. 1785) concluded that "the visual system is able to access low- and high-frequency channels, depending on the demands of the task, i.e., the spectral location of the signal" (see also Morgan, 1992; Morgan & Fahle, 1992;

The aspect-ratio discrimination threshold for a rectangle that was rendered visible by short-range motion is qualitatively comparable with the corresponding threshold for an LD rectangle that was created by removing all dots outside the central rectangles area of the dot pattern (D. Regan, unpublished observations), but whether these thresholds are quantitatively similar to those shown in Figure 5.13C,D is not known. I have been unable to find any report on orientation discrimination for spatial form that is rendered briefly visible by short-range motion.

The Relation between Motion-Defined Form and Relative Depth

There is a proliferation of laboratory demonstrations that binocular relative disparity alone can create a compelling impression that two objects are at different distances. Indeed, the three-dimensional illusion created by the stereoviewers available in every airport depends on this fact. But in everyday conditions it is often the case that binocular relative disparity is by no means the most effective depth cue. This is because the left and right eyes are only approximately 6 cm apart. Consequently, for objects more than about 10 meters away, stereoscopic depth perception grows ineffective (p. 348). Nevertheless, it is the case that distant objects can be seen in vivid relative depth when viewed from, for example, the cockpit of a low-flying helicopter or fixed-wing aircraft. In such situations it is *relative motion information* that is being utilized by the visual system to generate the impression that the objects are at different distances.

Two kinds of relative motion information about relative depth

So far I have focused on the topic foreseen by Helmholtz in the first part of the quotation at the beginning of this chapter, namely the human ability to detect and discriminate spatial form that is rendered visible by relative motion. But the quotation ends with the words, "just as if he were looking at a good stereoscopic view of it." In this section I will review research on the visual system's ability to recover, from the information provided by self–motion, the relative depths of objects in the environment.

Information about the relative distances of objects that is carried by the relative rates of expansion of their retinal images.   If they were viewed binocularly from sufficiently close range, relative disparity information would immediately reveal that object O_N was nearer than object O_F in Figure 5.2B. But when one eye is

---

Morgan & Mather, 1994; Yang & Blake, 1994). Taking a different line altogether, Cavanagh & Mather (1989, p. 103) argued that "the differences between the short-range and long-range motion phenomena are a direct consequence of the stimuli used in the two paradigms and are not evidence for the existence of two qualitatively different motion processes."

closed, there is no static monocular information to reject the possibility that what could be a separate object (i.e., O_N) is in fact a mark on the surface of object O_F. (I assume that objects are sufficiently far away that a younger observer whose lens still retains some flexibility could not use accommodation to resolve the problem.) But two things happen if the observer moves directly forward.

First, the boundaries of the textured retinal image of O_N expand outwards across the differently textured retinal image of O_F. As discussed earlier, this will cause the image of O_N to segregate from its immediate background (that is, from the retinal image of O_N).

The second consequence of the observer's self-motion can be understood in term of an equation derived by the distinguished astronomer Fred Hoyle as a footnote in his novel *The Black Cloud*, published in 1957. He showed that the time to collision (TTC) with a rigid spherical object that is approaching the eye at constant speed is given by Equation (5.1):

$$TTC \approx \theta / (d\theta / dt) \qquad (5.1)$$

where θ is the instantaneous angular subtense of the object and $(d\theta/dt)$ the instantaneous rate of increase of angular subtense.

We have found evidence that the human visual system contains a mechanism that is sensitive to the ratio $\theta / (d\theta / dt)$ independently of θ and of $(d\theta / dt)$ (Regan & Hamstra, 1993). The relevance of this point is that if we consider the retinal image of stationary object O_N as a whole, and the retinal image of stationary object O_F as a whole, then the following is true.

> Because of their different distances, the values of $\theta / (d\theta / dt)$ are different for O_N and O_F. Furthermore, the relative values of $\theta / (d\theta / dt)$ for O_N and O_F give their ordering in depth ("closer" is signaled by lower $\theta / (d\theta / dt)$) (Beverley & Regan, 1980).

(This topic falls into an area often called *optic flow*.)

The sliding of objects' retinal images across each other provides information about the relative distances of the objects. Figure 5.2A illustrates a situation in everyday life in which the relative distances of objects are represented by an ordered relationship within the velocities of their retinal images (whether or not the retinal images are completely superimposed). (This topic also falls into an area often called *optic flow*).

Figure 5.2A shows a moving observer (e.g., an observer in a railway train or a car) who briefly fixates some fixed object (F) while looking at right angles to the direction of self-motion. The sketch shows why retinal images of objects closer than F will move in the direction opposite to retinal images of objects more distant than F.

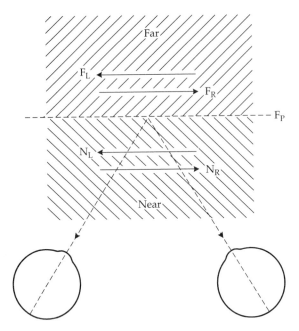

5.17 Hypothetical disparity coding of motion channels into "near" and "far" pools. Channels for unidirectional motion are segregated on the basis of crossed and uncrossed disparities. After Regan and Beverley (1973).

The organization depicted in Figure 5.17 would provide an initial processing of retinal image information that would allow the relative distances of objects to be recovered from dynamic information in their retinal images.*

Psychophysical evidence that motion-sensitive mechanisms are segregated with respect to relative disparity

When the left and right eyes view identical patterns in binocular fusion, and the two patterns are caused to oscillate sinusoidally from side to side at the same frequency, the resulting percept depends on the temporal phase difference between the two oscillations. When the phase difference is zero, the binocularly fused target appears to move entirely within a frontoparallel plane. When the phase difference is 180 degrees, the target appears to move back and forth in depth along a line passing between the eyes. When the phase difference is 45 degrees, the tar-

---

* Single cells in the visual cortex of monkey have been reported that respond preferentially to the kind of stimulus depicted in Figure 5.2B. (Roy et al., 1992).

get appears to follow an elliptical orbit in depth. The sense of the rotation round this orbit is that the target appears to be moving from left to right when it is perceived to be nearest to the eyes (largest crossed disparity) and from right to left when it is perceived to be furthest from the eyes (largest uncrossed disparity). When the phase difference is 315 degrees, the target appears to follow the same orbit in depth as for a 45 degree phase difference, but in the opposite direction.

In an experiment using the temporal phase manipulations just described, both eyes viewed identical random-dot patterns, each of which subtended 5 × 5 degrees, and each of which had a circular hole of diameter 2 degrees at its center. Immediately behind the holes were two identical random-dot patterns that were considerably larger than the holes and that could be oscillated from side to side with the same frequency but with any desired relative phase or relative amplitude. When the relative temporal phase was 45 degrees or 315 degrees, the central dot-covered area of the pattern bodily appeared to follow an elliptical orbit in depth.

When we adapted to one direction of rotation in depth, visual sensitivity was depressed for test stimuli with the same direction of rotation, but for test stimuli with the opposite direction of rotation, visual sensitivity was either unaffected or increased (Regan & Beverley, 1973b).

We concluded that mechanisms sensitive to the direction of motion within a frontoparallel plane are selectively sensitive not only to the direction of motion (as was already well known), but also to the disparity of the particular frontoparallel plane. This hypothesis is illustrated in Figure 5.17.

Further evidence for the hypothesis illustrated in Figure 5.17 was provided by Anstis and Harris (1974), who reported movement aftereffects contingent on binocular disparity. Findings reported by Fox et al. (1982), Webster et al. (1988), and Verstraten et al. (1994) can also be explained in terms of this hypothesis.

The hypothesis illustrated in Figure 5.17 leads to the following questions:

1. Is visual sensitivity to the relation between two MD targets different when they are both located within the same fronto-parallel plane compared with the case when one is located at a near disparity and the other at a far disparity? For example, is the just-noticeable difference in the separation between two bars along a line parallel to the frontal plane different in the two conditions?
2. Suppose that we superimpose two sheets of sparse random dots and that one sheet has a near disparity and the other sheet has a far disparity. Now to each sheet we add many additional random dots with randomly selected disparities so that the perceived distinction between the two planes is severely degraded. Now move the original sparse sheets of dots in opposite directions. Does the ordered motion information facilitate the degraded disparity information?

A study that may relate to item (2) was reported by von Grünau et al. (1993).

Experimental comparison of the effectiveness of motion parallax and binocular disparity as stimuli for the perception of spatial structure in the depth dimension

In a series of studies, Rogers and Graham compared motion parallax and binocular disparity as stimuli for producing the perception of relative depth. Their optical arrangement was similar to that depicted in Figure 5.10. They manipulated motion parallax by presenting one display screen to the observer's left eye and a different display screen to the right eye. Both screens were covered with random dots. When there was no relative motion between the observer's head and the display screen, the identical random-dot patterns on the two screens appeared to lie on a flat sheet when viewed in binocular fusion (see pp. 310–312).

Rogers and Graham first compared the effects of motion parallax produced by motion of the observer with the effects of motion parallax produced by motion of the stimulus display. The perceptions of relative depth (depth corrugations across a pattern of random dots) were similar in the two cases. This experiment showed that relative motion was the crucial variable, and the motion of the observer's head is not necessary (Rogers & Graham, 1979).

In a later study, Rogers and Graham (1982) replicated Tyler's contrast sensitivity curve for DD gratings shown as Figure 6.6, and they went on to show that the contrast sensitivity curve for depth corrugations produced by motion parallax had a similar shape to that shown in Figure 6.6 (see also Graham & Rogers, 1982).

Disordered Processing of Motion-Defined Form in Patients

The psychophysical procedures used to investigate the processing of MD form in the basic research studies just described are not convenient for studies on patients or even on large populations of control observers; they are lengthy and require complex equipment and considerable observer cooperation. These were the reasons for developing a simple test for assessing visual acuity and sensitivity to MD form along the lines of the familiar Snellen letter reading test (Regan & Hong, 1990). To a normally sighted observer, a letter "Z" is clearly evident in the display shown in Figure 5.3E. Such an observer sees the letter through the part of the visual system sensitive to relative motion.

The MD letter test procedure is as follows. Ten different letters are presented in random order, each of which is paired with a reference presentation that does not contain a letter, because all dots move in the same direction. The reference and the letter presentation are in random order. The observer is instructed to signal whether the letter was presented first or second (detection task) and which letter was presented (recognition task). The 10 letters are presented in random order, first at the fastest available speed, then at the second fastest speed, and so on. Speed thresholds for detection and for recognition are estimated from plots of percent correct detections and percent correct recognitions versus dot speed.

A substantial proportion of patients with multiple sclerosis show elevated thresholds for recognizing MD letters. Some patients cannot read MD letters even when motion contrast is so high that, in control subjects, letter visibility is not improved by further increases in speed. These patients are effectively blind to MD letters. The following conclusions have been drawn from studies on patients with multiple sclerosis (Regan et al., 1991; Giaschi et al., 1992).

1. Because the failure to read MD letters spared the ability to read LD letters, patients had not experienced a general loss of shape recognition.
2. Because the ability to read luminance-defined (LD) letters of low as well as high contrast was spared, the processing of MD and LD shape is mediated by different neural mechanisms.
3. The hypothesis that motion information is processed hierarchically is supported by the following three findings: some patients failed to read MD letters but detected them normally; other patients failed to both detect and read MD letters; both types of patients had normal thresholds for detecting dot motion. The hierarchical hypothesis is further supported by the findings that manipulating either presentation duration or dot lifetime dissociated the detection of MD form from orientation discrimination for MD form (Regan & Hamstra, 1992b).

Because multiple sclerosis is associated with the presence of multiple, widely distributed plaques in white matter, we were left with the following questions: Could the selective pattern of loss just described be caused by a single, discrete, white matter lesion? If so, does the lesion have some unique cerebral location and extent?

These questions were addressed by a study on 13 patients with a unilateral cerebral hemispheric lesion following neurosurgery (Regan et al., 1992b). Visual acuity was excellent for all patients (between 6/6 and 6/3). Speed thresholds for recognizing MD letters were abnormal in seven patients, all of whom retained normal ability to detect the presence and direction of dot motion. The lesion was located in the left hemisphere for three of the seven patients, and in the right hemisphere for the other four, but for clarity all are represented in the same hemisphere in Figure 5.18. Figure 5.18A–F illustrates that all seven patients had extensive lesions in parieto-temporal *white matter* underlying Broadman cortical areas 18, 19, 37, 39, 21, and 22. The black areas indicated by arrows in B and C are the regions of overlap of five lesions. Four of the seven patients failed to recognize MD letters, but the ability to detect them was spared, while the other three failed to either recognize or detect.

The ability to read MD letters was normal in the remaining six patients, and in none of the six did the lesion extend into the area of overlap shown in Figure 5.18. This study added the following conclusion to the three listed above.

4. A specific loss of ability to detect and/or recognize MD form was produced by lesions that involved the cerebral region (indicated by hatching in Figure 5.18), but not by lesions outside that region.

It has been proposed that, *in monkeys*, a predominantly M-stream (magnocellular) pathway that passes through cortical area V1 and then through cortical areas MT and MST to cortical area 7a is important for the perception of motion, while a predominantly P-stream (parvocellular) pathway that passes into the temporal lobe through cortical areas V1 and V4 is important for the perception of color and form (Van Essen & Maunsell, 1983; Desimone et al., 1985; Van Essen, 1985; Maunsell & Newsome, 1987; De Yeo & Van Essen, 1988; Merigan & Maunsell, 1990; Merigan et al., 1991a,b) There are several analogies between this hypothesis, based on monkey neurophysiology, and the hypothesis that the *human visual pathway* contains two parallel pathways passing through striate cortex, one of which (the dorsal pathway) processes the "where" while the other (the ventral pathway) processes the "what" of stimulus attributes (Ungerleider & Mishkin, 1982).

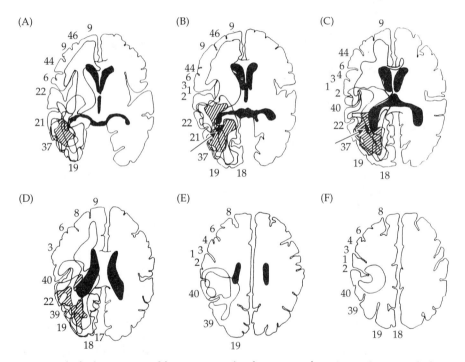

5.18 Brain lesions mapped by computerized tomography. The outlines mark the lesion boundaries delineated by CT in seven patients with unilateral cerebral hemisphere damage who had abnormal speed thresholds for recognizing motion-defined letters. Lesions are plotted onto six templates of axial brain anatomy. The templates represent slices approximately 8 mm apart, oriented 15 degrees above the orbito-meatal line. Ventricles are marked in black. Brodmann numbers of adjacent cortical areas are marked. For explanatory purposes all lesions are plotted onto one hemisphere. The black areas indicated by arrows in B and C indicate overlap between lesions in five patients. From Regan et al. (1992b).

How to reconcile our findings on brain-damaged patients with the monkey-based M-stream and P-stream dichotomy? The problem is that neurons sensitive to oppositely directed motion are required to extract MD form, and such neurons are not found before area MT. This is far along the so-called motion pathway, and long after the branching off of the so-called form/color pathway. Our proposal was as follows (Regan et al., 1992b, p. 2208):

> One way of linking our present findings to animal evidence for the parallel processing of motion and form rests on the evidence that there are many interconnections between cortical areas in the so-called motion and form pathways, some of which descend from prestriate areas in the motion pathway to striate cortex (Desimone et al., 1985; Van Essen, 1985; Van Essen et al., 1990). In particular, we suggest that interconnections between the two pathways may be important for the detection and recognition of MD form. In all seven patients who lost ability to recognize MD letters, the responsible lesions involved white matter and may have interrupted connections between the homologs of areas in the MT/MST/7a pathway and of areas in the V1/V4/IT pathway.

As well, the lesions may have interrupted connections descending from homologs MST/MT to V1.

> However, these suggestions can only be tentative, because part of the animal evidence is lacking.The monkey data just cited is restricted to neural properties in areas of monkey visual CORTEX, and with the interconnections between cortical areas. It is known, however, that at least 20 subcortical structures project directly to visual cortex and that in some cases (e.g., the connections between claustrum and cortex) the connections are reciprocal and organized in a precise point-to-point fashion, thus preserving the retinotopic projection (Tigges & Tigges, 1985; Sherk, 1986). In view of these facts it seems unlikely that a complete understanding of the relation between structure and function in primate visual pathway will be achieved without taking into account the reciprocal interconnections between cortex and subcortical structures. In particular, the (at least) nine visual areas and the (at least) 20 subcortical structures constitute a distributed system, whose system properties presumably underlie visual perception (Mountcastle, 1979). . . . The relevance of this point is that, with the possible exception of the interconnections between cortex and the LGN and superior colliculus, our current knowledge of the role of cortical-subcortical visual connections in visual perception is sparse (Regan et al., 1992b, p. 2208).

See pp. 26–30 and Appendix A for further discussion of the relation between structure and function.

Psychophysical Models of the Processing of Motion-Defined Form: Local Signals and Distant Comparisons

Detection of local motion

The hypothetical Reichardt detector is a local-motion detector that prefers a particular direction of motion (Reichardt, 1961, 1986). The basic idea is that the visual pathway compares the signals that arise from different points on the retina after delaying one of the signals.

The operation of a Reichardt detector can be simulated by electronic hardware as illustrated in Figure 5.19. Suppose two electronic photocells (P) separated by distance Δx, are connected to a comparator (e.g., a multiplier), and that the signal from the left photocell is subjected to a delay of τ seconds. The comparator will give a strong output when the signals arriving from the two photocells are identical at every instant. This situation is achieved when, for example, a spatial noise pattern is moving over the photocells from left to right at the particular speed that causes it to reach the first photocell exactly τ seconds before it reaches the second photocell.* This speed is equal to $(\Delta x / \tau)$. Spatial noise patterns moving faster or slower will generate a lower running-average output from the comparator, and spatial noise patterns moving in the opposite direction will produce no running average output at all. A complete Reichardt detector comprises a section for rightward motion (Figure 5.19) plus a mirror-image section for leftward motion.

The detector's output is the difference between the running-average outputs of the two sections.

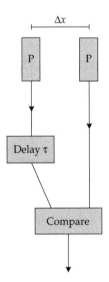

5.19 The "delay and compare" principle of a Reichardt motion detector. The rightwards-motion subunit only is shown.

---

* The autocorrelation function of the pattern must obey certain restrictions discussed on p. 428.

As originally described, the two input receptive fields of a Reichardt detector were essentially point receptive fields. Consequently, although the original detector provided a good description of motion processing in the compound eye of the fly (as was intended by Reichardt), it provided a poor description of motion processing in humans (not included in Reichardt's original aim). The original Reichardt detector suffered from aliasing in that a change in the spatial frequency of a moving grating could cause it to signal a change in the direction of motion, even though the grating's direction of motion remained constant. This aliasing effect is not observed in human vision. In their so-called *elaborated Reichardt detector*, Van Santen and Sperling (1984, 1985) avoided this aliasing problem by replacing the point receptive fields by bandpass spatial-frequency filters (see Figures 2.1 and 2.12), and by appropriately controlling the temporal phase shifts within the model (see p. 428). Models that are applicable to more general kinds of velocity field have also been proposed (Reichardt & Schlögl, 1988; Reichardt et al., 1988; Zhang, 1995).

Turning from theory to experiment, evidence that the human visual system contains mechanisms that are selective for the direction of motion was reported by Levinson and Sekuler (1980). They found that adapting to a pattern of random dots moving uniformly in one direction elevated the luminance-detection threshold for patterns of uniformly moving test dots; that the threshold elevation was largest when the test and adapting directions were the same; and that the threshold elevation was zero when test and adapting directions of motion were opposite. The half-width of the directional tuning curve was between 40 and 60 degrees.

In a subsequent study, Williams et al. (1991) ingeniously exploited the concept of metamerism (see first paragraph of the footnote starting on page 214). Their motion stimuli were random dot patterns in which each dot took an independent two-dimensional random walk of constant step size. The direction in which any given dot moved between successive frames was independent of its previous moves and independent of the directions of motion of other dots. For any stimulus, the set of directions in which all dots moved was chosen from the same probability distribution, which could be either a *uniform* distribution or a *multimodal* distribution. With the uniform distribution, the spectrum of directions was virtually continuous, but with the multimodal distribution, only a few discrete directions of dot motion were allowed. Williams et al. found that a range of uniformly distributed directions that covered 180 degrees out of 270 could be matched by a dot pattern that contained only 6 to 10 discrete directions of motion. The two patterns of motion looked alike. They concluded that "the outputs of 12 direction-selective mechanisms, each with a half-bandwidth of 30 deg, are combined nonlinearly to produce the percept of motion" (Williams et al., 1991, p. 275).

And Stromeyer and his colleagues have reported evidence that the direction-selective motion channels are based on opponent-movement processing (Stromeyer et al., 1984; Zemany et al., 1998).

Experimentally measured receptive field size for motion detector units in humans ranges from 2 minutes of arc at high spatial frequencies (30 cycles/deg.) to 7 degrees at low spatial frequencies (0.01 cycles/deg.) (Anderson and Burr [1985, 1987]); but see Fredericksen et al.[1997] for caveats).

Processing of motion-defined form by comparing the local velocities in two separate regions I:
Boundaries defined by compressive/expansive motion

Next I discuss how the visual system might detect the two kinds of MD boundary illustrated in Figure 5.4A–C. First I shall discuss the early visual processing of a boundary that is rendered visible by a difference of the component of velocity perpendicular to the boundary (e.g., Figure 5.4C).

We proposed that the human visual pathway contains compressive/expansive relative-motion filters ($RM_{C,E}$ in Figure 5.20A). Each relative-motion filter receives inputs from local-motion filters (LM in Figure 5.20A) that signal the component of the local velocity of light/dark (or dark/light) contours resolved along a line passing through the centers of their receptive fields (Regan & Beverley, 1978a, 1980; Beverley & Regan, 1979a; see also Morrone et al., 1995).*

The kind of relative-motion filter illustrated in Figure 5.20A was originally hypothesized to explain the early processing of retinal image expansion (Regan & Beverley, 1978a; Beverley & Regan, 1979a). The crucial finding was that, after adapting to oscillation in the width of a bright, solid, untextured bar, threshold for detecting oscillations of the width of a subsequently presented test bar were raised considerably, but a constant-width bar that oscillated from side to side produced essentially no such threshold elevation *even though the movements of any given edge were identical for the two adapting bars.*

The effect transferred from a bright adapting bar on a dark background to a dark test bar on a bright background. Results were similar when the changes in width were repetitive unidirectional ramps rather than sinusoidal oscillations.

I consider next the spatial spread of the changing-size aftereffect. The difference between the threshold elevations for the two kinds of test target ("TED") fell as the test bar's width was increased. Threshold elevation difference ("TED") was localized to the region near the adapting bar's edges, falling off according to the decay equation

$$(\text{TED})_x = (\text{TED})_{x=0} \exp(-x/L) \tag{5.2}$$

---

* Evidence for a distinction between the $RM_{C,E}$ relative-motion filters and the motion-in-depth (MID) stage included the following finding. After adapting to a rectangle whose height remained constant but whose vertical edges repetitively ramped towards each other, observers noted that a subsequently viewed, static rectangle appeared to be expanding. This changing-size aftereffect died away, whereupon the test rectangle appeared to move in depth. The decay of both aftereffects followed an exponential time course. The decay time constant (in seconds) for the changing-size and motion-in-depth aftereffects, respectively, for four observers were as follows: 9.5, 54; 7.5, 24; 6.4, 34; 8.1, 30 (Regan & Beverley, 1979c).

(A)

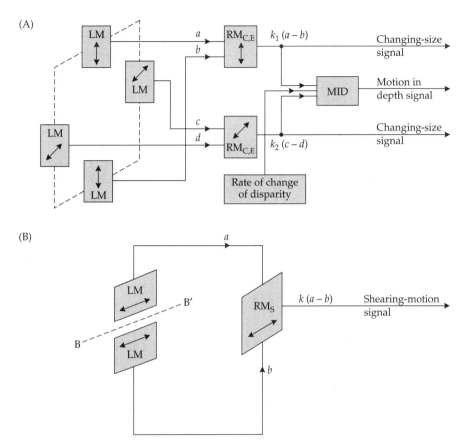

(B)

5.20 Hypothetical relative-motion detectors. (A) Expansion or contraction of an object's retinal image (dotted) excites local-motion detectors (LM) whose outputs are subtracted by relative-motion detectors (RM$_{C,E}$) sensitive to compressive/expansive motion. These relative-motion detectors generate a changing-size signal and in addition feed a motion-in-depth stage (MID) that generates a motion-in-depth signal whose amplitude is inversely proportional to time to collision. The motion-in-depth signal is optimal if $k_1(a - b) = k_2(c - d)$, where k_1 and k_2 are, respectively, inversely proportional to the instantaneous height and width of the retinal image. (B) The velocity component of moving texture elements parallel to the boundary BB' excites local-motion detectors (LM) whose outputs are subtracted by a relative-motion detector (RM$_S$) sensitive to shearing motion. Part A after Beverley and Regan (1979a). See also Regan and Hamstra (1993).

where (TED)$_x$ and (TED)$_{x = 0}$ were, respectively, the threshold elevation differences for test bars whose widths differed from the width of the adapting bar by x degrees and zero degrees. The distance constant L was 1.2 degrees for test bars wider than the adapting bar (Beverley & Regan, 1979b).

Figure 5.21 shows that the aftereffect specific to changing-size (TED) was evident only for a bar whose width was less than about 1.5 degrees.

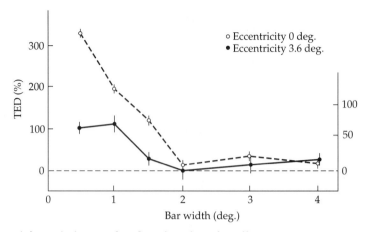

5.21 Spatial restriction on the changing-size aftereffect. The observer adapted to
a bar whose opposite edges oscillated in antiphase with a peak-to-peak amplitude of
0.1 degrees. The test bar's width was the same as the adapting bar's, and its opposite
edges oscillated either in antiphase or in-phase. (Antiphase oscillations caused the
bar's width to vary while it remained constant in position. In-phase oscillation
caused the test bar to move from side to side while its width remained constant.)
Ordinates are "threshold elevation differences" (TEDs) defined as the threshold elevation for an antiphase test bar minus the threshold elevation for an in-phase test bar.
The width of the bar is plotted as abscissa. After Beverley and Regan (1979b).

Subsequent studies showed that the hypothetical relative-motion filter operates by subtracting the velocities of the two edges, and is essentially blind to any
common component of the velocities of the edges, so that when stimulated by an
object moving along an arbitrary direction of motion in depth, it selectively
extracts the retinal image correlate of the velocity component directed along a
line passing through the observing eye (Regan & Beverley, 1980).*

* There is some asymmetry between the mechanism sensitive to expansion and the mechanism sensitive to contraction. Although the motion-in-depth aftereffects caused by adapting to expansion and by adapting to contraction both obeyed the equation $V_N = kV_A^n$, the
value of k was larger after adapting to expansion than after adapting to contraction,
although n was approximately 1.0 in both cases. (V_N was the edge speed of the test rectangle required to null the motion-in-depth aftereffect, V_A was the adapting edge speed, and k
and n were constants [Regan & Beverley, 1978b].) Takeuchi (1997) offers a review of recent
work on distinctions between the visual processing of expansion and contraction, and
reported the following: (1) visual search for expanding targets among distracters is a parallel process; (2) there is a search-speed asymmetry between expansion and contraction;
(3) two-dimensional expansion/contraction is found faster than one-dimensional expan-
sion/contraction.

There is evidence that relative-motion filters that prefer orthogonal directions of motion are combined so as to extract a rough physiological equivalent of div **V**, the local *divergence* in the velocity field of moving texture elements; see Appendix I (Regan & Beverley, 1978a, 1979b, 1982; Regan et al., 1986). I mention this point because the local value of div **V** is zero over the entire velocity field shown in Figure 5.4C except for the boundary BB'. For the compressive motion shown, div **V** would assume a large negative magnitude along the exact location of the boundary; if the direction of vectors V_1 and V_2 were reversed, div **V** would assume a large positive magnitude along the exact location of the boundary BB'.

I suggested that, because of its sensitivity to div **V**, the two-dimensional changing-size filter ("looming detector") proposed by Regan and Beverley (1978a) plays a role in detecting compressive/expansive MD boundaries (Regan, 1986b).

It has also been suggested that the one-dimensional relative-motion filters ($RM_{C,E}$) sketched out in Figure 5.20A also play a role in detecting MD boundaries defined by compressive/expansive motion such as, for example, boundary BB' in Figure 5.4C and the component of motion contrast at right angles to BB' in Figure 5.4A.

Processing of motion-defined form by comparing the local velocities in two separate regions II: Boundaries defined by shearing motion

Next we consider the early visual processing of a boundary that is rendered visible by a difference across the boundary of the component of velocity parallel to the boundary (e.g., Figure 5.4B). The relative-motion filter RM_S depicted in Figure 5.20B differs from the kind of relative-motion filter depicted in Figure 5.20A in that the two local motion filters that feed an RM_S filter are fed from different locations along a line perpendicular to their common preferred direction of motion rather than a line parallel to their preferred direction of motion, as is the case for the $RM_{C,E}$ filter. Consequently, the RM_S filter detects a boundary defined by shearing motion (dashed line in Figure 5.20B), whereas the $RM_{C,E}$ filter detects a boundary defined by compressive/expansive motion.

Resolution of a relative velocity vector into orthogonal components by the two kinds of relative-motion filter

Reichardt detectors (elaborated or otherwise) respond best to motion along a particular direction (or in the opposite direction) but give no response to motion at right angles to that direction. Therefore, if the local-motion detectors that feed the $RM_{C,E}$ and RM_S relative-motion filters in Figure 5.20(A,B) are Reichardt detectors, the $RM_{C,E}$ and RM_S relative-motion filters driven from any given small region of the visual field will achieve a rough physiological equivalent of the mathematical process of resolving the relative velocity vector into orthogonal components, a process that retains complete information about the magnitude and direction of the original vector. For example, if an $RM_{C,E}$ filter receives inputs from local motion filters fed from two retinal locations on opposite sides of boundary BB' in Figure 5.4A and an RM_S filter receives the same two inputs, then the outputs of the two relative motion filters will, respectively, signal compressive/expansive relative motion ($V_2\cos\theta_2 - V_1\cos\theta_1$) and shearing relative motion ($V_1\sin\theta_1 - V_2\sin\theta_2$) across boundary BB' in Figure 5.4A.

Processing of motion-defined form on the basis of local signals

As mentioned earlier, the kind of hypothetical relative-motion filter just discussed falls into the general class that compares motion signals from two local regions some distance apart. But just as was the case of modeling the processing of LD form discussed on pp. 140–171, the processing of MD form can be modeled in terms of signals from a single region of the visual field.

The convexity cell. As described next, it is possible to build an orientation- and size-tuned filter for MD form whose receptive field has a spatially opponent organization analogous to the organization of the receptive field illustrated in Figure 2.1. In principle, such a filter could detect objects on the basis of motion parallax. It could detect MD objects that match its size preference (by means of the regional binding principle), or, alternatively, act as a boundary detector for sharp-edged MD objects that are much larger than its preferred size.

The circularly symmetric receptive field of the hypothetical convexity cell of Nakayama and Loomis (1974), illustrated in Figure 5.22, has the following double-opponent organization. The center of the receptive field (dashed circles in parts A and B) and the surround of the receptive field receive inputs from local-motion detectors, all of which respond most strongly to motion along the same direction. But their inputs to the receptive field center excite the cell, whereas their inputs to the surround inhibit the cell. Consequently, the pattern of texture-element motion indicated by the arrows in Figure 5.22A produces the convexity cell's weakest response, whereas the pattern of motion shown in Figure 5.22B causes the convexity cell to respond most strongly.*

As mentioned earlier, a Reichardt detector does not respond to motion perpendicular to its preferred direction of motion. Consequently, if the local-motion filters that feed a convexity cell are Reichardt detectors, then two superimposed convexity cells that are fed by local-motion filters that prefer orthogonal directions of motion will perform a rough physiological equivalent of the mathematical operation of resolving a velocity vector of arbitrary magnitude and direction into its orthogonal components (see Figure 5.4A).

---

* The receptive field of a *"higher convexity cell"* is created by summing the outputs of several convexity cells, all of which are driven from the same visual field location but prefer different directions of motion round the clock (Nakayama & Loomis, 1974). Double-opponent neurons with the velocity-opponent and spatially opponent properties of the hypothetical higher convexity cell have been found in the visual pathways of both primates and non-primates (Frost et al., 1981; Frost & Nakayama, 1983; von Grünau & Frost, 1983; Allman et al., 1985). In humans there is psychophysical evidence for detectors sensitive to differential motion within a small (< 1.0 deg.) region of the visual field (Regan & Beverley, 1978a, 1979b, 1980; Beverley & Regan, 1979b, 1980a; Murakami & Shimojo, 1996).

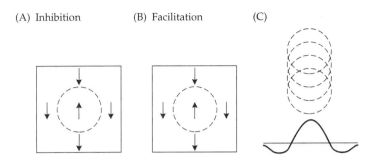

5.22 Functional model of an orientation- and frequency-tuned spatial filter for motion-defined form. (A, B) The double-opponent receptive field consists of an excitatory center (shown by the dashed circle) with an inhibitory surround. The preferred direction of motion within the excitatory part of the receptive field is arrowed. (C) If, as illustrated, the receptive field is circularly symmetric, an elongated spatial filter can be built by summing the outputs of many such receptive fields whose field centers fall along a straight line so as to give a receptive field whose velocity sensitivity profile is shown by the continuous line.

As originally described by Nakayama and Loomis, the convexity cell had concentric receptive field organization depicted in Figure 5.22A,B and, therefore, is insufficient to account for the finding that observers can discriminate the orientation of an MD bar, and still less that orientation discrimination threshold is as low as 0.5 degrees (Figure 5.13A). One approach to this problem would be to propose that at least some convexity cells have elongated receptive fields; another approach would be to propose that the outputs of several similarly organized convexity cells that are served from different locations along a straight line across the visual field (dashed circles in Figure 5.22C) are summed, so as to create a filter for MD form that is selective for orientation and has a velocity tuning profile similar to the profile depicted by the continuous line in Figure 5.22C.

A spatial filter for MD form of this kind would respond to an MD bar-as-a-whole that was positioned directly over the excitatory region of its receptive fields (as indeed would a convexity cell with an elongated receptive field). The response would be strongest when: (a) the bar's width and orientation matched the excitatory receptive field; and (b) the texture elements whose motion renders the bar visible move at equal speeds but in opposite directions along the preferred line of motion inside and outside the bar. If we assume that the filter profile has inhibitory flanks, the flat low-frequency segment of Figure 5.7 would indicate that there are filters that prefer spatial frequencies of 0.2 cycles/deg. and lower.

Encoding the location of a motion-defined boundary and edge sharpening. It is an apparent paradox that, although receptive field size for detecting MD form is large (> 0.4 deg., see pp. 306–307), the edges of suprathreshold MD target appear to be sharp, far sharper than the mean distance between the moving texture elements (Regan & Beverley, 1984), and both Vernier acuity and aspect-ratio acuities for MD form are very fine. A proposed explanation for this observation can be understood as follows. I will first discuss the processing of an MD boundary that is defined by shearing motion before going on to a boundary that is defined by compressive/expansive motion.

Figure 5.23A shows a hypothetical elongated receptive field. When stimulated by an area of texture elements that is considerably larger than the entire receptive field and that is moving at the same speed along the direction preferred by the field center (vertically upwards in this case), the field center provides an excitatory signal and the surround provides an equal and opposite signal: thus, the net output is zero.

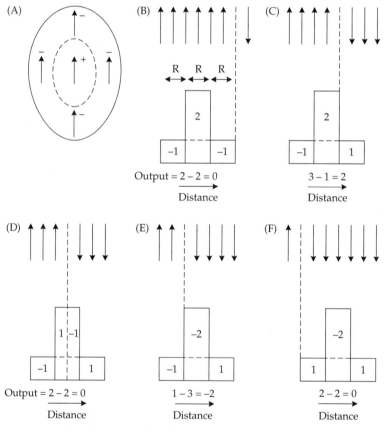

5.23 How a Mexican-hat receptive field for motion-defined form responds to a boundary defined by shearing motion. (A) Elongated double-opponent receptive field. (B–F) Effect of the location of the motion-defined boundary (vertical dashed lines) on the output of the detector. For ease of explanation the Mexican-hat profile of the receptive field is squared off.

For ease of explanation, in Figure 5.23B–F, I have depicted the profile of this receptive field as a square-edged "Mexican hat." Figure 5.23B–F explains how to predict responses of this receptive field to a sharply defined boundary that is created by equal and opposite dot speeds (as, for example, the MD target in Figures 5.3E, 5.13 and 5.14). In arbitrary units, the output of the Mexican-hat receptive field is zero when the receptive field is located entirely to the left of the boundary (Figure 5.23B), +2 when the velocity discontinuity (i.e., the MD boundary) is located along the dashed line in part C, zero when the boundary bisects the receptive field (part D), –2 when the boundary is located along the dashed line in part E, and zero when the entire receptive field is to the right of the boundary (part F). A receptive field whose center prefers motion directed vertically downwards will give a mirror-image pattern of responses to that depicted in Figure 5.23B–F. Thus, the pattern of activity among a parallel array of such filters will represent the location of a motion-defined boundary with considerably greater accuracy than the width of any given receptive field. *Here I assume that the output of any given filter carries a "location" label.*

When a receptive field organized along the lines depicted in Figure 5.24A is stimulated by a boundary of the kind shown in Figure 5.24B, the predicted response is also as illustrated in Figure 5.23B–F.

Encoding the width and location of a motion-defined bar. Figure 5.25A,B depicts MD bars of width Δx that are defined by shearing motion and by expansive/compressive motion, respectively. Figure 5.25C,D shows the predicted response patterns of a parallel array of Mexican-hat filters of the kind depicted in Figure 5.23B–F when stimulated by the bar depicted in Figure 5.25A. The response pattern shown in Figure 5.25C is for filters whose width is matched to

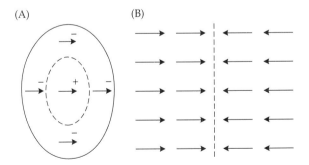

5.24 How a Mexican-hat receptive field for motion-defined form responds to a boundary defined by compressive/expansive motion. (A) Elongated double-opponent receptive field. (B) The dashed lines mark a motion-defined boundary defined entirely by compressive/expansive motion contrast. The location of the boundary has the same effect as that depicted in Figure 5.23B–F.

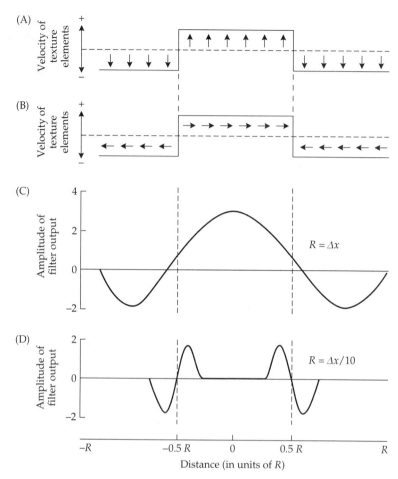

5.25 The response of a parallel array of local relative-motion filters to a motion-defined bar. (A, B) Velocity cross-sections of bars defined by motion contrast (shearing motion contrast in part A and compressive/expansive motion contrast in part B). Bar width is Δx. (C, D) The pattern of outputs within a parallel array of filters (wide filters in part C and narrow filters in part D).

the bar width. In particular, the width (R) of the central excitatory region is equal to Δx, the width of the bar. These filters respond to the bar as a whole.

If the output of any given filter carries a *position label*, the pattern of activity shown in Figure 5.25C will represent both the location and the width of the bar. And if any given filter also carries a *width label*, additional information about the width of the bar will be represented in the pattern of excitation among filters of different widths that are driven from one location. A relevant discussion of these issues is to be found on pp. 144–151.

The response pattern shown in Figure 5.25D is for a parallel array of filters whose width is considerably narrower than the width of the bar. In particular, R = (bar width)/10. These filters respond to the edges of the bar rather than to the bar as a whole, and the polarity of an edge is signaled by the positive–negative versus negative–positive spatial ordering of the output peaks.

When a parallel array of the kind of receptive fields illustrated in Figure 5.24A is stimulated by the kind of bar depicted in Figure 5.25B, the predicted responses are exactly as shown in Figure 5.25C,D.

> The location of the MD edge is represented within the pattern of activity shown in Figure 5.25D with a precision far higher than the width ($3R$, see Figure 5.23B) of any individual filter. In particular, the precision with which the boundary can be located depends on both the noise level of the filters and their width ($3R$ in Figure 5.23B). We suggested that this could explain the perceived sharpness of MD edges (Regan & Beverley, 1984; Regan, 1986,a, b)

It is not known whether the visual pathway contains *coincidence detectors* for boundaries defined by shearing motion. Figure 5.26A,B illustrates how detectors of this kind could, in principle, be created along the lines of Figure 2.53 by replacing the filters for LD form by filters for MD form.

For example, if two filters of $R = \Delta x/10$ that were separated by distance Δx were connected together to form a detector whose output carried a separation label, then, when the edges of the MD bar depicted in Figure 5.25A fell exactly on their centers, they would signal the width (Δx) of the bar as well as its presence. There is evidence that the visual pathway contains filters that, though not

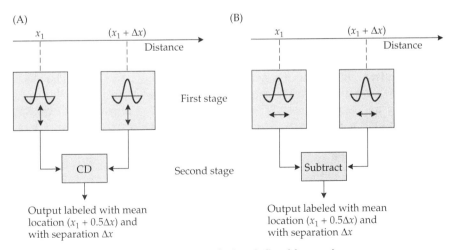

5.26 Hypothetical detectors for boundaries defined by motion contrast. (A) Detector for shearing motion contrast. (B) Detector for compressive /expansive motion contrast.

necessarily fulfilling the definition of a coincidence detector, are sensitive to compressive/expansive relative motion. These hypothetical entities are the *changing-size detectors* or *looming detectors* illustrated in Figure 5.20 and discussed on pp. 330–333 (Beverley & Regan, 1979a, 1980a; Regan & Beverley, 1978a, 1979a, 1980). Figure 5.26B illustrates this hypothesis. The two first-stage filters are double-opponent as in Figure 5.24A. The difference between Figure 5.26A and B is that the preferred direction of motion is perpendicular to separation Δx in Figure 5.26A and parallel to separation Δx in part B.

Beverley and Regan (1979b) provided estimates of the shapes of the receptive fields depicted in Figure 5.26B. The relation between the widths of the receptive fields and their separation Δx is much exaggerated in Figure 5.26B; experimentally, there seems to be considerable overlap.

Encoding the orientation of a motion-defined bar. For ease of explanation, the double-opponent receptive field in Figure 5.27A is shown as rectangular and I assume that its Mexican-hat velocity sensitivity profile is squared off as illustrated in Figure 5.23B–F. The MD bars depicted in Figure 5.27B,C are similar to the bars used to collect the orientation discrimination data shown in Figure 5.13A,B. The elongated receptive field shown in part A will be maximally excited when the bar shown in part B is centered on the receptive field, but will be unresponsive when the bar shown in part C is centered on the receptive field. Similarly, the elongated receptive field shown in part D will be maximally excited when the MD bar shown in part E is centered on the receptive field, but will be unresponsive when the bar shown in part F is centered on the receptive field.

To account for the very low orientation discrimination thresholds shown in Figure 5.13A,B, I suggested that the human visual pathway contains orientation-tuned mechanisms that respond to MD form, and that orientation discrimination threshold is determined by the pattern of activity within a population of such mechanisms (Regan, 1989b).

A hypothetical detector for a rate of change of size of an object's retinal image. An alternative possible explanation for the kind of data shown in Figure 5.21 is that the threshold elevations for detecting size changes result, not from adapting a mechanism that receives velocity signals from two regions within the visual field, but from adapting a mechanism that receives input from only one region of the visual field. We have already encountered this dichotomy between local signals and distant comparisons in the context of modeling the early processing of LD form. This alternative proposal can be stated as follows: The aftereffect is caused by adapting a processing stage that is sensitive to a unidirectional rate of change of spatial frequency.

Figure 5.28A is a schematic of how, by analogy with Reichardt's motion detector, sensitivity to a rate of change of retinal image size could be created from the outputs of spatial filters fed from the same location. If, for example, the output of the narrower filter is delayed by τ seconds, the multiplier will give a stronger

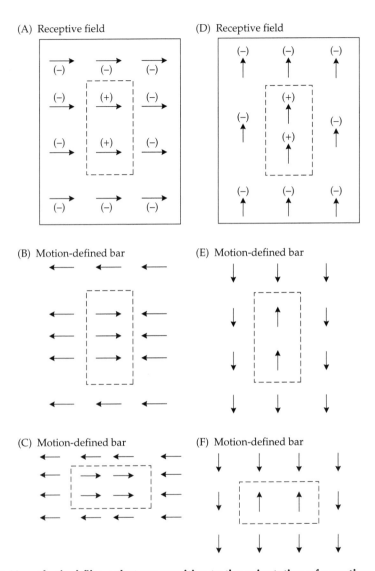

5.27 Hypothetical filters that are sensitive to the orientation of a motion-defined bar. (A, D) Receptive fields of hypothetical filters. The preferred direction of motion of texture elements (arrowed) produces excitation when texture elements are within the receptive field center (dashed rectangle) and inhibition when they are within the surround. (B, C, E, F) Motion-defined bars similar to the bars used to obtain the orientation-discrimination data shown in Figure 5.13A, B.

output when the spatial frequency of the stimulus grating is decreasing than when it is increasing.

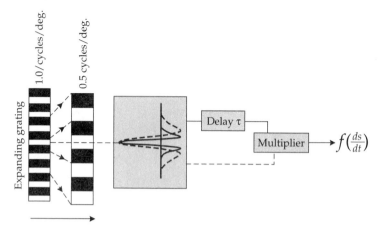

5.28 Hypothetical local filter sensitive to expansion or contraction of an object's retinal image. Two filters for luminance-defined form whose widths differ but are driven from the same retinal location feed a comparator (e.g., a multiplier). The output of the narrower filter is delayed before it reaches the comparator. If a bright bar within an expanding grating is centered on the filters, the output of the comparator will be some function of the rate of decrease of grating spatial frequency.

An experiment by Anstis and Rogers would seem to have rejected this candidate "local signal" explanation for the changing-size aftereffect. They created a grating by impressing a sinusoidal variation of dot luminance across a dynamic random-dot display. (A static random-dot pattern is a randomly scattered array of dots. A dynamic random-dot pattern is created by re-randomizing the pattern on each frame so that the observer sees twinkling dots rather like the display on a de-tuned television set.) When the magnification of the grating was zoomed upward, its spatial-frequency content zoomed downwards just as in Figure 5.28A.

Anstis and Rogers adapted to an expanding grating of this kind whose magnification was zoomed upwards from 1.0 cycles/deg. to some higher value, then abruptly returned to 1.0 cycles/deg., and the process repeated. The center of expansion of the grating stayed at the center of the display, as is the case in Figure 5.28A. After adapting to this stimulus for about 30 seconds, the spatial frequency of a subsequently presented test grating appeared to be shrinking even though the test spatial frequency was, in fact, constant at a little less than 1.0 cycle/deg. But Anstis and Rogers observed no such effect when they caused the location of the adapting grating's center of expansion to vary randomly in position along a direction at right angles to the bars of the grating. Because the spatial frequency power spectrum of the adapting grating zoomed downwards identically for the two adapting stimuli, Anstis and Rogers concluded that they had failed to find evidence for any mechanism that is sensitive to a rate of change of spatial frequency while being insensitive to spatial phase. They concluded that the changing-size aftereffect required the presence of smoothly moving LD contours (Anstis, 1997).

CHAPTER 6

Disparity-Defined Form

Preamble

Animals with eyes placed on opposite sides of the body enjoy the advantages of a wide field of view that encompasses almost the whole of the surrounding environment. Animals who have evolved front-facing eyes with extensive binocular overlap lose a large part of this advantage and are vulnerable to a stealthy attack from the rear. However, by creating binocular disparity, front-facing eyes provide a basis for stereoscopic vision.

When a three-dimensional object is viewed binocularly, the left and right eyes' retinal images are, geometrically, slightly different. This geometrical difference is called binocular disparity. But the binocular disparities created by an interocular separation of only a few cm (about 6 cm in humans) are very small, and to utilize them requires a formidable investment in neural machinery to control ocular vergence, and also to render disparity processing independent of the comparatively large variations of vergence angle associated with a moving head in everyday life (Steinman et al., 1985).

What survival advantages might be gained by exchanging for binocular depth perception both the security of near-panoramic vision, and the reduced neural demands of nonstereo vision, has long been a puzzle. One easily demonstrated advantage is a somewhat greater facility in judging the distances of nearby objects. A second advantage is that binocular information can be used to judge the trajectory of an approaching object and also its time of arrival (Beverley & Regan, 1975; Portfors-Yeomans & Regan, 1996; Gray & Regan, 1998b). This is especially useful when monocularly available information is either absent (e.g., for small objects, Gray & Regan, 1998b) or corrupted, as for nonrigid or rotating nonspherical objects (Gray & Regan, 1999b).

On the other hand, many individuals have defective binocular vision, and this seldom seems to cause handicap. For example, even the loss of one eye in adult life did not prevent Wiley Post from establishing solo aviation records (Mohler & Johnson, 1971). And one of the most striking things about stereoscopic depth perception is the large interindividual differences (Richards, 1971b; Russell, 1979; Julesz, 1971).

One suggestion, put forward by several authors including Julesz (1971), is as follows. As illustrated in Color Plates 1–6, many animal species who are subject to the attention of carnivorous predators have evolved a remarkable match of their reflectance, color, and texture to their everyday surroundings so that, by remaining still, they achieve almost perfect camouflage. "Almost perfect" camouflage, however, may not be enough when in the close proximity of a predator with binocular depth perception. Only those creatures whose three-dimensional shape closely matches their immediate surroundings (e.g., as shown in Color Plates 3 and 5) can have confidence that they will not be the victim of a predator with binocular depth perception.

Although, following Wheatstone (1838), the vivid depth created by a stereoviewer was commonly attributed to binocular disparity, the stereo line drawings that Wheatstone used contained monocular as well as binocular cues to depth, as do almost all stereo photographs. A demonstration that binocular disparity alone can create image segregation was not available until Julesz isolated neural processing that occurs after convergence of signals from the left and right eyes by creating computer-generated patterns that contain no monocular cues to the camouflaged form (Julesz 1960, 1971).

A Julesz static random-dot stereogram (RDS) consists of randomly located elements such as dots. One eye views such a pattern while the other eye views a second pattern that is identical to the first except that part of the pattern is shifted bodily to the left or right (Figures 5.15, 5.16, and 6.1). In monocular view the shifted area is not visible: each pattern looks like a flat array of random dots. In binocularly fused vision, however, normally sighted observers see the camouflaged form. Furthermore, the shifted area appears to be a different depth from the rest of the pattern. Because there are no monocular clues to either form or relative depth, the perception of the form and the relative depth of the shifted area can be attributed entirely to neural processing at and/or subsequent to the stage at which the left and right eyes' signals converge.* Many fine examples are to be

---

* The fact that a particular observer can see and recognize a cyclopean form indicates that the observer's visual pathway contains a binocularly driven neural mechanism but does not necessarily imply that the observer has a neural mechanism sensitive to disparity. This point can be demonstrated by viewing a cyclopean target generated by the red–green analglyph

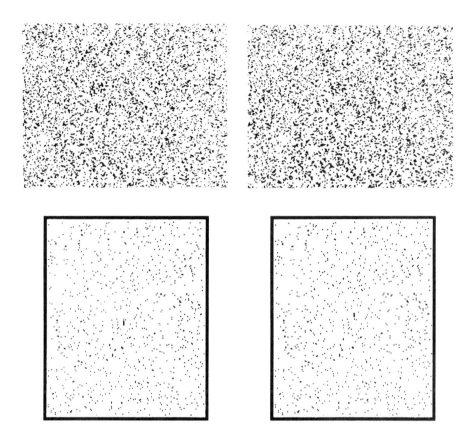

6.1 Illustrations of cyclopean forms. (Upper half) A cyclopean grating. View the stereogram from arm's length. Hold a pencil in front of the page at such a distance that with the left eye closed the point is at the center of the left dot pattern, and with the right eye closed the point is at the center of the right dot pattern. Now open both eyes and look at the pencil point. After a few moments you will see three rather than two dot patterns. The central dot pattern is binocularly fused and the camouflaged target will slowly emerge. The pencil can now be removed. (Note that sinusoidal cyclopean gratings are necessarily horizontal: a vertical grating has a monocular cue to spatial form. Sharp-edged [squarewave] cyclopean gratings, however, may have any orientation.) (Lower half) A sharp-edged cyclopean rectangle. Lower half from Regan and Hamstra (1994).

---

technique. First observe that a shape is seen in vivid depth and that the shape can be recognized, but when one eye is closed, the shape is no longer visible. Now remove the red–green goggles. The shape is immediately visible. The same point can be made by increasing the relative disparity of a cyclopean target to a point where the target can no longer be fused, then

found in Julesz's (1971) book. Figures 5.15 and 6.1 allow the reader to experience this so-called cyclopean depth perception.

A critical review of binocular vision and stereopsis is provided by Howard and Rogers (1995).

Corresponding Points, the Horopter, Relative Disparity, and the Correspondence Problem

In this section I discuss the geometrical theories of binocular single vision and of stereopsis. Under the headings *empirical horopter*, *psychophysics of absolute and relative disparity*, and *correspondence problem*, I discuss major problems in reconciling the facts of stereopsis and binocular vision with the geometrical theory of stereopsis and binocular vision.

The geometrical theory of stereopsis

Howard and Rogers (1995, pp. 4–24) provide a thorough overview of the history of the geometry of binocular vision from the time of the Greeks—many of whom, including Plato (c. 427–347 B.C.), Euclid (c. 300 B.C.) and Ptolemy (c. 150 A.D.) believed that the eyes radiate light—up to the modern random-dot stereogram.

Because the left and right eyes are about 6.5 cm apart, the left and right retinal images of a three-dimensional object are geometrically different. For example, the left eye sees more of the left side of a three-dimensional object than does the right eye, while the right eye sees more of the right side than does the left eye.

Imagine two idealized identical eyes, each with a fovea. Further, imagine that the two retinae are superimposed so that the foveae and horizontal meridians coincide. *Corresponding points* on the two retinae now coincide.

Veith (1818) and Müller (1826) used classical theorems of Euclid's geometry to show that object points that lie on a circle that cuts through both the fixation point and the second nodal point (p. 444) of each eye are imaged onto corresponding points (Howard & Rogers, 1995, pp. 17–18). This *Vieth–Müller circle* is called the *geometrical horizontal point horopter* (Figure 6.2A). The images of object points that lie on the *geometrical vertical point horopter* by definition also fall on corresponding retinal points. Ideally, this horopter is a line that lies within a vertical plane that cuts through both the center of the Veith-Müller circle and a point midway between the eyes. Readers can find a thorough discussion of this topic in Howard and Rogers (1995, pp. 48–52) and Tyler (1991).

Objects closer than the fixation point produce retinal images that are said to have *crossed horizontal absolute disparity*, while objects farther than the fixation point produce retinal images that are said to have *uncrossed horizontal absolute dis-*

---

increasing the disparity further. Two copies of the target are seen, and the target's shape can be recognized, but it is not seen in depth (Hamstra & Regan, 1995; see Figure 6.10).

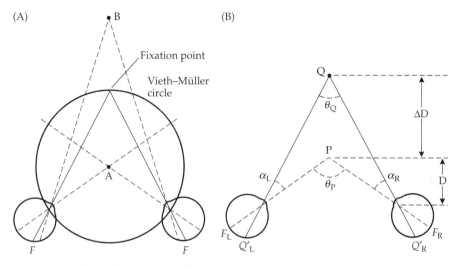

6.2 The Vieth–Müller circle and absolute disparity. (A) The images of any point on the Vieth–Müller circle fall on corresponding points on the left and right retinae and thus have zero absolute disparity. The images of point A are said to have a crossed horizontal absolute disparity, and the images of point B are said to have an uncrossed horizontal absolute disparity. (B) Definition of absolute disparity.

parity. This terminology can be understood as follows. Point one finger downwards and one finger upwards and align them tip to tip. Now move one sufficiently farther away than the other so that when you fixate on one finger the other finger is seen double (i.e., diplopic). Now fixate on the nearer finger. If you open and close your left eye you will see that the right eye's image is the right component of the further finger's diplopic image. Now fixate on the further finger. If you open and close your left eye you will see that the right eye's image is the left component of the nearer finger's diplopic image. Figure 6.2A brings out the geometric reason for this observation.

In this section I will call crossed absolute disparities *near disparities* and uncrossed absolute disparities *far disparities.*

Figure 6.2B illustrates the geometrical definition of *horizontal absolute disparity.* Lines passing through the two foveal centers (F_L and F_R) converge onto a point of zero absolute disparity. A point object (Q) that is more distant than this fixation point is imaged at Q'_L on the left retina and at Q'_R on the right retina. The *absolute disparity* of the retinal images of point object Q is ($\alpha_L + \alpha_R$). Note that this is the absolute disparity of point object Q even if there is no other object in the visual field. If there is a second point object P in the visual field and if P is located at the point of intersection of the two dashed lines in Figure 6.2B so that the two eyes fixate on point object P, then angle ($\alpha_L + \alpha_R$) is also the *relative disparity* of object Q with respect to object P.

It is straightforward to show that $(\alpha_L + \alpha_R) = (\theta_P - \theta_Q)$. A simple geometrical proof shows that, for objects in the straight-ahead position, as in Figure 6.2B, $(\alpha_L + \alpha_R) \approx I\Delta D/D^2$ where I is the interpupillary separation, $\Delta D << D$, and $(\alpha_L + \alpha_R)$ is expressed in radians. In words, the relative horizontal disparity of the images of two points that differ in distance by a given small amount decreases with the square of their mean distance. This is the geometrical reason why the binocular perception of relative depth fails rapidly when viewing distance is increased beyond 10 m or so.*

The empirical horizontal point horopter and the psychophysics of absolute and relative disparity

Now we step from the theoretical (geometrical) theory of stereopsis into the different world of what the human visual system actually does.

The empirical point horopter. Among the several psychophysical criteria for measuring the empirical horopter are equal perceived depth, binocular fusion, and nonius line alignment.† These different procedures do not give the same horopter and none of them give the theoretical (Vieth-Müller) horopter. Furthermore, the empirical horopter depends on the angle of binocular convergence. These issues are discussed by Ogle (1964) and by Howard and Rogers (1995).

The psychophysics of absolute and relative disparity. There is another difference between theory and reality. When a single luminous point is viewed in a dark room, the perceived distance of the point is by no means determined by its absolute disparity. Suppose that one views a bright point of light in a dark corridor. If viewing is monocular, the object is perceived to be about two meters away, whatever its actual distance (Gogol, 1965). More to the point, when viewing is binocular, placing that point of light at a distance far greater than two meters shifts the perceived distance to only a little greater than two meters, and placing the point of light far closer than two meters shifts its perceived distance to only a little closer than two meters (Gogol & Tietz, 1973).

---

* The situation is somewhat different for stereomotion because the rate of change of disparity associated with an approaching object falls off with V_Z/D^2, where V_Z is the component of the object's linear velocity directed along a line passing midway between the observer's eyes. Thus there is a tradeoff between approach speed and distance, so that, for geometrical reasons, visual sensitivity to a rate of change of relative disparity can extend to greater distances than visual sensitivity to static disparity. Numerical examples that bring out this point are given in Regan, Kaufman, and Lincoln (1986).

† A short vertical line is presented to one eye and a second short vertical line is presented to the other eye. The two lines lie one above the other so that they cannot be binocularly fused, and their distance is adjusted so that, when the observer converges exactly on the desired plane of fixation, they appear to be aligned vertically. These are *nonius lines*. The short black lines in the stereogram shown in the lower half of Figure 6.1C,D are nonius lines. By fusing this stereogram, readers can see the instability of their own binocular convergence.

And when an extended pattern of dots is viewed in a dark room, oscillations of the pattern's absolute disparity produce absolutely no sensation of motion in depth (Erkelens & Collewijn, 1985a,b; Regan et al., 1986a). The pattern appears to be stationary, even though large side-to-side oscillations are visible when one eye is closed.* Yet when a small stationary object is introduced into the field of view, the small object is immediately seen to be moving back and forth in depth relative to the large dot pattern.

> The binocular stimulus for the perception of static depth is relative disparity rather than absolute disparity, and the binocular stimulus for the perception of motion in depth is a rate of change of relative disparity rather than of absolute disparity.

The role of absolute disparity in stereopsis is more indirect than the role of relative disparity. Ogle (1953) and Blakemore (1970) found that the just-noticeable difference in horizontal absolute disparity between two targets (i.e., the relative disparity threshold) was lowest when the mean absolute disparity of the two targets was zero, and that the threshold rose as absolute disparity was increased in either the near (crossed) or far (uncrossed) direction (Figure 6.3A). In other words, as absolute disparity increases, sensitivity to a difference in static disparity decreases.

Note that the largest absolute disparity in Figure 6.3A is about 1.7 degrees, and that, over most of the range of absolute disparities in Figure 6.3A, the target lines were not binocularly fused: they were seen as double. Observers can make crude judgments of relative depth (in particular, whether a stimulus is closer or farther away than the fixation point) up to about 4 to 7 degrees of absolute near disparity and up to 9 to 12 degrees of far disparity (Westheimer & Tanzman, 1956; Mitchell, 1966, 1969, 1970; Blakemore, 1970).

Complementing the static disparity data shown in Figure 6.3A, we showed that, as absolute disparity increases, sensitivity to stereomotion decreases. The observer's left and right eyes were presented with stimulus patterns that could be manipulated independently while the two patterns were viewed in binocular fusion. Both eyes viewed a pattern of tightly packed dots that acted as a reference plane. This pattern had nonius lines at its center to allow the observer to check that he was accurately converging onto the dotted plane. A dichoptically presented line was centered 1.0 degrees to the right of the nonious lines. When the left and right eyes' images of the lines were oscillated at 0.1 Hz in antiphase, the binocularly fused line appeared to oscillate in depth at 0.1 Hz (stereo condition). And when the left and right eyes' images of the line were oscillated in phase at 0.1 Hz, the binocularly fused line appeared to oscillate from side to side at 0.1 Hz.

Figure 6.3B brings out the effect of absolute disparity on the binocular processing of changing relative disparity (the corresponding percept is motion in

---

* If a single bright dot rather than an extended pattern is viewed in a dark room, oscillations in depth can be detected, but they are very weak (Regan et al., 1986a).

(A)   (B)

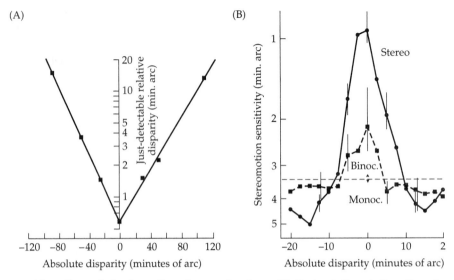

6.3 The effect of absolute disparity on visual sensitivity to static relative dispari-
ty and to oscillations of relative disparity.(A) The just-noticeable difference in horizontal disparity between two lines as a function of the mean absolute horizontal disparity of the two lines. The straight-line plot on log–log axes indicates a power law
relationship. (B) The continuous line shows the effect of absolute disparity on visual
sensitivity to oscillations of relative disparity. Part A after Blakemore (1970); part B
from Regan and Beverley (1973d).

depth) and of motion parallel to the frontal plane. When absolute disparity was
less than about 10 minutes of arc, sensitivity to oscillations in depth ("stereo")
was higher than in the "binocular" condition. But the converse obtained when
absolute disparity was greater than about 10 minutes of arc. Then sensitivity in
the stereo condition was *lower* than in the binocular condition.

In the "monocular" condition, either the right (upright triangle) or the left
(inverted triangle) eye was occluded. The horizontal dashed-line marks the mean
monocular sensitivity. This brings out the point that the perception of oscillation
would fail if the observer closed one eye while viewing just-detectable oscillations in the stereo situation at an absolute disparity of near-zero. In contrast, if
the absolute disparity were about 15 minutes of arc and the observer turned
down the amplitude of stereo oscillations until they were just not detectable, then
closing one eye would render the oscillations visible.

The effective region of stereomotion sensitivity for the binocularly fused target
in Figure 6.3B was restricted to about 10 minutes of arc on either side of the fixation plane. In contrast, the relative disparity thresholds for static targets are plotted out to ± 1.7 degree in Figure 6.3A but, as already mentioned, the stimulus

lines were seen double (not binocularly fused) over much of that range, thus extending measurements beyond the range of *patent stereopsis* into what Ogle called *qualitative stereopsis*.

Binocular retinal image motion during active head rotation. So far I have discussed stereopsis on the assumption that the observer's head was absolutely still. And, indeed, in the research discussed so far, the observer's head was held still with a head/chin rest and, in many cases, by a bite bar as well. But in everyday life we do not observe the world from a bite bar. For example, our heads move and oscillate when we walk and even when we try to stand still. For many years it was assumed that this was not a problem; it was assumed that "the oculomotor system compensates almost perfectly for motions of the body when visual as well as vestibular stimulation is available to the subject as he moves. Second, it was assumed that compensating oculomotor activities are almost perfectly yoked in the two eyes. Once these two assumptions are made, the fusion, stability and clarity of the visual world during normal activity can be explained" (Steinman & Collewijn, 1980, pp. 427–428).

But these assumptions are quite wrong. When the sensor-coil rotating-magnetic-field technique was used to obtain precise measurements of the eye movements of observers while they actively (but not violently) rotated their heads about a vertical axis and maintained fixation on a distance target: "Eye movement compensation of such head rotations was far from perfect and compensation was different in each eye. Average retinal image speed was of the order of 4 deg./sec. within each eye and the speed of changes in retinal image position between the eyes" (i.e., vergence speed) "was on the order of 3 deg/sec. Vision, subjectively, remained fused, stable and clear" (Steinman & Colleweijn, 1980, p. 415).

Later experiments showed that the standard deviation of vergence increased from about 0.05 degree when the head was supported on a biteboard to about 0.5 to 1.0 degree when the head was freely moving (Steinman et al., 1985).

Thus, *relative disparity* rather than *absolute disparity* is the major determinant of stereopsis (Collewijn et al., 1991). As well, the sluggishness of the stereo mechanism presumably provides some smoothing of the effects produced by noisy variations of vergence. (See pp. 360–362.)

Disparity contrast. Visual sensitivity to relative disparity is usually explained in terms of the just-noticeable difference of disparity between two targets. But the data shown in Figure 6.3A,B suggest that the concept of *disparity contrast* might prove to be useful, where disparity contrast is defined as $(\delta_N - \delta_F)/(1 + |0.5[\delta_N + \delta_F]|)$, where δ_N is the absolute disparity of the nearer of two targets, and δ_F is the disparity of the further target (near [crossed] disparities are signed positive and far [uncrossed] disparities are signed negative). This definition can be compared with the definition of *motion contrast* given on pp. 301–304 and with Michaelson's definition of *luminance contrast* given on pp. 53–60 and 470–476.

The correspondence problem

Figure 6.4 depicts the so-called *Keplerian grid* and brings out an immediate problem that arises even for the simple stimulus of two (identical) dots or vertical lines at different depths, a stimulus that is popular in laboratory studies of stereoacuity. Images at location a_L and a_R of line A and images at locations b_L and b_R of line B are thrown onto left and right retinae, respectively. In practice, normally sighted people see what is actually there: two identical lines A and B at different depths. Within the Keplerian framework this means that the brain has first selected the corresponding images on the left and right retinae and then calculated the correct relative disparity δ (where $\delta = (a_L - b_L) - (a_R - b_R)$). How is this possible? *The four retinal images a_L, b_L, a_R, and b_R are all identical.* This is the correspondence problem.

The basic Keplerian model predicts that all combinations of a_L, b_L, a_R, and b_R would be matched, thus assigning object lines to points $G1$ and $G2$ in space as well as to A and B. But in fact we do not see lines at $G1$ and $G2$.

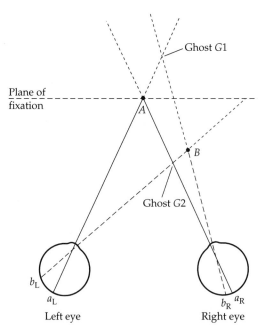

6.4 Basic Keplerian model of binocular vision. If the external geometry of binocular space is assumed to correspond to a neural organization such that each intersection between the two continuous lines drawn through point objects A and B corresponds to a neural disparity-detector, then we should see "ghost" images at $G1$ and $G2$ in addition to the images at A and B. But we do not see ghost images at $G1$ and $G2$. From Regan (1989a).

The correspondence problem becomes even more critical when the visual system is confronted with a Julesz random-dot stereogram, because it is possible to match any given dot in one eye's retinal image with any given dot in the other so that an enormous number of different depths is possible. Yet the brain does solve this problem and solves it effortlessly—or so it seems when one sees a Julesz random-dot form floating in space. Although experiments with random-dot stereograms are sometimes taken to suggest that the brain solves the correspondence problem before form detection, neurons that merely summed the input from both eyes could, in principle, detect the monocularly camouflaged form (see footnote on page 322).

Does the Visual System Contain Different Mechanisms for Processing Static (Positional) Disparity and for Processing a Rate of Change of Disparity?

A bright vertical bar oscillating in depth between 0 and 0.4 degrees of near disparity or between 0 and 0.4 degrees of far disparity at a frequency of 2 Hz was slowly moved into different positions in the visual field while the observer fixated a stationary mark. The observer was required to indicate when he perceived the target to oscillate in depth (Richards & Regan, 1973). We investigated the stereo visual fields of an observer with clinically normal vision and stereopsis (the author D. R.). This observer had large areas of the left visual field that were essentially blind to stereomotion (*stereoscotomas*).* The stereomotion-blind areas were quite different for near and far disparities. (Areas of the visual field that are stereomotion-blind generally retain normal sensitivity to motion parallel to the frontal plane [Regan et al., 1986b; Hong & Regan, 1989].)

Findings were quite different when we explored the binocular visual field using a static-disparity target. We briefly presented (for 0.1 sec.) a pair of lines whose disparity was either 0.4 degrees near (crossed) or 0.4 degrees far (uncrossed). Visual field defects were almost absent.

The difference between the stereo fields when tested with changing-disparity and when tested with static disparity suggested the following:

> Within the human visual system, changing-disparity and static disparity are processed by different mechanisms.

* Such findings are not uncommon. Roughly 20% of the population has stereomotion-blind areas within the visual field. At any given location within the visual field, stereomotion blindness can be specific for approaching versus receding motion or vice versa (Regan et al., 1986b; Hong & Regan, 1989). This finding may at least partially explain why some strongly right-handed individuals (like the author) bat the "wrong way round" (left-handed) in games such as cricket and favor the backhand in games such as squash. For at least some people, this behavior may reflect a visual rather than a motor peculiarity. The ramifications of left or right half-field stereomotion blindness in games such as soccer remain to be explored, as do the implications for highway safety.

The finding that, in some observers, regions of the visual field are blind to static disparity yet sensitive to changing disparity (Rouse et al., 1989) is consistent with this hypothesis. Further psychophysical evidence for the above hypothesis is reviewed elsewhere (Regan, 1991d, 1998; Regan et al., 1979, 1986a,b; 1998; Portfors-Yeomans & Regan, 1996; Portfors & Regan, 1997).*

Although the absence of a currently known physiological correlate of a psychophysical hypothesis does not necessarily weigh against a psychophysical hypothesis (pp. 26–30 and Appendix A), it may be relevant to note that some neurons in the visual cortex of animals are sharply tuned to the direction of motion in depth ("hitting the head" cells and "missing the head" cells) while being comparatively insensitive to static disparity (Cynader & Regan, 1978, 1982; Regan & Cynader, 1982; Poggio & Talbot, 1981; Spileers et al., 1990), and that these cells seem to be distinct from the classical *binocular depth cells* in that the binocular depth cells are sharply tuned to static disparity (Barlow et al., 1967; Nikara et al., 1968; Hubel & Wiesel, 1970; Poggio & Fischer, 1977) and prefer motion parallel to the frontal plane (Cynader & Regan, 1978). This distinction may relate to the psychophysical finding just discussed that humans can lose visual sensitivity to stereomotion and to static disparity independently of one another.

Furthermore, the electrophysiological finding that some single neurons in the brains of animals prefer approaching motion while others prefer receding motion may relate to the electrophysiological finding in humans that approaching motion and receding motion produce different brain responses (Regan & Beverley, 1973c) and may also be related to the psychophysical finding that a single location in the visual field can be blind to approaching motion while retaining sensitivity to receding motion, or vice versa (Hong & Regan, 1989).

Richards' Pool Hypothesis of Stereopsis

Whitman Richards' observers monitored the accuracy of their convergence onto a screen by means of nonius lines. When they reported accurate convergence, he presented a pair of 2×0.25 degree vertical lines, one to the left eye, the other to the right. The presentations were brief (0.08 sec.) to prevent eye movements from contaminating the data. The bars had one of several disparities, and the observer's task was to signal whether the bar appeared in front or behind the screen. Richards plotted percent correct responses versus the relative disparity of the briefly presented bars. *Note that the bars were often seen double, so that Richards was*

---

* Consider a transparent sphere covered in random dots and back-illuminated by a parallel beam of light that throws its shadow on a back-projection screen. When the sphere is stationary, observers report a flat two-dimensional pattern of dots. But when the sphere is rotating, the dots appear to lie on the surface of a three-dimensional rotating sphere, even though the dots in the screen all lie on a flat surface. (Nowadays, this well-known phenomenon is usually studied by generating the dots on the screen of a computer monitor.)

Much of my left visual field is stereomotion-blind. (My stereomotion fields are shown in Richards and Regan [1973] and Regan et al., [1986b].) I have informally observed that *investigating the kind of depth perception that Ogle called qualitative stereopsis as well as depth perception for binocularly fused targets, which Ogle called patent stereopsis.* In a second experiment Richards instructed his observers to match the perceived depth of a variable-depth probe to the bar (Richards 1970, 1971b).

The two procedures led to the same conclusions. Figure 6.5A indicates that observer A had a strong perception of relative depth when presented with near disparities but only a weak perception of relative depth when presented with far disparities, and that observer B showed the converse behavior. In contrast, observer C (who had normal stereo vision) experienced strong perceptions of relative depth when presented with both near and far disparities (Figure 6.5B).

Note that observers A and B experienced the maximum perceived relative depth when presented with bars whose disparity was about one degree. These bars were seen double rather than in binocularly single vision.

Richards concluded that "... normal or complete stereoscopic depth perception may be reduced to at least two, and possibly three basic mechanisms ... roughly corresponding to the crossed, uncrossed, and near-zero disparities. In order to interpret the nonmonotonic relation between depth and disparity, it is proposed that there is a pooling of the activities of the disparity detectors that sample any one of these regions of disparity. Thus the magnitude of the depth sensation would be based upon the (relative) activity in one or more of these three pools of binocular activity: crossed, near zero, or uncrossed. Anomalous stereoscopic depth perception would result if one or more of these pools were absent" (Richards, 1971b, p. 414).

If stereoacuity is determined by the difference in the slopes of the tuning profiles for the near and far pools of disparity detectors, we would expect that stereoacuity would be finest at zero disparity Figure 6.3A shows that this is indeed the case.

Some correspondence has been noted between Richards' psychophysical concept of near and far pools and single-cell properties in monkey visual cortex in that the visual cortex of monkey contains neurons that are excited by a broad range of far disparities and inhibited or unaffected by a broad range of near disparities or vice versa (Regan et al., 1979). On the other hand, near-zero disparities seem to be served by a complex arrangement of sharply tuned neurons that prefer different depths, some of which are very sensitive to the spatial correlation between the patterns presented to the left and right eyes (Poggio & Fischer, 1977; Poggio et al., 1985, 1988; Poggio, 1991; Gonzalez et al., 1993).

---

the illusion of the three-dimensional rotating sphere is clearly evident when I view the dot pattern in my right visual field, but when I use a stereomotion-blind area, the depth illusion collapses and the dots appear to move within a fronto-parallel plane. This is the case whether viewing is monocular or binocular.

> But such attempts to relate physiological findings at the single-cell level to Richards' hypothesis are not relevant to the point that Richards' hypothesis is about function, and if cast in physiological terms would be framed in terms of how the pooled activities of large populations of neurons affect behavior.

The visual processing of changing-disparity also seems to be segregated into near and far pools: visual field areas that are selectively blind to stereomotion commonly assume quite different shapes for near and far disparities (Richards & Regan, 1973; Regan et al., 1986b; Hong & Regan, 1989).

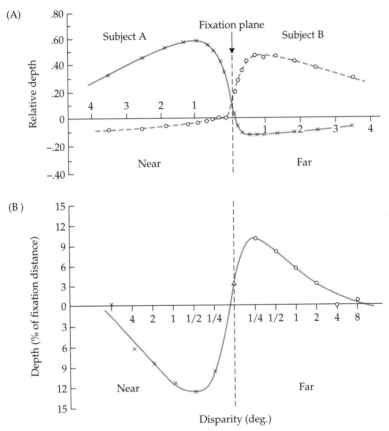

6.5 Experimental basis for Richards' pool hypothesis of human stereopsis. (A) Matched distance from the fixation target versus the relative disparity of a bar for two stereoanomolous observers. (B) Corresponding data for an observer with normal stereoscopic vision. After Richards (1971b).

Do Laboratory Data Obtained with Random-Dot Stereograms Give Us the Correct Impression of How the Visual System Processes Stereoscopic Depth in Everyday Conditions?

The chief feature of the random-dot stereogram technique is that the camouflaged form is not visible when one eye is closed but is clearly visible in binocular vision. It has been argued that the technique allows visual processing that occurs after convergence of retinal image information for the two eyes to be studied in isolation from processing that occurs before convergence.* But is this really so? The argument implicitly assumes that interactions between the monocular and binocular stages of processing can be neglected.

Addressing this issue directly, Whitman Richards concluded that: "Depth perception elicited from random-dot stereograms devoid of monocular cues is severely impaired when compared with similar stereograms that reveal the monocular contours. For transient stimuli, monocular contours appear necessary to elicit a range of depth sensations for different disparities, suggesting that monocular cue analysis is an integral component of the stereomechanism" (Richards, 1977, p. 967). "Considering the fact that in the real world the brain is seldom presented with the task of correlating random dot patterns, but rather almost always relies on the pairing of vivid feature objects, our result may not seem surprising. Given a set of redundant cues, certainly the greatest economy in building and operating an information processing machine can be achieved by utilizing first those cues that are the most common" (Richards, 1977, p. 969).

Rather than varying the correlation between the spatial characteristics of cyclopean and monocular processing, we varied the correlation between the temporal characteristics of cyclopean and monocular processing and came to a similar conclusion (see pp. 364–367).

> The two studies call into question the relevance of the results of laboratory experiments using random-dot stereograms to human visual performance in the everyday world. This would seem to be an issue that requires resolution one way or the other, but has received surprisingly little attention.

Detection of Disparity-Defined Form

Just as for the four kinds of form already discussed, cyclopean form has its own contrast sensitivity function (CSF), though contrast detection threshold is usually expressed in terms of relative disparity. In any given luminance-defined stereo stimulus (e.g., a Julesz random-dot pattern), the texture elements must be detect-

---

* This does not necessarily mean that cortical activity has been isolated. There are heavy descending connections from cortex to each lateral geniculate body, some of which come from contralateral cortex (Singer, 1977; Marrocco & McClurkin, 1985).

ed before relative disparity is processed; therefore it is not surprising that luminance contrast can affect stereo depth perception.

The disparity-contrast sensitivity function for cyclopean gratings

Tyler (1973, 1974) measured the disparity-contrast sensitivity function for disparity-defined (DD) form using a stereograting. In binocular fusion, normally sighted observers see a dotted surface that is sinusoidally corrugated in depth. But the dotted surface appears to be flat when one eye is closed. Thus, the percept of depth corrugations is generated entirely by neural processing that occurs after the signals from the two eyes have converged. With this device, Tyler reasoned, the contrast sensitivity function of cyclopean vision could be isolated and studied. The upper half of Figure 6.1allows the reader to experience a cyclopean grating.

Figure 6.6 indicates that visual sensitivity starts to roll off at a spatial frequency of only 0.5 to 1.0 cycles/deg. Tyler's arguments that this low bandwidth was a characteristic of cyclopean vision rather than being due to poor spatial sampling in the stimulus display were as follows: that a 10-fold reduction in dot density had only a slight effect on the maximum frequency at which the grating could be resolved (about 4 cycles/deg.), and that the depth resolution limit in (noncyclopean) line stereograms was 3 cycles/deg. The bandwidth of the filter characteristic in Figure 6.6 is about 10 times smaller than the corresponding bandwidth for the luminance-defined gratings used to collect the Figure 1.19 data. On the other hand, a better comparison would be between cyclopean and LD grat-

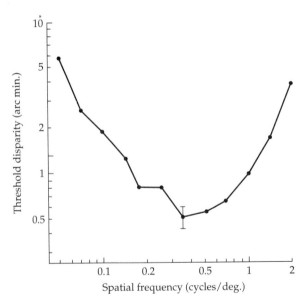

6.6 The contrast sensitivity curve for cyclopean form. The peak-to-peak disparity required to just detect the depth corrugations of a cyclopean grating (ordinate) are plotted versus the grating's spatial frequency. From Tyler (1974).

ings that had the same number of samples per cycle. *This comparison is not yet available.*

The reduction of sensitivity at low spatial frequencies evident in Figure 6.6 is difficult to interpret. Low-frequency attenuation would be expected if, as suggested by several authors, the receptive fields for cyclopean form have inhibitory flanks (Schumer & Ganz, 1979; Tyler, 1991; Cormack, et al., 1993), and if there are no filters that prefer spatial frequencies below about 0.4 cycles/deg. On the other hand, the cyclopean grating used to obtain the data of Figure 6.6 subtended 20 degrees so that the grating would contain only one cycle at 0.05 cycle/deg. on the abscissa. One full cycle across a 20 degree display gives a spatial-frequency distribution that extends from almost zero spatial frequency to 0.1 cycles/deg. (pp. 415–416, and see Figure B.7). As discussed earlier (on pp. 53–60), the leakage of power to low spatial frequencies would tend to produce an artifactual fall in sensitivity as the total number of cycles was reduced below about 3, even if the cyclopean receptive fields had no inhibitory flanks.

It would be no easy task to determine cyclopean sensitivity at very low spatial frequencies. At a frequency of 0.05 cycles/deg., three full cycles require a field size of 60 degrees. (A difference of Gaussians [DOG] stimulus would also be very wide. The exact width would depend on the ratio of space constants in the DOG equation, but for a peak frequency of 0.05 cycles/deg., the cyclopean equivalent of the DOG shown in Figure 1.21 would be about 32 degrees wide.) To ensure that the effective field size really was equal to the size of the display, it would be necessary to arrange that depth corrugations were equally visible across the entire field of view. Presumably, this would require at the least that dot size be scaled with viewing eccentricity, so as to allow for the variation of visual acuity across the visual field.

The effect of luminance contrast on stereoacuity

The just-noticeable difference (JND) in depth falls according to a power law as luminance contrast is increased, so that a plot of the JND versus contrast is linear on log–log axes (Halpern & Blake, 1988; Legge & Gu, 1989; Rohaly & Wilson, 1999). (This JND is also called the disparity increment threshold, or *stereoacuity*.) In this respect the behavior of the JND resembles that of Vernier acuity for LD form (pp. 98–106), but is quite different from the behavior of spatial frequency, orientation, and line-separation discrimination thresholds, all of which are independent of contrast for contrasts more than 2 to 3 times above detection threshold (see pages 108–115, 115–123, and 156–169).*

Given that stereoscopic depth mechanisms are affected by both luminance and disparity, it is not surprising that the perceived depth created by a given relative disparity can be affected by luminance contrast. And, indeed, perceived depth increases as contrast is reduced (Fry et al., 1949; Lit et al., 1972; Schor & Howarth,

---

* The effect of luminance contrast on the disparity at which binocular fusion breaks down is quite different from its effect on stereoacuity. The disparity at which a fused image is replaced by a double image (diplopia) is independent of contrast (Schor et al., 1989).

1986). Furthermore, a low-contrast target whose disparity is zero (i.e., a target on the horopter) appears to be more distant than a high-contrast target of zero disparity. According to Rohaly and Wilson (1999), perceived depth is a power function of contrast whose exponent ranges from 0.17 to 0.58, depending on spatial frequency. It seems that this effect of luminance contrast has a dual origin: interactions that take place both before and after the stage at which information from the two eyes converges (Halpern & Blake, 1988; O'Shea et al., 1994).

Rohaly and Wilson (1999) pointed out that the effect of luminance contrast on perceived depth weighs against the hypothesis that perceived depth is determined by the most excited neuron among a population of neurons, each of which is tuned to a narrow range of disparities (see Marr & Poggio, 1976, 1979). They argued that a change in contrast would not alter the identity of the most excited neuron. They noted that Richards' pool theory (pp. 354–356) could be made to account for the effect of contrast on perceived depth by making the ad hoc assumption that for both the *near pool* and the *far pool* a weakening of the output signal indicates "farther away."

So far I have reviewed data obtained using targets whose disparity information is carried by the difference in the luminance profiles of the images on the left and right retinae (the so-called *first-order* stimuli). The effect of luminance contrast on the just-noticeable difference in disparity is quite different for the so-called *second-order* stimuli. For second-order stimuli, the JND is almost independent of contrast (Wilcox & Hess, 1998). (Second-order disparity information is the disparity information carried by the contrast envelope of the stimulus as distinct from the luminance envelope of the stimulus.)*

Channels for Disparity-Defined Form

Even though the cyclopean form that is so strikingly evident when viewing a Julesz random-dot stereopair in binocular single vision disappears as soon as one eye is closed (see Figure 6.1), the luminance-defined texture elements that comprise the pattern must be detected before cyclopean processing can take place. For this reason, early spatial filtering of luminance information as well as the spatial filtering of disparity information is involved in the processing of cyclopean form.

Cyclopean channels

As discussed next, there are several lines of evidence that, by analogy with the case for luminance gratings, support the hypothesis that the contrast sensitivity

---

* Note, however, that we are talking about the *stimulus*. At an early stage of visual processing, both monocular retinal images are processed nonlinearly. The luminance profile within each of the retinal images of a first-order stereo stimulus will be distorted, as will the luminance profile within each of the retinal images of a second-order stereo stimulus. In addition, the contrast envelope within each retinal image of a second-order stereo stimulus will be demodulated (see pp. 93–98, 423–427, and 461–466).

function for disparity modulation can be regarded as the envelope of multiple overlapping channels that prefer different depth corrugation frequencies. First, Schumer and Ganz (1979) measured cyclopean contrast sensitivity curves (Figure 6.6) before and after adapting to a stereograting of spatial frequency S cycles/deg. They found that adaptation produced a threshold elevation that was maximal for a test grating of S cycles/deg., and fell off above and below the adapting frequency with a bandwidth of between two and three octaves at half-amplitude, thus providing evidence for cyclopean size-tuned channels. This evidence is analogous to the classical evidence for spatial-frequency channels in the luminance domain (see Figures 2.8 and 2.9A) and the evidence for spatial-frequency channels in the color domain (Figure 2.9B).

Second, authors using the masking paradigm have provided evidence for frequency-tuned cyclopean channels (Julesz & Miller, 1975; Tyler, 1975, 1983). Yang and Blake (1991) concluded that at least two broadly tuned channels are present in cyclopean vision.

A third line of evidence for cyclopean spatial-frequency channels is that adapting to a stereograting of spatial frequency S cycles/deg. increases the perceived spatial frequency of a test stereograting of slightly higher spatial frequency while decreasing the perceived spatial frequency of a test stereograting of slightly lower spatial frequency (Tyler, 1975). This experiment was analogous to the frequency-shift experiments of Blakemore and Sutton (1969) for luminance gratings (but see pp. 48–53 and Figure 1.16 for caveats), and of Favreau and Cavanagh (1981) for chromatic gratings. The existence of a tilt aftereffect for cyclopean form provides evidence that cyclopean channels are tuned to orientation as well as spatial frequency (Tyler, 1975; Cavanagh, 1989).

What is the relation between the early spatial filtering of luminance information and the spatial filtering of disparity information?

What are the spatial characteristics of the monocular processing of luminance contrast that precedes the analysis of binocular disparity? This question has attracted the attention of many researchers over the last thirty years. The question can also be framed in terms of the idea that the luminance signal in the left and right retinal images is the *carrier* of the disparity signal. (Pp. 423–427 review the topic of carriers, modulation, and demodulation.)

Using random-dot stereograms whose luminance distributions had been passed through a narrow-bandwidth spatial filter, Julesz and Miller (1975) found that stereopsis is not impaired if the spatial frequency of masking noise is more than two octaves away from the spatial frequency of the disparity signal. They concluded that independent and parallel channels for luminance-defined form carry the different frequency components of a broad-bandwidth disparity signal. Further support for this idea is provided by the finding that stereopsis fails if the spatial frequency content of the patterns viewed by the left and right eyes do not overlap (Mayhew & Frisby, 1976).

Pulliam (1981) provided further experimental evidence for a relationship between disparity spatial frequency and luminance spatial frequency. He measured the threshold for detecting sinusoidal disparity corrugations (upper half of Figure 6.1), but rather than the kind of dot pattern used in Figure 6.1, his left and right retinal images were one-dimensional luminance gratings whose bars were at right angles to the bars of the disparity grating. His two main findings were as follows:

1. Sensitivity to depth corrugations increased progressively as luminance spatial frequency was increased from 0.3 to 7 cycles/deg.
2. The depth corrugation sensitivity maximum moved towards higher spatial frequency as luminance spatial frequency was increased.

Pulliam concluded that channels for disparity-defined form that prefer high spatial frequencies of disparity variation also prefer the luminance-defined *carrier* pattern in the left and right retinal images to have a high spatial frequency. This conclusion may well be related to the previous report of Felton et al. (1972, p. 349) who concluded that *"narrow bar detectors feed small disparity mechanisms whereas wide bar detectors feed large disparity mechanisms."*

In a more recent study, Lee and Rogers (1997) used patterns of randomly scattered dots whose luminance distributions had been passed through narrow-bandwidth spatial filters. They showed that the cause of the shift of the depth corrugation sensitivity peak reported by Pulliam was that sensitivity to depth corrugations of low spatial frequency is reduced when the spatial frequency of the luminance carrier is increased. They also found that one subset of filters responded to a combination of depth corrugation frequencies in the range of 0.25 to 1.0 cycles/deg. and luminance frequencies in the range 1 to 4 cycles/deg., while a second subset of filters responded to a different combination: depth corrugation frequencies less than 0.25 cycles/deg. and luminance frequencies above 4 cycles/deg.

Finally, they noted that these interactions between luminance spatial frequency and disparity spatial frequency seem not to exist when depth corrugations are clearly visible, that is, at suprathreshold magnitudes of disparity variations. They attributed this finding to "the operation of a scaling mechanism at supra-threshold levels which equates the stereo-efficiency of the different luminance channels feeding stereopsis." (Lee & Rogers, 1997, p. 1776).

A Comparison of the Temporal Characteristics of Visual Processing before and after Binocular Convergence

In the preceding sections of this Chapter I compared the spatial characteristics of processing that takes place before and after the convergence of binocular information. In the next section I compare the temporal characteristics of these two stages of processing.

Selectivity for temporal frequency

The continuous line in Figure 6.7A shows how monocular threshold for detecting sinusoidal side-to-side oscillations of a bar moving within a fronto-parallel plane depends on oscillation frequency. Realizing that this temporal tuning characteristic is not necessarily the tuning characteristic of the monocular channels that feed the disparity-processing stage, we adopted a different approach. We stimulated the left eye with a bar whose horizontal position varied according to a sinusoidal waveform of frequency F_1 Hz while the right eye viewed a similar bar whose horizontal location varied according to a sinusoidal waveform of frequency F_2 Hz (Regan & Beverley, 1973a). When $(F_2 - F_1)$ was much less than either F_1 or F_2, observers perceived a single binocularly fused bar that oscillated in depth at a frequency of approximately $0.5(F_1 + F_2)$ Hz. The amplitude of these depth oscillations waxed and waned with a periodicity of $(F_2 - F_1)$ Hz.

The rationale of this approach was that the left monocular channel received stimulation at frequency F_1 Hz and the right monocular channel received stimulation at frequency F_2 Hz. Activity at frequency $(F_2 - F_1)$ Hz could not occur until the signals from the two eyes had converged. Thus, the $(F_2 - F_1)$ *beat frequency* was a "signature" of signals that had passed through the stage at which disparity was

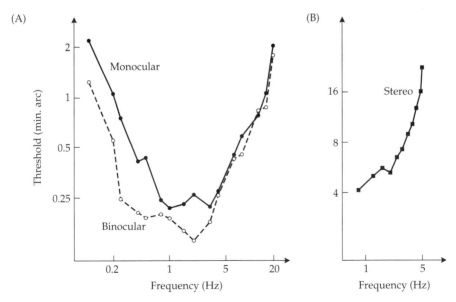

6.7 A comparison of the temporal frequency tuning characteristics of monocular signals and of the signals that feed the disparity-processing stage. (A) The continuous line shows the effect of temporal frequency on monocular sensitivity to oscillation within a fronto-parallel plane. (B) The effect of temporal frequency on sensitivity to the monocular signals that feed the disparity-processing stage. After Regan and Beverley (1973a).

processed. When we held the value of $(F_2 - F_1)$ at a constant low value (0.1 Hz) and measured the effect of F_2 on threshold for detecting the 0.1 Hz variations, we obtained the curve shown in Figure 6.7B. With the value of $(F_2 - F_1)$ held constant, the post-convergence processing of binocular information could not contribute to the frequency dependence of the "stereo" curve.

> The curve shown in Figure 6.7B can, therefore, be regarded as the isolated temporal tuning characteristic of the input to the binocular disparity-processing stage. Clearly, it is very different from the tuning characteristic shown in Figure 6.7A.

We estimated the tuning characteristic for the processing of binocular disparity by holding F_1 constant at a low value and measuring the effect of $(F_2 - F_1)$ on threshold for detecting the $(F_2 - F_1)$ Hz variation in the depth signal. The temporal tuning curve thus obtained had an even steeper high-frequency attenuation than that shown in Figure 6.7B. The perception of depth oscillations failed completely at 2 Hz for one observer, indicating that binocular processing adds even further high-frequency attenuation to that already imposed upon the monocular signals that reach the stage of binocular processing (Regan & Beverley, 1973a).

Temporal integration

To investigate the temporal integration of disparity information we replaced the sinusoidal oscillation described in the previous section with squarewave oscillations: the left eye was presented with a target that oscillated from side to side at F Hz while the right eye's target oscillated from side to side at $(F + \Delta F)$ Hz (Figure 6.8A). In binocular fusion the observer saw a pattern of random dots that subtended 5 degrees whose 2 degree central region appeared to move irregularly backwards and forwards in depth (Figure 6.8B).

The timing of the irregular changes of disparity had no counterpart in the monocular stimulation of either eye. (Compare the three traces in Figure 6.8.) There were no monocular cues to the time course of depth movements.*

In one experiment we measured the just-noticeable excursion of disparity as a function of F (from 0.5 to 8 Hz) with ΔF held constant, and as a function of ΔF (from 0.2 to 8 Hz) with F held constant. The curves obtained were similar in the two conditions. This finding was completely different from our findings described in the previous section where we used sinusoidal rather than squarewave oscillations and found that threshold was considerably more sensitive to ΔF than to F.

---

* There is some analogy between this approach to isolating cyclopean processing and the Julesz random-dot stereogram. The random-dot stereogram operates in the spatial domain; there is no monocular cue to the spatial form that is visible in binocular fusion (Figures 5.15 and 6.1). In contrast, the technique illustrated in Figure 6.8 operates in the temporal domain.

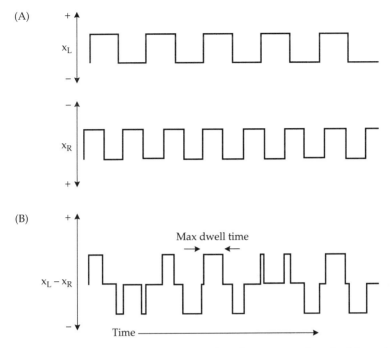

(A)

x_L

x_R

(B)

Max dwell time

$x_L - x_R$

Time

6.8 Method for dissociating visual processing that occurs after the binocular convergence of information from left and right eyes from processing that occurs before binocular convergence. The stimulus was a pattern of black dots of 2 minutes of arc diameter that were randomly scattered on a brightly illuminated 5 × 5 degree square. Dots within a central circular area of 2 degrees diameter could be moved horizontally from side to side in opposite directions for the patterns presented to the left and right eyes, dot density remaining constant over the entire 5 × 5 degree pattern. (A) Squarewave horizontal displacement of the positions (X_L and X_R) of the dots presented to the left and right eyes. Oscillation frequency was F Hz for the left eye's image and $(F + \Delta F)$ Hz for the right eye's image. The way in which binocular disparity changed with time is illustrated in part B. Note that only three values of binocular disparity were possible, and that the maximum disparity dwell time was $(F + \Delta F)^{-1}$ sec. After Beverley and Regan (1974a).

The similarity of both sets of curves suggested that they could both be described in terms of a single variable, and this was indeed the case. The two sets of data could be collapsed by plotting thresholds versus $(F + \Delta F)$.

Figure 6.8B brings out the physical meaning of $(F + \Delta F)$. Only three values of retinal disparity were possible; the longest time spent in any one of these three states (*the maximum disparity dwell time*) was $(F + \Delta F)^{-1}$ seconds.

The data points shown at the right of Figure 6.9 were obtained from the 112 data points shown in Beverley and Regan (1974a). (Each of the 112 points was based on 10 settings of threshold.) The format of Figure 6.9 is based on a standard

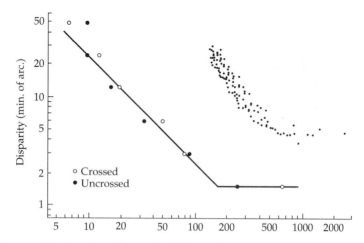

6.9 Temporal integration of disparity information. Open and filled circles plot the just-detectable pulsed increment of disparity for a monocularly visible target that started at zero disparity and moved toward either crossed or uncrossed disparities. The instant of disparity change was available monocularly, and the critical duration was 100–200 msec. Data points in the upper right of the figure show that critical duration was much longer when the instant of disparity change was not available monocularly. After Beverley and Regan (1974a,b).

format used to demonstrate *Bloch's law* for detecting a luminance increment (Graham, 1965). To the extent that the data points at the left side of the graph fit a line of 45 degree slope, disparity change was integrated (i.e., threshold disparity excursion multiplied by maximum disparity dwell time was constant). Integration ceased at a maximum disparity dwell time of 0.5 to 0.6 seconds. Within the *Bloch's law* framework of interpreting this kind of data, 0.5 to 0.6 seconds would be regarded as the *critical duration* for the temporal integration of disparity change (see footnote on page 307 for an alternative view). Figure 6.9 can be compared with comparable treatments of the integration of luminance and color, and of MD form information (Figures 3.11 and 5.9).

The continuous line in Figure 6.9 indicates that the 0.5 to 0.6 second critical duration is much longer than the duration over which a pulsed movement in depth is integrated, roughly 0.1 to 0.2 seconds (Beverley & Regan, 1974b). It is also much longer than the longest interval (0.10 to 0.18 seconds) that can elapse between brief monocular presentations to the two eyes if depth is still to be perceived (Efron, 1957; Ogle, 1963; Godel & Lawson, 1973). One reason for this difference might be that, in the experiments just cited, monocularly visiible stimulus changes occurred simultaneously with changes of disparity (as is, of course, invariably the case in everyday life outside the laboratory), whereas for the technique illustrated in Figure 6.8, disparity changes were not systematically related to the monocular movement signals from either eye.

If this explanation is correct, it might be that data obtained by totally isolating cyclopean processing from monocular processing—whether by the time-domain method illustrated in Figure 6.8 or by the Julesz space-domain random-dot stereogram technique—do not correctly represent the visual processing that occurs in everyday vision after information from the two eyes has converged. In other words:

> Isolated monocular processing plus isolated cyclopean processing does not necessarily equal combined monocular and binocular processing in everyday visual conditions where there are strong correlations between the spatial and temporal characteristics of monocularly available and binocularly available form.

This issue was also discussed earlier in the chapter (p. 357).

Orientation Discrimination for Disparity-Defined Form

A bar-shaped area within a random-dot pattern was rendered visible entirely by binocular disparity so that the bar could not be seen when one eye was closed. The bar resembled the rectangle illustrated in the lower half of Figure 6.1, except that the bar's aspect ratio was considerably higher (5.75:1). Figure 6.10A,B shows how orientation discrimination threshold was affected by the disparity of the dots within the bar relative to the dots surrounding the bar. The bar could not be seen at very low disparities. As disparity was increased through bar detection threshold (vertical arrows), orientation discrimination threshold fell to about 0.6 degrees for both near and far disparities (Hamstra & Regan, 1995). This compares closely with a lowest value of 0.5 degrees reported by Mustillo et al. (1988), even though they used a much larger bar (16×0.8 deg. compared with 2.3×0.4 deg.). The lowest value of orientation discrimination threshold was not significantly different from the lowest value for an LD bar with matched spatial sampling that was created by switching off all the dots outside the bar.

In a separate experiment, we found that perceived depth increased smoothly as disparity was increased through a range over which orientation discrimination threshold first fell and then leveled out (Hamstra & Regan, 1995). This finding suggests that the processing of the depth of a cyclopean form is dissociated from the processing of the orientation of that same form.

Positional Discrimination, Width Discrimination, Separation Discrimination, and Spatial-Frequency Discrimination for Disparity-Defined Form

In this section we return once more to the theme that was encapsulated by the quotation from Matin on pages 98–106. Just as in the case of luminance-defined form, the spatial order of an array of cyclopean forms is correctly preserved in perception. Another parallel with luminance-defined form: positional discrimination

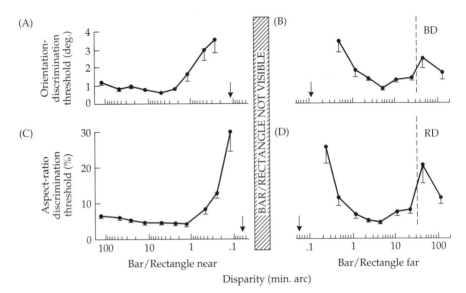

6.10 Orientation discrimination and aspect-ratio discrimination for cyclopean form. (A, B) Orientation-discrimination threshold for a cyclopean bar (ordinate) is plotted versus the disparity of the bar. (C, D) Aspect-ratio discrimination threshold for a cyclopean rectangle (ordinate) is plotted versus the disparity of the rectangle. Vertical bars indicate ±1 SE. Vertical arrows indicate disparity thresholds for detecting the bar or rectangle. Vertical dashed lines demarcate disparity ranges in which the bar (BD) or rectangle (RD) was seen double. For all other disparities, the bar or rectangle was fused. Parts A and B from Hamstra and Regan (1995); parts C and D from Regan and Hamstra (1994).

for cyclopean boundaries is far more acute than would be expected from the spatial tuning properties of cyclopean filters. We will see that the concept of *local sign* discussed on pages 98–106 can usefully be extrapolated to the perception of cyclopean form.

Positional discrimination

Readers who inspect the cyclopean rectangle in the lower half of Figure 6.1 will be struck by the remarkable sharpness of the rectangle's edges. "Remarkable," because the clearly visible edge is far sharper than the mean distance between the dots. Clearly, the sharpness is created after the signals from left and right eyes have converged (try closing one eye), that is, at or beyond the cyclopean level of processing. And it does not seem to be a "cognitive contour." It has the flavor of early, "preattentive" visual processing: provided you view the cyclopean rectangle in binocular fusion, the edges are sharp independently of cognitive variables, just as for a sharp-edged LD rectangle.

Can the relative position of a cyclopean edge be discriminated with a precision corresponding to the subjective sharpness of the edges in the lower half of Figure 6.1? Or is the sharpness a mere illusion? This is an empirical question that was addressed by Morgan (1986a), who found that Vernier offset threshold for a cyclopean bar is roughly 40 seconds of arc. This might seem poor compared with the 2 to 5 seconds of arc Vernier offset threshold that some observers can attain when viewing LD lines of very high spatial sampling frequency. On the other hand, Vernier offset threshold for an LD target whose spatial sampling matched the cyclopean target was little lower than the corresponding cyclopean threshold. Morgan noted that a 40 second Vernier offset threshold is some 10 times better than the 3 cycles/deg. resolution for a cyclopean grating (Figure 6.6), thus paralleling the roughly 10-fold mismatch between Vernier offset threshold and grating acuity for both LD and MD form. As well, cyclopean Vernier offset thresholds were about four times less than the size of the rather large pixels (160×80 seconds of arc) of Morgan's random-dot display, paralleling the finding that the 27 seconds of arc Vernier offset thresholds for dotted bars defined by motion parallax were considerably smaller than the 360 seconds of arc mean separations of dots (Regan, 1986a).

If the spatial-frequency channels for cyclopean form are as broadly tuned as the experimental evidence suggests (as discussed on pp. 360–361), with its implication that the corresponding receptive fields are very wide, we are left to account not only for the perceived sharpness of the edges of the cyclopean rectangle in Figure 6.1, but also for Morgan's finding that position discrimination threshold is so low. One candidate proposal is that the subjective sharpness of a cyclopean edge as well as threshold for the relative position of the edge is determined by the pattern of activity among an array of receptive fields that serve different receptive field locations along a line perpendicular to the edge. By analogy with a proposed explanation (Regan, 1986b, p. 143) for the finding that Vernier acuity for motion-defined (MD) form is far better than would be predicted on the basis of the contrast sensitivity curve for MD form, a candidate explanation for Morgan's finding that Vernier acuity for DD form is far better than would be expected from the contrast sensitivity function for cyclopean form (Figure 6.6) is that the edge-sharpening lateral-interaction process proposed to account for the high acuity for the relative position of an *isolated* steep gradient of disparity (i.e., a cyclopean edge) has an extensive spatial-summation field, whose functioning is disrupted when there is more than one disparity gradient within its summation field (Regan, 1991b; Howard & Rogers, 1995).

Bar-width and bar-separation discrimination

We have recently completed a cyclopean version of the experiment whose rationale is described on pp. 156–157 (see Figure 2.37). After each single presentation, observers were required to compare the two cyclopean test bars in order to make the following four discriminations: (1) their mean orientation; (2) their orientation difference; (3) their separation; (4) their mean location. Between the two test bars was a "noise" bar, whose orientation, width, and location were varied independently of the four task-relevant variables. A cyclopean masker pattern was presented immediately following each trial. We found that observers could discriminate each of the four variables while ignoring all task-irrelevant variables. This was the case even when presentation duration was sufficiently short (82 msec) to deny the possibility of fixating the two test bars in succession.

We (Kohly & Regan, unpublished data, 2000) concluded that:

1. The human visual system contains long-distance cyclopean comparator mechanisms (cyclopean *coincidence detectors*) whose outputs are labeled orthogonally with the mean orientation, orientation difference, separation, and mean location of a pair of cyclopean bars.
2. These mechanisms are "blind" to any cyclopean stimuli located between the two test lines.

These findings cannot be explained in terms of responses from spatial filters for DD form that are driven from the same retinal location.

Spatial-frequency discrimination

I have been unable to find any report of spatial-frequency discrimination thresholds for DD gratings.

Aspect-Ratio Discrimination for Two-Dimensional Disparity-Defined Form

We measured aspect-ratio discrimination threshold for DD form using a cyclopean rectangle of mean area 1.0 deg.^{2} similar to that illustrated in the lower half of Figure 6.1 (Regan & Hamstra, 1994).

To ensure that neither the height (a) nor width (b) of the rectangle provided a reliable cue to aspect ratio, we varied randomly the rectangle's area by up to ±40% from trial to trial. Figure 6.10C,D show that aspect-ratio discrimination threshold fell to a minimum as the rectangle's disparity was progressively increased above rectangle detection threshold (arrowed). The lowest thresholds were 3.1, 3.4, 4.0, and 7.4% for four subjects.

If we assume that first a and b are encoded, then the ratio a/b is computed, a 3.1% discrimination threshold implies that the precision with which a and b are encoded is better than 1.0 minutes of arc—considerably better than the 9 minutes mean separation between dots in the stereopair (Figure 6.1C,D), but in line with Morgan's (1986a) estimate of 0.7 minutes of arc Vernier acuity for cyclopean form.

To explain the findings just described, I propose that the aspect ratio of a DD rectangle is processed according to the schematic shown in Figure 2.63A, but with broadly tuned receptive fields sensitive to DD form rather than LD form and with the coincidence detectors sensitive to the separation between two narrowly tuned receptive fields for DD form rather than, as in Figure 2.53, the separation between two narrowly tuned receptive fields for LD form. The processing of aspect ratio information for a DD rectangle would be along the same lines as illustrated in Figure 2.63B–F for an LD rectangle.

In a separate experiment, we found that the perceived difference in depth between the cyclopean rectangle and its surroundings increased approximately linearly with relative disparity up to a point just before the onset of diplopia. Over the same range of disparities, aspect-ratio discrimination threshold first decreased, then leveled out, then rose again. One possible explanation for this finding is that it reveals a distinction between two classes of mechanisms, one that supports depth perception, the other involving spatial interactions among disparity-sensitive mechanisms (Regan & Hamstra, 1994).

By switching off all dots outside the cyclopean rectangle we created a rectangle that was rendered visible by a combination of disparity contrast and luminance contrast, but had the same spatial sampling as the cyclopean rectangle. The lowest aspect-ratio discrimination threshold for the (DD + LD) rectangle was significantly (though only slightly) lower than for the DD rectangle, even though the rectangle's boundary was subjectively sharper for the DD rectangle than for the (DD + LL) rectangle. (This point is demonstrated photographically in Regan and Hamstra [1994].) For near disparities, the lowest threshold was 4.0 ± 0.5% in Figure 6.10C, compared with 3.0± 0.4% for the (DD + LD) rectangle; for far disparities, the lowest threshold was 4.3 ± 0.5% in Figure 6.10D, compared with 3.3 ± 0.4% for the (DD + LD) rectangle.

Figure 2.61D shows the effect of aspect ratio on the percentage of "elongated vertically" responses for an observer who was viewing the DD rectangle illustrated in Figure 6.1C,D. The aspect ratio at the 50% point on the psychometric function was 1.02 (SE = 0.01); that is, squareness was judged to an accuracy of 2%. The psychometric functions shown in Figure 2.61E,F were collected using the same test aspect ratios as in Figure 2.61D, but the data in parts E and F were collected after adapting to a DD rectangle of aspect ratio either 1.5 (in Figure 2.61E) or 1/1.5 (in Figure 2.61F). The area of the test rectangle was randomly varied by up to ±40% in all cases. Oppositely directed aspect-ratio aftereffects are evident in Figure 2.61E,F. In particular, after adapting to a vertically elongated rectangle, a horizontally elongated rectangle of aspect ratio 0.87 appeared square, while after adapting to a horizontally elongated rectangle, a vertically elongated rectangle of aspect ratio 1.11 appeared square. Thus, the mean aftereffect was 12% (Hamstra, 1994).

An aspect-ratio aftereffect was also observed when the adapting rectangle was cyclopean and the test rectangle was luminance-defined, though the size of the aftereffect (5.1%) was smaller than in the other two cases. The existence of a cyclopean-to-LD aspect-ratio aftereffect shows that the processing of aspect ratio for DD rectangles is not entirely separate from the processing of aspect ratio for LD rectangles. On the other hand, the information about aspect ratio carried by disparity contrast and luminance contrast seems to have converged only partially at the aspect-ratio processing stage: the ratio between the magnitudes of the cyclopean-to-LD aftereffect and the LD-to-LD aftereffect was only 0.29, 0.30, and 0.47 for the three subjects studied (Hamstra, 1994).

Stereopsis at Isoluminance

Scharff and Geisler (1992) found that some (3 of 6) of their observers could discriminate between far (uncrossed) and near (crossed) disparities at equiluminance when all detectable chromatic aberration artifacts had been removed.

They used the *ideal observer* approach to compare discrimination performance for equiluminant and achromatic stereograms. (The concept of the ideal observer is discussed on pp. 142–143 and 245–250.) A detailed description of their calculations is given in Jordan et al. (1990). They found that chromatic information was used with the same efficiency as luminance information for two of the three observers who could perform the task, and with less efficiency for the third observer, Scharff and Geisler (p. 874) concluded that "the same or similar stereo mechanisms are processing color and luminance information." They offered explanations for previous claims that observers cannot see stereo depth at equiluminance.

Disordered Processing of Disparity-Defined Form in Patients

A partial or complete loss of stereoscopic depth perception is a common result of disordered control of eye position (strabismus or turned eye) that prevents binocular fusion of the retinal images, but this tells us little about the central processing of DD form. Again, some infants are born with, or develop, unequal refraction in the two eyes. For example, one eye may be long-sighted and the other normally sighted, so that if one retinal image is in sharp focus, the other is blurred. If this imbalance is left uncorrected for too long, visual acuity in the long-sighted eye falls to a low level that cannot be corrected by wearing glasses. It is widely thought that this condition (anisometropic amblyopia) is a result of unequal competition for space on binocular cells in the developing primary visual cortex; the cell bodies and dendrites become covered by tightly packed synapses driven by the good eye, leaving no room for connections from the long-sighted eye. Even after treatment that restores acuity to the bad eye and establishes binocular single vision, it is often found that stereoscopic depth perception is absent. Again, this finding tells us little about the central processing of DD form.

A complete loss of stereoscopic vision associated with damage to the visual cortex is seldom reported and, particularly in the earlier reports (Riddoch, 1917; Critchley, 1953, pp. 329–330), it is not clear that disordered control of ocular vergence was ruled out as a possible cause of the perceptual loss. It has been claimed that damage to the right rather than the left cerebral hemisphere is more often associated with defective stereoscopic depth perception (Carmon & Becholdt, 1969; Benton & Hecean, 1970), though this conclusion has been challenged (Ross, 1983). A problem in the interpretation of studies in which observers have been required to identify the shape of a cyclopean target (Durnford & Kimura, 1971) or in which evoked potentials to cyclopean stimuli have been recorded (Lehmann & Julesz, 1978) is that these procedures do not necessarily test the processing of stereoscopic depth. The shape of a cyclopean target may be clearly visible to an observer who has no sensitivity to binocular disparity, but who does possess binocularly driven neurons (see footnote on page 322). By the same token, the presence of cyclopean evoked potentials does not necessarily indicate the presence of neurons sensitive to stereoscopic depth, unless the stimulus is an abrupt change between equal disparities on either side of the fixation plane, i.e., an abrupt change between equal but opposite binocular correlations (Norcia et al., 1985).

Psychophysical Models of the Processing of Disparity-Defined Form

All the psychophysical models of the early processing of disparity-defined form discussed in this section have been framed by analogy with the spatial filtering approach to the processing of luminance-defined form (described on pp. 415–416). A challenge to modellers that has not so far been addressed is that discussed on page 357. However, there is a second problem that cannot be ignored even when modeling is restricted to *cyclopean* disparity-defined form where no monocular cue to the form is available.

The correspondence problem again

Those who seek to model the processing of binocular disparity run jarringly into a famously knotty problem. As mentioned on pp. 352–353, the problem assumes its most challenging aspect in the context of the random-dot patterns introduced by Bela Julesz that are so instructively set out in his 1971 book. All dots are identical. Therefore, any individual dot in the left eye's retinal image can be matched with any individual dot in the right eye's retinal image. (Note, however, that the same does not hold for randomly occurring clusters of dots.) How does the brain know which dot in the left eye's retinal image should be matched with any given dot in the right eye's retinal image? This is called the *correspondence problem.*

By binocularly fusing the left and right images in Figure 5.15 or Figure 6.1, the reader can demonstrate that the human brain does not regard the correspondence problem as a real problem. It is the human mind that has a problem.

One proposed explanation has it that the matching process starts with the lowest spatial frequencies (i.e., the widest spatial filters), so that the search for correct matches is conducted over a large range of disparities. (The correspondence problem is less severe at this coarse level, because random clusters of dots are more visible than individual dots.) The coarse matches obtained are used to shift the left and right retinal images into closer correspondence, thereby restricting the range of disparities over which a search must be conducted. This procedure is then conducted at finer and finer scales, the processing at each successively finer scale being governed by the results of the preceding processing at the coarser scale

(Marr & Poggio, 1979; Nishihara, 1987; Quam, 1987). This attractive hypothesis has the advantage of plausibility. But according to Badcock and Schor (1985) and Rohaly and Wilson (1993), it is, nevertheless, wrong.*

It has been suggested that exploratory eye movements play an important role in solving the correspondence problem (Marr & Poggio, 1979). But, according to Rohaly and Wilson (1993), this hypothesis also is incorrect.

One candidate explanation is framed in terms of Whitman Richards' pool theory of stereoscopic depth perception (see Figure 6.5). He proposed that disparity detectors are organized into three pools, one sensitive to near disparities, one sensitive to far disparities, and one sensitive to a narrow range of near-zero disparities close to the fixation plane (Richards, 1971b). It has been suggested that Richards' pool theory might explain the correspondence problem: "[N]ear and far pools both respond to a wide range of possible disparities so they signal a weighed sum of all possible matches: multiple 'ghosts' are not produced because the amount of perceived depth is uniquely determined by the *relative* activity of the near and far pools" (Regan et al., 1990, p. 324). This suggestion was developed quantitatively by Wilson et al. (1991). According to this line of argument, the correspondence problem does not require global (full-field) processing; it is solved by relatively local processing (Rohaly & Wilson, 1993).

Modeling the processing of disparity-defined form

Models of the detection and discrimination of DD form have been reviewed in detail by Tyler (1991,1995). In brief, there is evidence for a visual processing stage that can be modeled as an array of frequency- and orientation-tuned filters for cyclopean form (Julesz & Miller, 1975; Schumer & Ganz, 1979; Tyler, 1983; Cavanagh, 1989; Yang & Blake, 1991; Cormack et al,. 1993). Presumably these are located at or central to the stage of global stereopsis of Julesz. To account for the perception created by cyclopean patterns of small dots (e.g., Figure 6.1A–D), I conventionally assume that the receptive-field profiles of any given narrow-width luminance-contrast spatial filter as "seen" by the monocular inputs for the right and left eyes, respectively, are slightly displaced horizontally. This horizontal displacement creates the filter's selectivity to the disparity of a local luminance-defined texture element or boundary. Following the proposal of Schumer and Ganz (1979), I assume that these local-disparity signals feed spatially opponent excitatory and inhibitory inputs into the receptive fields of orientation-tuned filters (labeled SF_{DDF} in Figure 7.1). See also Cormack et al. (1993) and Tyler (1991). This nonlinear spatial pooling extends over different spatial extents, thus creating spatial filters that prefer different spatial frequencies. None of these filters, however, is as narrow as the narrowest SF_{LDF} filter. Note however, that no current model can account for the findings described on p. 369–370.

---

* In any case, if this process is conceived in terms of starting with a lowpass-filtered version of the Fourier power spectrum of the dot pattern, important shape information about irregularly shaped clusters of dots in the left and right eyes' dot patterns may be lost, because the phase spectrum is necessary to recover this information.

CHAPTER 7

Integration of the Five Kinds of Spatial Information: Speculation

According to Helmholtz, the processes that underlie visual perception are inductive and are learned—though below the level of consciousness.

> [B]y their peculiar nature they may be classed as *conclusions*, inductive conclusions, unconsciously formed. We are not simply passive to the impressions that are urged on us, but we *observe*.
>
> H. von Helmholtz, *Physiological Optics*, 1909

> The surprising tendency for attributes such as form, color and movement to be handled by separate structures in the brain immediately raises the question of how all the information is finally assembled say for perceiving a bouncing red ball.
>
> D. H. Hubel, *Eye, Brain and Vision*, 1988

Preamble

This section focuses on the integration of spatial information carried by the five kinds of spatial contrast and addresses three questions that emerge from the experimental data reviewed in the previous five chapters. First, given that any neuron in primary visual cortex is sensitive to variations in more than one visual submodality (though see the footnote on page 33), how is it that observers can almost perfectly unconfound simultaneous variations in orientation, spatial frequency, temporal frequency, and contrast? Second, why are orientation and spatial-frequency

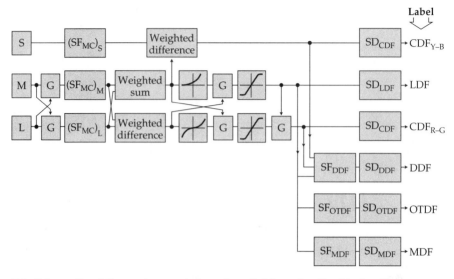

7.1 Schematic of the early processing of spatial form for five kinds of form.
$(SF_{MC})_S$, $(SF_{MC})_M$, $(SF_{MC})_L$: Spatial filters for monochromatic contrast fed by short-, medium-, and long-wavelength cones. SF_{DDF}, SF_{OTDF}, SF_{MDF}: Spatial filters for, respectively, disparity-defined form, orientation-texture-defined form, and motion-defined form. G: Variable-gain stage. SD_{CDF}, SD_{LDF}, SD_{DDF}, SD_{OTDF}, SD_{MDF}: spatial discrimination stages for the five kinds of spatial form.

discrimination thresholds for OTD, MD, CD, and DD form low compared with the bandwidths of the most sharply tuned spatial filters for LD form? Third, why is it that, when spatial sampling is matched, spatial discrimination thresholds are the same or only a little different for the five kinds of form (provided that the number of spatial samples per degree is not too high)?

A fourth problem is less obvious. As stated earlier, spatial information about any given object can be encoded in terms of any one of five kinds of spatial contrast, and the early processing of any one of these different kinds of contrast is to some extent independent of the processing of any of the other kinds of contrast. Nevertheless, in everyday life we usually see only one version of any given object rather than several versions of the same object. Registration fails so seldom that it is easy to overlook the fact that registration poses a problem at all.* Treisman (1996) has reviewed the considerable literature on registration and "binding."

---

* As mentioned on pp. 314–316, the perceived location of an MD target can be grossly inaccurate. Furthermore, the misperception of *absolute* location exists simultaneously with normal discrimination of *relative* location and with the perceived sharpness of its boundaries. In the fluttering heart phenomenon, the color-defined boundaries of a target become dynamically dissociated from its luminance-defined boundaries. Again, a central lesion can cause an LD object to be perceived as having several locations at the same time (Teuber, 1963).

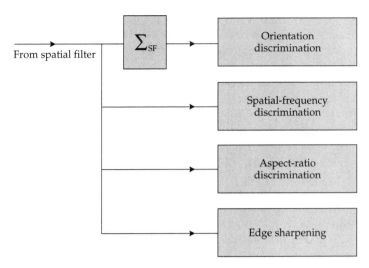

7.2 Schematic of the spatial discrimination stage of processing. This figure illustrates the contents of the SD boxes at the right of Figure 7.1.

I have discussed functional models of the detection and the several kinds of spatial discrimination of targets defined by the five kinds of spatial contrast in the previous five chapters. In this chapter I will attempt to integrate those five discussions. I will start with the information-processing schematics shown in Figures 7.1 and 7.2.

Independence of Spatial Discriminations

On pp. 30–33, in the section on sets of filters I reviewed the hypothesis that a limited number of visual dimensions are processed through independently functioning "sets of channels" that have low crosstalk, and I pointed out the importance of this independence for generalizing skills of eye–hand coordination learned in one visual environment to other visual environments. Figures 7.1 and 7.2 illustrate a functional rather than structural hypothesis, and in that context it is valid to assign to the spatial-filter stage the independence between the processing of different kinds of spatial information (see Appendix A and pp. 30–33).

In the physiological (structural) context, however, the human organism is faced with the problem that any given neuron in primary visual cortex changes its firing in response to a wide variety of visual inputs. For example, a neuron that responds to a change in orientation may also respond to changes in spatial frequency. Yet observers can unconfound variations of spatial frequency from simultaneous variations of orientation as well as contrast (Burbeck & Regan, 1983a; Bradley & Skottun, 1984; Heeley & Timney, 1988; Chua, 1990; Heeley et al., 1993; Vincent & Regan, 1995). And discrimination thresholds for spatial frequency, orientation, and contrast are closely similar when the grating changes along all three dimensions simultaneously rather than one at a time, so that the observer has three tasks instead of only one (Vincent & Regan, 1995). (The same is true when the three variables are orientation, spatial frequency, and temporal frequency [Vincent & Regan, 1995, unpublished data].) Clearly, this performance cannot be explained in terms of the firing of a single cortical neuron, because the firing of any given neuron confounds changes in orientation, spatial frequency, temporal frequency, and contrast (but, see the footnote on page 33).

A possible physiological explanation for the psychophysical (i.e., functional) finding that several pairs or triplets of variables are encoded independently with negligible crosstalk has been proposed previously (Regan & Beverley, 1985a; Regan & Price, 1986). In brief, I suppose that the visual pathway contains a population of neurons whose dependence on orientation, spatial frequency, contrast, color, velocity, and so on vary independently and randomly from neuron to neuron. Suppose that within this population there is a neural subpopulation that shows a neuron-to-neuron variation in preferred *orientation*, but all neurons within the subpopulation are similarly affected by all other variables. Relative activity within this first subpopulation will represent a change of stimulus orientation while rejecting covarying changes in spatial frequency and so on. Further suppose that there is a second subpopulation that shows a neuron-to-neuron variation in preferred *spatial frequency*, but every neuron within this subpopulation is similarly affected by all other variables. Relative activity within this second subpopulation will represent a change in stimulus spatial frequency while rejecting covarying changes in orientation and so on. In other words, although responses to a change of stimulus orientation, spatial frequency (and many other variables) are confounded at the level of firing of any given cell within the population, I propose that these two visual dimensions are unconfounded by *two different connectivities* within the population. I assume that a similar line of argument can be used to explain the approximately independent processing of the 11 pairs or triplets of features listed in the discussion on p. 35.

In terms of the distinction between functional and structural models of the visual system, the idea just reviewed is that the proposed connectivity between striate cortical neurons is at one and the same time the physiological basis for both the orthogonality created by the Figure 1.10 "sets of filters" and the fine-grain discriminations supported by the opponent stages in Figure 1.10.

It is not yet known whether observers can unconfound and separately discriminate simultaneous trial-to-trial variations in several stimulus variables for OTD, MD, CD, or DD form.

Spatial Filters

The hypothesis that information about the low and medium spatial-frequency content of images carried by all five kinds of contrast converges before the stage of frequency- and orientation-tuned filtering would provide a simple explanation for the finding that, except for targets with high spatial sampling frequencies, all the spatial discrimination thresholds that have been compared are not greatly different for the various kinds of form. It would also provide a simple explanation for registration. However, as discussed earlier (e.g. p. 250), this possibility can be rejected (see also Cavanagh, 1989).

For our present purpose, a major point brought out in the previous four chapters is that the narrow-width orientation- and frequency-tuned filters for LD form are located earlier in the sequence of information-processing stages than are the corresponding spatial filters for OTD, MD, and DD form. This is necessarily so, because the processing of individual texture elements (e.g., short lines or dots) must precede the processing of OTD, MD, or DD form. Therefore, in all these three cases a comparison of the outputs of narrow-width spatial filters for luminance-defined form that serve different visual field locations must precede the detection of DD, MD, or OTD form. Consequently, the spatially integrative filters tuned to both orientation and width for DD, OTD, and MD form pass moderate and low spatial frequencies only. These filters—labeled SF_{DDF}, SF_{OTDF}, and SF_{MDF} in Figure 7.1—have moderately wide spatial profiles. (There are, of course, orientation- and frequency-tuned spatial filters with moderately wide as well as narrow profiles for LD form.)

The hypothesis illustrated in Figure 7.1 is that each kind of contrast has its own orientation- and frequency-tuned filter. As well, in Figure 7.1 the spatial filters for motion-defined form (SF_{MDF}) feed a spatial discrimination stage for motion-defined form (SD_{MDF}), and so on. Each of these five SD stages is assumed to be organized as in Figure 7.2.

Next I review the proposed explanation, discussed on pp. 174–184, for the observation that we recognize solid shapes or outline drawings with equal facility (see first footnote on page 40). I propose that information about an LD target from wide filters that respond to any given target as a whole and information from *coincidence detectors* (see pp. 156–169) that process the target's edges feed similar spatial discrimination stages. More speculatively, I raise the possibility that the same might hold for spatial filters and coincidence detectors sensitive to OTD form, MD form, and DD form (though no direct evidence for this speculation has, as yet, been published).

Moving on to spatial discriminations, I next discuss Figure 7.2. Specific models of orientation discrimination and size discrimination and, in particular, opponent-process and line-element models, have been discussed in the previous five chapters (also see Appendix D). Although aspect-ratio discrimination thresholds for OTD (2.8 to 5.3%), MD (2 to 3%), and DD (3.1 to 7.4%) form are significantly (though not greatly) higher than for solid high-contrast sharp-edged LD rectangles (1.6 to 2.9%), they are little different from thresholds for LD squares whose spatial sampling is matched (Regan & Hamstra, 1991, 1994; Regan et al., 1996). The distinction between "regional binding" and "boundary detection" models was discussed on pp. 39–40. Stages 2–4 in Figure 2.63A set out a kind of model of aspect-ratio discrimination that can utilize either one or both of these modes of action. I propose that corresponding models that involve the appropriate kinds of spatial filters and coincidence detectors might describe aspect-ratio discrimination for OTD, MD, CD, and DD shapes. One possible explanation for the finding that the aspect-ratio aftereffect cross-adapts between DD and LD rectangles (Figure 2.61D–F) and between CD and LD shapes (see second paragraph of footnote on page 177) is that some convergence of disparity and luminance information and of color and luminance information occurs before aspect ratio is encoded in Figure 7.2. It is not yet known whether there is similar convergence of texture, and motion information.*

Finally, as discussed in the previous five chapters, it has been proposed that edge-sharpening information for any one of the five kinds of target is carried by the relative activation of the relevant kind of spatial filters that serve adjacent retinal locations and that the operation of an edge-sharpening mechanism is degraded when there is more than one gradient of the relevant kind of contrast within its receptive field.

The hypothesis that there are spatial filtering and spatial discrimination stages for each kind of contrast can account for the following findings: A brain lesion can degrade the ability to recognize MD letters while sparing not only the ability to detect MD spatial contrast but also the ability to read LD and OTD letters; a brain lesion can degrade the ability to read OTD letters while sparing the ability to read LD and MD letters; a brain lesion can degrade the ability to read low-contrast LD letters while sparing the ability to read MD or OTD letters (Regan et al., 1991, 1992b; Giaschi et al., 1992; Regan & Simpson, 1995).

So far as spatial-frequency discrimination is concerned, a prediction of the hypothesis under discussion is that spatial-frequency discrimination threshold for any given one of the five kinds of test grating would *not be elevated* by any of the other four kinds of masker grating (see Figure 2.26). This prediction has not yet been tested.

Similarity of Orientation and Spatial-Frequency Discrimination Thresholds for the Five Kinds of Form

As discussed in the previous five chapters, although the idea that spatial discrimination thresholds are determined by the relative activity within a population of filters can explain why both orientation and spatial-frequency discrimination thresholds are hyperacuities for all five kinds of form (in the sense that wavelength discrimination is a hyperacuity), it does not of itself account for the finding

---

* Gorea, Papathomas, and Kashi have investigated and modeled image segregation produced by combinations of color, texture, and motion contrast (Gorea & Papathomas, 1991a,b; Papathomas & Gorea, 1990; Kashi et al., 1995; Papathomas et al., 1997).

that orientation-discrimination and spatial-frequency discrimination thresholds are *approximately the same* for all five kinds of form.

In Figure 7.1, each kind of form has its own spatial filter and spatial discrimination stage. To account for the similarity of thresholds, it would be necessary to assume that the relevant noise levels as well as the tuning profiles of all six kinds of spatial filter were matched (see pp. 36–39, 108–115, 115–123, and Figure 2.29). This matching might have come about during early visual development—driven by the human infant's persistent attempts to achieve eye–hand coordination. Since an object is an object independently of how it is detected by the eye, the precision of orientation discrimination required of the organism would be the same for LD, OTD, MD, CD, and DD form. In terms of Figures 1.10, 7.1, and 7.2, I propose that feedback signals descending from the motor system would, during early visual development, modify the filters (arrowed dashed lines in Figure 1.10) and/or spatial discrimination stages until orientation discrimination thresholds were approximately the same for targets defined by all five kinds of spatial contrast (Regan & Price, 1986; Regan, 1991b).

To the extent that orientation-discrimination threshold is determined by the maximum slope of the orientation-tuning profiles of the relevant filters (see pp. 36–39 and 115–123), the suggestion just discussed is consistent with the finding that the orientation tuning bandwidth of the postadaptation threshold elevation curve for LD gratings is not greatly different from the corresponding bandwidths for OTD and CD gratings (compare Figures 2.10A, 2.28D, and 4.6). For cyclopean filters, on the other hand, Tyler (1975) estimated orientation-tuning bandwidth to be considerably wider than orientation-tuning bandwidth for LD filters.

An alternative explanation for the finding that orientation, spatial-frequency, and aspect-ratio discrimination thresholds for different kinds of spatial form is the Figure 7.1 schematic modified as follows. Spatial filter outputs are collapsed across different kinds of contrast before reaching the processing stage that determines spatial discrimination (i.e., there is only one spatial discrimination [SD] stage for orientation, only one for spatial frequency, and only one for aspect ratio rather than the five shown in Figure 7.1). According to this idea, illustrated in Figure 7.3, orientation-discrimination threshold would be limited by noise at the spatial discrimination stage rather than by noise at spatial filter stage. This would also be the case for spatial frequency and aspect-ratio discrimination threshold (see pp. 98–107 and see footnote on page 120).

According to this alternative hypothesis:

> The outputs of the spatial discrimination stages carry an orientation label or a spatial frequency label and so on, but any given label is collapsed across the five kinds of spatial contrasts. This hypothesis predicts that spatial-frequency discrimination threshold for any given one of the five kinds of test grating *would be elevated* by any one of the five kinds of masker grating (see Figure 2.62). An experimental test of this prediction has not so far been reported.

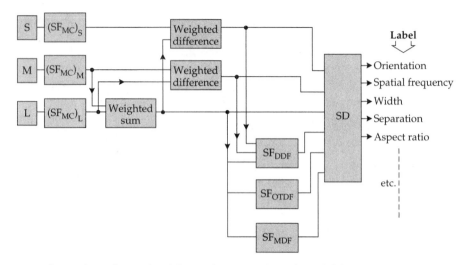

7.3 Alternative schematic of the early processing of spatial form. In this extreme variant, information about all five kinds of form converges before the spatial discrimination stage. For clarity, certain details present in Figure 7.1 have been omitted.

Are there, as depicted in Figure 7.3, separate output lines for orientation, spatial frequency, and so on, or does one line carry two or more labels? This question also remains to be answered (see the footnote on page 33).

In Figure 7.2, orientation information is collapsed across spatial frequency before reaching the orientation-discrimination stage. Collapsing across spatial frequency explains the finding that orientation-discrimination threshold is the same between gratings of the same spatial frequency and between gratings of quite different spatial frequencies (Burbeck & Regan, 1983a; Bradley & Skottun, 1984; Olzak & Thomas, 1991, 1992, 1996; Heeley et al., 1993). Spacial-frequency information is not collapsed across orientations for reasons described on pp. 173–174.

Orientation discrimination has a claim for uniqueness among the spatial discriminations in that orientation-discrimination threshold is little, if at all, lower for high-contrast, solid, sharp-edged LD bars than for OTD, MD, or DD bars, even though their boundaries are less precisely defined than the boundaries of a high-contrast sharp-edged, solid LD bar.

Registration

In this book I have reviewed psychophysical evidence for the following three theoretical constructs:

1. Spatial filters whose outputs carry labels for location, width, and orientation, some of which encode the spatial features of a target on the basis of regional binding, others of which encode the boundaries of a sharp-edged target by virtue of their sensitivity to a steep gradient of contrast.
2. Five classes of the filters just described, corresponding to the five kinds of spatial contrast.
3. Second-stage mechanisms that compare the outputs of two spatial filters served from spatially separated locations in the visual field. These second-stage mechanisms (*coincidence detectors*) are "blind" to stimuli located between the two first-stage receptive fields. Their outputs signal orthogonally the mean orientation, orientation difference, separation, and mean location of a pair of lines or bars. There is evidence that such mechanisms exist for LD form (pp. 156–169) and DD form (pp. 369–370). It is not known whether they exist for MD and OTD form.
4. An encoding stage for aspect ratio (e.g., Figure 2.63A).

This theoretical framework leaves to be explained why normally sighted people seldom report that an object's location is misperceived (see the footnote on page 376). As well, it is necessary to explain why normally sighted people seldom perceive any conflict between the spatial information carried by the five different kinds of contrast. The schematic shown in Figures 7.1 and 7.2 calls for separate registration processes for orientation, size, aspect ratio, and location.

The evidence that each of the five kinds of contrast has its own orientation- and size-tuned spatial filter forces us to place the registration process at a later stage than spatial filtering. One function of the cross-connections between the processing of chromatic contrast and luminance contrast (Figures 2.16 and 7.1) might be to maintain in register the information about an object's orientation and size carried by chromatic contrast and luminance contrast. It is not known whether there are corresponding cross-connections for the other three kinds of spatial contrast. *This question could, perhaps, be answered by extending to OTD, MD, and DD form the masking experiments of Switkes et al. (1988) and Mullen and Losada (1994).* A further possibility, illustrated in Figure 7.3, is that spatial information carried by the five kinds of contrast converge before the discrimination stage, thus providing a possibility for holding in register the five kinds of spatial information. As mentioned earlier, this hypothesis is open to experimental test.

The discussion of Figure 2.63A proposes a possible explanation for the finding that the aspect-ratio aftereffect transfers from a solid sharp-edged rectangle to an outlined ellipse (pp. 174–184) and, furthermore, may account for the common observation that we recognize solid and outlined shapes with equal facility (see the first footnote on page 40).

An explanation for the accurate registration of the five kinds of information about an object's aspect ratio is suggested by the finding that the aspect-ratio aftereffect shows cross-adaptation between LD and DD rectangles (pp. 174–184 and 370–372) and between LD and CD shapes (see second paragraph of footnote on page 177). In terms of Figure 7.1, this finding could be explained if spatial information carried by the five kinds of contrast converges to some extent before the "aspect-ratio processing " stage in Figure 7.2.

A final point on the boundary registration problem. It is true that luminance contrast has a unique advantage in encoding the boundary of sharp-edged, high-contrast, solid targets. Such boundaries stimulate narrow LD filters, so that the boundary can be defined more precisely by LD contrast than for the other four kinds of contrast. However, the suggestion that luminance contrast generally overrides the other four kinds of contrast in encoding boundary location (Gregory, 1977; Gregory & Heard, 1979; Livingstone & Hubel, 1984; Yeh et al., 1992) seems not to be valid except, perhaps, in the special case just described. Rivest and Cavanagh (1996) concluded that, when its special advantage of high resolution at high contrast is removed, luminance contrast does not play an over-riding role in the encoding of boundary location. In particular, they found that the precision of contour localization is better for a boundary defined by luminance plus other forms of contrast than for a boundary defined by luminance contrast alone. This conclusion is in accord with the finding that Vernier step threshold is lower for a Vernier target defined by disparity contrast plus luminance contrast than for a target defined by luminance contrast alone (Morgan, 1986), and the finding that Vernier step threshold is lower for a target defined by texture contrast plus luminance contrast than for a target defined by luminance contrast alone (Gray & Regan, 1997).

APPENDIX A

Systems Science and Systems Analysis

Signal Analysis Is Not Systems Analysis

Students are sometimes puzzled by scientific reports whose authors seem to assume that, because the temporal-frequency domain description of any given signal can be derived from the time-domain description of that signal (and vice versa), and because the spatial-frequency domain description of any given pattern of luminance can be derived from the spatial description of that luminance distribution (and vice versa), then it necessarily follows that a similarly unique equivalence holds between the inputs and outputs of a system. An egregious example of this line of thought is offered in electrophysiology by authors who assume that the temporal frequency characteristic of the electrical response of the human brain can be predicted theoretically by calculating the Fourier transform of the brain's response to a flash of light. And in psychophysics, some authors fail to point out why psychophysical responses to an arbitrary two-dimensional isolated target (a *spatial transient*) are not *necessarily* straightforwardly predictable from a knowledge of psychophysical responses to sinusoidal gratings. (Empirical evidence shows that, in general, they most certainly are not; see pages 171–184.)

"One size fits all" predictability at this elementary level holds only for linear systems and, even in small-signal conditions (e.g., at contrast detection threshold), the visual system falls far short of obeying the linearity criteria set out on

385

page 391. Figure E.2 shows that even a grossly nonlinear neuron whose behavior approximates that of a rectifier (see Figure A.5) can mimic linear behavior under small-signal conditions. And some favored psychophysical procedures such as adaptation and masking owe their effectiveness to nonlinear behavior (see requirement #2 on p. 391, and Figure 2.15).

The role of signal analysis

In the context of visual psychophysics the chief role of signal analysis is the description of the input to the visual system, i.e., the description of the visual stimulus. When physiological methods such as evoked electrical or magnetic fields are used to study the visual system as a whole, signal analysis commonly takes on two additional roles: analysis of the system's outputs, and output data reduction. Although attempts to analyze the visual system's output are rare in psychophysical research, there are a few examples, including Crawford's (1947) classic study of the time course of excitability following a brief stimulus flash.

The typical stimulus used by psychophysical researchers who study spatiotemporal vision is one of the following: a temporal variation of luminance, i.e., a time series; a spatial variation of luminance, i.e., a spatial pattern; a combination of the two.

Basis functions

Signal analysis allows a stimulus to be specified as the linear sum of a few *basis functions*. In signal analysis there are several criteria for choosing a particular set of basis functions including: (1) orthogonality; (2) ease of mathematical manipulation; (3) a well-developed mathematical basis, and a literature on applications to the solution of many different problems; (4) ease of computation with available equipment.

There are two main classes of basis functions. The first class is fixed basis functions that do not depend on the signal to be analyzed. They include sine/cosine (Fourier), Gabor, Cauchy, Walsh, Haar, polynomial, and Bessel functions. The second class of basis functions depends on the signal to be analyzed, and can be created by multivariate procedures such as principal component analysis. A hybrid approach is also possible.

The sine/cosine pair used in Fourier analysis* has the following features: orthogonality; mathematical manipulation is convenient; the mathematical basis of Fourier analysis is well-developed; and there is an enormous literature on the application of Fourier methods to the analysis of time series and spatial patterns.

---

* Fourier's masterpiece did not have an easy birth. During the French Revolution and the period of the Terror, Fourier's outspoken criticisms of public officials led to the issue of a decree in 1794 demanding his arrest and summary guillotining, and he was actually in prison on July 28, 1794, when Robespierre was arrested and executed. Fourier was released during the subsequent general amnesty. His mathematical work was again interrupted in 1798 when he was appointed secrétaire perpétual of the Scientific Institut d'Egypte by Napoleon who, on departing Egypt in 1799 to become First Consul, left Fourier responsible for virtually all nonmilitary affairs including being leader of an expedition to investigate

The description of a signal in the time domain is completely equivalent to its description in the temporal-frequency domain. The same holds for the descriptions of a spatial pattern in the spatial and spatial-frequency domains. In the time domain, the forward Fourier transform allows the temporal-frequency domain description of a signal to be obtained from the time-domain description of that signal, while the inverse Fourier transform allows the time-domain description of any given signal to be obtained from the temporal-frequency domain description of that signal (Aseltine, 1958; Bracewell, 1965; Hsu, 1970; Papoulis, 1962). Forward and inverse Fourier transforms, respectively, can also be used to go from the spatial domain to the spatial-frequency domain description of a spatial pattern and back again.

It is remarkable that a formal attempt to reconcile the total exclusiveness of the time domain and the frequency domain in the context of the theory of communication was not published until Gabor's (1946) paper. Gabor traced his line of thought back to early work on quantum mechanics and especially to Heisenberg's principle of indeterminacy, published in 1927. This principle states that there is a tradeoff between the precisions with which we may know simultaneously the momentum and the location of a particle. From Heisenberg's insight, Pauli was able to redefine observable physical quantities in such a way that the uncertainty relationship between them appears as a direct consequence of the mathematical identity $\Delta f \Delta t = K$, where Δf is the uncertainty in the frequency of a sinusoidal oscillation of duration Δt, and K is a constant that depends on how we define the uncertainty Δf. (If we define Δf as follows, then $K = 1$. Consider the amplitude spectrum of a sinusoidal oscillation of duration Δt; Δf is the distance between the two zero crossings on either side of the central lobe, see Figure B.7A.) The equation $\Delta f \Delta t = 1$ implies that the maximum possible frequency resolution in the power spectrum of a sinusoidal oscillation of duration Δt is Δt^{-1}, and that no recording device can ever transcend this limitation. Thus. the maximum resolution in the spectrum of a 1.0 second sample of a sinusoidal oscillation is 1.0 Hz, so that if one wishes to clearly separate two frequencies that differ by only 1.0 Hz, it is necessary to record for more than 1.0 seconds. The uncertainty relationship $\Delta f \Delta t = 1$ has, perhaps, received less attention in the vision research literature than its significance deserves. As originally stated, the equation reconciles the time and temporal frequency domains, but an analogous relationship exists between the uncertainty of in the spatial frequency of a sinewave grating and the spatial width of that grating. A minimally mathematical discussion of this and related issues is

---

and document the monuments of upper Egypt. After Fourier's return to France, Napoleon refused to let such a diplomatic talent be wasted on education and research and in 1802 appointed him as Préfect of Isère. It was in the time he could spare from his onerous duties that he indulged his interest in mathematics. He had developed the analytic method named for him by 1807 but, due to severe problems with peer reviewers, his method was not published until 1822 (in book form), and the original 235-page handwritten manuscript was not published in full until 1972, 165 years after submission (Gratton-Guiness, 1972).

given in Regan (1989b, pp. 34–39 and 98–108). Formal treatments are available in Gabor (1946), Thrane (1979, 1980), and Jenkins and Watts (1968).

Among the several issued discussed by Gabor in his 1946 paper was how to achieve the optimal compromise in the unavoidable tradeoff between the precision with which a signal is defined simultaneously in temporal frequency (Δf) and in time (Δt). He stated that Gaussian signals provide the best compromise, because the product of their uncertainties in time and frequency is a minimum. This is also the case when a Gaussian waveform is multiplied by a sine or a cosine. Marceltja (1980) extrapolated this pair of orthogonal time-domain functions to the spatial domain (see Figure 2.49). Some researchers have used spatial Gabor functions as visual stimuli in psychophysical studies on the grounds of their compromise between localization in space and localization along the spatial-frequency axis.

Klein and Levi (1985) discuss the orthogonal pair of basis functions called the symmetrical and antisymmetrical Cauchy functions (see Figure 2.50). They go on to argue for their superiority over Gabor functions as stimuli in visual psychophysics.*

First, note that neither Walsh nor Haar functions are merely a pair of square waves with 90 degree phase difference. Beauchamp (1975) reviews Walsh and Haar functions and their applications and compares these two kinds of analysis with Fourier analysis. Walsh functions involve only two states (+1 and –1), thus matching the internal symbolism of digital computers, and yet possess many of the attractive manipulative properties of the sine and cosine series. The functions form a complete orthonormal set. Each function has a constant amplitude (+1 or –1), but a variable mark-to-space ratio. Each functions is defined over a limited time interval called a time base.

Haar functions were described by A. Haar in 1910. These functions can represent any given waveform to a high degree of accuracy with only a few constituent terms. The functions form a complete orthonormal set. Each function has three possible states (0, +A, and –A), where the magnitude of A is a function of $\sqrt{2}$. Unlike the Walsh functions, the amplitude of a Haar function varies with its place in the series.

Certain polynomials can be rendered orthogonal by multiplying by a weighting factor. These orthogonal polynomials consist of a series $f_n(x)$ ($n = 0,1,2\ldots$), where n is the degree of the polynomial. This class includes many special func-

---

* Note that their argument applies to system analysis rather than signal analysis. Although all orthonormal sets of basic functions are equivalent in linear systems analysis, when studying a nonlinear system (such as the visual system) one particular set may provide greater insight [see Regan (1991a) and Westheimer (1998) for a discussion of this point]. Ideally, the basis functions used in psychophysics or physiology should match the properties of the physiological mechanism(s) being studied. Note, however, that mathematical methods, signal analysis machines, and software packages that are designed for the study of human-designed systems may not be the best choice for studying the visual pathway. (See pp. 399–401.)

tions commonly encountered in practical engineering, for example Chebychev, Hermite, Laguerre, Jacobi, and Legende polynomials (Beauchamp, 1975).

Bessel introduced the functions named for him in 1824. The function $J_n(z)$, known as "Bessel's function of the first kind of order n and argument z" may be defined as follows:

$$J_n(z) = \frac{1}{2\pi} \int_0^{2\pi} \cos(n\theta - z\sin\theta)d\theta \qquad\qquad \text{(A.1)}$$

(McLaughlan, 1961, pp. 1–7)

The Bessel function of order zero (i.e., $n = 0$) resembles a damped cosine curve. The curve is not strictly periodic. If z is a radius in polar coordinates, the resulting circularly symmetric Bessel function takes the form of a set of circular bars (Figure 2.58A). Kelley (1960) introduced to psychophysics the use as visual stimuli of Bessel functions of order zero (see the footnote on the previous page).

Fourier methods, along with the Gabor and all the other functions just discussed, came to vision research from physics and mathematics already fully developed. The difference of Gaussians (DOG) stimulus (Figure 1.21), however, had a different history (see pp. 53–60). Rather than being chosen for its mathematical properties, this stimulus was originally introduced as a quantitative description of the Mexican-hat sensitivity profile of cat retinal ganglion cells (Rodieck, 1965; Rodieck & Stone, 1965a,b). Figure 1.22A,B shows examples of DOG stimuli.

Human-Designed Systems: Linear Systems and the Wide and Wild World of Nonlinear Systems

People who live in industrial countries base many of their expectations and demands on the assured linear performance of a wide variety of systems. Even though no physical system is truly linear, human engineers respond to these demands by designing systems whose behavior is approximately linear over the range of input or output amplitudes that is adequate for the system's purpose. But for many requirements of industrialized humankind, linear systems are useless. Such requirements can only be fulfilled by using a system whose behavior is nonlinear. Although there is only one kind of linear behavior, the number of kinds of nonlinear behavior is indefinitely large. Nonlinear behavior is even more crucial to the effective operation of systems that are not designed by human engineers—biological systems.

Human-designed systems: Functional versus structural analysis

I will first briefly review the analysis and functional characterization of human-made systems before drawing attention to some features of biological systems that raise the question whether analytic approaches that are valid for human-made systems are necessarily entirely valid for biological systems.

We can represent a human-made system as shown in Figure A.1. In general, the system will have many inputs and many outputs (at least some of which may be recordable responses).

The first step in studying a system is to compare the system's output with its input for a variety of inputs. Our aim is to identify the function F in Equation (A.2).*

$$O_i(t) = F[I_1(t), I_2(t), \ldots, I_n(t)] \qquad (A.2)$$

Equation (A.2) indicates that, in general, any given output (O_i) may depend on every one of the n inputs and that any or all of the dependencies may be nonlinear.

The point of this endeavor is that, given F, we can predict the outputs of the system for any arbitrary input. In that sense we *understand* the system even though we may have no idea how the system functions. In many contexts this complete predictability of behavior may be quite adequate and a knowledge of how the system achieves this function, obtained through a structural analysis of the system, may well be unnecessary.

To illustrate this point, consider a particular system: an electronic pulse sequence generator. To know that it will generate a particular sequence of pulses when appropriately triggered is an elementary level of understanding that, nevertheless, may be adequate for many purposes. Hidden within the black chips and little metal cans of such an electronic system there are many interconnected solid-state circuit elements. The physics of these elements is not simple (Kittel, 1953), and only a small fraction of those who use the device have a firm understanding of the basic solid-state physics. (Forty years ago the circuit elements of a pulse sequence generator were vacuum tubes, resistors, and capacitors, often in plain view, and to that extent reassuringly familiar and seemingly less mysterious than whatever is hidden within a chip. But the physics of the vacuum tube is not all that simple either!) To pursue this metaphor further, the function of the pulse generator *as a unit* is, by the designer's intent, rather independent of the properties of the components that, together, do the job. Indeed, if all one saw were the input and output terminals of an electronic pulse sequence generator, one might

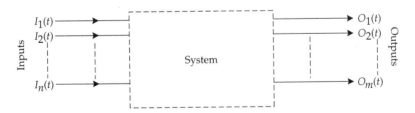

A.1 A system with multiple inputs and multiple outputs.

---

* In mathematics, a function is an operator or operation which, applied to a number, yields a number. Thus function F applied to the instantaneous numerical values of inputs $I_1, I_2, \ldots, I_n$ at time t yields the value of output O_i at time t. The distinguished philosopher Quine (1987) is illuminating on this and on many other related points.

not know or even care whether the active elements were solid-state semiconductor junctions or glowing vacuum tubes. Suppose, for example, that an eighteenth century clockmaker, miraculously transported to the present day were given the components of a radio set, a circuit diagram, wiring instructions, and all necessary tools. He might well construct a working receiver, and even go on to establish a successful business, making hand-crafted radios. But without further instruction the operation of the radio would remain magical to the clockmaker. Understanding the functional principle demands a knowledge of resonant circuits, heterodyning, feedback-controlled amplification, automatic gain control, and other abstract concepts that are not given by familiarity with, or even understanding of, the circuit elements. *One "understands" a radio in terms of these intermediate-scale functions and, at this functional level of understanding, a vacuum-tube radio and a solid-state radio are rather similar.* Our eighteenth century clockmaker's attention would focus on the circuit elements. His failure in understanding would be a failure to "see" the radio at an abstract level in terms of functional subunits, an abstract level that *without a knowledge of the purpose of the system* is exceedingly difficult to relate to the physical structure of the radio that is visible to the eye. This discussion is intended to bring out the significance of "purpose" or "goal" in the formal definition of "system" (see footnote on page 26).

Linear systems

A system or part of a system is said to behave *linearly* if the relation between its output and its input obey the following requirements:

1. If input I_a produces output O_a and input I_b produces output O_b, then input $(I_a + I_b)$ produces output $(O_a + O_b)$. (This requirement is sometimes called the superimposition requirement.)
2. The output does not depend on the previous history of input. (This is called an instantaneous or zero-memory system.)
3. The output does not depend on the time at which the input is applied. (This is called time invariance [Bracewell, 1965, p. 185]).

Any system that does not obey these requirements is said to be nonlinear (Bracewell, 1965, pp. 185–186).

> The crucial point about linear behavior is that the same method of linear systems analysis can be used with any linear system, be the system electronic, mechanical, hydraulic, acoustical, optical, or whatever.*

A very convenient feature of linear system behavior is that, if a sinusoidal input is applied to a linear system and the amplitude and phase of the steady-state output is recorded over the range of input frequencies that produce an output, then the time-domain output produced by a single input pulse or any other transient waveform can be computed by means of the inverse Fourier transform. (The converse calculation

---

* A minimally mathematical discussion of a minimum phase shift linear system is provided in Regan (1989a, pp. 2–5).

can be carried out by means of the forward Fourier transform.) Furthermore, the minimum possible phase shift produced by any linear system can be calculated if the effect of input frequency on output amplitude is known (Aseltine, 1958; Bracewell, 1965).

For these reasons, engineers often find ways of applying linear systems analysis to real physical systems, even though no physical system is perfectly linear. For example, many physical systems whose behavior is quite nonlinear when the input or output amplitude is large, nevertheless behave approximately linearly over a limited range of input amplitudes, and linear systems analysis is approximately valid over that range. A coil spring provides a familiar example of this point. The relation between the length of the spring and the compressive force applied to it may be tolerably linear, but only up to the point that the individual coils hit each other. If approximately linear behavior is required, the engineering design should constrain the system to operate always within the approximately linear range. A system of this kind that behaves linearly provided that the range of input (or output) variation is restricted is called *piecewise linear* (DiStefano et al., 1967, pp. 46–47).

It is easy to think of example of systems whose approximately linear behavior becomes, either abruptly or gradually, nonlinear as the input (or output) amplitude grows large. But the approximately linear behavior of some systems becomes strongly nonlinear when the amplitude of the input signal becomes too *low*. A psychophysical illustration of this point is that the visual processing of the expansion of a small target becomes strongly nonlinear when the target's trajectory simulates a direction of motion that just grazes the observing eye. Our proposed explanation for this finding was that the retinal image of one edge of the target is stationary for that particular trajectory, and that a plot of detector output versus retinal image speed for a local motion detector becomes strongly nonlinear in the immediate vicinity of zero speed (Regan & Beverley, 1980).

We found that the effect of this nonlinearly could be abolished (so that the system operated linearly) by adding a small amount of positional jitter to the target's motion. Interestingly, the amplitude and temporal frequency of the optimal jitter were about the same as that produced by the jitter of eye fixation that occur in everyday life when the head is not on a bite bar (Regan & Beverley, 1980). This procedure for reducing the effect of this kind of nonlinearly is called *linearizing*, and is used very widely to improve the performance of man-made devices such as magnetic tape recorders and servo-operated mechanical controls. Physiological examples of linearizing are discussed in Appendix E.

So far I have discussed systems that obey the superimposition requirement with respect to a particular input variable over some finite range of that variable, and whose linear behaviour degrades more or less gradually as the range is extended. On finding that a system obeys linearity requirement #1, a researcher might be lulled into a false sense of certitude and confidence, and might even be tempted to label the system "linear." But requirement #1 is only one of the linearity requirements. Many kinds of animals roam the field of vision research, some of whom are by no means as tamely linear as our hypothetical researcher might wish them to be, and indeed how they superficially seem to be. An example of this potential pitfall is provided by Figure 4 in Regan et al. (1975). This shows a physiological response that, over a considerable range of the input variable, obeyed linearity requirement #1 tolerably well in near-equilibrium static conditions. But in a nonstatic situation, the response exhibited gross deviations from all three linearity requirements. This dramatic dynamic nonlinearity included a large dependence on the starting point. I well remember how we were startled to see how a physiological system could show such exceedingly different natures in different situations. It was as though one had picked up a kitten and found it transformed into a rattlesnake. And the same transformation could be reproduced time and again.

The creation of a linear system from nonlinear parts

A simple illustration of how engineers can build an active* system using a grossly nonlinear system element follows. In Figure A.2 the system element AE is a voltage-amplifying element. We assume that a plot of output voltage versus input voltage for element AE is monotonic, though it may be grossly nonlinear. However, the system within the dashed box is almost perfectly linear. Linear behavior is achieved by negative feedback: a fraction (β) of the output voltage (V_O) is inverted and fed back to the input. Therefore, the input to AE is ($V_I - \beta V_O$). The open loop gain (A) of AE is defined as $V_O/(V_I - \beta V_O)$. By definition, the gain (G) of the system within the dotted box is V_O/V_I. It follows that $G = A/(1+A\beta)$ so that, if $A\beta >> 1$, $G \approx 1/\beta$. The fraction β can be set by high-stability resistors. Thus, the negative feedback creates a linear amplifier (Fink. 1975).†

Note that the linear behavior is created by the connectivity within the system enclosed within the dashed box; this linearly is a *system properly* that cannot be assigned any discrete location within the system (see the second footnote on page 29).

> The above is only one of many possible illustrations that different kinds of feedback can create system properties that are not intuitively obvious and, importantly, are not revealed by inspection of the structure of the system unless one has prior knowledge of the purpose of the system and a mathematical understanding of its principle of operation.

And if we would try to investigate this behavior in reductionist style by cutting the system into pieces, the act of cutting may well destroy the very property

---

* An *active system* contains a power source whereas a *passive system* does not.

† We assume that the phase shift within the feedback loop is negligible. In particular, if there is appreciable time delay within the feedback loop the feedback, though negative at low frequencies, can become positive at some higher frequency where the phase shift is exactly one-half cycle; the circuit will tend to oscillate at that frequency.

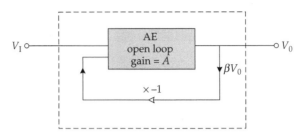

A.2 The use of negative feedback to create a linear amplifier from a nonlinear amplifying element AE.

we seek to study.* Graeme et al. (1971) offer illustrations of this point in the context of man-made artifacts, while Milsum (1965) gives biological examples.

Quite apart from the point just discussed, it is, in principle, possible that, by placing in sequence two nonlinear elements whose nonlinearities are equal and opposite, a system that obeys linearity requirement #1, and even obeys all three linearity requirements, might result. For example, the effect of some particular nonlinearity in the visual system might be cancelled by a second nonlinearity in the motor system, so that the combined eye–hand system behaved linearly.

The sequence of subsystems within a system

Consider the system depicted in Figure A.3 that consists of a sequence of three different subsystems A, B, and C, all of which are linear. A study of the system as a whole using methods of functional analysis (by comparing $O(t)$ with $I(t)$) will show that the system as a whole is linear. But without access to points inside the system it is not possible to establish the different properties of the three subsystems, nor their sequence, nor even the presence of the three subsystems (Jenkins & Watts, 1968, p. 45).

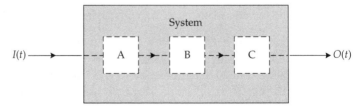

A.3 A system that consists of three sequential linear subsystems.

---

* Furthermore, ". . . it may, in fact, be illusory to think that the smaller the pieces into which a system is dissected the better we will understand it" (Marmarelis & Marmarelis, 1978, p. 5).

The situation is different for certain simple nonlinear systems. Suppose, for example, subsystem B is a zero-memory rectifier, while subsystems A and C are linear (a so-called sandwich or LNL system). In the context of electrophysiology, Spekreijse (1966, 1969) showed that the sequence of the three subsystems could be demonstrated and their individual characteristics established (see also Spekreijse & Oosting, 1970; Spekreijse & Reits, 1982; Korenberg & Hunter, 1986). A similar nonlinear systems analysis approach was subsequently adopted in psychophysical studies (Regan & Beverley, 1980, 1981).

More generally, by recording nonlinear cross-modulation components up to high (e.g., the tenth) orders, the characteristics and sequence of multiple nonlinear stages can be established, even when the inputs are initially processed in parallel, as in binocular vision (M. P. Regan and D. Regan, 1988, 1989a). In the context of physiological systems, when compared with the well-known white noise (time domain) method of nonlinear systems analysis (Marmarelis & Marmarelis, 1978), this frequency domain approach has the advantage of being considerably more resistant to physiological noise.

Nonlinear behavior

Although any linear system can be analyzed by the same method of linear systems analysis, there is no single method of analysis that can be applied to all nonlinear systems. For nonlinear systems, the method of analysis depends on the type of nonlinear behavior. And the number of different kinds of possible nonlinear behavior is indefinitely large. For the engineer, this offers an indefinitely large range of nonlinear behaviors to be exploited—while at the same time challenging him or her with mathematical and conceptual problems that are seldom straightforward and may even exceed the competence of any living mathematician.

Next, I will discuss several kinds of nonlinear behavior that are familiar to engineers, and point out their relevance for understanding biological systems.

Nonessential nonlinearities.

The behavior of a nonessential nonlinearity approximates linear behavior more and more closely as the amplitude of the input signal is progressively reduced.

In Figure A.4A–D, the heavy lines are the input–output characteristic of nonlinear (parts B–D) systems and a linear (part A) system. The input to any given system is plotted along the x-axis, and the output is plotted along the y-axis. Parts B and C show that the waveform distortion (clipping) that is evident when the peak-to-peak amplitude of the input is large (B) is largely eliminated when the peak-to-peak amplitude of the input is small (C), so that the system's behavior approximates that of a linear system (A). Part D illustrates a different kind of waveform distortion to that shown in part B. This kind of distortion also is largely eliminated when the input signal is small.

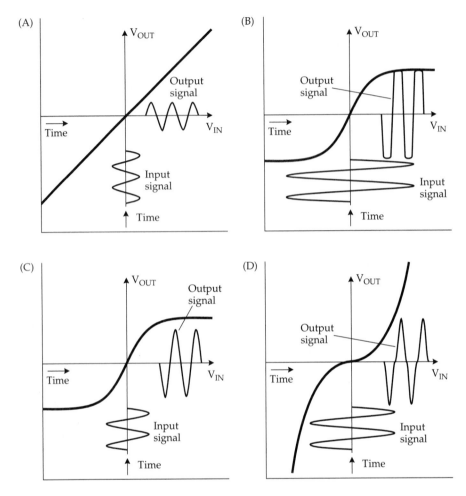

A.4 Example of a nonessential nonlinearity. The input to the system is plotted along the *x*-axis and the system's output is plotted along the *y*-axis. (A) The input-output behavior of a linear system. This behavior is independent of the amplitude of either the input or the output signal. A compressive nonlinearity produces a distorted output when fed by a sinewave whose peak-to-peak amplitude is large (B), but distortion is much less when the amplitude of the input signal is small (C). (D) A different kind of large-signal distortion from that illustrated in part B.

Nonessential nonlinearity can be understood at an intuitive level in terms of smooth curvature of the input–output characteristics. In Figure A.4B,C, as the input sinusoid traverses a shorter and shorter segment of the input–output characteristic, so does the segment traversed more and more closely approximate a straight line. (This is called small-signal conditions.)

The input–output characteristic of retinal cones is one familiar example of the class of compressive characteristics that behaves as illustrated in Figure A.4B,C. There is evidence that the shape of the cone characteristic causes a sinusoidal grating of high contrast to look nonsinusoidal, i.e., as illustrated in Figure A.4B. The characteristic generates higher harmonic components, so that an observer who adapts to a high-contrast sinusoidal grating is adapting visual pathway neurons that prefer higher harmonics of the stimulus grating's spatial frequency in addition to neurons who prefer the grating's spatial frequency (Maudarbocus & Ruddock, 1973).

Essential nonlinearities. The point on the input–output characteristic addressed by the mean value of the input is called the *operating point*. In Figure A.4A–D the operating point is at the origin. In Figure A.5A the operating point is marked *a*. An input of large amplitude gives a distorted output (asymmetric about zero in this case) but, just as in Figure A.4A–D, the output becomes progressively less distorted as the peak-to-peak amplitude of the input signal is progressively reduced (Figure A.5B). The explanation is the same, as in Figure A.4. Figure A.5C,D shows that, when the operating point is centered on the discontinuous change of slope, the output remains distorted even for very small amplitudes of the input signal (see the footnote on page 140).

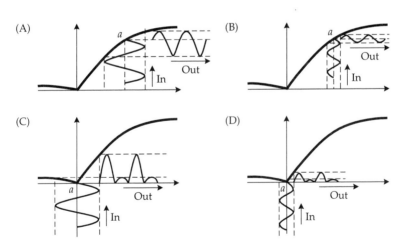

A.5 Example of an essential nonlinearity. The input to the system is plotted as abscissa and the output is plotted as ordinate. The heavy curve is the system's input–output characteristic. Parts A and B show that, when the operating point *a* is located so that the input waveform never crosses the abrupt change of slope in the characteristic, the waveform distortion seen when the peak-to-peak amplitude of the input is large (A) is almost eliminated when the peak-to-peak amplitude is small (B). Parts C and D show that, when the operating point is centered on the abrupt change in the slope of the characteristic, the output is strongly distorted for small as well as for large peak-to-peak amplitude of the input signal.

A nonlinearity whose behavior does not progressively approach linear behavior as the peak-to-peak amplitude of the input is progressively reduced is called an essential nonlinearity. Essential nonlinearities include rectification, multiplication, and division.

In practical vision research the simple concept illustrated in Figure A.5C,D is complicated by the fact that small amounts of noise at the input to a rectifier can cause the neuron to behave approximately linearly for small signals. That is, the noise can "mask" the nonlinearity (van der Tweel, 1961). Figure E.2 illustrates this phenomenon in the case of a retinal ganglion cell. The phenomenon, called linearizing, has been studied in the context of the visual system by Spekreijse (see Appendix E).

A static zero-memory rectifier is a nonlinear system element familiar to engineers. As discussed on pp. 420–422, an amplitude-modulated waveform can be demodulated by a rectifier. The crystal in a radio "crystal set" of the early 1920s was such a rectifier. Another example: for low-loss distribution of electrical power over long distances it is necessary to use voltages as high as one million; to allow these voltages to be efficiently reduced to safe values it is necessary to use AC rather that DC. But many domestic devices require DC. The conversion from AC to DC is achieved by a "DC power supply" built from four rectifiers that form a part of very many domestic appliances.

In biology there are many example of subsystems that, to some extent, function like a rectifier. For example, rectifier-like behavior has been identified in the human visual system (Spekreijse & van der Tweel, 1965) and, at single-unit level, in the retinae of goldfish, monkeys and other animals—see Appendix E. The auditory hair cell transducer function resembles a rectifier (Hudspeth, 1983). (Without this early rectifier stage, membrane capacitance would restrict our range of hearing to low frequencies.) And the use of systems science in physiological studies of Y cells led to a model in which the Y cells' receptive field contains many parallel rectifiers, rectifiers that correspond to inputs from simple cells. (Here the rectifier property corresponds to the fact that, though a simple cell can fire at different positive rates, it cannot fire at a negative rate [Hochstein & Shapley, 1976; Victor & Shapley, 1979].) Rectifiers are used widely in visual psychophysics to model the ON and OFF retinal subsystems (see pp. 93–98, 256–258, and Figure 4.12).

Gain control. Among the many annoying features of early radio sets was that the loudness varied as the strength of the radio signal varied. Modern sets are fitted with automatic gain control. After the user has set the volume control to achieve the desired loudness, a circuit within the radio set alters its gain so as to maintain the desired loudness in the face of fluctuations in the amplitude of the carrier wave arriving at the radio's input. It has been proposed that an approximation to the behavior of some biological subsystems can be modeled as automatic gain control For example, if firing is regarded as a output and spatial contrast as input, the characteristic of many neurons in the magnocellular layers of the primate lateral geniculate nucleus has a steep slope at low contrasts and flattens at higher contrasts. There is evidence that the ambient level of contrast shifts this characteristic along the contrast axis so as to center the steep section of the characteristic at the local ambient contrast level (Ohzawa et al., 1982). Psychophysical and objective evidence for contrast gain control in human vision is reviewed on pages 83–91.* A psychophysical study of the relevance of local gain control to the perception of spatially sampled targets is reviewed on pp. 470–476.

Memory and hysteresis. If a response of a system to an input applied at time t depends on inputs applied before time t, then the system is said to have memory. If past inputs over a finite period of time only are important, then the system is said to have finite memory (Cooper & McGillem, 1967, p. 14). (In psychophysics, adaptation is a commonly encountered effect of this kind.)

One particular kind of memory is called hysteresis. A system is said to exhibit hysteresis when the response to input $I(t_1)$ depends on whether the rate of change of I was positive or negative at $t < t_1$. The manifestations of hysteresis may not be intuitively obvious even in simple nonlinear systems. For example, a system might have more than one possible output for a given input (the jump effect). Nonlinear oscillations in simple human artifacts are shown in Regan, 1989a, Figure 1.6. In physiological systems, the manifestations of hysteresis can be even more dramatic and surprising (e.g., Figures 4-6 in Regan et al., 1975). Formal discussions of nonlinear oscillations and the jump effect are available (Stoker, 1950; Hayashi, 1964; Blaquière, 1966; Hagedorn, 1982).

What is nonlinearity good for? What use is linearity?

A high-quality audio amplifier exhibits remarkably linear behavior. It can transduce the minute fluctuations of power generated by a CD player into large fluctuations of electrical power with very little distortion of the amplitude and phase spectra of the signal leaving the CD player. Many people are willing to pay highly for the linear behavior of such an electronic system.

But in a certain sense, linear systems are "tame" and somewhat boring: both the static and dynamic behavior of a linear system is severely restricted and its range of possible behaviors is narrow (Hirsch & Smale, 1974). As noted by Reichardt and Poggio (1981, p. 187), writing on the topic of neural information processing: "[E]very nontrivial computation has to be essentially nonlinear, that is, not representable (even approximately), by linear operations."

Linear systems are not enough—not even within the highly controlled, artifact-filled environment that (at least in peacetime) the human race devotes great effort to create. Engineers have learned to control and exploit many different

---

* This kind of nonlinear behavior is not restricted to the visual system: There is evidence that the similarly shaped hair cell transducer function behaves analogously, as mean sound intensity changes from moment-to-moment (Hudspeth, 1983).

kinds of nonlinear behavior, though the choice of possibilities has been largely restricted to those that are tolerably well understood at a mathematical level. For example, if it is required that a circuit should rest in one state when the input voltage is below a certain well-defined level and rapidly switch to a second resting state as soon as the input voltage rises above this well-defined level, a linear system is of no value. To achieve such behavior, the engineer ensures that the nonlinearity of the amplifying element AE in Figure A.2 is much exaggerated rather than being eliminated as in the system shown in Figure A.2. The resulting nonlinear electronic system is called a Schmitt trigger. Two Schmitt triggers are used in the window discriminators familiar in single-unit electrophysiology.

The domestic water closet (WC) is a homely example of a particular class of nonlinear system. The system's output triggered by a single movement of a lever (the input) is one cycle of a sawtooth waveform (called a *relaxation oscillation*). And when stimulated with an appropriate forcing frequency (e.g., by a playful cat), a WC can demonstrate forced nonlinear oscillations including an excellent illustration of *entrained subharmonic oscillations* of order $N/2$, $N/3$, etc. Formal treatments of nonlinear forced oscillations are provided in Stoker (1950), Hayashi (1964), and Hagedorn (1982).

To What Extent Are Methods Developed for Studying Human-Designed Systems Valid for the Study of Biological Systems?

Before comparing biological systems with human-designed systems, we should note the following points about human-designed systems. Each is designated with an (H):

1(H). The efforts of engineers to exploit nonlinear behavior has been marked by caution and hesitancy. This caution and hesitancy has been mandated by the requirement to create only those systems whose behavior can reliably and accurately be predicted. The requirement of predictability reflects the requirement that (beyond certain limits) injuries and loss of life are not acceptable consequences of adopting new technologies.*

---

* In 1966 a total of 41,907 people were killed on the roads of the United States and 3.511 million were injured (NHTSA). A comparison with U.S. losses in war conveys a context for the numbers of highway casualties. Throughout the entire Vietnam War approximately 55,000 were killed and died of wounds and about three times that number were wounded; during the three years of the Korean War approximately 25,000 were killed and died of wounds and about three times that number were wounded. Thus, the annual losses on the roads of this medium-sized country are considerably larger than those sustained in a medium-sized war. It is evident that the tolerance of risk associated with a technology is considerably greater for the automobile than for other technologies, such as, for example, commercial aircraft and children's playgrounds. Again, although the tolerable level of deaths and injuries associated with new technologies may be higher when a nation is desperately engaged in a major war, the tolerable level is not much higher.

Although the predictability requirement can be satisfied to an important extent by empirical testing, it is often felt that the system's behavior should be well understood in terms of mathematical analysis and in terms of simulation. The problem here is that only a limited number of the indefinitely large number of kinds of nonlinear systems have been fully analyzed. And the required mathematics may be difficult or even currently intractable.

2(H). Human technology has a history of, at most, a few thousand years.

3(H). Humans design systems by exercising abstract intellectual thought and depend on mathematical analyses and numerical methods that are, at this time, severely limited in their capabilities.

4(H). Human engineers are limited to the principles of physics, materials science, chemistry, and so on that are known during their time.

Next we discuss the corresponding issues for biological systems. Each is designated with a (B).

1(B). The pressure on modern humans to exploit inventiveness in order to create artifacts that will even further improve the level of comfort and quality of life in the industrialized world can hardly be compared with the survival pressures exerted on nonhuman life forms, and especially on those who are a food source for another species. For example, the astonishing achievements of animal flight remained beyond human grasp until the present century. And animal camouflage anticipated our current understanding of spatial vision by, perhaps, hundreds of millions of years.

Evolutionary history is characterized by what, in human terms, is prodigious inventiveness, most dramatically evident in the Cambrian "explosion" of new forms of life some 570 million years ago. As already mentioned, human inventiveness is constrained by the fear that, by using a new technology, even a single individual might suffer injury or death. In contrast, the biological analog of inventiveness is unrestrained by such a consideration—as exemplified by the fierce competitions between the males of many mammalian species that leave the losers outcast, and often grievously injured also. Evolutionary history exhibits what in human terms would be regarded as a callous disregard for life far beyond anything in human history; but it also exhibits an ability to fight on, continuing the innovation of new life forms in the face of catastrophes that dwarf the catastrophes experienced by humans.

"Survival of the fittest" is the well-accepted core of evolutionary doctrine, but how the mutations come about at the right time has always been somewhat of a mystery. But recent findings suggest that (at least in flies) environmental stress (e.g., a large increase of ambient temperature) produces a large increase in the rate of mutations, thus offering a greater chance that one of the mutated organisms will be better adapted to the new environment than the original organism so that life will continue—albeit in a changed form.

Very large numbers of entire species have been lost over evolutionary time. The long-term survival of an entire species seems never to have been assured, and the level of insecurity has at times been very high. There have been five so-called mass extinctions. The late Cretaceous mass extinction some 65 million years ago that famously removed dinosaurs from Earth also eliminated many other life forms, but even that extinction was considerably less severe than the late Permian event of some 225 million years ago, in which an estimated 96% of all marine species were lost (McGhee, 1996).

2(B). Even if we consider only multicellular biological systems, evolution has continued over some 570 million years, compared with a few thousand years during which humans have designed systems.

3(B). However biological systems came to be, it seems unlikely that the process discussed in 3H above provides any useful analogy.

4(B). Obviously, the creation of new biological systems is not affected by restriction 4H.

5(B). The narrative on pages 390–391 brings out the significance of "purpose" or "goal" in the formal definition (see page 26) of a human-designed system. To the extent that it is a valid concept in the context of biological systems, "purpose" may well be unknowable. This thought carries us to the next section.

Levels of Difficulty

Many people have remarked that it is helpful to have a rough idea of the level of difficulty of any given problem before launching a serious attack on that problem. Elementary conceptual tools that are adequate for solving an elementary problem may well be inadequate when one is faced with a conceptually difficult problem. If one has no way of avoiding a physical encounter, it is as well to know whether the encounter will be with an injured and angry kitten or with an injured and angry bear; the necessary methods will be different, and to choose inappropriate methods could be shaming in the first case and fatal in the second.

In vision research, the analysis of physical stimuli (*signal* analysis) requires some acquaintance with such undergraduate-level topics as differential and integral calculus, vector calculus, Fourier analysis, and Bessel functions. The analysis of simple man-made nonlinear *systems* such as an oscillating pendulum, an oscillating cart spring or an oscillating modern bow is more demanding (Hayashi, 1964; Stoker, 1950; Hagedorn, 1982). The analysis of complex man-made nonlinear systems presents a further escalation of conceptual and mathematical difficulty, and may call for mathematical methods that are not yet available.

Although it is difficult to assess the level of difficulty presented by the simpler nonlinear systems that are not man-made (e.g., a living single neuron), the level may well be more severe that that presented by even the most complex system designed by humans. And the functional analysis of the visual system of the brain presents a level of difficulty that is so severe that it cannot be estimated with any confidence. In terms of complexity—even if we focus only on neural firing—the visual system contains more than 10^9 neurons, and each neuron has up to tens of thousands of synapses on its surface. In terms of conceptual difficulty it is not unlikely that areas of physics and mathematics as yet unknown are required for the functional understanding of the visual system. And as already mentioned, although the purpose of a human-designed system is embedded in the formal definition of *system*, "purpose" may not even be a valid concept in the context of biological systems.

A Simplifying Assumption: "Sets of Filters"

Readers who have endured the theoretical discussion of Appendix A to this point and examined Figure A.1 and Equation (A.2) might well feel that to pursue psychophysical research on the human visual system is an intimidating and even foolhardy endeavor. But in the academic context, "philosophy leads to pessimism, research to understanding" (Selverston, 1980, p. 561). The history of research into color vision is instructive. Guild and Wright independently adopted the strategy of progressively simplifying their stimuli until they obtained interpretable results that were similar for different observers. Their final stimulus was a centrally viewed patch of light that was sufficiently small (2 × 1.5 degrees) to fall on a rather homogeneous area of the retina, had no spatial structure when the two halves of the field were matched, and was the only light visible in a dark room (Wright, 1946, 1991). In this same spirit of simplifying a difficult problem to the point where the problem can, in principle, be addressed rationally, and it can be established whether anything useful has been achieved by the simplification, a reduced and special-case version of Figure A.1 is presented as Figure 1.10 and discussed on pp. 30–33.

Outline of Fourier Methods and Related Topics

Fourier Series

Because everyone has grown up with the concept of temporal frequency and because illustrations can be taken from the familiar stuff of everyday life, it is easier to start thinking about Fourier theory in terms of temporal patterns rather than spatial patterns. Furthermore, this approach retraces the historical sequence of Fourier theory development. This too may be helpful for the readers who, as I do, find that the historical approach can aid understanding. My experience is that to see *how a thing came to be* can give a deeper understanding than being provided only with a description of the finished article; and, for me at least, this is the case whether the thing is a human-engineered device* or a mathematical method.

Fourier showed that any waveform that is repeated F times per second can be described as the sum of a series of sinusoids whose frequencies are F Hz, $2F$ Hz,

---

* Twenty years ago, most bicycles looked rather similar. The design seemed to be so obvious that one would not suspect that the first one had been made much differently. But the elegant simplicity of the bicycle's design did not come all of a piece. It slowly evolved through trial and error. At one time dinosaurs ruled the road: the ordinary bicycle (the "penny farthing") was the only design, so it was called simply "the bicycle." Andrew Ritchie's account of how the bicycle evolved to its present form leads to a deeper understanding of why it is as it is than can be attained by looking at one or even by taking one to pieces.

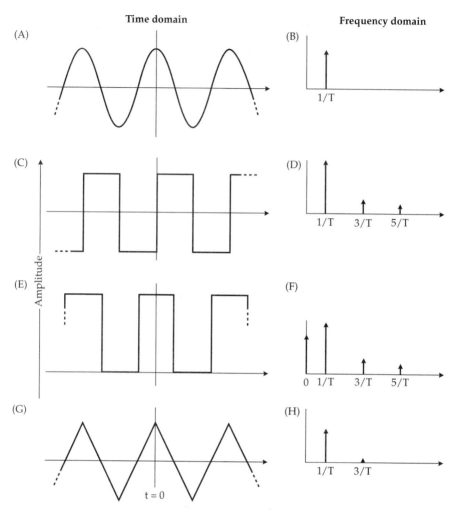

B.1 Time-domain and frequency-domain representations of extremely long repetitive (i.e., periodic) wavetrains. (A, C, E, and G) Time-domain representations of a cosine wave, square wave, positive square-wave pulsetrain, and triangular wave, respectively. If each wavetrain extends very far into past and future time, then their frequency-domain representations are spectra composed of very thin lines as illustrated in Parts B, D, F, and H, respectively. Only the first few harmonic components are shown. From Regan (1989a).

3F Hz, 4F Hz, and so on. Putting this another way, any repetitive waveform of frequency F Hz can be synthesized by adding together a series of sinusoids whose frequencies are given by nF Hz, where n is an integer. The F Hz frequency component is called the *fundamental* or *first harmonic* component, the 2F Hz component is called the second harmonic component, the 3F Hz component is called the *third harmonic* component, and so on. (But Fourier was not using "frequency" in its everyday meaning, and this can lead to confusion.)

There are, of course, an indefinitely large number of different waveforms with the same repetition frequency F Hz, but any one of them can be synthesized by adding together harmonics of exactly the same frequencies F, $2F$, $3F$, and so on. The different waveforms are created by altering the relative amplitudes and/or the relative phases of the individual harmonics. Figure B.1 illustrates this point.

Figure B.1A shows the time-domain representation of a cosine wave of period T seconds and amplitude $y(t)$ that extends infinitely into past and into future time, and Figure B.1B illustrates that in the frequency domain this same wave is represented by an infinitely narrow line. Figure B.1C shows the time-domain representation of a square wave of period T seconds and amplitude $y(t)$ that extends infinitely into past and future time. In the frequency domain, this same wave can be expressed as the sum of an indefinitely large series of sinusoids:

$$y(t) = 4/\pi[\sin(\omega_0 t) + 1/3 \sin(3\omega_0 t) + 1/5 \sin(5\omega_0 t) + \cdots] \qquad (B.1)$$

where $\omega_0 = 2\pi/T$.

Figure B.1D illustrates that the fundamental component of a square wave has a higher amplitude than the fundamental component of a sinusoid of the same amplitude as the square wave (approximately one and one-third times larger). Note that the amplitudes of successive harmonics fall off rapidly, so that a close approximation to the square wave can be obtained with only a few harmonics. The first three are illustrated in Figure B.1D.

The train of square wave pulses in Figure B.1E is always positive rather than being balanced about zero, and is equivalent to the train of square waves in Figure B.1C riding on a constant (DC) term. Accordingly, the Fourier series in Figure B.1F is the same as the series in Figure B.1D plus a zero-frequency (i.e., DC) term.

Figure B.1G,H show, respectively, the time-domain and frequency-domain representations of a triangular wave. The higher harmonics fall off even more rapidly than for a square wave. In this case, the Fourier series is

$$y(t) = 8/\pi^2[\cos(\omega_0 t) + 1/9 \cos(3\omega_0 t) + 1/25 \cos(5\omega_0 t) + \cdots] \qquad (B.2)$$

Figure B.2 tabulates the first few terms of the Fourier series that represent several common waveforms.

Figure B.1 illustrates the crucial property of the transform from time to frequency:

> A repetitive signal that continues for an infinitely long time is equivalent to the sum of discrete, infinitely narrow frequency components, all of which are harmonically related, called a Fourier series.

Fourier went on to show how any complex repetitive waveform can be analyzed into a series of harmonic components. In brief, the nth harmonic is extracted by first multiplying the F Hz repetitive waveform by a sine and a cosine of

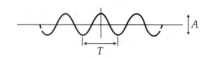

$$\frac{A}{2}\cos wt$$

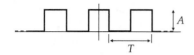

$$\frac{A}{2}+\frac{2A}{\pi}\left[\cos wt-\frac{\cos 3wt}{3}+\frac{\cos 5wt}{5}-\ldots\right]$$

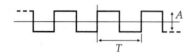

$$\frac{2A}{\pi}\left[\sin wt+\frac{\sin 3wt}{3}+\frac{\sin 5wt}{5}+\ldots\right]$$

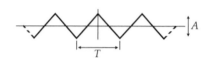

$$\frac{4A}{\pi^2}\left[\cos wt+\frac{\cos 3wt}{3^2}+\frac{\cos 5wt}{5^2}+\ldots\right]$$

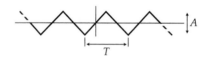

$$\frac{4A}{\pi^2}\left[\sin wt-\frac{\sin 3wt}{3^2}+\frac{\sin 5wt}{5^2}-\ldots\right]$$

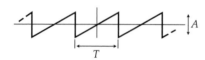

$$\frac{A}{\pi}\left[\sin wt-\frac{\sin 3wt}{3}+\frac{\sin 5wt}{5}-\ldots\right]$$

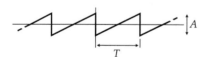

$$-\frac{A}{\pi}\left[\sin wt+\frac{\sin 3wt}{3}+\frac{\sin 5wt}{5}+\ldots\right]$$

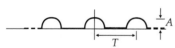

Half-wave rectified cosine wave

$$\frac{A}{\pi}+\frac{A}{2}\cos wt+\sum_{n=1}^{\infty}(-1)^{n+1}\frac{2A\cos 2nwt}{\pi\left(4n^2-1\right)}$$

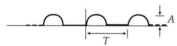

Half-wave rectified sine wave

$$\frac{A}{\pi}+\frac{A}{2}\sin wt-\sum_{n=1}^{\infty}\frac{2A\cos 2nwt}{\pi\left(4n^2-1\right)}$$

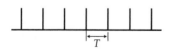

Equally spaced delta
functions of unit area

$$\frac{2}{T}\left[\frac{1}{2}+\cos wt+\cos 2wt+\cos 3wt+\ldots\right]$$

or $$\frac{1}{T}\sum_{n=-\infty}^{n=+\infty}e^{inwt}$$

frequency nF Hz, and then integrating the products over a duration of $1/nF$ seconds, where n is an integer.

Before going on to standard texts that provide a mathematical treatment of Fourier methods, some readers may find it helpful to acquire an intuitive insight into why it is that the Fourier spectrum of an F Hz repetitive waveform can be extracted by multiplying that waveform by sine/cosine pairs. A minimally mathematical explanation is provided next.

Fourier's procedure is explained in Figures B.3–B.5. Figure B.3A shows one cycle of a sine and Figure B.3D shows one cycle of a cosine, each of amplitude 1.0; these are called the reference waveforms. Suppose that the waveform to be analyzed (the test waveform), shown in parts B and E, is a sine wave of amplitude S with exactly the same frequency as the reference waveforms. This test

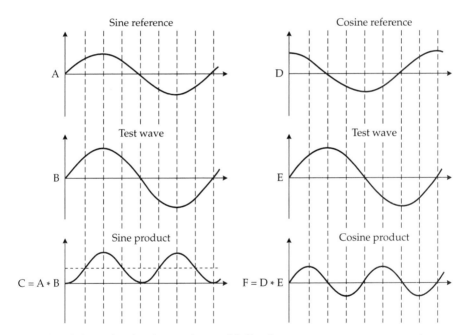

B.3 Signal detection by sine/cosine multiplication. Part A shows the sine reference waveform, and part D shows the cosine reference waveform. The test wave (B and E) is a sine wave with the same frequency as the reference waves. The horizontal dashed line in part C indicates that ordinate-by-ordinate multiplication of parts A and B gives a nonzero product when integrated over one cycle of the reference wave. On the other hand, part F shows that ordinate-by-ordinate multiplication of parts D and E gives a zero product when integrated over one cycle of the reference wave. From Regan (1989a).

◀**B.2 Fourier series for several repetitive (i.e., periodic) waveforms.** Only the first few terms are shown. From Regan (1989a).

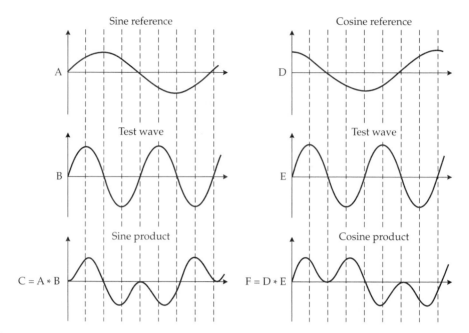

B.4 Selective rejection of harmonics by sine/cosine multiplication. Parts A and D show the sine and cosine reference waveforms. The test signal is a sine wave whose frequency is twice that of the reference waveforms. Part C illustrates that ordinate-by-ordinate multiplication of parts A and B gives zero product when integrated over one cycle of the reference wave, and part F shows that part D times part E also gives a zero integrated product. From Regan (1989a).

waveform (B) is multiplied by the reference sine wave (A), ordinate by ordinate. The product is a waveform (C) that is always positive, because when curve A is positive, curve B is positive, and when curve A is negative, curve B is negative. The waveform shown in part C can be separated into a constant amplitude (horizontal dashed line) plus a sinusoid that is as often positive as negative. Figure B.3A–C illustrates the following equation:

$$S \sin x \sin x = S \sin^2 x = S \left[(1 - \cos 2x)/2 \right] \tag{B.3}$$

where $S \sin x$ is the test waveform and $\sin x$ is the reference sine wave.

The effect of multiplying the same test waveform (E) by the reference cosine (D) is quite different from the effect of multiplication by the reference sine wave. Ordinate-by-ordinate multiplication gives a waveform that is as often negative as it is positive (F), so that over one full cycle of the reference sine wave, the area under the curve in part F is zero; that is, the integral over one full cycle is zero. Figure B.3D–F illustrates the following equation:

$$S \sin x \cos x = (S/2) \sin 2x \tag{B.4}$$

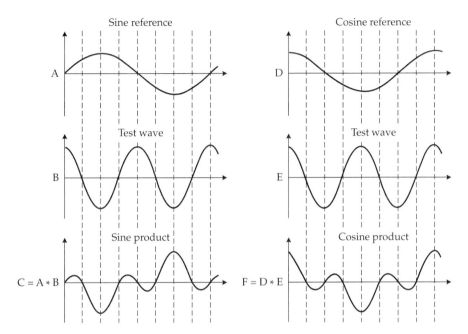

B.5 Selective rejection of harmonics by sine/cosine multiplication. This figure is the same as Figure B.4 except that the test wave is in cosine rather than sine phase. The conclusion is the same. After multiplication, both integrated products are zero (C, F). From Regan (1989a).

It is easy to see that if the phase of the test sine wave is changed by 180° (i.e., the test sine wave is inverted), the steady level in part C merely changes from $+S/2$ to $-S/2$, and the area under the curve in part F remains zero. The crucial point is that the area under the curve is not zero in part C; the mean level is equal to half the amplitude of the test wave in part B.

Now we consider the case in which the waveform to be analyzed is a cosine of amplitude S, and of exactly the same frequency as the reference sine and cosine. We have already seen that the result of multiplying a cosine by a sine wave is a sinusoid of frequency $2x$ that integrates to zero over one full cycle of the reference wave. On the other hand, the result of multiplying the test cosine wave by the reference cosine is a waveform that is always positive and never negative, because when the test is positive the reference is positive, and when the test is negative the reference is negative. This waveform can be separated into a constant amplitude and a sinusoid, just as in the case of Figure B.3C. This case can be understood in terms of the following equation:

$$S \cos x \cos x = S \cos^2 x = S\,[(1 + \cos 2x)/2] \qquad (B.5)$$

Again, it is easy to see that if the test wave is inverted by changing its phase by 180°, the steady level merely changes from +S/2 to –S/2, and the area under the curve in part F remains zero.

This takes us to the case of a test sinusoid $y = S \sin(x - \phi)$ that has exactly the same frequency as the reference waves, but whose phase (ϕ) is arbitrary. We write the familiar trigonometrical relation

$$\sin(A - B) = \sin A \cos B - \cos A \sin B \tag{B.6}$$

as

$$S \sin(x - \phi) = S(\sin x \cos \phi - \cos x \sin \phi) \tag{B.7}$$

$$= A\, sin\, x - B\, cos\, x$$

It follows from Pythagoras' theorem that $(\sin \phi)^2 + (\cos \phi)^2 = 1$. Hence

$$S = \sqrt{A^2 + B^2} \text{ and } \tan \phi = A/B.$$

In words, a test sinusoid of amplitude S and phase ϕ is equal to the sum of a sine and a cosine, and if we can find the amplitudes (A and B) of this sine and cosine, we can calculate the amplitude (S) and phase (ϕ) of the test sinusoid. In fact, we already know how to find amplitudes A and B. If we multiply the test sinusoid by the sine and cosine reference waves, then sine multiplication will give a steady level equal to $A/2$ and cosine multiplication will give a steady level equal to $B/2$, hence giving the amplitude and phase of the test sinusoid.

Fourier went on to consider nonsinusoidal repetitive test waveforms that contained multiple harmonic components. These different harmonic components can be treated one by one. Suppose, for example, that the sine and cosine reference waves are at the fundamental frequency and the test sinusoid is the second harmonic component. Figure B.4 is Figure B.3 redrawn with a second harmonic test sine wave (B and E), and Figure B.5 is Figure B.3 redrawn with a second harmonic test cosine wave (B and E). Figures B.4 and B.5 illustrate that in all four cases, multiplication gives waveforms that integrate to zero over one full cycle of the reference waveforms: the positive and negative areas in Figures B.4 and B.5 cancel both for sine products and for cosine products. It follows that the outputs will also integrate to zero for any arbitrary phase of the test sinusoid. Fourier showed that the same holds for the third harmonic, fourth harmonic, and so on, as can be illustrated visually along the lines of Figures B.4 and B.5; only when test and reference frequencies are equal does integration over one full cycle of the reference wave give a nonzero value.

Rather than this intuitive approach, a more formal approach can be taken via the following well-known trigonometrical equations:

$$\sin(A - B) = \sin A \, \cos B - \cos A \, \sin B \tag{B.8}$$

$$\sin A \sin B = \frac{1}{2}[\cos(A-B) - \cos(A+B)] \qquad (B.9)$$

$$\cos A \sin B = \frac{1}{2}[\sin(A+B) + \sin(B-A)] \qquad (B.10)$$

Suppose that the test waveform is a sinusoid

$$y = S \sin(Nx - \phi) \qquad (B.11)$$

where N is an integer greater than 1, and the reference waveforms are $\sin x$ and $\cos x$. Equation (B.8) implies that the test sinusoid can be synthesized by adding together a sine and a cosine. In particular,

$$y = S \sin(Nx - \phi) = C \sin(Nx) - D \cos(Nx) \qquad (B.12)$$

When the test sinusoid is multiplied by the sinewave reference we have

$$y \sin x = C \sin(Nx) \sin x - D \cos(Nx) \sin x \qquad (B.13)$$

Now, from Equation (B.9)

$$C \sin(Nx) \sin x = C/2[\cos(N-1)x - \cos(N+1)x] \qquad (B.14)$$

and from Equation (B.10)

$$D \cos(Nx) \sin x = D/2[\sin(N+1)x - \sin(N-1)x] \qquad (B.15)$$

Both of these product terms constitute the sum of two sinusoids. Clearly, the same applies when we multiply the test sinusoid by the cosine reference. Thus, if we multiply the harmonic of frequency NF Hz by either a sine wave or a cosine wave of frequency F Hz, then we obtain a mixture of two sinusoids, one at the sum frequency $(NF + F)$ Hz, the other at the difference frequency $(NF - F)$ Hz, and both integrate to zero over one full period (T) of the reference frequency (where $T = 1/F$). A steady (DC) product is obtained only when $N = 1$, so that $\cos(N - 1)x = 1$, the case illustrated in Figure B.3.

Next, a difficult concept: The "temporal frequency" in the spectrum shown in Figure B.1B, D, F, and H is not the familiar temporal frequency of everyday conversation. The "temporal frequencies" plotted as abscissae in Figure B.1B, D, F, and H refer to sinusoidal oscillations that have no end and no beginning in time; they extend infinitely into the past and infinitely into the future. Attempting to visualize such oscillations as a physical reality can lead to despair, for they are theoretical constructs rather than physically realizable entities.

This fact of Fourier theory can be difficult to digest and might cause one to be irritated with Fourier himself for what might seem his deliberate incomprehensibility (until one realizes that the problems encountered by Fourier during his lifetime dwarf one's temporary difficulties with his great legacy (see the footnote on page 386). A way of getting over this barrier is to realize *why* Fourier introduced this concept. His intent was that the time-domain and frequency-domain descriptions of an oscillation should be complementary—that they should, as it were, exist in different worlds. Thus, the sinusoidal oscillation shown in Figure B.1A that exists through infinite time has no location in time, but is specified by an infinitely thin vertical line along the abscissa in the temporal frequency domain description (Figure B.1B). And, conversely, an infinitely short instant in time has an equal representation at every point along the abscissa in the temporal frequency domain from zero to infinite frequency. For example, the power spectrum of an infinitely short click is flat from zero to infinite temporal frequency.

Now we leave the Fourier domain (that exists only in the mind) and return to the physical world. An excellent approximation to the Fourier domain description of a repetitive temporal waveform can be obtained by analyzing the waveform by means of sine/cosine pairs that exist for conveniently short (rather than infinite) periods of time. For example, if a violinist maintained middle C′ for one second, and this was analyzed with sine/cosine pairs of one-second duration, the amplitude and phase spectrum obtained would closely approximate that given in the sixth row of Figure B.2.* Although the harmonic components in the spectrum would not be represented by infinitely thin lines of frequencies 256 Hz, 768 Hz, 1280 Hz, . . ., almost all the power in the first harmonic would lie between 255 and 257 Hz, almost all the power in the third harmonic would lie between 767 and 769 Hz, and so on. If the note had been sustained for duration 10 seconds and it had been analyzed with the sine/cosine pairs of 10 seconds, power in the harmonic would have been even more sharply focussed: 255.9 to 256.1, 767.9 to 768.1, and so on. Admittedly, these are not infinitely thin lines, but they are close enough approximations for many practical purposes.

The approximation can be as close as one desires. For example, a repetitive electrical brain signal evoked by a grating that was counterphase-modulated at a little less than 8 Hz was analyzed by submitting a continuous 640 second sample of the signal to (in effect) multiplication by sine/cosine pairs of 640 second duration (M. P. Regan & D. Regan, 1989a). One of the frequency components had essentially all of its power within a range of 31.822 to 31.824 Hz along the frequency axis, i.e., the power was spread over a range of ±0.001 Hz, that is ±0.003% of the center frequency. This component was very poorly defined in time (within a range of ± 320 seconds) and, correspondingly, it was very precisely defined along the frequency axis: each of the two descriptions lay almost completely within one of Fourier's two complementary worlds.

Now we switch our focus from a repetitive *temporal* variation of some variable to a repetitive *spatial* variation of light intensity. Everything I have said so far about repetitive temporal variations can be said about repetitive spatial varia-

---

* The note emitted by a violin string approximates a sawtooth, because the bow pulls the string sideways until the static frictional force is suddenly overcome and the string snaps back to its original position, and so on in rapid succession.

tions if we substitute space (i.e., distance) for time and spatial frequency for temporal frequency. In particular:

> Any given point location within a spatial pattern contributes to every spatial frequency in the spatial-frequency spectrum of the pattern, while any given single spatial frequency in the spectrum contributes to the description of the entire pattern.

The Fourier Transform

Our next conceptual hurdle follows, as we grapple with the way in which an isolated event in time (as distinct from an infinitely repeated event) is described in the frequency domain. Consider, for example, a single pulse of voltage that has a rectangular shape in time and a duration of T_1 seconds. The frequency-domain description is reached in the following way. Imagine that the pulse is repeated very many times, rather than occurring only once. First suppose that the repetition period (T_2) is equal to the duration of the pulse as illustrated in Figure B.1E and in the second row of Figure B.2. This train of pulses is represented in the frequency domain by the Figure B.1F series of lines of frequency $1/T_2$, $3/T_2$, $5/T_2$, and so on, plus a line at zero frequency representing the mean DC level (see second row in Figure B.2). In our imaginary experiment, the separation of successive harmonics is $2/T_2$ Hz. If the pulse duration T_1 is held constant while the repetition period T_2 is progressively increased, then the separation of successive harmonics will progressively reduce until, as T_2 tends to infinity, the line spectrum becomes a continuous distribution: a continuous plot of amplitude versus frequency and a continuous plot of phase versus frequency. The *forward Fourier transform* converts a once-only temporal waveform (a *temporal transient*) into the frequency domain. The *inverse Fourier transform* converts a frequency-domain description of any given temporal transient (i.e., an amplitude spectrum plus a phase spectrum) into that temporal transient.

To anticipate, Figure B.6 shows the so-called *power spectrum* (actually the amplitude² spectrum) of a bar of fixed width.* Note that the phase spectrum is not shown in Figure B.6: the first zero in the power spectrum is, in fact, a zero-crossing in the amplitude spectrum, i.e., the first lobe has positive amplitude,

---

* To avoid confusion I chose to show a power spectrum in Figure B.6 (and in Figure B.7). Many students are puzzled by the fact that the amplitude spectrum given by the forward Fourier transform consists of two mirror-image sections, one with positive frequencies and one with negative frequencies (e.g., Figure 1.55 in Regan, 1989b). Suppose you wish to generate a cosine function of time. This can be done as follows. At time t = 0 you have two vectors of equal length both pointing along the y-axis. Now you start them rotating at the same angular speed, one rotating clockwise, the other anticlockwise. Their vector sum has an amplitude that varies about zero, following a cosine waveform. The anticlockwise direction of rotation is conveniently regarded as negative, and the clockwise positive (Stuart, 1961, pp. 48–51).

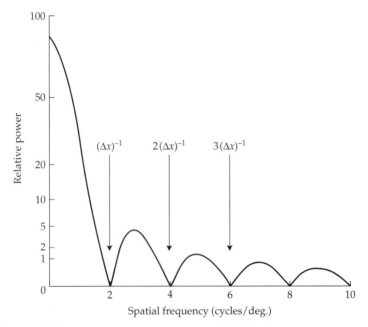

B.6 The spatial-frequency power spectrum of a bright bar. The spectrum was calculated along a direction perpendicular to the long axis of the bar. The bar's width (Δx) was 0.5 degrees.

while the second lobe has negative amplitude. The importance of the phase spectrum is most dramatically brought out by the following time-domain illustration: The power spectrum of a single brief click is the same as that of continuous white noise (white noise sounds like the hiss of escaping steam); the distinction between these two very different temporal waveforms is represented entirely in their phase spectra (see Figure 1.20 for a spatial-domain illustration). The next section takes us to the main point: the spatial frequency description of a localized non-repetitive image (a *spatial transient*).

Localized Images:
Spatial-Frequency Description along One Dimension

Any realizable spatial form can be described completely either in the spatial domain or in the spatial-frequency domain (where a power spectrum plus a phase spectrum are required for a complete description). In the spirit of Fourier's original time domain/temporal frequency dichotomy, the theoretical concept labeled *spatial frequency* is defined so that the description of a spatial form in the spatial domain and the description of the same form in the spatial-frequency domain are complementary (i.e., in different worlds) (Duffieux, 1946; Schade, 1948; Hopkins, 1956; Gaskell, 1978). Thus, as mentioned earlier, a limitingly narrow bar has a power spectrum that is flat from zero to an indefinitely high spatial frequency. In other words, a sharply defined location in space is located with zero precision in the spatial frequency domain. Conversely, the spatial form that corresponds to a limitingly narrow concentration of power along the spatial-frequency axis is a sinusoid that contains an indefinitely large number of cycles. In other words, any given spatial-frequency extends over infinite space, i.e., is located with zero accuracy in space.

Spatial frequency is a difficult concept when applied to an image of finite size. Attempting to grasp the concept in terms of the period* of a real grating can lead to misunderstanding. For example, the peak in the power spectrum of a grating of finite extent is, in general, not at a spatial frequency equal to the reciprocal of the grating's period.

A further point: the relation between edge sharpness and spatial frequency is not intuitively obvious. Consider, for example, a vertical, very long, sharp-edged bright bar whose width (Δx) is 0.5 degrees. Its power spectrum along the horizontal direction is shown in Figure B.6. Clearly, it would be a dubious enterprise to assign some unique or even dominant spatial frequency to the bar. But the crucial point here is that if the bar is blurred, the edges grow less sharply defined in the spatial domain, and the high frequency power in the spectrum is attenuated relative to the low-frequency power.

> Yet it is not meaningful to state that the high-frequency power is located at the bar's edges, because the power at any given spatial frequency belongs to the bar as a whole.

Many researchers have used sinusoidal grating stimuli to investigate spatial vision. In practice, physical gratings necessarily contain a finite number of cycles (each of angular subtense P degrees). A physically realizable luminance-defined grating can be regarded as a notional infinitely extended grating of period P whose luminance waveform (or whose contrast) is multiplied by a transient waveform (i.e., "*windowed*") so that the grating is truncated. Commonly used windows include a rectangular waveform (the grating starts and ends abruptly) and a Gaussian waveform (the grating starts and ends smoothly). When discussing the spatial-frequency content of such a grating, it is important to bear in mind the following:

> The spectrum belongs to the truncated grating as a whole, and the contribution of the notional, infinitely extended grating can be profoundly modified by the windowing function.

For simplicity, consider first a grating patch located at the center of an area of uniform luminance equal to the mean luminance of the grating, this surround

---

* The period of a real grating is the distance between adjacent bright bars (or adjacent dark bars).

area being very much larger than the grating patch. (The plot of luminance versus distance [x] inset in Figure B.7A illustrates such a grating. For clarity, only three cycles are shown.) Figure B.7A–E brings out the effects of windowing in the special case of a cosine grating whose bars are parallel to the y-axis, and is windowed along the x-axis by a rectangular waveform. Figure B.7A illustrates that when a grating of width Δx contains a sufficiently large number of complete cycles (15 in this case), the power spectrum consists of a central lobe of half-width $(\Delta x)^{-1}$ cycles/deg. whose peak lies close to P^{-1} cycles/deg. For a sharply truncated grating such as that shown in the inset, there is an appreciable "leakage" of power along the spatial-frequency axis. (Note that in part A the fourth root of power is plotted as ordinate in order to highlight the side lobes while retaining a zero value on the ordinate.) The width of the central lobe increases as the total number of cycles decreases. Figure B.7B depicts the situation for a grating that consists of five cycles. (Note that in part B the ordinate is linear so that the side lobes are less evident.) When the grating contains only one complete cycle, power is broadly distributed along the spectrum, extending downwards almost to zero cycles/deg., and the peak is appreciably displaced from the nominal spatial-frequency of P^{-1} cycles/deg. (Figure B.7C). If the grating contains a nonintegral number of cycles, there will be power at zero cycles/deg. (Figure B.7D). (Zero cycles/deg. represents the mean level of luminance, i.e., *zero contrast*.) When the number of cycles is less than one, it is not meaningful to assign a discrete spatial frequency to the grating (Figure B.7E).

Now we consider a grating patch located at the center of a very large dark region. The spatial-frequency power spectrum illustrated in Figure B.7A–E will be added to a power spectrum similar to that shown in Figure B.6, so that the power spectrum of the grating patch will look different from that depicted in Figure B.7A–E. This complication will be severe for gratings with less than about two cycles, and will become less and less marked as the number of cycles is increased beyond two.

There are many examples in the literature where the low-frequency segments of contrast sensitivity functions have been obtained with grating stimuli that contained only a small number of cycles—even less than one in some cases. When you are thinking about the shape of such low-frequency segments, it may be helpful to bear in mind the points brought out in Figure B.7C–E.

A second point brought out in Figure B.7A–E is that, even when an abruptly truncated grating contains as many as 15 cycles, some power is not at the nominal spatial frequency of P^{-1} cycles/deg. When the grating contains only few cycles, most of the power is not at P^{-1} cycles/deg., whatever the windowing function. It

B.7 The spatial-frequency power spectrum of a sinusoidal grating. The period of ▶ the grating is P degrees, and the spectrum is along a direction perpendicular to the bars. The grating is truncated abruptly, as illustrated by the inset in part A. The grating's width (Δx) contains 15 cycles in part A, 5.0 in part B, 1.0 in part C, 1.5 in part D, and 0.5 in part E. The ordinate is scaled as the fourth root of power in part A, and is linear in parts B–E. All plots are normalized to a maximum of 1.0.

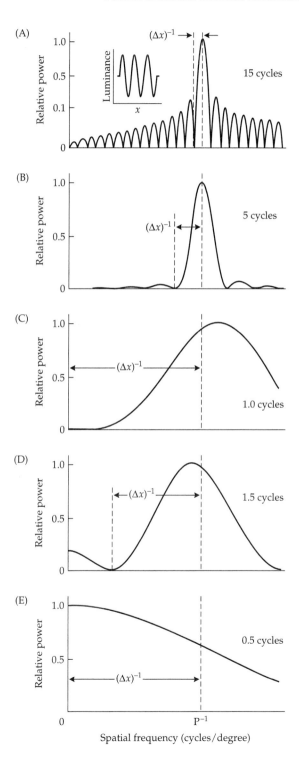

(A) Relative power — 15 cycles, $(\Delta x)^{-1}$, Luminance vs x

(B) Relative power — 5 cycles, $(\Delta x)^{-1}$

(C) Relative power — 1.0 cycles, $(\Delta x)^{-1}$

(D) Relative power — 1.5 cycles, $(\Delta x)^{-1}$

(E) Relative power — 0.5 cycles, $(\Delta x)^{-1}$

P^{-1}

Spatial frequency (cycles/degree)

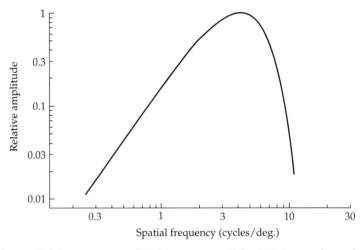

B.8 The spatial-frequency amplitude spectrum of the DOG waveform shown in Figure 1.17. This figure kindly supplied by H. Wilson.

is important to note that this is not a quirk of the mathematics. On the contrary, Figure B.7A–E indicates where the physical power really is.

> When a grating is windowed by waveforms of different spatial widths it is, in general, incorrect to assume that what one has is a grating of constant frequency P^{-1} cycles/deg. contained within envelopes of different widths.

The physical reality illustrated in Figure B.7C–E is not greatly different for a Gaussian window.

Figure B.8 shows the spatial-frequency description of the DOG stimulus depicted in Figure 1.21. The peak of the spatial-frequency distribution is altered by magnifying the Figure 1.21 along the horizontal axis. Widening the DOG stimulus shifts the peak spatial frequency downwards, and narrowing it shifts the peak spatial frequency upwards without changing the shape of the plot in Figure B.8. Wilson and his colleagues have used the sixth spatial derivative of a DOG waveform on the grounds of its better fit to their masking data (Figure 2.12). The sixth derivative has a second excitatory lobe flanking the inhibitory lobes in Figure 1.21 (see Figure 3.3 in Wilson [1991b]).

Can Complex Patterns Be Synthesized by Superimposing Sinusoidal Gratings?

It is sometimes said that any spatial light distribution, for example, a photograph of the Statue of Liberty, could be synthesized by superimposing many sinusoidal gratings of appropriate frequencies, orientations, and phases. In principle this statement is correct for gratings that are created by interference of coherent light (see pp. 433–434). But for the commonplace kind of grating (e.g., a grating displayed on a monitor) this is not really so, though a fair approximation can be made to some rather simple patterns. The reason is simple: as illustrated in Figure 1.18, a sinusoidal grating is not a sinusoidal distribution of light power, but rather a sinusoidal distribution plus a mean (DC) level that can never be less than half the peak-to-peak amplitude of the sinusoid.

An "imaginary experiment" can help clarify the basic physics at an intuitive level. Imagine that we generate sinusoidal voltages of frequency $F, 3F, 5F, 7F, 9F$, and so forth. Now we feed an F Hz sinusoid of appropriate amplitude to the Z axis of an appropriately triggered CRT to produce a pure sinusoidal grating. As we successively add the higher harmonics (with appropriate amplitudes and temporal phases, see pp. 433–434) to the Z axis input, the sinusoidal grating displayed in the CRT will progressively change until we have a square wave grating of 100% contrast with edges as sharply defined as we please (assuming that we have chosen a CRT of high resolution with fast electronics).

Alternatively, suppose that we attempt to synthesize a squarewave grating by optical rather than electronic superimposition. We use the F Hz sine wave to generate a sinusoidal grating on one CRT, then generate the $3F$ grating on a second CRT, and so on. Now we optically superimpose, onto the F Hz grating, first the $3F$ Hz grating with appropriate spatial phase, then the $5F$ Hz grating, and so on. (Bodily moving the position of the grating's bars through one cycle is equivalent to a phase change of 360°.) As the successive gratings are superimposed, the resulting pattern becomes more and more like a square wave grating, but at the same time the contrast progressively falls because more and more DC levels of mean light intensity are being added to dilute the contrast of earlier patterns. Before we achieve the sharp-edged square wave grating we synthesized in the first "imaginary experiment," the pattern's contrast has fallen so low that it disappears altogether!

In addition to the nonexistence of negative light energy, spatial patterns of light differ from time series in a second, more subtle way. Time goes forward but not backward. In spatial Fourier optics, the time dimension is replaced by the spatial dimension, and opposite directions in space are treated equally. The following illustration can assist at an intuitive level.

A time series can be completely described either in the time domain or, in Fourier terms, in the frequency domain. If a time series is subjected to physical low-pass filtering (e.g., with an R-C filter) the phases, as well as the amplitudes, of the constituent frequency components are necessarily affected. This is because real time does not go backward. In particular, a physical low-pass filter cannot respond to an input until the input is applied to the filter. The practical consequences are illustrated in Figure 1.19 in Regan (1989a) (compare the effects of a 15 Hz and a 250 Hz upper corner frequency). Turning from temporal to spatial dimensions, the equivalent of low-pass filtering a time series is blurring a spatial image. The consequence of this fundamental difference between time and space is that blurring can, in principle, merely attenuate high with respect to low spatial frequencies without necessarily altering their relative phases. This occurs because any spatial direction is treated in the same way as the opposite direction. (A similar effect can be achieved in the time domain—though not in real time—by digital filtering that treats negative and positive time as equivalent. See Regan [1989], pp. 27–29, for a minimally mathematical account.)

Localized Images: Spatial-Frequency Description along Two Dimensions

Although only their power spectra along the x direction are shown, the gratings in Figure B.7A–E are, or course, two-dimensional. Their power spectra along the y direction is uninteresting (they resemble Figure B.6). A one-dimensional Fourier spectrum provides a quite inadequate description of the commonly used windowed checkerboard stimulus shown in Figure B.9A. The two-dimensional power spectrum of a (very large) checkerboard stimulus is shown in Figure B.9B. It can be seen that there is no power parallel to the edges of the checkerboard. This point can be demonstrated by blurring the checkerboard. Kelley and Magnuski (1975) provide a brief introduction to the 2D Fourier transform and provide references for further reading.

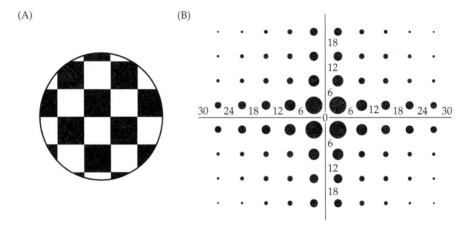

B.9 Fourier spectrum of a checkerboard. (A) A circular area of a checkerboard pattern. (B) Two-dimensional Fourier spectrum of a checkerboard pattern that contains many more checks than the pattern shown in part A. The term at zero spatial frequency is omitted. The area of each spot indicates the magnitude of the frequency component. The numbers are cycles/degree for a spatially extensive pattern of checks whose side length is 10 minutes of arc. Note the absence of components parallel to the sides of the checks. Note also that this figure does not imply that a checkerboard pattern could be synthesized by superimposing sinusoidal gratings. After Kelly (1976).

Modulation

Amplitude-modulated (AM) patterns have been used in numerous studies of spatial vision (and also of motion perception). Figure 2.17B shows an AM sinusoidal grating in which the contrast-modulating waveform is itself a sinusoid that modulates the contrast (as distinct from the luminance) of the *carrier wave* shown in Figure 2.17A. A Gaussian or a half-sinewave has been used as the contrast-modulating waveform in a number of studies. Figure 2.17D shows an AM sinusoidal grating where the contrast-modulating waveform is a half-sinewave.

Many students find it easier to attain an intuitive understanding of modulation by first considering modulation in the time domain rather than modulations in the spatial domain, because examples of modulations in time-domain signals are an everyday experience. So we will first consider temporal waveforms before turning back to spatial waveforms.

Suppose we feed a sinusoidal function of time $x(t) = A \cos(2\pi f_c t)$ of frequency f_c Hz to one input of an electronic analog multiplier and into the other input we feed a second temporal waveform $y(t) = 1 + a \cos(2\pi F_m t)$ that comprises the sum of a DC voltage and a modulating sinusoid of frequency F_m. Suppose further that $F_m \ll f_c$. The output of the multiplier will be an AM waveform described by the equation

$$z(t) = A \cos(2\pi f_c t)[1 + a \cos(2\pi F_m t)] \tag{B.16}$$

where a is the *modulation depth* and $z(t)$ is the instantaneous amplitude. Suppose that we feed this waveform through a linear amplifier to a loudspeaker so that we hear a sound (an AM tone) described by equation (B.16). By definition, the modulation depth of the tone is equal to the fraction $(A_{max} - A_{min})/(A_{max} + A_{min})$, where A_{max} and A_{min} are, respectively, the maximum and minimum amplitudes of the waveform's envelope.

Equation (B.16) can be rewritten as :

$$z(t) = (a/2) \cos 2\pi(f_c - F_m)t + \cos(2\pi f_c) + (a/2)\cos 2\pi(f_c + F_m)t \tag{B.17}$$

Equation (B.17) demonstrates that the amplitude-modulated stimulus is equivalent to the sum of three tones with frequencies $f_c - F_m$, F_c, and $f_c + F_m$ with specific amplitude and phase relationships. The first term is called the *lower sideband*, the second the *carrier*, and the third the *upper sideband*.

Note that the waveform contains no term of frequency F_m, the modulation frequency that one clearly hears.

Figure B.10 parts B and C are time-domain and frequency-domain representations of an AM sinusoid of modulation depth 0.2. Figure B.10 parts C and F show that the effect of increasing modulation depth to 1.0 is that the power of two sidebands increases. If the modulation depth is progressively increased beyond 1.0, the amplitude of the carrier progressively falls relative to the sideband amplitude until, in the extreme case shown in Figure B.10G–I, the carrier is eliminated ("suppressed carrier, two sidebands").

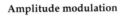

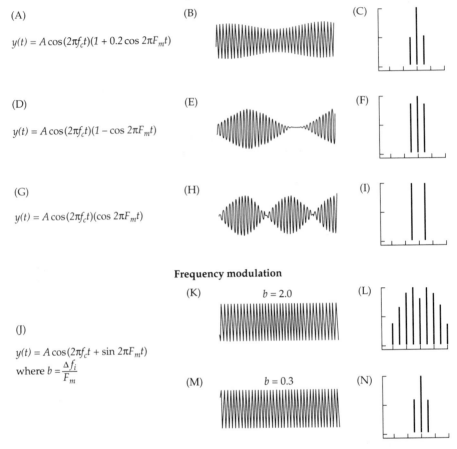

B.10 Amplitude and frequency modulation by a sinusoidal modulating wave-form. The equation (A), time-domain waveform (B), and spectrum (C) of a 150 Hz sinusoid that was amplitude-modulated (AM) by a 5 Hz sinusoid to a modulation depth of 0.2. Parts D–F are the same as parts A, B, and C, but for a modulation depth of 1.0. Parts G–I are the same, but for suppressed-carrier, two-sideband AM. (J) Equation for a frequency modulated (FM) sinusoid. (K, L) 150 Hz sinusoid, frequency-modulated by a 5 Hz sinusoid to a modulation index (b) of 2.0; (M, N) for $b = 0.3$. From Regan (1989a).

The waveform in Figure B.10H can be generated by feeding the f_c Hz carrier to one input of our multiplier and an F_m Hz sinusoid (with no added DC) to the other input. Note that the envelope in Figure B.10H goes through a maximum amplitude twice in each cycle of the modulating F_m Hz waveform. One can see intuitively why there is no carrier component in the Figure B.10I spectrum—the carrier changes phase by 180° every time the envelope in Figure B.10H passes through a minimum amplitude. (Turning back to the spatial-frequency domain,

Figure B.10I shows why the sum of two gratings of closely similar spatial frequencies looks like a grating whose contrast is amplitude-modulated. According to Graham and Robson (1987), the beat pattern in the AM grating considerably reduces spatial probability summation, thus accounting for the discrepant narrow estimates (0.3 octaves) for the bandwidths of spatial-frequency channels when the subthreshold summation technique is used [Sachs et al., 1971; Kulikowski & King-Smith, 1973].)

A frequency-modulated (FM) tone can be generated by feeding a modulating waveform to the appropriate input of a voltage-controlled oscillator (VCO) that has been adjusted to generate an f_c Hz carrier wave. If the modulating waveform is a sinusoid of frequency F_m Hz, the FM waveform can be written:

$$y(t) = A \cos(2\pi f_c t + b \sin 2\pi F_m t) \qquad (B.18)$$

where $y(t)$ is the amplitude of the FM signal as function of time, f_c Hz is the carrier frequency, F_m Hz the modulation frequency, and b is the *modulation index*, a ratio defined by the equation

$$b = \Delta F_i / F_m \qquad (B.19)$$

where ΔF_i is the maximum departure of instantaneous frequency from the carrier frequency f_c. In other words, instantaneous frequency oscillates between $f_c + \Delta F_i$ and $f_c - \Delta F_i$. Figure B.10L illustrates that when the modulation index b is large, the FM equation (B.18) can be rewritten as a series that contains many more than the three frequency terms of the AM equation (B.17). However, when b is much less than 1.0 then, as shown in Plomp (1976, p. 59), Equation (B.18) can be approximated as

$$y(t) = (b/2)\cos2\pi(f_c - F_m) + \cos(2\pi f_c - \pi/2) + (b/2)\cos 2\pi(f_c + F_m)t \quad (B.20)$$

Equation (B.20) is called *quasi-FM* and closely approximates the case of genuine FM for small modulation index illustrated in Figure B.10N. Note the close relationship between the AM waveform of Equation (B.17) and the quasi-FM waveform of Equation (B.20). The AM and quasi-FM waveforms have the same power spectrum (compare Figure B.10 parts C and N): the only distinction is a phase shift of π radians (i.e., 90°) for the carrier frequency.

The strident noise produced by police cars in many countries provides an illustration of an FM tone. The slow modulating frequency is very clearly heard, so it may seem surprising that:

For neither high (Figure B.10L) nor low (Figure B.10N) values of modulation index does the FM waveform contain any power at the modulating frequency.*

---

* Anyone surprised by this fact is in good company. Having obtained for the first time the spectrum of an FM sinusoidal waveform and found that there was no energy at the modulating frequency, Carson (1922) wrote: "The foregoing solutions, though unquestionably

Parts K and L of Figure B.10 bring out the point that, even when large-amplitude sidebands are present in the frequency domain, the time-domain envelope of an FM signal is nearly flat. Compare this with the large ripple in the envelope of an AM signal, clearly evident in parts B, E, and H of Figure B.10.

Turning back to the spatial domain, Figure B.10 describes AM and FM spatial distributions of luminance if we replace time by distance and ensure that the ordinate (luminance) in parts B, E, H, K, and M is always positive by adding a constant luminance level to the waveform shown. Parts C, F, I, L, and N will describe the spatial-frequency power distributions of these spatial patterns if we plot spatial frequency rather than temporal frequency along the abscissae and add a term at low spatial frequency corresponding to Figure B.6. *But there will be no power corresponding to the modulating envelope.*

Demodulation

Returning to the time domain, Figure B.11 illustrates how a half-wave rectifier can demodulate a waveform such as that shown in Figure B.10E. The output waveform contains a component at the modulating frequency in addition to high-frequency components. A low-pass filter can be used to extract the modulating frequency from the high-frequency residue. Thus, the rectifier has recovered the modulating waveform, even though it was not present in the spectrum of the input. (According to our current understanding, this is the process that explains why the modulation of an AM sinusoidal tone is clearly audible.) A formal mathematical treatment of the demodulation of one or the sum of two AM or FM waveforms is available (Regan & Regan, 1993; Regan, 1996).

I mentioned earlier that there is no power corresponding to the modulating waveform in the spectrum of an AM spatial grating. It therefore following from the definition of "linear system" (see pp. 389–391) that, *if one can see the modulating waveform, a nonlinear process in one's visual system is necessarily responsible.* The fact that modulating waveforms are often quite visible is hardly surprising; the visual pathway abounds with rectifier-like processes. (Two examples can be mentioned: excitatory and inhibitory synapses; a neuron cannot fire at a negative rate.) Even the nonessential nonlinearity of a curved transducer characteristic (e.g., the cone characteristic) can demodulate an AM spatial waveform. Appendix E discusses this topic, and Figure E.2 shows the rectifier-like performance of a cell in the lateral geniculate nucleus.

---

mathematically correct, are somewhat difficult to reconcile with our physical intuitions, and our physical concepts of such 'variable frequency' mechanisms as, for example, the siren." The reason why we hear the modulating spatial of an FM or AM tone is that the rectifier-like characteristic of the ear's hair cell transducer function demodulates the waveform (see pp. 426–427).

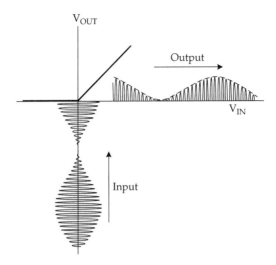

B.11 Demodulation of an amplitude-modulated waveform. The AM waveform that enters the rectifier has zero power at the modulating frequency. The rectifier's output has power at the modulating frequency.

In research into spatial vision, one point that is sometimes forgotten is that a spatial filter may precede the nonlinearity that is responsible for demodulating the waveform. If the carrier spatial frequency lies outside the passband of the spatial filter, the nonlinearity will have no chance to recover the modulating waveform because the modulated wave does not reach the nonlinearity.*

A rigorous discussion of the possible roles of demodulation in visual processing is provided by Daugman and Downing (1995).

Autocorrelation, Cross-correlation, and Convolution

Some acquaintance with *autocorrelation* is requisite for understanding the principle of Reichardt's motion detector, and for understanding the modification required to enable the detector to signal accurately the motion of a periodic luminance variation (Reichardt, 1961; van Santen & Sperling, 1984).

The degree to which one pattern resembles a second pattern can be quantified by *cross-correlating* the two patterns. This topic takes us on to *convolution*. When employing a digital computer to calculate the effect of passing the luminance distribution in a retinal image through a parallel array of spatial filters, some modelers have

---

* In the case of modulated temporal waveforms, this point has been exploited to measure the properties of the first-stage filter (Spekreijse, 1966; see also Regan & Beverley, 1981).

found it convenient to use the mathematical method of convolution (e.g., Watt & Morgan, 1985). To avoid possible confusion, students should bear in mind that to take advantage of this convenience is not to suggest that the visual system actually performs convolution.

Autocorrelation

Suppose we have a time-varying voltage $f(t)$. Its autocorrelation function is defined as

$$\phi_{ff}(\tau) = \lim_{R \to \infty} \frac{1}{2R} \int_{-R}^{R} f(t)f(t - \tau)dt \tag{B.21}$$

In words, the signal $f(t)$ is shifted by τ seconds, multiplied by the unshifted $f(t)$, and then averaged over a signal duration (R) that tends to infinity. Thus, $\phi_{ff}(\tau)$ is a measure of how similar $x(t)$ is with its value t seconds earlier *on the average*.

Now we turn from functions of time to functions of distance. The autocorrelation function for a luminance distribution that varies as a function $f(x)$ of distance x is obtained as follows. First calculate, at any given point x the value of

$$\phi_{ff}(\Delta x) = \lim_{D \to \infty} \frac{1}{2D} \int_{-D}^{D} f(x)f(x - \Delta x)dx \tag{B.22}$$

for all values of Δx (positive and negative). Then obtain the mean of $\phi_{ff}(\Delta x)$ for all locations within the luminance distribution.

The original *Reichardt detector* illustrated in Figure 5.19 would correctly signal the speed and direction of motion of any moving luminance distribution whose autocorrelation function fell to near-zero over a distance smaller than the separation between the two inputs to the detector. But the autocorrelation function of a sinusoidal grating is a periodic function of distance. A Reichardt detector cannot reliably signal the speed and direction of motion of a luminance distribution whose autocorrelation function is periodic. It was to circumvent this problem that van Santen and Sperling (1985) proposed their *elaborated Reichardt detector*.

Cross-correlation

Suppose that we have two time-varying voltages $f(t)$ and $F(t)$, and we record the two voltages from time $t = 0$ to time $t = R$. The cross-correlation function between the two signals is defined as

$$\phi_{fF}(\tau) = \lim_{R \to \infty} \frac{1}{2R} \int_{-R}^{R} f(t)F(t - \tau)dt \tag{B.23}$$

The cross-correlation function is a measure of how similar *on the average* are the values of $F(t)$, τ seconds into the past, with values of $f(t)$ at the present time. If functions $f(t)$ and $F(t)$ are independent, then the cross-correlation function is zero for all values of τ. If $f(t)$ and $F(t)$ are identical random processes, then the cross-correlation function will assume a large positive value for $\tau = 0$, and be negligible for all other values of τ.

Convolution

Cross-correlation is closely related to *convolution*. Consider a linear electrical circuit (a linear *system*). The relation between $x(t)$, the input to the system, and $y(t)$, the system's output, is given by a linear transformation of the input called the *convolution integral*.

$$
y(t) = \int_{\tau=0}^{\tau=\infty} h(\tau)\, x(t-\tau) d\tau \tag{B.24}
$$

where the function $h(\tau)$ is called the *impulse response* of the system. (The impulse response provides a complete functional description of the input–output relation of a linear system.)

In the digital computer realization of convolution, both the input function and the impulse response are broken into sets of samples at (in the case of a time series) discrete intervals of time. The integral product is replaced by a summation of products. This is a procedure used in *time series prediction* as, for example, when a financier tries to establish the memory characteristic of the stock market from daily reports in the past in order to predict future behavior.

Convolving means folding back, and this is precisely what has been done to the system's impulse response. The geometrical meaning of convolution is illustrated in Figure B.12(A-C). Function $f(s)$ is said to "scan" across function $F(s)$, creating the product $f(s)F(s)$ for every value of s.

When the function $f(s)$ is wide (as illustrated in Figure B.12E), the effect of convolving $f(s)$ with $F(s)$ is, of course, to lose much of the fine details in $F(s)$ (Figure B.12F). In the case that function $F(s)$ is piecewise linear (as illustrated in Figure B.12A), and $f(s)$ is narrow (as illustrated in Figure B.12B) then, as illustrated in Figure B.12C, the result of this convolution will be to transform a piecewise-linear function to a closely similar function that is, however, continuously differentiable. (The first spatial derivative is finite at all points.)

I will now state without proof an important theoretical result.

The Fourier transform of the convolution of two functions is equal to the product of the Fourier transforms of the two functions. In other words, convolution in the space domain is equivalent to multiplication in the Fourier domain.

For dynamic systems: "In summary, the convolution integral expresses mathematically the physical process by which a dynamic system weights or remembers its past history of inputs in generating its current output. This weighting function is identically the impulse response $h(t)$ which we use more frequently for manipulative purposes in its Laplace-transform version as the transfer function $H(s)$"(Milsum, 1966, p. 136). (s is the Laplace operator or variable.)

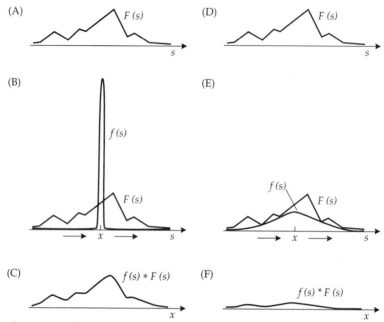

B.12 The geometrical meaning of convolution. (A–C) Function $f(s)$ scans across function $F(s)$, thus creating the product $f(s)F(s)$ in part C. (D–F) When function $f(s)$ is wide, much of the fine detail in $F(s)$ is lost. After Walker (1988).

I refer readers who wish to pursue this topic further to Walker (1988, pp. 247–251), Jenkins and Watts (1968, pp. 4–7, 34–45, 155–162), and for a biological context, Marmarelis and Marmarelis (1978, 19–29), and Milsum (1966, 135–136, 389–392).

Coherent Light, Incoherent Light, Interference, and Diffraction

Some acquaintance with a sub–area of physics called *physical optics* is necessary for a thorough grasp of why the wave nature of light limits the sharpness of the retinal image, and of how *interference fringes* are created on the retina. In writing the following brief review my aim was to convey to students an intuitive understanding of the relevant physics.

Huygens' theory of secondary wavelets

Huygens (1629–1695) considered that each point in front of a light wave can be regarded as a local source of light that produces *secondary wavelets*. In pre-university physics classes, Huygens' principle is commonly demonstrated by means of water waves. A stroboscopic flash lamp is placed on the floor with a long glass-bottomed tank above it so as to cast shadows of waves onto a white ceiling. A wire fitted to one prong of an electrically driven tuning fork is dipped into the water at one end of the tank so as to produce waves whose shadows can be rendered stationary by appropriately adjusting the flash frequency. In Figure B.13 the waves are shown moving from the left towards a barrier AB that contains an opening S that is somewhat narrower than the wavelength. At all points except S the waves will be either reflected or absorbed but, because there is a gap, there is a disturbance in the space to the right of the barrier. This demonstration shows that, rather than forming a narrow pencil of waves of width S, the waves spread out from S in semicircles as though they were generated at S. This is the meaning of the statement that "S acts as a source of secondary wavelets."

Huygens proposed that the location of the wavefront at some later time is the envelope of the secondary wavelets that originated from every point on the original wavefront. Figure B.14 illustrates the way in which Huygens' construction predicts the future location of a plane wavefront. The position of the wavefront at time t_0 is represented by a plane through AB at right angles to the plane of the paper. If we draw spheres centered on different points along AB, all of which have the same radius ct, the envelope of these circles defines a plane that is perpendicular to the paper and cuts through $A'B'$ and indicates the location of the wavefront at time $(t_0 + t)$, where c is the speed of light.

Huygens postulated that the effect of the secondary wavelets is restricted to the points that touch their envelope. He further postulated that only those parts of the envelope along the direction of propagation need be considered (otherwise they would produce an equally strong wave in the backward direction). This amounts to the assumption that the secondary wavelets do not have uniform amplitude in all directions. This *obliquity factor* calls for amplitude to be proportional to $(1 + \cos\theta)$, where θ is the angle with the forward direction.

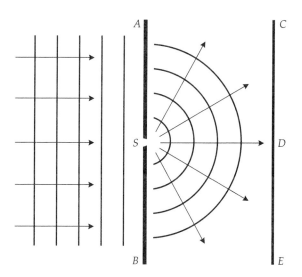

B.13 Diffraction of waves at a small aperture. From Jenkins and White (1957).

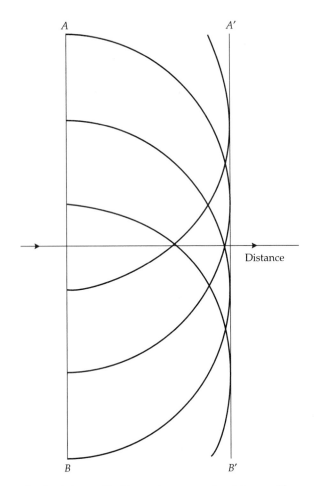

B.14 **Huygens' principle applied to a plane wavefront in a uniform medium.**
After Ditchburn (1976).

Although Huygens had no direct physical or mathematical justification for his decision to ignore the inconvenient parts of the secondary wavelets, his construction remains a useful "aid to thinking," and is used as such in many degree-level and even postgraduate-level texts on physical optics. For example, "Huygens's theorem was later extended by Fresnel and led to the formulation of the so-called Huygens–Fresnel principle, which is of great importance in the theory of diffraction . . . and which may be regarded as the basic postulate of the wave theory of light" (Born & Wolf, 1959, p. 131). Huygens' construction offers predictions that are correct in many simple cases. For example, it predicts correctly the laws of reflection and refraction. But Huygens' theory by itself is insufficient to calculate the distribution of light within a diffraction pattern.

Huygens' theory can be regarded as an intuitive feeling, anticipating by more than a century the fact that a complete knowledge of the electromagnetic field at all points on a wavefront at one instant is sufficient to calculate the location of the wavefront at a later time. In essence this is what Fresnel (1788–1827) and Kirchoff (1824–1887) formally proved, while at the same time providing a natural account of the obliquity factor. Kirchoff showed that a knowledge of the electromagnetic disturbance within a small area is sufficient to predict, using the electromagnetic wave equations, the future effects of this disturbance at a distant point. (See Born & Wolf for a rigorous development of this point.)

Interference of light

The interference phenomenon was observed by Thomas Young (1773–1829), who used the arrangement illustrated in Figure B.15. As commonly encountered in undergraduate-level university physics classes, a near-monochromatic light source (such as a sodium gas discharge lamp) is placed behind a narrow slit S_0 that is perpendicular to the plane of the drawing. As illustrated, the slit acts as a secondary source of spherical wavefronts. In their turn, the narrow slits S_1 and S_2 in the thin metal barrier B act as secondary sources of spherical wavefronts. Since S_1 and S_2 are exactly the same distance from S_0, the waves emerging from them are exactly in phase with one another.

Young discovered that the light falling on the screen was not uniform. On careful examination he found a series of bright and dark fringes on the screen. The fringes disappeared when he removed the barrier B, leaving screen C uniformly illuminated.

In pre-university physics classes the fringes are usually explained along the following lines:

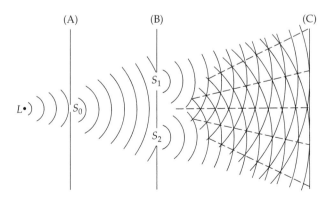

B.15 Young's two-slit experiment demonstrating interference of light. From Ditchburn (1976).

1. Monochromatic light is an oscillation of electric field strength along one direction of space accompanied by an oscillation of magnetic field strength along a perpendicular direction, and the associated energy propagates along a direction at right angles to the plane that contains the two oscillations. At some instant during any given cycle of oscillation, the electric field vector **E** assumes its maximum amplitude along a particular direction and one half-period later it attains the same amplitude in the opposite direction. The amplitude of the magnetic field vector **H** similarly oscillates between positive and negative values. The only difference between light and radio waves is that the electromagnetic oscillations of light have frequencies some 100 million times higher (a little less than 10^{15} Hz compared with roughly 10^6 Hz).

2. The light emitted from slit S_1 or slit S_2 is an indefinitely long train of sinusoidal oscillations.

3. Any points on the screen for which the distance to S_1 differs from the distance S_2 by either zero or an integral number of wavelengths will be at the center of a bright fringe, while any point on the screen for which the difference in distances is an odd number of half-wavelengths will be at the center of a dark fringe. The dark fringes are dark because the electromagnetic oscillations arriving from S_1 are exactly 180 degrees out of phase with the oscillations arriving from S_2. The two electric field vectors, for example, are always equal in magnitude but opposite in direction and, therefore, cancel to zero. This is called *destructive interference*. At points on the screen where the electromagnetic oscillations from S_1 and S_2 arrive exactly in phase (dashed lines in Figure B.15) the two oscillations add rather than canceling. This is called *constructive interference*.

This account is correct so far as it goes, and will do for the present. I will defer a more advanced account until pp. 436–439.

Interference fringes on the retina

The "Young's two-slit principle" just described was used by Bryam (1944) and by Westheimer (1960) to create interference fringes on the retina at a time when fully coherent laser light was not available.

The blurring effect of spherical aberration is reduced by placing two tiny apertures in front of the cornea. It is intuitively obvious that the effect of spherical aberration will be merely to displace (i.e., cause a fixed shift of spatial phase) of the fringe pattern as a whole. (For a formal treatment, see Saleh, 1982.) However, although this procedure is sometimes referred to as "bypassing the eye's optics," this is not an entirely correct description. The eye's optics are not completely bypassed, because light scatter within the eye cannot be entirely avoided. Nevertheless, fringe contrast on the retina can be considerably higher than when the naked eye views a grating display of 100% contrast: fringes on the retina whose spatial frequency is as high as 110 cycles/deg. can have a contrast of 20% (Williams, 1985). The results of experiments using this technique are reviewed at pp. 245–253. With the availability of lasers, the procedure has become routine.

The optical quality of the eye

Although the angular subtense of stars (other than our sun) is very small indeed, the image of a distant star formed on the retina is not a miniscule point of light, but rather a nonuniform blob. Part of the reason is the wave nature of light and is, therefore, inescapable. I will discuss that problem at pp. 439–440. What we are concerned with here are the imperfections of the retinal image formed by the eye.

As discussed at pp. 441–444, one way of describing lens aberrations is as the terms in a mathematical series. This formalism lists the following primary monochromatic aberrations: spherical; astigmatism; coma; distortion; field curvature.* In addition, there are the primary chromatic aberrations: longitudinal chromatic aberration (i.e., a variation of focal length with wavelength) and transverse chromatic aberration (i.e., a variation of magnification with wavelength).

Along the optic axis (i.e., a line passing through the centers of curvature of the glass surface of the lens) the only aberrations are spherical aberration and longitudinal chromatic aberration. (All the other aberrations listed above are *off-axis aberrations*.) Spherical aberration can be defined as a variation of focus with aperture (Smith, 1966, p. 50). Figure C.1B shows a *thin lens* imaging a distant star. The rays that pass close to the center of the lens, and that emerge almost parallel to the optic axis, converge onto the *paraxial focal point* of the lens (F_P). A ray that passes through the outer parts of the lens and that emerges steeply inclined to the optic axis comes to a focus at F_A, some distance from F_P (exaggerated in Figure C.1). Thus, the image of a distant star is contained within a volume whose circular cross-sectional area is large within planes perpendicular to the paper and to the optic axis that cuts through F_P and F_A, and falls to a minimum somewhere between F_P and F_A. This minimum area is called the *circle of least confusion (CLC)*.

Spherical aberration can be conveniently demonstrated by holding a glass of red wine some distance from an electric light bulb. Image quality can be improved by placing a hole in a piece of cardboard in front of the glass so as to reduce the aperture of the red-wine lens.

Primary spherical aberration increases with the fourth power of the distance from the center of the lens (Hopkins, 1950). In terms of human vision, this means that spherical aberration increases very rapidly indeed as the diameter of the pupil increases (e.g., in dim light or after administration of a mydriatic).

A curious feature of the human eye is that the foveal center is not on the optic axis. The foveal center lies about 5 degrees nasal and 1.5 degrees superior to the

---

* An alternative formalism for describing the imperfections of an imaging system, the *wavefront aberration* approach, is reviewed at pp. 441–444.

axis. This means that the foveal image is degraded by off-axis as well as by on-axis aberrations.

But the human eye is not a human-designed imaging device. In point of fact, it is very different from a human-designed imaging device. Spherical aberration is less than it would be with an equivalent imaging system that used a simple spherical-surfaced glass lens, because the eye's optical surfaces (cornea and lens) are aspherical, and the refractive index of the lens varies across its thickness rather than being constant. (Advances in computer-aided design and optical fabrication techniques have recently allowed human lens designers to adopt this approach.) As well, the Stiles–Crawford effect* indicates that cones weigh the light passing through the center of the lens more heavily than light passing through the outer parts of the lens (Metcalf, 1965). And the retinal image falls onto a curved retina rather than onto a flat camera film, so that the deleterious effects of field curvature are much reduced (Guidarelli, 1972).

According to Charman (1991) the major off-axis aberration of the human eye is oblique astigmatism: the image of a distant star is a pair of perpendicular lines at different distances from the lens with a *circle of least confusion* between them; the length of the lines increases with both the angle from the optic axis and the diameter of the pupil.

For readers who wish to learn more of this topic, I suggest Charman (1991). He provides an incisive, lucid, and well-referenced review.

Coherence, coherence length, coherence time, and incoherence

The explanation of Young's discovery given on pages 433–434 is correct so far as it goes. But it does not explain why the contrast of the fringes falls progressively to zero as we move the screen so as to increase the difference in the distances of S_1 and S_2 from any given point on the screen (i.e., increase the *difference in path length*). This failure is a consequence of the assumption numbered (2) on page 434 —and of an oversimplified conception of the nature of light.

To investigate this question Michaelson (1852–1931) invented a device (the Michaelson interferometer) that was more suited to his purpose than Young's double-slit arrangement. He found that what he termed the *visibility (V)* of the fringes† fell off with the difference in path length. This effect is shown in Figure B.16. Michaelson's near-monochromatic light source was a low-pressure gas discharge lamp that provided the cadmium red line at a wavelength of 6,428 Angstrom units (i.e., 643.8 nm) where one Angstrom unit (Å) is 10^{-8} cm and one nanometer (i.e., 10^{-9} m) is 10Å.

---

* The Stiles–Crawford effect (of the first kind) is the difference in brightness of two narrow pencils of light, both of which fall onto the same retinal location, but one of which passes through the center of the pupil and the other near the edge of the pupil.

† Michaelson defined V as follows: $V = (E_{max} - E_{min})/(E_{max} + E_{min})$, where E_{max} was the relative energy of a bright fringe and E_{min} was the relative energy of a dim fringe. A similar equation framed in terms of luminance gives C, now called *Michaelson contrast, luminance contrast, spatial contrast*, or just *contrast*.

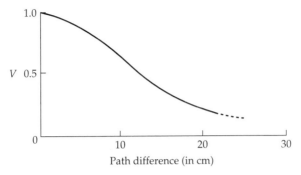

B.16 Variation of fringe visibility (*V*) with path difference. From Ditchburn (1976).

There are two complementary and entirely equivalent explanations for this progressive reduction of fringe contrast with increasing path length difference. The first explanation can be understood by referring to Figure B.17, which shows the distribution of power with wavelength within the cadmium red line. The fact that the energy is spread out across a range of frequencies can be expressed as follows:

> The source of the near-monochromatic light does not emit electro-magnetic oscillations of only one wavelength. On the contrary, it emits a very large number of different wavelengths, and the relative power carried by these different oscillations falls off steeply with wavelength on either side of the central wavelength.

This interpretation of the effect shown in Figure B.16 explains the progressive reduction of fringe contrast with increasing length of path difference. For small path-length differences, each of the many wavelengths in Figure B.17 forms fringes that are slightly displaced from each other—though only very slightly displaced. But for larger path-length differences, the fringes associated with the different wavelengths in Figure B.17 fall on considerably different locations on the screen, thus reducing the contrast of the fringes.

Now for a completely different explanation. It is, of course, not the case that the light radiated by the source of near-monochromatic light consists of an infinitely extended train of sinusoidal electromagnetic oscillations. The real question is: To what extent does the radiated light depart from this idealization?

> The radiated light can be regarded as a wavetrain* of finite length followed by a second wavetrain of finite length whose phase is random with respect to the phase of the preceding wavetrain, and so on.

---

* The term *wavetrain* refers to the profile along the time axis. A *wave group* is the resultant of a set of sinusoidal waves closely grouped around a mean wavelength. Thus, a long wave train can also be called a wave group (Ditchburn, 1976, p. 71).

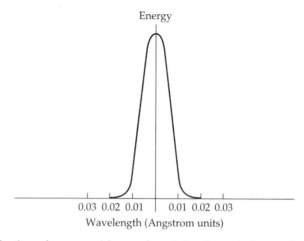

Energy

0.03 0.02 0.01 | 0.01 0.02 0.03
Wavelength (Angstrom units)

B.17 Distribution of energy with wavelength for the cadmium red spectral line produced by a low-pressure gas discharge lamp. Ordinate: Energy. Abscissa: Wavelength in Angstrom units. Zero on the abscissa corresponds to the center wavelength of the red line (6428 Angstrom units). From Ditchburn (1976).

The implication is as follows. The *power spectrum* of a sinusoidal wavetrain of infinite duration consists of infinitely narrow lines (Figure B.1B). But when that infinite wavetrain is cut, so that it starts abruptly at time t, and stops abruptly at time $t + \Delta t$, its power spectrum is not a line but rather a central lobe with smaller sidelobes (see Figure B.7A). The width of the central lobe (from zero to zero) is ΔF Hz where $\Delta F = 2/\Delta t$. The corresponding width expressed in terms of wavelength ΔF is given by $\Delta \lambda = c/\Delta F$, where c is the speed of light. The length of the wavetrains will vary about some mean, called the *coherence length,* and the mean value of Δt is called the *coherence time* of the light (Born & Wolf [1959], pp. 318–319). Fringe visibility will drop to near-zero when the path-length difference in the interferometer considerably exceeds the coherence length, because the amplitudes of two successive wavetrains can add to give a resultant magnitude between zero and the sum of the two magnitudes.*

As illustrated in Figure B.16, light whose coherence length is as long as a few tens of centimeters can be produced by low-pressure gas discharge lamps. (Laser light can have a considerably greater coherence length and is, therefore, considerably more monochromatic than the light of a low-pressure gas discharge lamp.)

Why are the wavetrains so short? An emission-line spectrum is produced by passing an electrical discharge through a low-pressure gas. Sodium, for example, emits two closely spaced lines in the yellow region of the spectrum, and Cadmium emits a strong red and a strong green line. Figure B.17 illustrates that such lines

---

* *Magnitude* is sign-free *amplitude.*

are very narrow. When gas pressure is raised to a few atmospheres the lines broaden, and when the pressure is made considerably higher still, the lines run together to form a continuum. The spectra of lines from hot solids are also continuous.

A continuous spectrum (as distinct from a line spectrum) is usually produced in conditions in which each atom is strongly affected by its neighbors, and they are disturbed so often that instead of emitting long sinusoidal wavetrains they emit irregular pulses. This kind of light is entirely *incoherent*. Domestic light bulbs produce incoherent light, and the light emitted by standard computer monitors is almost entirely incoherent.

To summarize, incoherent light can be described in the following two equivalent ways:

1. The light is the sum of very many wavelengths, so that a plot of power versus wavelength is essentially continuous. In the case of sunlight, the distribution is roughly flat across the entire visible spectrum.
2. The alternative explanation is that the excited atoms radiate light in very short bursts whose coherence time is so short that, as explained by Figure B.7E, the light energy is distributed across a very wide range of oscillation frequencies (and, hence, wavelengths).

Diffraction and the Airy disc

The propagation of light is not truly straight-line when a beam of light passes close to the edge of an opaque obstacle. For example, some light penetrates into its geometrical (i.e., straight-line) shadow, and bright–dark fringes may be present. Phenomena of this kind have long been known: they were described by Grimaldi (1618–1673) and by Hooke (1635–1703). *Diffraction* means a departure from straight-line propagation.

In general, diffraction is produced by any arrangement that causes a change in amplitude (or phase) which is not the same over the entire area of the wavefront. In all optical experiments, the width of the beam is limited by the dimensions of the apparatus, so that some diffraction is always present, though often concealed by imperfections in optical imaging. Diffraction sets an inescapable limit to the sharpness of optical images.

Diffraction is explained in terms of the interference phenomenon described earlier in this section. For our present purpose, the significance of the diffraction phenomenon is chiefly in the limit it sets to the sharpness of the retinal image. Figure B.18 shows the diffraction pattern produced by a circular aperture, such as, for example, the iris of the human eye. The illustration depicts the distribution of light power within the image of a very small point of light formed by a lens whose optical defects are negligible (a *diffraction-limited* image). Approximately 84% of the light power falls within the central area (the *Airy disc*). The radius of the first dark ring is equal to $1.22\lambda/2R$, where λ is the wavelength of the (monochromatic) light and R is the radius of the aperture.

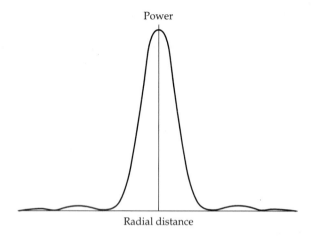

Power

Radial distance

B.18 The Airy disc. The light power in the image of a distant star formed by an aberration-free lens is plotted as ordinate versus radial distance across the image.

Readers who wish to investigate physical optics beyond the skeletal content of this appendix are referred to Ditchburn (1976) and Jenkins and White (1957) for undergraduate-level treatment, and to Born and Wolf (1959) for more advanced discussions.

Imaging

Lens Design and the Geometrical Theory of Aberrations

Figure C.1A illustrates the result of applying Huygens' theory of secondary wavelets (pp. 430–433) to image formation by a perfect (i.e., aberration-free) lens. When the lens receives parallel light from a distant star, it transforms the flat wavefronts that hit the lens into spherical wavefronts that converge onto a very tiny point. For the present, I will ignore the effects of diffraction that, as shown in Figure B.18, will actually cause the image to assume the form of an Airy disc rather than an indefinitely small point. (That is why the heading for this section is the *geometrical* theory of aberrations. The *diffraction* theory of aberrations is discussed rigorously in Born and Wolf [1959, Chapter 9].)

In addition to the theoretical construct of the *wavefront*, a second theoretical construct will be useful: the *ray*. A ray is a line pointing along the direction of propagation of the wavefront and therefore, by definition, is normal (i.e., perpendicular) to the wavefront at the point that it intersects the wavefront.

The rays in Figure C.1B that are almost parallel to the optic axis are called *paraxial* rays. They come to the *paraxial focus* F_P. As mentioned earlier, the rays from the outer parts of the lens come to a focus closer to the lens than F_P. This aberration is called a *positive spherical aberration*. In a lens with positive spherical aberration, the farther from the center of the lens a ray originates, the closer to the lens does it cross the optic axis.

441

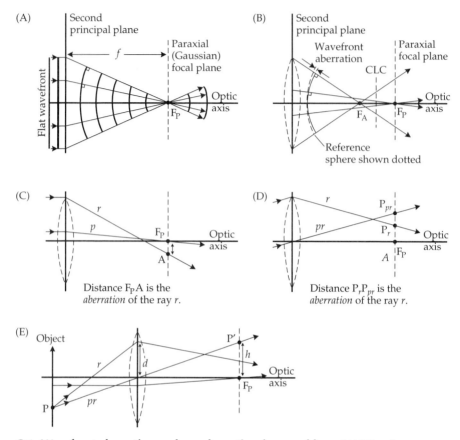

C.1 Wavefront aberration and ray aberration for a real lens. (A) Wavefront prop-agation for an aberration-free lens (ignoring diffraction). (B) Definition of *wavefront aberration*. (C–E) Definition of *ray aberration*. Key: The curved bold lines in part A are cross-sections of the wavefront. The dashed arc of a circle in part B is a cross-section through the *reference sphere* that is centered on the paraxial focus F_P. CLC is the circle of least confusion. (C) F_PA is the ray aberration for a ray r that enters the lens parallel to the optic axis. (D) P_rP_{pr} is the ray aberration for a ray r that enters the lens at an angle to the optic axis, pr being the principal ray. (E) The aberration of ray r depends on d, h, and distance F_PP' at right angles to the paper.

The continuous circular line in Figure C.1B shows that a simple *thin lens** is not a perfect imaging device: the refracted wavefront is not perfectly spherical. The path difference between the real wavefront and the *reference sphere* (dotted line centered on the paraxial focus F_P) is called the *wavefront aberration*, usually expressed in terms of wavelengths of monochromatic light. As illustrated in

---

* A thin lens is a lens whose thickness is far smaller than its focal length.

Figure C.1B, the amplitude of the wavefront aberration generally varies over the surface of the lens. (An outline of this approach to quantifying optical performance is given by Ditchburn [1976, pp. 282–283]. Rigorous treatments are available in Hopkins [1950] and Born and Wolf [1959, Chapters 5 and 9]).

Figure C.1C illustrates an alternative to the wavefront aberration formalism of quantifying lens aberrations. Suppose that a flat wavefront is incident on the lens (i.e., the incident rays are parallel.) Distance F_PA is defined as the *aberration of the ray* or simply the *ray aberration*. The ray aberration will depend on how far its point of origin is from the center of the lens. (This statement, of course, is equivalent to saying that the wavefront aberration varies over the surface of the lens.) For an image of a distant object located off the optic axis, the *aberration of ray r* is defined as distance P_rP_{pr} (Figure C.1D), where P_{pr} is the point of intersection of the principal ray *pr* with the paraxial focal plane, and P_r is the point of intersection of ray *r* with the paraxial focal plane.

In brief, for an aberration-free imaging system, all the rays from a given point on the object will pass through a corresponding point in the image plane. In other words, the aberration of the ray is zero for every ray. But for a real lens, the *aberration of the ray* will not be zero for every ray. For any given ray *r*, the ray aberration will in general depend on the following: the distance (h) between P' (i.e., the Gaussian image of point P) and the paraxial focus F_P in the plane depicted in Figure C.1E; the distance between the Gaussian image of point P and the paraxial focus in a plane orthogonal to the plane of the paper; the distance d in Figure C.1E (*aperture dependence*). The aberration of the ray *r* can be expressed as a function of these three variables and rearranged as a power series containing five different combinations of the variables. The different combinations have been given the following names: spherical aberration (positive or negative); coma; astigmatism; distortion (pincushion or barrel); field curvature. For each of the aberrations there is a primary aberration (any given variable is raised to the lowest power, e.g., squared), secondary aberration, and so on. The primary aberrations are often called Seidel aberrations, after von Seidel.* For an introduction to lens aberrations I recommend Ditchburn's book. "The detailed theory of aberrations involves laborious algebra, and it is easy to lose sight of the physical principles. In the following paragraphs wave theory is used with a minimum of formulae to classify the aberrations and the effects (on the image) of the different types of aberration are described" (Ditchburn, 1976, pp. 283–284).

The discovery of photography in 1839 by Daguerre (1789–1851) was chiefly responsible for early attempts to extend the Gaussian theory. Practical optics, which until then was mainly concerned with the construction of telescope objectives, was confronted with the new task of producing objectives with large apertures and large fields. J. PETZVAL, a Viennese mathematician attacked with

---

* H. H Hopkins (1950) developed a method for quantifying imaging performance that is quite different from that of von Seidel: the wavefront aberration approach.

considerable success the related problem of supplementing the Gaussian formulae by terms involving higher powers of the angles of inclination of rays with the axis. Unfortunately, PETZVAL's extensive manuscript on the subject was destroyed by thieves; what is known about this work comes chiefly from semi–popular reports. PETZVAL demonstrated the practical value of his calculations by constructing in about 1840 his well–known portrait lens (shown in Figure 6.3B) which proved greatly superior to any then in existence. The earlier systematic treatment of geometrical aberrations which was published in full is due to SEIDEL [in 1856]. (Born & Wolf, 1959, p. 202)

A simple thin lens suffers from chromatic aberrations as well as the monochromatic aberrations. In high-quality instruments (e.g., cameras, telescopes) this is not acceptable. High-quality lenses contain many elements, some separated, some in contact, some made of one kind of glass, others made of a different kind of glass. Lens designers, in effect, pit one aberration against another so as to reduce the net aberration. The resulting lenses are by no means thin; thickness may amount to an appreciable fraction of focal length.

The imaging system of the human eye is not equivalent to a thin simple lens. For example, the cornea is not spherical.* Furthermore, the imaging apparatus of the eye is not *thin*, and certainly not simple in any sense of the word. So before reviewing the imaging performance of the human eye, I should step aside to define the cardinal points of a thick lens.

Cardinal Points

In Figure C.2A, the ray entering the thick lens from the left is parallel to the optic axis, as is the ray exiting the lens in Figure C.2B. Any ray that was directed towards the first nodal point in Figure C.2C before entering the lens will exit the lens parallel to its initial direction along a line that cuts the optic axis at the second nodal point N'. Thus, if the lens is rotated about an axis that passes exactly through N', the incident ray shown will continue to exit the lens exactly as illustrated. (A camera whose lens is slowly rotated about its second nodal point and whose film plane is curved was commonly used to capture wide-field images, as in photographs of an entire high school.)

Note that the actual path of the ray within the lens is not as shown by the heavy dashed lines. In general, the ray will change direction at every one of the many surfaces (at least 10 in a good camera lens) that it encounters. This path can, of course, be calculated by using elementary (but very tedious) algebra. But a specification of the locations of the cardinal points with respect to the outer surfaces of the lens provides a complete summary of the characteristics of the lens.

---

* Because it is far easier to make high-quality spherical surfaces than high-quality aspheric surfaces, most human-engineered lenses have spherical surfaces.

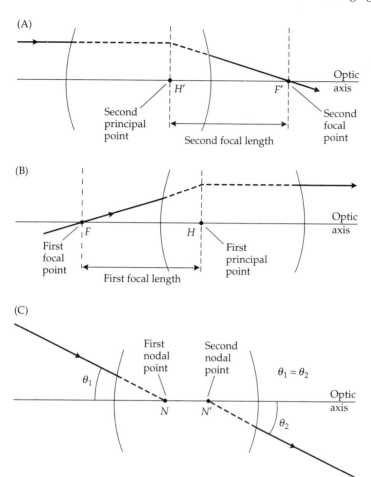

C.2 The cardinal points of a lens. The two curved fine lines conventionally represent a multi-component lens whose thickness is not negligible with respect to its focal length (i.e., a *thick* lens). Parts A–C define the first and second principal points, the first and second focal points, the first and second focal lengths, and the first and second nodal points.

Gaussian Optics

Gaussian optics is the elementary theory of imaging by lenses, mirrors, and their combinations. Only those rays that are almost parallel to the optic axis (paraxial rays), and only those points that lie in the immediate neighborhood of the optic axis are considered. Thus, all monochromatic aberrations are neglected.

Figure C.3A shows how the image formed by a thin converging lens can be obtained geometrically. In the case of a thin lens, the Gaussian formulae are as follows.

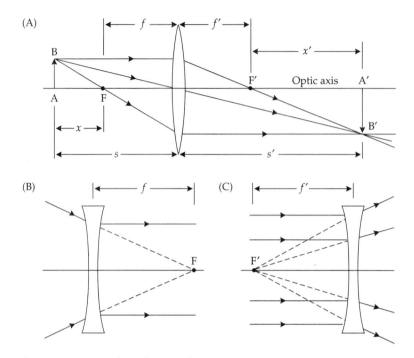

C.3 Elementary (Gaussian) theory of image formation by a thin lens.
(A) Geometrical method for obtaining the image formed by a thin converging lens.
(B, C) Definition of the first and second focal points of a thin diverging lens.

$$\frac{1}{s}+\frac{1}{s'}=\frac{1}{f} \tag{C.1}$$

and
$$M = -s'/s = -f/x = -x'/f \tag{C.2}$$

where M is the lateral magnification. Equation (C.3) gives the *Newtonian* form of the lens equation:

$$xx'= f^2 \tag{C.3}$$

Figure C.3B,C indicates how the image formed by a thin diverging lens can be obtained geometrically. Note that, in the lens formulae, the focal length of a diverging lens is a negative quantity.

Fourier Optics

Fourier developed the method that is named for him as an aid to solving problems such as the time course of diffusion of heat along a bar. The extension of his methods from the time/temporal frequency domains to the space/spatial-frequency domains was driven by the wartime need for improved methods of lens design. The imaging behavior of a lens is linear to a very close approximation. But the human visual system falls far short of fulfilling the linearity conditions set out on pages 389–391, and attempts to apply spatial Fourier methods to psychophysics have been bedeviled by a number of misunderstandings and misinterpretations that can confuse and puzzle students. On pages 416–422, I discussed two such misunderstandings. In the following section I discuss more misunderstandings, and point out some properties of imaging systems (such as the human eye's imaging structures) that are not intuitively obvious, and that might be mistaken for neural properties.

The historical background

As mentioned earlier, to design "fast" lenses that gave a wide, crisply defined field at high aperture, early lens designers who worked from the Seidel formulae balanced one aberration against another. Before large computers were available, successful lens design required a rare intuitive gift. Even so, the lens designer's ambition did not extend beyond a sharply defined flat image, that is, high resolution with a flat field. To compare the theoretical performance of different lenses in imaging a low-contrast target whose size was well above the resolution limit was impractical. Although the optical transfer function (see below) can, in principle, be derived from the distribution of light within the image of a point target, the calculation is difficult and empirical measurement is inconvenient.

In 1946, 124 years after Fourier's work became widely available, Duffieux published a book that extended Fourier methods to the analysis of spatial distributions of light, and showed that any physically realizable spatial pattern of light can be completely described as a sum of multiple sinusoidal components plus a constant term. Unfortunately, this pioneering work was published privately and was not widely available. Shortly afterward, working at the RCA company in the United States, Schade (1948) applied Fourier methods to specifying the optical performance of TV systems. Regrettably, initial publication was through a series of papers in the *RCA Review* and subsequent publication in 1956 was through the *Journal of the Society of Motion Picture and Television Engineers*, neither of which vehicles reached the wide scientific audience of the major scientific journals, and Schade's work went unnoticed for many years. Meanwhile, Fourier optics was being vigorously advanced at Imperial College, London, by H. H. Hopkins and his colleagues, who developed the mathematical and conceptual basis of Fourier methods as applied to the design of imaging systems. By the mid-1950s Hopkins was giving an advanced course on the topic every summer at Imperial College that was attended by optical engineers and physicists from the United States and the Far East as well as from Europe. The publication of Hopkins' work in the *Proceedings of the Royal Society* and the *Proceedings of the Physical Society* brought Fourier optics to the attention of a much wider audience, and today it has become standard practice to specify and design optical systems in Fourier terms. Details of how this is done are given in Hopkins (1956, 1962) and Goodman (1968).

The optical transfer function

Before the advent of Fourier methods, the imaging performance of a lens was specified entirely by its resolution for gratings of 100% contrast. As the number of lines per millimeter in the object plane is increased, the grating image grows progressively less visible until eventually no grating can be seen at all. Grating resolution is defined as the maximum number of lines per millimeter that can just be detected.

The demands of aerial photography during the Second World War highlighted the fact that resolution is an incomplete description of an optical system's performance. A more complete description is illustrated in Figure C.4. This description might be obtained as follows. A sinusoidal grating is used as a target because, as pointed out by Hopkins (1956), the image of a sinusoidal grating produced by a linear system is always a sinusoidal grating (Figure 1.17). With a sinusoidal grating of fixed contrast as target, the modulation and spatial phase of the image are measured over a range of spatial frequencies. Figure C.4 illustrates typical plots of modulation and of phase versus spatial frequency for a practical lens system.

In 1961 the International Commission for Optics met in London and recommended that the left plot in Figure C.4 be called *the modulation transfer function* (MTF)* of the imaging system, the right plot the *phase transfer function* (PTF), and the two together the *optical transfer function* (OTF). The optical transfer function is the Fourier transform of the line-spread function.† A single OTF does not specify

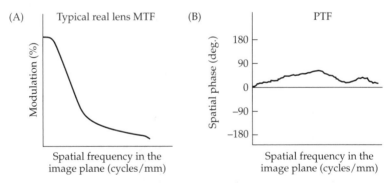

C.4 Optical transfer function for a real lens. (A) Modulation versus spatial frequency in the image for real lens. In the optical industry, spatial frequency is often expressed in cycles per mm of distance across the image. (B) The phase transfer function for the same lens. The variation of phase with spatial frequency is due to lens aberrations. From Regan (1989a).

* The term "transfer function" is used only for linear systems. Therefore it is not correct to call curves such as those shown in Figure 1.19 "modulation transfer functions." Less loaded terms such as "contrast sensitivity curve" or "contrast sensitivity functions" are preferable.

† Consequently, the OTF of the imaging structures of the human eye can be calculated from the measured line-spread function shown in Figure 1.13A.

an imaging system, because the OTF depends on several factors including aperture, field angle, orientation of test grating, focal setting, and object distance.

The use of sinusoidal gratings to investigate human spatial vision was pioneered by Schade in 1956, but it was not until Campbell and Robson proposed that the visual system contains parallel spatial-frequency channels that the application of spatial Fourier methods to vision research attracted widespread attention.

Modulation transfer functions of real lenses: Relevance to vision research

Figure C.5 illustrates that specifying the resolution of a lens in lines per millimeter tells us much less about its performance than does the MTF. Figure C.5A compares the MTFs of two camera lenses of equal resolution but of different performances. Lens *a* would be the better choice with high-resolution film (e.g., in aerial reconnaissance), whereas lens *b* would be superior for TV use. In optical engineering it is now technically possible to match the lens MTF to the detector characteristics. Figure C.5B shows the MTF for typical *f*/1.3 lens. When such a lens is used in low-light-level applications it can be redesigned in such a way that reducing the resolution actually improves performance at low spatial frequencies. In this application, the design with the best resolution is not the best lens for the job. Clearly, these aspects of lens physics are relevant to our understanding of the imaging components of the human eye, whose optical "design" can presumably be assumed to conspire with the contrast and resolution characteristics of the retina and visual pathway to give us optimal vision in everyday conditions, even though our remote ancestors evolved this design without any conscious awareness of Fourier optics.

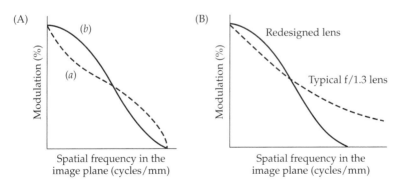

C.5 Resolution and modulation transfer function of a lens can be manipulated independently. (A) Modulation transfer functions for two lenses with the same resolution. Lens *a* is suitable for aerial photography and lens *b* for a television camera. (B) Redesign of a lens can improve contrast performance at low spatial frequencies at the expense of resolution, all without affecting focal length or aperture. From Regan (1989a).

Figure C.6A illustrates the effect of defocus on a "perfect" (i.e., diffraction-limited) lens. As defocus (i.e., blur) is increased, the high-frequency end of the perfect lens MTF progressively drops. In other words, fine detail disappears first, as would be expected. But at high levels of defocus there is a remarkable phenome-

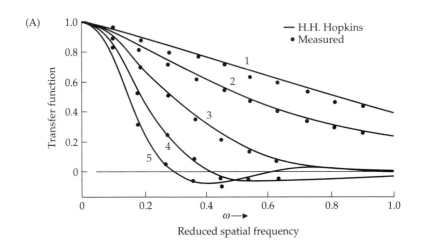

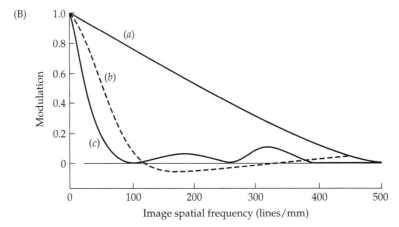

C.6 Contrast reversal, "notches," and spurious resolution produced by a real lens. (A) Effect of defocus on the modulation transfer function (MTF) of a "perfect" (i.e., aberration-free) lens. Ordinates plot the image contrast, and the abscissa is a measure of the sine wave grating target's spatial frequency. Numbers indicate increasing defocus. Filled circles plot measured data. Continuous lines are theoretical predictions calculated by H. H. Hopkins. (B) Effect of defocus on the MTF (continuous line, a) of a "perfect" lens (dashed line, b) and a lens with spherical aberration (continuous line, c). Part A is modified from Hopkins (1955); part B is from Lindberg (1954).

non. As spatial frequency increases, the MTF falls to zero, then crosses zero contrast and becomes negative (Figure C.6A, curve 4). This effect can be demonstrated with a regular slide projector.

Figure C.6B illustrates a further effect relevant to human vision research. As we have just seen, the MTF of a "perfect" lens (continuous line, *a*) can become negative (dashed line, *b*) under defocus. But for a lens with spherical aberration, defocus can create ripples in the MTF (continuous line, *c*). In other words, if the grating's spatial frequency is progressively increased, the defocused image becomes less visible until its contrast falls to zero, as would be expected. But if spatial frequency is further increased, a spatial pattern is seen beyond the resolution limit, but the spatial pattern in the image *does not necessarily resemble the object being imaged*. This deceptive imaging by a slightly defocused system beyond the resolution limit is called "spurious resolution." The effect is well known to microscopists who must be alert to the possibility that detail in the image might not be present in the object being viewed.

In the context of both basic and clinical vision research, when distinguishing between the properties of visual pathway neurons and the properties of the imaging structure of the eye (i.e., the lens and cornea), it is important to realize that lenses themselves show effects such as those illustrated in Figures C.5 and C.6. There are at least three possible consequences.

1. Figure C.5B (dashed line) underlines the point that a subject with comparatively good acuity might have comparatively low sensitivity at low spatial frequencies because of the cornea and lens rather than neural factors.
2. Figure C.6A,B illustrates that it is, in principle, possible for a ripple in the human visual contrast sensitivity curve to be produced by inaccurate accommodation or refraction in addition to the intermediate-frequency loss produced by selective damage to size-tuned visual neurons or by monocular diplopia (pp. 191–203 and 203–205).
3. Figure C.6A,B illustrates that when viewing an acuity test target (e.g., a grating) whose spatial frequency is beyond the resolution limit of the eye's optics, it might be possible to see pattern that is not actually present in the target. (Note that this effect is quite different from the aliasing patterns discussed in Appendix F.) In principle, this spurious resolution might be mistakenly thought to represent the eye's real resolution, if, for example, the psychophysical method of two-alternative forced choice is used to measure acuity. The subject would be able to distinguish a grating target from a blank field beyond the resolution limit, but this is a spurious response because the target would not be seen correctly. By the same token, Figure C.6B shows that it is, in principle, possible to record electrophysiological responses to spatial patterns that are beyond the eye's resolution limit, but this would be less a measure of vision than a demonstration of an arcane effect in physical optics.

It remains to be shown whether any or all of these optical artifacts can be important in psychophysical or electrophysiological studies of human spatial vision.

A final note: It was shown experimentally that so-called simple cortical cells linearly sum the light flux from different parts of the receptive field. When the firing rate was plotted versus the spatial frequency of a grating stimulus, the tuning curve was sharper than when the firing frequency was plotted versus the width of a single bar stimulus. This empirical finding was taken by some authors to mean that the cell preferred a grating stimulus to a bar stimulus. This argument is erroneous because, if a system is linear, then, just as with lenses, the spatial-frequency description of its behavior is equivalent to the spatial-transient description of its behavior. If spatial summation is linear, the difference between tuning for bar and grating necessarily follows; measuring the difference merely confirms linearity. In this respect, one linear cell behaves like any other linear cell.

> It is only if the cell is nonlinear that the two descriptions are not equivalent, and in that case a comparison of the two descriptions can provide insights into the type of nonlinearity (Hayashi, 1964; Blaquière, 1966).

To say that a neuron analyzes the retinal image terms of spatial frequency is to imply far more than that its behavior can be described in terms of responses to sinewave grating stimuli. Otherwise, one could argue that camera lenses and TV systems are spatial-frequency analyzers also. The claim implies that the cell is nonlinear, so that its spatial-frequency tuning cannot be predicted from its responses to isolated bar stimuli without taking the special properties of the particular cell into account.

Is Human Visual Acuity Limited by Diffraction, or by the Eye's Imaging Performance?

The *waveform aberration* approach (Figure C.1B) offers an alternative to the von Seidel expansion and the optical transfer function methods for specifying optical imaging performance. Figure C.7 depicts the wavefront aberration of an individual human eye. The contour lines, drawn at one-wavelength intervals, indicate the amount of optical path length by which the wavefront lies in front of the reference sphere. As a "rule of thumb" guide to lens designers, Rayleigh suggested that the defect of an image caused by a wavefront aberration of one-quarter of a wavelength should be less than the inescapable unsharpness resulting from diffraction (Ditchburn, 1976, p. 283). This estimate of permissible tolerance (the *Rayleigh limit*) is used by lens designers to calculate acceptable limits for monochromatic and chromatic aberrations.

According to the Rayleigh limit for monochromatic light on the visual axis, the quality of the foveal image is determined by diffraction for pupil diameters up to about 2.5 mm. Since the width of the Airy disc (Figure B.18) is inversely pro-

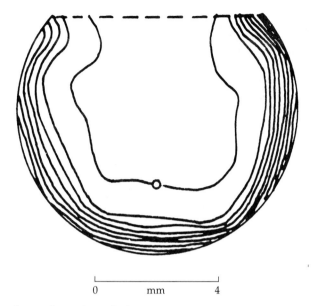

C.7 The wavefront aberration of a human eye. The contour lines, drawn at one-wavelength intervals, indicate the amount of optical path length by which the refracted wavefront departs from the reference sphere for monochromatic light of wavelength 580 nm. The pupil was dilated to a diameter of 7.6 mm by administering drops of a mydriatic to the eye. The upper part of the pupil was cut off by the eye lid. From Smirnov (1962).

portional to the aperture of the lens, imaging quality is poor for very small pupil sizes, and improves progressively up to 2.5 mm. Beyond 2.5 mm, optical aberrations exert an increasing effect on image quality in the human eye. Spherical aberration is the most important and, at the edge of a 5 mm diameter pupil, spherical aberration is equivalent to a one diopter defocus* (van Meeteram, 1974). In summary, the sharpest retinal image is obtained when the pupil diameter is about 2.5 mm (Campbell & Green, 1965).

The Development of the Eye's Optics through Early Life: Why Are We Not All Short-sighted or Long-sighted?

> The cone mosaic is set by biological needs while the optical image quality is the comparatively flexible component in the visual chain. (Snyder, Bossomaier, and Hughes, 1986.)

---

* The optical power of a lens is measured in diopters, defined as the reciprocal of focal length, focal length being expressed in meters. Thus a lens of focal length 1.0 m has a power of 1.0 diopter.

The keen eye of what Rousseau called the "noble savage" is no myth.* Indeed, far from the luxurious lifestyle of what we proudly call our advanced post-industrial civilization, the visual acuity of the Australian aboriginal can reach an unparalleled 6/1.5 (see footnote on p. 192) while, in our towns and cities, short sight (myopia) is very prevalent.

Is the increased incidence of myopia caused by something in the water? Or is it, as Parkinson's disease has been suggested to be, a result of some so-far unidentified industrial pollutant(s)? Has our soft lifestyle caused our genes to rot?

The belief that reading ("too much close work") causes short sight used to be dismissed as an "old wives' tale" by the medical profession. But "old wives' tales" are (like much of our knowledge of the physical world) based on the attentive observation, over long tracts of time, of things that seem to go together.†

Even in large cities it is possible to find many people who do not need glasses. They are neither short-sighted nor long-sighted; they are *emmetropes*. How is it that the length and the focal power of their eyes conspire so perfectly that a sharply focused retinal image is placed exactly onto the photoreceptor layer of the retina? And, more to the point, how is this balance maintained as the eye grows progressively larger during early life?

It had long been known that the incidence of refractive error within the general population does not follow a normal (i.e., bell-shaped) distribution: there is a marked peak centered on zero error. Recent findings suggest that the maintenance of a sharp image on the retina controls the development of the eye's optics and in particular that the retina is part of a feedback loop that controls the increase in eye length so as to maintain a sharp retinal image. Here is the grain of truth in the "old wives' tale."

The eye of the recently hatched free-range chicken is close to the ground as it walks around in search of tasty vegetation, worms, and grit. And the optics of its eye develop so that the close ground is sharply imaged onto the upper part of the retina while, simultaneously, more distant objects are sharply imaged onto the lower part of the retina.

> The optics of the adult eye are the outcome of a growth process in which the requirements of the retina determine the development of the optics.

When chickens were raised wearing small hoods that carried lenses whose optical effects could be compensated for by accommodation, the chickens devel-

---

* The Academy of Dijon offered a prize for the best essay on the question: "Have the arts and sciences conferred benefits on mankind?" The social philosopher Rousseau argued "No," introducing the notion of the noble savage and, in 1750, won the prize (Russell, 1961, p. 662). Rousseau had in mind the native people of North America.

† To assume that, because A is highly correlated with B it necessarily follows that A causes B (or that B causes A) is, or course, a notorious fallacy. But although this conclusion does not necessarily follow, "old wives' tales" not infrequently contain a grain of truth.

oped a refractive disorder (short sight or long sight) in the direction required to compensate for the lens. And this refractive disorder was not caused by any change in the curvature of the cornea (Schaeffel et al., 1988).

> The eyeball was longer in eyes that had looked through negative lenses during visual development than eyes that had looked through positive lenses during visual development.

In the context of a feedback loop, the experiment of Schaeffel et al. provided *closed loop* condition (i.e., a chicken could restore the optical quality of its retinal image by a compensating growth process). When *open loop* conditions were created (by total occlusion), enormous amount of myopia (up to 30 diopters) resulted (Wallman & Adams, 1988; Gottlieb et al., 1988; Schaeffel et al., 1990; Wildsoet & Wallman, 1995).

The relevance to us of this research on the visual development of the optics of the chicken's eye is that short sight in humans is associated with elongation of the eyeball, an elongation that in people with extreme short sight can cause damage to the retina. Young and Leary (1991) provide a review of this topic.

Why Is the Retina Backwards?

> The immediate utility of an organic structure often says nothing at all about the reason for its being. (Gould & Lewontin, 1979)

The vertebrate retina offends sound optical design. As illustrated in Figure 1.9, light must pass through the ganglion cells, horizontal cells, bipolar cells, and amacrine cells before reaching the photoreceptors. The associated scatter will degrade the image formed in the plane of the photoreceptors. A further unfavorable feature of the awkward design is that the axons of the ganglion cells find themselves on the wrong side of the retina, and must gather themselves together at the *blind spot* before exiting through a hole in the retina.

It does not need to be like this. The eyes of cephalopod molluscs are not compromised in this way (Goldsmith, 1991). Plate 1 in Weale (1968) illustrates the eye of the snail *Haliotis*, a creature whose retina is not backwards. According to Goldsmith (1991, p. 62), "The reasons for this awkward structure of the vertebrate retina have to do with its embryological origins, in which the eyecup is formed by the collapse and invagination of a ventricular cavity of the developing brain. In fact, the design of the fovea is (in part) an adaptation to deal with the clumsy result of this embryological heritage."

APPENDIX D

Opponent-Process and Line-Element Models of Spatial Discriminations

Opponent-process and line-element models were originally developed in the context of color vision as alternative theoretical approaches to data on wavelength (hue) discrimination. Both approaches have subsequently been used in attempts to model several different kinds of spatial discrimination and several different kinds of motion discrimination (e.g., Campbell et al., 1970; Beverley & Regan, 1975; Westheimer et al., 1976; Regan, 1982; Regan & Beverley, 1983b, 1985; Wilson & Gelb, 1984; Wilson & Regan, 1984; Wilson, 1986, 1991b).

The two kinds of models have in common the basic idea that, at the first stage of visual processing, the visual variable of interest excites a limited number of broadly tuned filters. As described on pages 8–40, visual variables for which this seems to be the case include the following: wavelength; spatial frequency; orientation; the direction of motion within a fronto-parallel plane; the direction of motion in depth. Fine discriminations of the variable in question are determined by the *relative activity* of the relevant broadly tuned filters (see pp. 33–34, 36–39, 75–91, and 115–123).

It has been suggested that the point of passing visual information through an array of broadly tuned filters is to encode visual information in a compressed form at an early stage for efficient transmission to more central regions of the brain. Remarkably, passing retinal image information through a few broadly tuned filters does not necessarily destroy information.

Provided that the broadly tuned filters have overlapping sensitivities and also that their noise levels are low, information about differences much finer than the bandwidth of a filter is encoded in terms of the relative activities of the set of filters, and can be recovered at a later stage of processing .

See pp. 30–33. Both opponent-process and line-element models are concerned with this implicit representation of fine-grain information (reviewed in Regan [1982]).

A distinction between the two kinds of model is as follows. A line-element model demonstrates that the visual information necessary for the experimentally measured discrimination response is encoded in terms of relative activity within the relevant set of broadly tuned filters, but the model does not specify a mechanism to read out a visual signal whose form is congruous with an observer's yes/no discrimination response. This is sufficient if the aim of the model is to account for the perception of a difference between two values of, for example, wavelength. One need only adapt the widely accepted view that a particular sensation corresponds to a particular spatio-temporal pattern of brain activity (Mountcastle, 1979; Szentagothai, 1978; Sperry, 1980). One could argue, however, that a psychophysical model should go further, because a psychophysical discrimination threshold is based on an observer's yes/no discrimination response. In contrast to line-element models, an opponent-process model specifies a discrete mechanism that is sensitive to the relative activity of the set of filters, and whose bipolar response is congruent with the kind of yes/no motor response collected during a psychophysical procedure such as a 2AFC or d' measurement (see pp. 8–17).

By specifying multiple discrete bipolar mechanisms, opponent models create for themselves the problem that if every possible combination of filter has its own hard-wired opponent mechanism, the total number of opponent mechanisms might be implausibly large. Possible ways around this problem include the following: hard-wired opponent mechanisms exist only for adjacent pairs of channels; opponent mechanisms are not hard-wired but rather are the temporary creation of task-dependent, attention-driven descending signals, perhaps along the lines of the hypothetical shifter circuits proposed by Andersen and Van Essen (1987)—see the dotted arrowed lines in Figure 1.10. Line-element models avoid this problem by not specifying how the pattern of activity within the multidimensional response space is translated into a bipolar discriminative signal.

The line-element concept is, perhaps, most easily understood in the context of color vision. It is well known that the color of a uniform patch of light is encoded in terms of the responses of the three types of cone photoreceptors, so that any spectral distribution can be represented as a point in a three-dimensional space. Any given one of these three dimensions corresponds to the excitation of one of the three types of cone photopigment. Line element models assume that the discrimination process has direct access to these levels of excitation.

Equation (D.1) gives the distance ds between two neighboring points whose coordinates are (U_1, U_2, U_3) and $(U_1 + dU_1, U_2, + dU_2, U_3 + dU_3)$:

$$ds = [(dU_1)^\gamma + (dU_2)^\gamma + (dU_3)^\gamma]^{1/\gamma} \tag{D.1}$$

In ordinary Euclidean space Pythagoras' theorem holds, and $\gamma = 2$ in Equation (D.1). The crucial assumption is that two colors within the three-dimensional space are just-noticeably different if the length of the line element ds has some fixed value, and that this value is the same for all pairs of colors. To ensure that this is the case it has been found necessary to distort the space so that it is no longer Euclidean but rather some form of three-dimensional Riemannian space (Eisenhart, 1960). Equation (D.2) gives an example of such a line element:

$$(ds)^2 = g_{11}(dU_1)^2 + 2g_{1,2}\, dU_1\, dU_2 + g_{22}(dU_2)^2$$

$$+ 2g_{2,3}\, dU_2\, dU_3 + g_{3,3}(dU_3)^2 + 2g_{3,1}\, dU_3\, dU_1 \tag{D.2}$$

where the coefficients $g_{i,k}$ are any continuous functions of the coordinates U_1, U_2, and U_3 which make the expression positive at all points in the three-dimensional Riemannian space.

To avoid complexities of non-Euclidean geometries, several authors have attempted to construct Euclidean spaces in which the coordinates (V_1, V_2, V_3) are nonlinear functions of the cone outputs rather than being simple cone outputs. The line element ds then reverts to the form

$$ds = [(dV_1)^\gamma + (dV_2)^\gamma + (dV_3)^\gamma]^{1/\gamma} \tag{D.3}$$

where the space is Euclidian if $\gamma = 2$, and the problem is reduced to finding the three functions that will ensure that the just-noticeable difference in color is represented by a line element of constant length through the three-dimensional space. This has proved to be a challenging problem. Detailed reviews of the role of line-element models in color theory are available (Wyszecki & Stiles, 1967; Wandell, 1982).

In the spirit of the classical work on color theory, Wilson and Gelb (1984) developed a line-element model of spatial discriminations (Figure 2.48). Their model was more complicated than color models in that the response space had considerably more than three dimensions. They assumed that spatial information from any small area of the retina was processed by an array of spatial filters tuned to six different ranges of spatial frequency, and perhaps 12 preferred orientations. Wilson and Gelb based the response profile of the spatial filters on the oblique masking data reported by Wilson et al. (1983), shown in Figure 2.12. The neural representation of any local, vertically extended target along the horizontal direction is given by the outputs of the six spatial filters that are most excited by the target, and their nearest neighbors along the horizontal direction. To allow for the nonlinear effect of stimulus contrast, the outputs of the filters is passed through the "dipper" characteristic depicted in Figure 2.15. The spatial target is represented as a point in a multidimensional space, whose dimensions correspond to the nonlinearly transduced outputs of the spatial filters. According to Wilson (1991b), in most cases this space is a higher-dimensional version of Equation (D.3) with $\gamma = 2$, i.e., a Euclidean space, but when high-frequency temporal modulation is involved, the value of γ is greater than 2, so that the space is non-Euclidean. Related models have been developed by Watson (1983), Klein and Levi (1985), and Nielson et al. (1985).

A line element in a multidimensional *filter* response space does not account for the findings that spatial-frequency discrimination threshold is the same between orthogonal and between parallel gratings, and that orientation discrimination threshold is the same between gratings of the same spatial-frequency and between gratings of very different spatial frequencies (Burbeck & Regan, 1983a; Bradley & Skottun, 1984). Such pairs of gratings are represented by locations that are far apart in filter response space.

In addition to the finding just mentioned, knotty problems that challenge current models of early spatial vision for LD form include the following: (1) discrimination threshold for orientation, spatial frequency, and contrast are closely similar whether all three variables change simultaneously or only one changes at a time (Vincent & Regan, 1995); (2) line interval discrimination threshold is little affected by the presence of nearly flanking lines (Morgan & Ward, 1985); (3) aspect-ratio discrimination threshold for either an outlined or a solid shape is as low as 1.6 %, even when height and width are removed as reliable cues (Regan & Hamstra, 1992a). These problems are discussed at pages 156–169 and 184–191.

Rectification, Linearizing "ON" and "OFF" Physiological Systems, and Clynes' Theory of Physiological Rein Control

ON and OFF Cells

Bipolar cells in primate retina include those that depolarize to light (ON bipolars) and those that hyperpolarize to light (OFF bipolars). These cells approximate half-wave rectifiers in their responses to temporal changes of local light intensity.

As illustrated in Figure 1.9, bipolar cells feed retinal ganglion cells. In 1938 Harline reported that the receptive fields of retinal ganglion cells have an antagonistic, concentric center-surround organization, some with an excitatory center with an inhibitory surround, others with an inhibitory center and excitatory surround (see Rodieck & Stone [1965a,b] and Gouras & Zrenner [1981]). Center-on and center-off retinal ganglion cells receive their inputs from the corresponding class of bipolar cell, and the connections are segregated anatomically (Nelson et al., 1978; see Schiller, 1986).

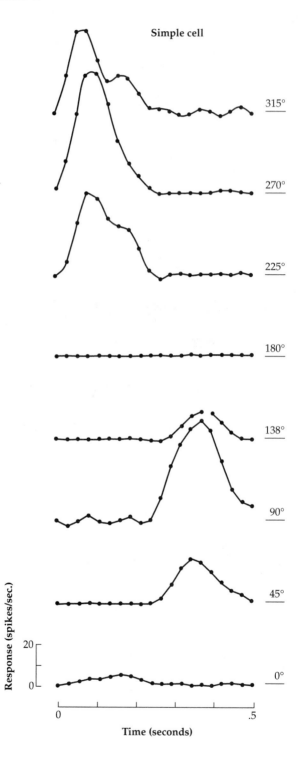

Although sensitivity to temporal variations of contrast falls off steeply at high spatial frequencies, it falls only shallowly as spatial frequency is reduced, so that ganglion cells do respond to temporal variations in the intensity of an unpatterned patch of light. The behavior of both on-center and off-center retinal ganglion cells is roughly equivalent to that of a half-wave rectifier. Full-wave rectification can be approximated by taking into account both on-center and off-center cells.

The classical *simple cells* in primary visual cortex of primates resemble cells in the lateral geniculate nucleus in that a spot stimulus reveals a receptive field with separate excitatory and inhibitory regions (Hubel & Wiesel, 1968). However, instead of being arranged approximately concentrically, these antagonistic regions form parallel strips in the cortical cells. Simple cells respond strongly to a moving bar when the bar is oriented parallel to the parallel strips within the receptive field. Most simple cells sum the contributions from different parts of the receptive field approximately linearly so that the response to an extended pattern (e.g., a grating) can be tolerably well predicted from the receptive field mapped out using a spot of light. But a simple cell is far from linear: in its firing response it approximates the behavior of a half-wave rectifier. Figure E.1 shows the responses of an excitatory-center simple cell to a counterphase-modulated grating (see Figure 2.5A). The cell responded strongly when one of the bars of the grating was centered on the excitatory center of the receptive field. This was the case for spatial phases of 270 degrees and 90 degrees in Figure E.1. But in both cases the cell responded only when the bar centered on the excitatory part of the receptive field was bright and adjacent bars were dim. During the next temporal half-cycle, the bar centered on the excitatory part of the receptive field was dim and adjacent bars were bright. The cell did not respond during this temporal half-cycle. Thus, the responses at 270 degrees and 90 degrees in Figure E.1 occurred during opposite temporal half-cycles.

Linearizing ON and OFF Cells

Figure E.2 shows how the firing frequency of a cell in the lateral geniculate body of a macaque monkey varied when the eye was stimulated with a light whose luminance was modulated sinusoidally. The cell acted approximately like a half-wave rectifier when the luminance modulation depth was high (75% in part A, 50% in part B): firing occurred during positive half-cycles, but no information

◀ **E.1 Linear and nonlinear aspects of the firing response of a cortical simple cell.** The traces are poststimulus time histograms of a representative simple cell in monkey striate cortex. These responses were produced by stimulating the eye with a counterphase-modulated sinusoidal grating presented at eight different positions, each separated by a 45 degree spatial phase, where 360 degrees of spatial phase is the distance between adjacent bright bars. There are two null positions, indicating approximately linear spatial summation of luminance changes. But the cell fails to fire on alternate half-cycles, indicating highly nonlinear behavior that resembles half-wave rectification. After DeValois, Albrecht, and Thorell (1982).

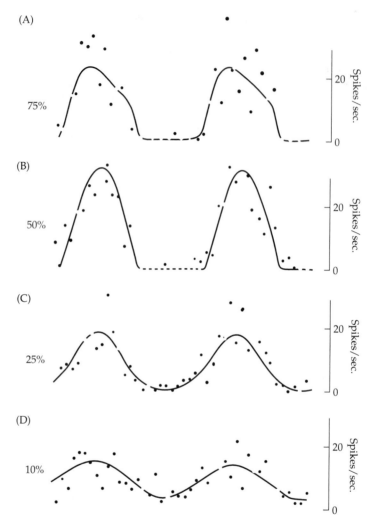

E.2 Rectifier-like behavior in the lateral geniculate body linearized by neural noise. Average spike firing frequencies for a green +, red – cell in the lateral geniculate nucleus of a monkey recorded while the animal's eye was being stimulated with a homogenous sinusoidally modulated flickering light. The modulation depth in percent is defined as $100(L_{max} - L_{min})/(L_{max} + L_{min})$, where L_{max} and L_{min} are, respectively, the maximum and minimum luminances during the flicker cycle. After Spekreijse, van Norren, and van der Berg (1971).

was signaled about negative half-cycles because the cell could not fire at a negative rate. The flattening of the response peak that was evident at the highest modulation depth (compare parts A and B) could be modeled in terms of a compressive rectifier characteristic (see Figure A.5). Figure E.2 also demonstrates the *lin-*

earizing phenomenon. The average response of the cell to low flicker modulation depths was much more sinusoidal than the response at high flicker modulation depths (compare parts D and A). The cause of this linearizing effect is explained in Figure A.5. Because of neural noise at the input to the cell, the operating point was not always located at the origin. Rather, it moved randomly along the characteristic to the left and right of zero on the abscissa. There was, of course, zero output when the operating point shifted sufficiently far to the left of the origin. But the probability was considerable that the small excursion of the signal fell entirely on the smoothly curving characteristic to the right of the origin. Consequently, the average response of the cell became approximately linear (see Figure A.5B). Spekreijse and van der Tweel (1965) pointed out that:

> One implication of this effect is that it is difficult to distinguish between a hard threshold and a smooth accelerating slope near the origin, because neural noise would mask a true hard threshold by linearizing it when signal amplitude was very small.

In an ingenious exploitation of the linearizing effect, Spekreijse showed that physiological rectifiers can be linearized, even when the input signal is large, by adding an *auxiliary signal*. The auxiliary signal need not necessarily be noise. A sinusoidal auxiliary signal allows the linear filter characteristic of the stage before the rectifier to be measured. Spekreijse and his colleagues have carried out such measurements at single-cell level in monkey and goldfish retinae (Spekreijse, 1969; Spekreijse et al., 1971) and at cortical slow wave level in human (Spekreijse & van der Tweel, 1965; Spekreijse, 1966; Spekreijse & Oosting, 1970; Spekreijse & Reits, 1982).

The basic idea is as follows. Consider an idealized "sandwich system" in which the first and last stages are linear frequency filters and the middle stage is a rectifier. Suppose that the input is a flickering light—a luminance that is modulated at a frequency of F Hz. Suppose further that the output waveform comprises a weak F Hz component of frequency F Hz plus a harmonic component, the strongest being at frequency $2F$ Hz. It was Spekreijse (1966) who first saw the crucial point:

> The harmonic distortion does not exist until the input signal reaches the nonlinearity.

With this insight he was able to design the following method for isolating and measuring the properties of the two linear filters. He kept the F Hz input signal constant, and measured the amplitude of the $2F$ Hz distortion term in the output. When a second input (the *auxiliary signal*) was added, the amplitude of the $2F$ Hz term was reduced because of the linearizing effect that the auxiliary signal exerted on the rectifier's abrupt change in slope. Reasoning that a constant linearizing effect means the amplitude of the auxiliary signal *on its arrival at the rectifier* is constant, Spekreijse adjusted the amplitude of the auxiliary signal while varying its frequency so as to maintain a constant linearizing effect. The reciprocal of the amplitude of the auxiliary signal gave the attenuation characteristic of the filter that preceded the rectifier. The attenuation characteristic of the entire sandwich system could then be obtained by comparing the amplitude of the output and input over a range of input signal frequencies (in the absence of an auxiliary signal). The attenuation characteristic of the second linear filter could be derived straightforwardly from the two characteristics already obtained (Spekreijse, 1966).

This rationale has been applied to human psychophysics in the context of motion perception (Regan & Beverley, 1980, 1981).

The Function of the ON/OFF Distinction

It seems reasonable to assume that the clear physiological distinction between the rectifying ON and OFF systems within the retina has some functional role. Schiller et al. (1986) pointed out that a neuron whose resting discharge rate was low could signal (say) light increment, but could not signal a wide range of light decrements. If a neuron is to signal both increments and decrements, the resting discharge rate would have to be rather high, and a high resting activity might be metabolically disadvantageous to the organism. But if some cells fire for decrement while others fire for increment, the resting rate for all cells can be very low, thereby achieving metabolic efficiency. Schiller et al. suggested that some purposes of the ON/OFF organization are: (1) to provide equal sensitivity and rapid information transfer for light increments and decrements (information transfer is rapid because increments and decrements are both transmitted centrally by means of an excitatory process); (2) to facilitate high sensitivity to spatial contrast.

Clynes' Theory of Physiological Rein Control

A third, and perhaps, equally important point was emphasized by Clynes (a pioneer in the development of the analysis of nonlinear biological systems) in his mathematical theory of physiological "rein control." In 1964, Clynes pointed out that the drift of the zero point can be far less in an ON/OFF (push–pull in electronic parlance) system than in a system that represents zero as a nonzero signal (reviewed in Milsum, 1966; see also Clynes, 1969).

A Note on Spatial Sampling and Nyquist's Theorem

Nyquist's Theorem and Aliasing

Aliasing is a potential problem in any sampled data system. The effect is often illustrated in terms of Western movies. The film camera samples the visual scene at some fixed rate, each sample occupying one frame of the film. If a wagon wheel is rotating slowly enough, the motion is reproduced faithfully. But at higher rates of rotation the wheel may appear to rotate more slowly than its actual rate, may appear not to rotate, or may even appear to rotate backward. The false rotation speeds are generated because the movie camera's sampling rate is too low to accurately record high rates of rotation. For example, if the speed of rotation is such that any given wheel spoke occupies the position occupied by another spoke one twenty-fifth of a second earlier and the camera takes twenty-five exposures per second, then the wheel will appear not to rotate. (This is the same principle that allows rapidly rotating machinery to be examined when "frozen" by illumination with a flashing strobe light.)

Errors will result unless the sampling rate is more than twice the highest temporal frequency present in the visual scene. This minimum sampling rate requirement is known as the Nyquist criterion. Temporal frequencies above half the sampling rate will be represented as spurious low-frequency components that were not present in the original scene signal; these higher frequencies are said to be "folded back," and they appear as noise of lower frequency.

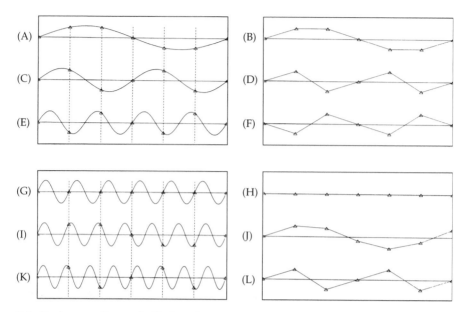

F.1 Undersampling and aliasing. Six samples per cycle of a sinusoidal waveform (A) give a tolerably faithful representation of the original waveform (B). Three samples per cycle (C) still provide a correct representation of the frequency of the sinusoid (D). But two or fewer than two samples per cycle (E–K) incorrectly represent the frequency of the sinusoid (F–L) as a frequency that is lower than the true frequency or even (G, H) as a constant level. From Regan (1989a).

Figure F.1 illustrates how a too-low sampling rate (i.e., "undersampling") creates spurious frequency components. A sampling rate six times higher than the frequency of a sine wave signal (A) correctly represents the sine wave's frequency, and even without low-pass filtering (i.e., when the points are joined with straight lines), the sampled waveform approximates the original sine wave (B). At a sampling rate of less than two per cycle, however, the true frequency of the sine wave signal is not represented, and in addition spurious frequencies are introduced (E–L). For example, although a sampling rate of F Hz represents an $(F/3)$ Hz sine wave correctly as an $(F/3)$ Hz waveform (C, D), the same sampling rate also represents a $(4F/3)$ Hz sine wave as an $(F/3)$ Hz waveform rather than as the $(4F/3)$ Hz waveform that it really is (K, L). Undersampling can even represent a sine wave (G) as a straight line (H)—the "stationary wagon wheel" effect. (This occurs when samples are taken at alternate zero-crossings.)

We can now see intuitively that sampling at less than twice per cycle will wrongly represent the frequency of a sine wave signal, and that even when sampling at a rate of exactly twice per cycle, the sine wave signal may be represented erroneously as a straight line. What may be less obvious is that, in principle, sampling at a rate just higher than twice per cycle and then suitably low-pass filtering the sampled waveform will restore the original sine wave signal. But this is, theoretically, the case. In practical instruments, any input frequencies higher than half the sampling rate are effectively removed by an "anti-aliasing" filter. An ideal anti-aliasing filter would look like Figure F.2A. It would pass all the desired input frequencies with no attenuation and completely reject any frequencies higher than half the sampling frequency. Such an ideal filter is, however, theoretically and practically impossible. Real filters look like Figure F.2B, with a gradual rolloff and finite rather than infinite attenuation of unwanted signals. Large input signals that are not sufficiently attenuated in the transition band (Figure F.2B) might still alias into the desired frequency range. To avoid this problem, the sampling rate is in practice set at 2.5 to 4 times the maximum desired input frequency and anti-aliasing filters are designed to produce a very large attenuation beyond the transition band.

For our present purpose, first consider a long train of sinewaves that is windowed so that its duration is only a few cycles. The frequency content of a long train of sinewaves is narrowly centered on P^{-1} Hz (where P sec. is the period of the sinewave) so that the Nyquist frequency is $2P^{-1}$ Hz. However, if we restrict the sinewave to only a few cycles, this act broadens its power spectrum, so that power is extended to frequencies that can be considerably higher than P^{-1} Hz (this effect is discussed at pp. 415–416). Consequently, for a windowed sine wave, the Nyquist frequency can be considerably higher than P^{-1} Hz.

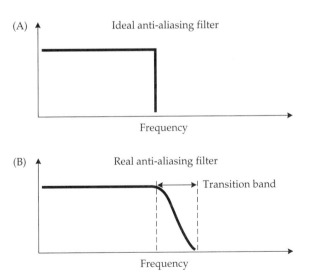

F.2 Practical anti-aliasing filters require sampling rates that are considerably higher than the theoretical minimum requirement. (A) Ideal anti-aliasing filter. (B) Practical anti-aliasing filter. From Regan (1989a).

As discussed in the next two sections, sampling theory can be extended from temporal to spatial waveforms. Later in this appendix (pp. 477–481) we discuss aliasing in human vision.

Spatial Sampling of the Stimulus and Its Effect on Grating Detection Threshold

Burr et al. (1985) measured the effect of *stimulus sampling frequency* on contrast sensitivity for a luminance-defined grating using the spatially sampled gratings illustrated in Figure F.3. There are four complete grating cycles in each of the four parts of Figure F.3, though the luminance profiles depicted in Figure F.4 show only two complete cycles. Burr et al. found that the greatest effect of sampling was for coarsely sampled stationary gratings of low spatial frequency. (The reader can informally check that conclusion by viewing Figure F.3 over a range of distances.) The effect was large: grating contrast threshold was as much as 10 times lower at a sampling rate of 64 samples/cycle than at 4 samples/cycle. This dif-

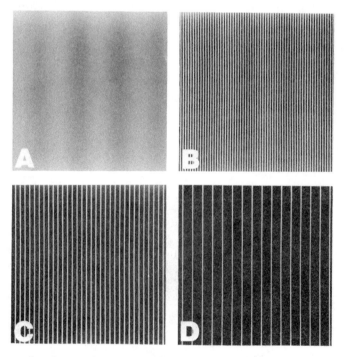

F.3 Photographs of a continuous (A) and sampled (B–D) luminance-defined grating. On very close viewing (with a positive lens to aid accommodation if required), only in part A is the grating visible. With increasing distance the gratings begin to emerge in the other photographs. From Burr, Ross, and Morrone (1985).

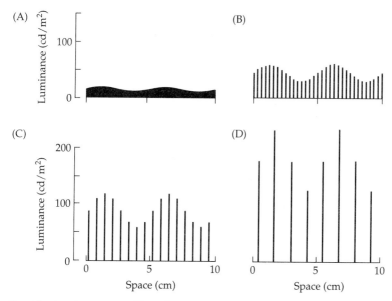

F.4 The luminance profiles of the four stimuli shown in Figure F.3. All four stimuli consist of four grating cycles in which the luminance has been compressed into narrow sample bars. The sampling rate is 64 samples/cycle in (A), 16 samples/cycle in (B), 8 samples/cycle in (C), and 4 samples/cycle in (D). As a result of the compressive sampling, both the local luminance and the local amplitude of modulation at the sampling points depend on the sampling rate. However, as shown in Figure F.6, the average luminance and peak-to-peak amplitude of the sampled grating is practically the same for the four stimuli. From Burr, Ross, and Morrone (1985).

ference became progressively smaller as the grating's spatial frequency was progressively increased until, at a grating frequency of about 10 cycles/deg., grating detection threshold was the same at all four sampling rates.

Harmon and Julesz (1973) had used the concept of *critical band masking* to account for their finding that the visibility of a coarsely sampled image can be improved by *blurring* the sampled image (Figure F.5). According to their proposal, the spurious high spatial frequencies that are introduced by the sampling (by the sharp edges of the sampling squares in Figure F.5) mask the lower frequencies that survive the sampling and that carry the content of the picture.

Burr et al. rejected this candidate explanation for their data by carrying out the following control experiments. They measured contrast sensitivity for a sinusoidal grating in the presence of a high-frequency mask that was equal in amplitude (but not matched in phase) to the spurious sampling frequencies. This mask was created from the Fourier transform (Figure F.6) of the sampled grating shown in Figure F.3, by scrambling the phase of the harmonic components. Burr et al. found that the effect of sampling frequency was essentially eliminated, thus rejecting critical-band masking as an explanation.

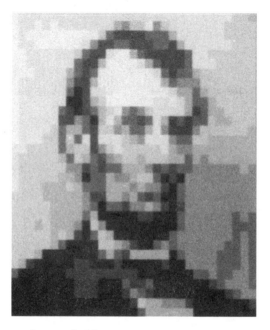

F.5 Blurring a coarsely sampled image improves recognition. Viewing from a distance has a similar effect. From Harmon and Julesz (1973).

A clue to a possible explanation was provided by the finding that contrast detection threshold for the sampled grating was proportional to the mean luminance of the sample bars. Thus, there was a Weber's law relationship between local bar luminance and global grating contrast threshold, but not between the luminance and the modulation amplitude of the same bars.

Burr et al. proposed the following:

> The response to any given line is regulated by local gain control that occurs before spatial summation and before the detection stage.

Burr et al. estimated the size of the summation pool for gain control to be very small, with a Gaussian space constant of no more than 0.5 minutes of arc, i.e., approximately the same size as the eye's line-spread function (see pp. 44–48).

After referring to the comment of Shapley and Enroth-Cugell (1984) that changes in visual sensitivity with luminance probably resulted from gain changes rather than compressive nonlinearity, Burr et al. pointed out that the combined action of many local spatial filters operating at different gains can be regarded as a global nonlinearity. (Contrast gain control is discussed at pp. 83–91.)

Burr and his colleagues went on to note that if gain control is as local as suggested by their data, mean or background luminance is not the most appropriate normalization factor in the definition of spatial contrast. In particular, the con-

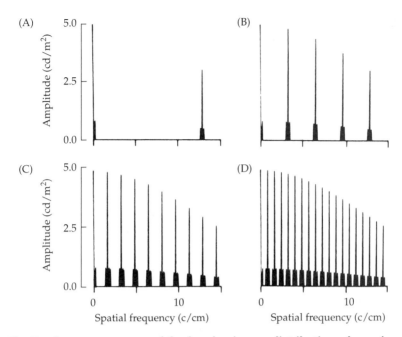

F.6 The Fourier power spectra of the four luminance distributions shown in Figure F.3. The term at zero spatial frequency (representing the mean luminance) and the component at the frequency of the sinusoid (0.2 cycles/deg.) are practically identical in the four conditions. (The mean luminance term is the tall spike at the far left in part A, and the spike at the grating frequency is the small spike next to it.) What sampling does is to introduce a string of spurious high-frequency terms at a repetition frequency determined by the sampling rate. From Burr, Ross, and Morrone (1985).

trast of a single target of luminance L_{max} surrounded by a uniformly illuminated area of luminance L_{min} is often defined as $(L_{max} - L_{min})/L_{min}$ (i.e., the Weber contrast). Burr et al. proposed that $(L_{max} - L_{min})/L_{max}$ is a superior definition, because the luminance that sets the local gain (L_{max}) is also the normalization factor for contrast. Burr et al. pointed out that, if the contrast of the sampled gratings shown in Figure F.3 were redefined as the amplitude of the sampled waveform divided by the local luminance of the bars carrying the contrast information, contrast sensitivity would be constant for all sampling rates, i.e., the effect of sampling would disappear.

Gray and Regan (1998a) measured the contrast sensitivity curve for spatially sampled OTD and LD grating of the kind illustrated in Figure 4.3A. Field size was 30 degrees (horizontally) × 7 degrees and the number of lines per degree along a line perpendicular to the (vertical) bars of the grating was 2.2. We measured detection thresholds using temporal 2AFC. In the case of OTD gratings, the test grating had one of four possible values of orientation contrast. The reference stimulus was an OTD grating of zero orientation contrast, i.e., parallel lines. Line orientation for any given reference stimulus varied from trial to trial, and could assume any value of line orientation (and with the same probability distribution) as in the OTD grating with which that reference stimulus was paired. This ensured that the only cue to the task (i.e., "was the grating presented first or second") was that the grating had an orientation gradient and the reference stimulus had not. The filled symbols jointed by a continuous line in Figure F.7 shows that the contrast sensitivity curve for the OTD grating peaked at about 0.13 cycles/deg., and fell off sharply at higher spatial frequencies. A similar curve was obtained for LD gratings with the same spatial sampling as the OTD gratings. These results replicated the findings of Kingdom et al. (1994).

The spatial frequency at which the number of texture lines per grating cycle fell to 2 is marked by the solid arrow. Inspection reveals that high-frequency rolloff started when the number of samples per grating cycles fell below about six. When the number of samples per cycles was increased to six over the entire range of spatial frequencies, we found that the contrast sensitivity curve extend-

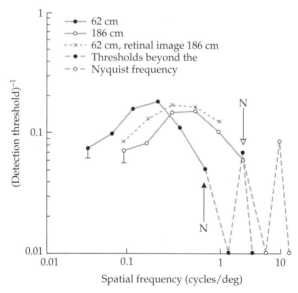

Spatial frequency (cycles/deg)

F.7 The high-frequency rolloff in the contrast sensitivity curve can be determined entirely by the spatial sampling of the stimulus grating. The data points show the effect of spatial frequency on orientation contrast detection threshold for a texture-defined grating similar to that shown in Figure 4.3A. The continuous and dashed lines join data points for which there were more than two and less than two, respectively, texture lines per grating cycle. When viewed from 62 cm, the grating had 2.3 texture lines per grating cycle and the number of texture lines per grating cycle fell to 2 at a spatial frequency of 1.1.4 cycles/deg. (solid arrow). After Gray and Regan (1998a).

ed to far higher spatial frequencies for both OTD and LD gratings. (Compare Figures 4.4 and F.7.) We concluded that the steep high-frequency rolloff in Figure F.7 was an artifact of undersampling. This might seem surprising given that Nyquist's theorem states that sufficient information to recover a continuous sinusoidal waveform is given by sampling the sinusoid just more than twice per cycle. The explanation we offered was that the steep degradation of both visual acuity and orientation discrimination with retinal eccentricity would have the effect that bars of the OTD grating, viewed extrafoveally, would be processed less effectively than the bars falling on the fovea, so that, in effect, the grating would be windowed even more severely than in the monitor display and its power spectrum thereby widened even more than expected from the number of cycles in the display (see pp. 415–416). This is one possible reason why spatial-frequency discrimination threshold starts to rise at a point where the number of spatial samples per grating cycle is considerably greater than two. A second possible reason is that the physiological filter that smoothed the sampled grating is unlikely to approach ideal performance (Figure F.2).

Our data on luminance-defined gratings might seem to disagree with the finding of Burr et al. (1985) that many more than six samples per cycle were required to attain maximum contrast sensitivity for LD gratings of low spatial frequency. The reason for this disagreement may be that Burr et al. used regularly spaced sampling bars, each of which extended across the entire grating (Figure F.3), whereas our sampling bars were short and irregularly spaced (Figure 4.3A).

The experimental conditions used to obtain the data plotted by the continuous line joining filled symbols approximated the experimental conditions of Kingdom et al. (1994). A weakness of this experimental design is that it allows thresholds to be measured for gratings for which the number of lines per grating cycle is considerably lower than two, even when the texture lines are spatially jittered or spatially randomized. This point can be understood as follows. The reference stimulus had zero orientation contrast over the entire display. But the aliasing present for spatial frequencies above the Nyquist frequency (i.e., when there were less than two lines per grating cycle) created patches of finite orientation contrast, so that the test and reference stimuli could be distinguished. For explanatory purposes, suppose that the texture lines had been spaced regularly rather than being spatially jittered. The dashed line joining filled symbols in Figure F.7 joins data points measured at spatial frequencies at and above the Nyquist frequency using a grating whose lines were not spatially jittered. (As already mentioned, the spatial frequency for which there were two texture lines per grating cycle is indicated by the solid arrow in Figure F.7.) Detection threshold was effectively infinite when there was exactly one line per grating cycle, one line per two grating cycles, and so on. However, grating threshold could easily be measured when there was one texture line per 1.5 grating cycles, one texture line per 2.5 grating cycles, and so on. As would be expected on theoretical grounds in these situations, threshold was approximately the same as for the spatial frequency for which there were 2 texture lines per grating cycle. When texture lines were irregularly spaced (as in Figure 4.3A), the amplitude of the peak-to-trough variation in threshold shown by the dashed line in Figure F.7 was reduced, but thresholds could still be measured when the number of lines per grating were far less than two. Such thresholds tell us nothing about visual sensitivity to the periodicity of the grating.

The reduction of sensitivity shown by the solid symbols in Figure F.7 for spatial frequencies below about 0.1 cycles/deg. also tells us nothing about visual sensitivity to OTD gratings. It was an artifact: the total number of cycles in the display fell from three cycles to one cycle as spatial frequency was reduced below 0.1 cycles/deg. (see Figure B.7C–E).

Spatial Sampling of the Stimulus and Its Effect on Spatial-Frequency Discrimination Threshold

Open symbols in Figure F.8 show that spatial-frequency discrimination threshold was flat from 0.07 cycles/deg. (three full cycles on the screen) up to about 0.4 cycles/deg., after which it rose sharply, and the task become impossible for spa-

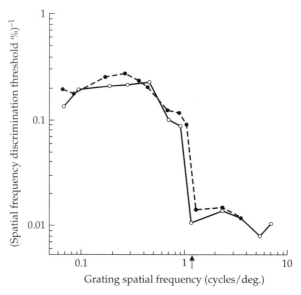

F.8 The high-frequency rolloff in the spatial-frequency discrimination curve can be determined entirely by the spatial sampling of the stimulus grating. The graph shows the effect of spatial frequency on spatial-frequency discrimination threshold for a texture-defined grating (open symbols) and for a spatially sampled luminance-defined grating (solid symbols). Each grating had 2.3 texture lines per degree of visual subtense along a direction perpendicular to the bars of the grating. The number of samples per grating cycle fell to two at a frequency of 1.14 cycles/deg. (solid arrow). After Gray and Regan (1998a).

tial frequencies higher than about 1 cycles/deg. Filled symbols show that spatial-frequency discrimination threshold for an LD grating with the same spatial sampling as the OTD grating behaved similarly; thresholds were not significantly different for the two kinds of grating.

How can we account for the steep degradation of visual performance at such low spatial frequencies? The number of lines per degree of visual angle is the most obvious suspect. In Figure F.8 the grating contained 96 (horizontal) × 16 lines on average and subtended 42 deg. (horizontal) × 7.5 deg., so that the mean number of lines per degree along a horizontal line perpendicular to the bars of the grating was 2.28. Looking at Figure F.8 in a different way, threshold started to rise when the number of lines per grating cycles fell below about 6 (i.e., at a spatial frequency of 0.4 cycles/deg.). The suspicion that the common shape of the OTD and LD discrimination curves in Figure F.8A was determined by a spatial sampling artifact rather than reflecting properties of the human visual system was confirmed when we repeated the experiment while ensuring that there were always six or more lines per grating cycle: quite different discrimination curves were obtained (Figure 4.9).

Aliasing in Human Vision Caused by Undersampling of the Retinal Image by Retinal Photoreceptors

In principle, visual acuity could be limited either by the optical quality of the retinal image (i.e., by the quality of the eye as an imaging device) or by the spacing of foveal cones. Several authors have attempted to find the relative importance of these two possibilities for visual acuity.

It is a commonly held view that the quality of the eye as an imaging device is well matched to the cone spacing. For example, visual acuity is not greatly improved when the image-degrading effect of the eye's optical aberrations are considerably reduced by creating interference fringes on the retina (Le Grand, 1937; Arnulf & Dupuy, 1960; Westheimer, 1960; Campbell & Green, 1965). Furthermore, the minimum spacing between foveal cones corresponds to a Nyquist frequency of 56 cycles/deg., and estimates of the modulation transfer function for the eye's optics (Campbell & Gubisch, 1966; van Meeteren, 1974) indicate that the contrast in the retinal image of a grating of 100% contrast is about 10 times less at 56 cycles/deg. than at low spatial frequencies (Williams, 1985).

Coming down on the side of oversampling, Snyder et al. (1986) showed that the eyes of several species produce a retinal image that is sharper than can be resolved by the photoreceptor mosaic. What in the evolutionary past of these animals might be the competitive advantage provided by this curious arrangement? One suggestion is based on the fact that the modulation transfer function of the eye's optics attenuates only gradually as spatial frequency is increased. Consequently, it would better retain spatial information at frequencies somewhat above the Nyquist frequency and thus allow the frequency spectrum of natural scenes to be processed more effectively (Snyder et al., 1986; Hughes, 1986;

Charman, 1991). According to Tolhurst et al. (1992), the spatial power spectrum of typical natural scenes attenuates approximately inversely with the square of spatial frequency—though there are considerable scene-to-scene variations. And both Helmholtz (1866/1962) and Bryam (1944) stated that they could detect the presence of gratings whose spatial frequencies exceeded 60 cycles/deg., even though they could not resolve the bars of the grating.* The anatomical work on human retinae reported by Hirsch and Curcio (1989) provides support for the view that cone spacing offers a "reasonable" prediction of visual acuity within the retinal region extending from slightly off the foveal center to about 2.0 deg. of retinal eccentricity. On the other hand, they drew attention to a "narrow peak of anatomical resolution at the foveal center where the acuity appears to be overestimated by cone spacing" (p. 1095), implying that "some potential spatial resolution in the foveal center may either be lost by the foveal optics or by the neural processing beyond the sampling stage" (p. 1101). The optimization of performance for the optics and retina taken as a whole is discussed further at pages 445–446.

Color Plate 7 and Figure F.9 illustrate how the arrangement of cones in the fovea of monkey is organized in a strikingly (though not perfectly) regular manner with hexagonal symmetry. In principle, therefore, a grating whose spatial frequency was appreciably greater than the Nyquist frequency should, through aliasing, generate visible moiré patterns.† Moiré patterns can be seen by creating on the retina interference fringes whose spatial frequency is considerably higher than 56 cycles/deg. (Bryam, 1944; Campbell & Green, 1965). Figure F.10A–C are sketches of the low-frequency aliasing patterns perceived in such condition (Williams, 1985): because the grating's spatial frequency was considerably above the Nyquist limit set by the distance between the regularly spaced cones, the high spatial-frequency information was represented by low spatial frequencies that *were not present in the retinal image, though clearly perceived by observers.*

At a grating frequency of 80 cycles/deg., observers reported an annulus of fine wavy lines whose outer diameter was about 2.5 deg. (Figure F.10A.) The center of the hole in the middle coincided with the line of sight (i.e., the central fovea). As the grating's spatial frequency was increased, the annulus of wavy lines shrank in diameter until at a frequency of 90 to 100 cycles/deg., observers reported a patch resembling zebra stripes or a fingerprint that subtended about 0.7 deg., and was centered on the line of sight (Figure F.10B,C). As grating frequency was further increased from 100 to 150 cycles/deg., the size of the striped patch progressively fell until at about 150 to 160 cycles/deg. it disappeared abruptly. At higher grating frequencies up to the limit of 200 cycles/deg. (set by the diameter of the eye

---

* On the other hand, this does not necessarily mean that the spatial patterning within the optical image at such high spatial frequencies would be of any value to the organism. Figure C.5 indicates that the modulation transfer function of an imaging system can ripple, but beyond the first zero, the spatial pattern of the image is spurious.

† Moiré patterns of low spatial frequency are seen when one fly screen is placed in front of another fly screen, or when someone on television is sufficiently ill-advised as to wear narrowly striped clothing.

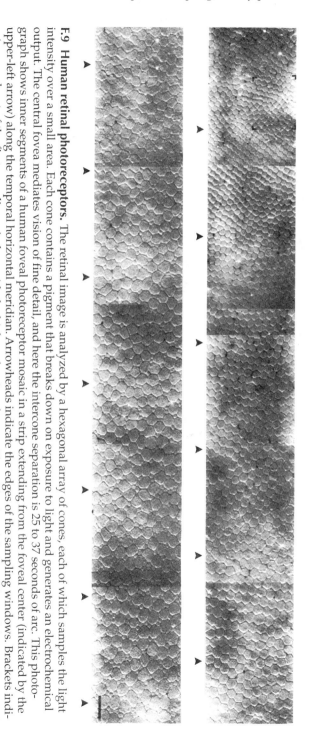

F.9 Human retinal photoreceptors. The retinal image is analyzed by a hexagonal array of cones, each of which samples the light intensity over a small area. Each cone contains a pigment that breaks down on exposure to light and generates an electrochemical output. The central fovea mediates vision of fine detail, and here the intercone separation is 25 to 37 seconds of arc. This photograph shows inner segments of a human foveal photoreceptor mosaic in a strip extending from the foveal center (indicated by the upper-left arrow) along the temporal horizontal meridian. Arrowheads indicate the edges of the sampling windows. Brackets indicate a quadrant of the first sampling window with the highest density of cones. The midpoint of the boundary of this quadrant and a quadrant adjacent to it in the temporal direction (to the right) with similar density and mean spacing was considered the point of zero eccentricity. The strip contains profiles of only cones up to the fifth window, where the profiles of rods (the small cells) begin to intrude, breaking the hexagonal symmetry of the cone lattice. Bar = 10 micrometers. From Hirsch and Curcio (1989). Photograph kindly supplied by Christine A. Curcio.

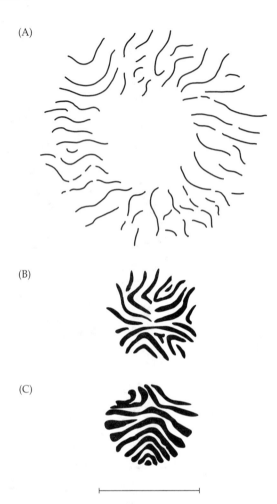

F.10 Moiré patterns caused by undersampling by foveal cones. Drawings of the
visual impressions caused by viewing sinusoidal gratings of spatial frequencies 80
(part A) and 100 (Parts B and C) cycles/deg. created on the observer's retina by
interference of coherent light. Parts A and B drawn by D. R. Williams; C drawn by a
naive observer. The scale bar at the bottom indicates 1.0 degree of visual angle. From
Williams (1985).

pupil), the interference fringes produced "a faint scintillating granular appearance of the field within the central fovea" (Williams, 1985, p. 200). Williams' conclusions were as follows:

1. The separation between cones is lowest in the central fovea, so the
   Moiré pattern within the central hole in Figure F.10A had a spatial
   frequency that was too high to see.

2. The zebra stripes in Figure F.10B,C were coarse because the spatial period of the grating approximated the distance between foveal cones.

3. Moiré patterns were difficult to observe at retinal eccentricities of more than about 1.25 degrees because the presence of rods renders the cone lattice less regular. Direct evidence for this degradation of lattice regularity is shown in Figure F.9.

APPENDIX G

The Measurement of Light

Photopic and Scotopic Vision

It is essential to make a clear distinction between physiological measurements of power or energy (radiometry) and measurements that relate to the characteristics of human vision (photometry).

Within a restricted high-intensity range, viewing conditions have only a small influence on the relative spectral sensitivity curve of the eye when compared with normal intersubject variability. The limits of this *photopic* range are that (a) the luminance should not fall below 3 cd/m^2 or so, and (b) the field should be viewed centrally and should be restricted to 2 to 3 degrees subtense. The stability of the eye's properties over the photopic range is the basis of the internationally agreed Commission Internationale de l'Éclairage (CIE) photopic system of light measurement.

At moderate light levels (about 3 to 0.003 cd/m^2) there is a transition range over which the eye's relative spectral sensitivity curve depends on light intensity. Photometric measurements in this mesopic range present special problems.

At very low light levels (below about 0.003 cd/m^2) there is a second range over which the relative spectral sensitivity curve of the eye is rather independent of light level. The stability of the eye's properties over this *scotopic* range is the basis of the CIE scotopic system of light measurement. It is a familiar experience that color vision is largely or completely lost at low levels of illumination (i.e., in scotopic vision), and because it is relatively rod-free, the fovea becomes less sensitive

483

than more peripheral retina. Furthermore, the eye's peak sensitivity shifts from the green in photopic vision to the blue–green in scotopic vision (the Purkinje shift), producing a striking subjective effect: white lettering and a red background that look equally bright in sunlight appear quite different under dim illumination; after sunset the white letters look far brighter than the red background.

Photometric Units

The quantification and measurement of physical quantities such as weight, temperature, and energy are familiar concepts. The quantification and measurement of a subjective quantity are less familiar, and less straightforward. Nevertheless, the amount of visible light can be quantified rather precisely even though it is essentially a subjective quantity. Indeed, the amount of visible light in particular working environments is specified by law.

The radiant power produced by a light source is called the *radiant flux*, is straightforwardly defined in *watts,* and can be measured with a radiometer. The amount of visible light corresponding to this flow of energy is called the *luminous flux* and is measured in *lumens.* Up to 1979 the lumen was defined in terms of an internationally agreed standard light source. At one time this standard light source was a standard candle (specially made from sperm whale oil, but a candle, nevertheless). After 1948 the standard light source was a special object (a *black body*) at the temperature of freezing platinum (2,042°K). In 1979, however, the definition of the lumen was changed by international agreement and the standard source was abandoned. The new definition is equivalent to the statement that one-watt power of monochromatic radiation whose wavelength is 555 nm provides 683 lumens. The size of the new lumen thus defined is effectively the same as the size of the old lumen. The human eye is less sensitive to light at the red and blue ends of the spectrum than at 555 nm (green) so that one watt of red or blue light provides less than 683 lumens. (And in the ultraviolet and infrared, one watt of power provides no lumens at all; that is, it cannot be seen.) The number of lumens given by one watt of power at any given wavelength λ nm is equal to K_λ. A graph of K_λ versus λ is called the V_λ curve or the "photopic spectral luminous efficiency" curve (or the "relative luminosity" or "relative visibility" curve) and is shown in Figure G.1. It peaks in the green at 555 nm.

The visual sensitivity curve for the dark-adapted eye is called the V'_λ curve. As already mentioned, peak sensitivity for the dark-adapted eye shifts from green toward the blue end of the spectrum. The V'_λ curve peaks at about 510 nm. Compared with the photopic (V_λ) curve, absolute sensitivity to blue and blue–green is increased while absolute sensitivity to red is reduced. The scotopic curve is defined so that K'_λ and K_λ have exactly the same value at 555 nm; therefore, the lumen has the same definition in scotopic and photopic vision (Figure G.1). At the peak sensitivity for the scotopic eye there are 1,700 lumens per watt.

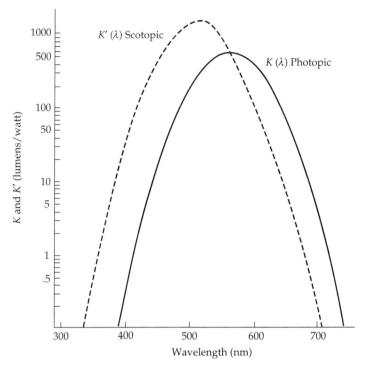

G.1 The spectral luminous efficiency curves for photopic (*K*) and scotopic (*K'*) vision.

The perceived brightness of a surface is largely determined by its *luminance.* Luminance is expressed in candelas per square meter (cd/m^2), where candela is the unit that expresses the "strength of a light source" in lumens per unit solid angle produced by the light source. Note that most light sources have different "strengths" in different directions—a searchlight is an extreme example—and this is documented for any given source by plotting a polar graph of candelas versus direction.

The amount of illumination received by a surface is called *illuminance* and is defined as the luminous flux falling per unit area in lumens per square meter (lumens/m^2).

There is no equivocation about the luminance of a surface: 1 cd/m^2 is the same in Europe, North America, Japan, and anywhere else. But it is not quite true to say that the physiological stimulation produced by a surface is entirely determined by its luminance. The retinal stimulus is determined by the amount of light falling per unit area on the retina, that is, the *retinal illuminance,* and for a surface of any given luminance the retinal illuminance depends on the size of the eye pupil. Prior to the present-day Système Internationale (SI) units, the unit of retinal illuminance was called the troland (cd/m^2/mm^2), defined as the retinal illuminance produced

Table G.1 Conversion between Obsolete Luminance Units and Système Internationale (SI) Luminance Units

Luminance unit[a]	Number of millilamberts
cd/m^2	0.314
cd/cm^2	3,140
cd/ft^2	3.38
cd/in^2	487
ft-lambert	1.08
lambert	1,000
International Apostilb	0.1

[a]1 lambert = 1/p (candela/cm2);
1 foot-lambert = 1/ p (candela/ft2).

by viewing a surface of luminance 1 cd/m^2 through a pupil of area 1 mm^2. The SI unit of retinal illuminance substitutes m^2 for mm^2; thus, it has the dimensions $cd/m^2/m^2$ and is equal to 10^8 trolands.

When calculating retinal illuminance, the Stiles–Crawford effect (of the first kind) should be borne in mind. Stiles and Crawford found that the luminous efficiency of light depends on its point of entry at the eye pupil. This is because rays that enter through the pupil center pass more or less up the axis of retinal cones, whereas rays that enter near the edge of the pupil strike retinal cones obliquely and thus pass through less cone pigment.

By international agreement, the SI system is the preferred system of units. Indeed, many scientific journals insist on the SI system. However, in the past there was a bewildering proliferation of light units in addition to the SI system that has now replaced them all. Although these older units are no longer used, readers may find the conversion table provided (Table G.1) useful when reading older scientific publications, and also when using photometers that are calibrated in non-SI units.

The Measurement of Radiant Power

Before embarking on attempts to measure radiant power, the experimenter is well advised to rethink whether it is really necessary to carry out the difficult measurement of absolute power, or whether relative power measurements or even photometric measurements would suffice.

Except within standards laboratories, the ultimate instrument for measuring radiant power is a calibrated bolometer or thermopile. Both thermopiles and bolometers have flat sensitivity curves through the invisible infrared, the visible spectrum, and the invisible ultraviolet regions. Therefore, when calibrating a visual stimulus one must ensure that no ultraviolet or infrared radiation reaches the measuring instrument. This point is worthy of attention even when there are interference filters in the stimulus beam.

Because thermopiles and bolometers are rather insensitive, it is often necessary to employ the absolute instrument to calibrate a photomultiplier tube that is sufficiently sensitive to detect the radiation falling on the position occupied by the subject's eye. It is sometimes possible to calibrate the photomultiplier by using the same light source and filter combinations that will be used in the physiological experiments. This method eliminates the need to allow for the bandwidths of interference filters and for the spectral distribution characteristics of light sources.

The Measurement of Color

It is often adequate to specify a stimulus color in terms of its *dominant wavelength* and *colorimetric purity*. In any case, this method of specifying a color has the practical advantage that it gives an immediate idea of what the color will look like. The two quantities can be measured by the following procedures: One-half of a bipartite 2° field is illuminated by the test stimulus. The other half of the field is illuminated by a mixture of white light (illuminant B) of luminance L_W and a narrowband monochromatic light whose wavelength is variable (wavelength λ and luminance L_λ). The test stimulus is then subjectively matched by varying L_W, λ, and L_λ. To match extraspectral purple colors to white it may be necessary to add the monochromatic light (in this case the complementary wavelength) to the test stimulus, rather than to the white stimulus. The dominant wavelength of the test stimulus is defined as λ and its colorimetric purity is approximately

$$p \approx L_\lambda \, / (L_W + L_\lambda) \qquad\qquad \text{(Eq. G.1)}$$

An exact expression is given in Williamson and Cummins (1983, p. 459). In most practical cases, for both narrow-bandwidth and medium-bandwidth (i.e., roughly 10 nm) interference filters, the colorimetric purity is approximately 100%, and the dominant wavelength is approximately the same as that for peak energy transmission, although the displacement of dominant wavelength for filters whose center wavelengths are in the deep blue or above roughly 630 nm may be significant in some circumstances. The dominant wavelengths and colorimetric purities of wideband pigment filters (e.g., Kodak Wratten filters), can be calculated from data given by the manufacturers.

The rigorous system of specifying color by three numbers and the notion of the unit of color-producing effect are thoroughly discussed by Wright (1946) and Wyszecki and Stiles (1967).

Linear and Logarithmic Scales: The Decibel

When a linear scale is used it is difficult to *see* both large and small signals simultaneously, let alone measure their amplitudes. Suppose that we wish to plot two ordinates, one of which is 1,000 times smaller in amplitude than the other. If we represent the larger one as a line 4 cm long, the smaller ordinate would be only 0.04 mm long, so that we could barely see it (Figure H.1A), much less estimate

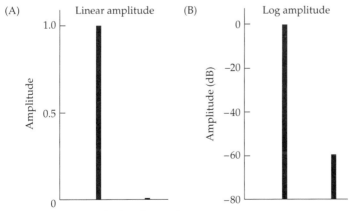

H.1 The value of logarithmic (dB) scale. The smaller of the two amplitudes is barely visible in the linear plot of part A, but is quite clearly measurable when displayed in the logarithmic (dB) plot of part B. Each 20 dB step corresponds to a 10:1 increase of amplitude. From Regan (1989a).

its size precisely. A logarithmic scale allows us to compare the two ordinates by compressing the larger amplitude with respect to the smaller one. For example, with the 80 dB logarithmic ordinate in Figure H.1B, the 1,000:1 amplitude ratio appears as a 4:1 ratio of height. Equal ratios are represented by equal distances on a logarithmic scale. In Figure H.1 all ratios are expressed relative to the larger ordinate.

Alexander Graham Bell discovered that the human ear responds approximately logarithmically to power difference, and he invented a logarithmic unit (called the bel) for measuring the sensitivity of the ear. In practice, the bel turned out to be an inconveniently large unit, and one-tenth of a bel, the decibel (dB), is more commonly used. A ratio is converted to the decibel scale as follows:

$$dB = 10 \log_{10} (\text{power ratio}) = 20 \log_{10} (\text{amplitude ratio})$$

The amplitude ratio might be, for example, a voltage ratio, a current ratio, or a frequency ratio. Thus, for example, 20 dB means a voltage ratio of 10:1 and (consequently) a power ratio of 100:1.

From Table H.1 we can see that our 1,000:1 ratio is expressed as our smaller signal's amplitude being 60 dB below the larger signal.

Table H.1 The Decibel (dB) Scale

dB[a]	Power ratio	dB	Voltage ratio
+20	100	+40	100
+10	10	+20	10
+3	2	+6	2
0	1	0	1
−3	0.5	−6	0.5
−10	0.1	−20	0.1
−10	0.01	−40	0.01

[a]$dB = 10\log(\text{power ratio}) = 20\log(\text{voltage ratio})$

Elements of Vector Calculus

For a minimally mathematical account of vector calculus I recommend Schey (1973): "I undertook to write this short text of vector calculus as a result of my experience several years ago in teaching electricity and magnetism to MIT undergraduates. The course began with elementary concepts, and culminated in a brief discussion of Maxwell's equations. It follows that en route we encountered a fair amount of vector calculus, and I was chagrined to find my students unequal to the challenge. (That puts it rather mildly; they took to hissing every time I said divergence, gradient or curl.) I tried to provide some of the mathematics in lectures, but couldn't do as much of this as necessary since my job was to teach physics not mathematics." Oh, how I would have welcomed Schey's book, had it been available 20 years earlier! In 1953 our first physics lecture at Imperial College was couched entirely in terms of vector calculus (even the name of which few of us had heard). And if we failed the year-end examination, the Army was eagerly waiting.

Scalar and Vector Functions

Taking (x, y, z) to be the Cartesian coordinates of any given point in three-dimensional space, the function $F(x, y, z)$ tells us how to associate a number with each point in space. For example, a function $T(x, y, z)$ gives the temperature at any point (x, y, z) within a room. This function is a *scalar function* and temperature is a *scalar quantity*: it has magnitude, but no direction.

A *vector function* **F**(*x, y, z*) tells us how to associate a *vector* with each point in space. For example, a function **V**(*x, y, z*) gives the local velocity of flow of a liquid at any point *(x, y, z)* within the liquid. Local velocity is a vector: it has a direction as well as a magnitude (i.e., speed).

A vector can be resolved into Cartesian components. In particular,

$$\mathbf{F}(x, y, z) = \mathbf{i}F_x(x, y, z) + \mathbf{j}F_y(x, y, z) + \mathbf{k}F_z(x, y, z) \qquad (I.1)$$

where **i**, **j**, and **k** are *unit vectors* whose directions are, respectively, along the *x*-, *y*-, and *z*-axes, and all of which have unit magnitude.

Vector Fields

When expressed in the notation of vector calculus, the equations of electromagnetism (Maxwell's equations) are far more compact than when expressed in a Cartesian format. Also, the vector notation helps students understand the physics at an intuitive level. For these reasons the notation of vector calculus has long been the format of choice when teaching electromagnetic theory. For reasons that will soon become clear, I will introduce the topic in terms of the three-dimensional flow of water.

> The vector field of local velocity within a volume of water can be specified fully by assigning an amplitude and direction to the velocity vector **V**(*x, y, z*) at every point *(x, y, z)* within the volume of water.

Although any given vector field can be specified and discussed in terms of Cartesian coordinates (Equation [I.1]), it is much less cumbersome to use an alternative way of specifying a three-dimensional (or two-dimensional) vector field: the notation of vector calculus. For example, rather than specifying Cartesian components of the velocity vector **V** at every point in space, this alternative notation specifies the values of div **V**, **curl V**, and **grad** *V* at every point in space.

Div, Curl, and Grad

For reasons that will become clear, I will restrict discussion to two-dimensional vector fields, and in particular the two-dimensional vector field of local velocity of a water surface.

Div and curl

Figure I.1A depicts a snapshot of the local velocity vectors on a water surface that lies immediately over an underwater output (e.g., the plug hole in a domestic bathtub). The speed and direction of motion at any point vary over the water surface and are indicated by the length and direction of the arrow. (The arrow refers to the velocity at the base of the arrow, rather than the point.) The dotted line in Figure I.1A encloses an arbitrary area, Δa. Figure I.1B shows the dotted line and the velocity **V** at one point on the line. At that point the component of velocity perpendicular to the dotted line is $V\cos\theta$, where V is the speed (i.e., the magnitude

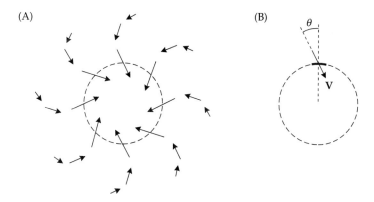

I.1 Two-dimensional velocity field. A snapshot of local velocity vectors on a water surface immediately above an outlet (A). An imaginary circle shown by the dashed line is redrawn in part B.

of **V**), and the component of velocity along the line is $V\sin\theta$. A small segment of the dotted line of length dl is shown in bold. In this two-dimensional case,

$$\text{div } \mathbf{V} = \frac{\lim}{\Delta a \to 0} \oint \frac{(V\cos\theta)dl}{\Delta a} \tag{I.2}$$

In words, we multiply the small length dl by the component of velocity **V** that is perpendicular to dl all the way around the dotted line, and sum all these products. Then we divide by area Δa. Finally we allow area Δa to tend to zero, and thus obtain the value of div **V** at one point in the flow field.

Div **V** is a scalar function of position: it has magnitude but no direction. It may be negative (as in our example of water running out of a bathtub) or positive (e.g., water rising out of the plug hole into a bathtub).

The value of **curl V** in the two-dimensional case is given by

$$\text{curl } \mathbf{V} = \frac{\lim}{\Delta a \to 0} \oint \frac{(V\sin\theta)dl}{\Delta a} \tag{I.3}$$

Curl **V** is a vector function of position: at any point it has a direction as well as a magnitude.*

The convention for assigning a direction to curl is as follows. Imagine that you are driving in a screw with a conventional right-hand thread. If the direction

* The term *rotation* (abbreviated **rot**) means the same as **curl**, but it has long dropped out of use.

around which the line integral in Equation (I.3) is calculated is the direction of rotation of the screwdriver, then the direction of the resulting **curl V** is the direction in which the screw travels.

Grad

In the special case of a two-dimensional velocity field, the *gradient* operator, often written **grad**, is defined as follows:

$$\textbf{grad } V = (\textbf{i}\frac{\partial}{\partial x} + \textbf{j}\frac{\partial}{\partial y})V \tag{I.4}$$

where V is the magnitude of velocity (i.e. speed) at any point (x, y), **i** and **j** are unit vectors, $\partial/\partial x$ signifies the rate of change along the x direction, and $\partial/\partial y$ signifies the rate of change along the y direction.

Grad V is a vector function of position.

Grad V at point (x, y) can be regarded as the rate of change of magnitude V at point (x, y). The direction of the vector **grad** V is the direction that gives the maximum rate of change.

The Retinal Image Flow Field

Translational motion of a nonrotating eye causes contours and texture elements in the retinal image to flow in a way that is jointly determined by the eye's motion and by the three-dimensional structure of the visual environment. In contrast, retinal image motion produced by eye rotation (e.g., by moving one's fixation from one object to another) is entirely determined by the rotation independently of the environment (Koenderink & van Doorn, 1976). To describe the retinal image flow pattern caused by a specified motion of the eye through a specified environment of stationary objects is a straightforward geometrical problem that has been worked out in detail (Gordon, 1965; Koenderink & van Doorn, 1976, 1981; Longuet-Higgins & Prazdny, 1980).

The converse problem, however, is comparatively little understood at an empirical level. In spite of considerable scientific effort, our knowledge of the ways in which the visual system actually does extract information about self-motion and about the three-dimensional structure of the environment is fragmentary.

If the effects of eye rotation can be allowed for or ignored, the three-dimensional structure of the environment can, in principle, be recovered from the retinal flow pattern produced by self-motion (Gibson, 1950; Lee, 1976; Longuet-Higgins & Prazdny, 1980). In practice, however, it seems that this simplifying assumption is not generally valid. The effects of eye rotation cannot always be ignored (Llewellyn, 1971; Regan & Beverley, 1982).

An advantage of specifying the retinal image flow field in terms of div **V**, **curl V**, and **grad** V rather than in terms of the velocity vector **V** is that the specification is unaffected by the bodily velocity of the retinal image as a whole that is caused by eye rotation, whereas the flow field expressed in terms of velocity **V** can change qualitatively (Koenderink & van Doorn, 1976; Longuet-Higgins & Prazdny, 1980). (This is because div **V**, **curl V**, and **grad** V are defined in terms of local relative motion.) The authors just cited pointed out that an organism whose visual system exploited this mathematical fact might gain advantage in analyzing retinal image flow patterns that contain components due to eye rotation in addition to components caused by self-motion. Longuet-Higgins and Prazdny (1980) noted that psychophysical evidence had been reported for div **V** detectors by Regan & Beverley (1978a).

Evidence That the Human Visual System Contains Filters for Rough Physiological Equivalents[*] of Div **V**, Curl **V**, and Grad V

We reported evidence that the human visual system contains filters sensitive to the difference between the local velocities at two retinal locations (Beverley & Regan, 1979b) that are insensitive to any common component of velocity at the two sites (Regan & Beverley, 1980), and later proposed that the outputs of such filters are scaled according to the distance between the locations at which velocities are sampled (Regan & Hamstra, 1993). In Figure 5.20A, k_1 and k_2 express the scaling. These filters seem to have receptive fields no larger than 1.0 to 1.5 degrees in diameter (Beverley & Regan, 1979b). Filters of this kind extract a rough physiological equivalent of **grad** V. We also reported evidence that the human visual system contains filters that extract a rough physiological equivalent of **curl V** (Regan & Beverley, 1985b) and div **V** (Regan & Beverley, 1978a, 1980; Beverley & Regan, 1980a).[†]

Expanding Retinal Flow Patterns and Div **V** Detectors

We generated a pattern of radial expansion in which div **V** was small at all locations except at the center of expansion. The bold continuous line in Figure I.2A shows how this was done. Short annular segments appeared at the focus and moved radially outwards at constant speed. The continuous line in Figure I.2B shows the variation of div **V** across the pattern. Observers adapted to the pattern while fixating on a point (M) to one side of the pattern (Figure I.3B). Then the

---

[*] The caveat "rough physiological equivalent" is necessary because these filters have finite receptive fields while **grad** V, div **V**, and **curl V** are point variables.

[†] Psychophysical evidence has been reported for filters sensitive to radial and circular motion that have very large receptive fields (Burr et al., 1998). Whatever their function may be, these filters do not approximate div **V** or **curl V** detectors: div **V** and **curl V** are point functions.

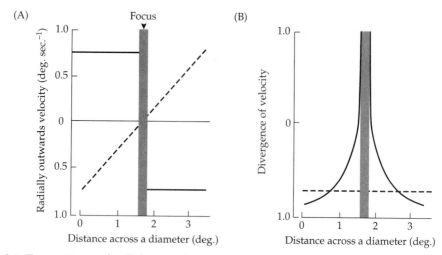

I.2 Two patterns of radial expansion. (A) The bold continuous and the dashed lines illustrate two patterns of radial expansion. (B) The continuous and dashed lines show the variations of div **V** across the two expansion patterns in part A.

adapting pattern was removed and we measured visual sensitivity to changes in the size of a small square (Figure I.3A). Figure I.3C shows that sensitivity to size changes was depressed when the test square was within about 0.5 degrees of the focus of expansion of the adapting pattern but not when the test square was located elsewhere. We found no such depression of visual sensitivity in a control experiment when the test square moved within a fronto-parallel plane rather than oscillating in size. We concluded that the changing-size test square was detected by a neural mechanism sensitive to div **V** (Regan & Beverley, 1979b).

Gibson (1950) stated that the focus of expansion produced by self-motion coincides with the moving observer's destination. Although this statement is correct when the observer's eye maintains a constant angle to the destination, it is not in general correct.* The kind of radial expansion produced by a zoom lens is depicted by the dashed line in Figure I.2A. In this kind of expansion, local speed is proportional to the distance from the focus of expansion. The dashed line in Figure I.2B shows that div **V** is uniform within such a pattern of expansion. A direct approach to a large vertical wall produces a retinal image pattern of retinal image flow that approximates this form of expansion. We generated a "zoom lens" pattern of retinal image expansion, simulating the retinal image flow pattern that would be produced by moving towards a flat picket fence (Regan & Beverley, 1982). Observers were unable to estimate accurately their projected point of collision with the fence. But observers could estimate their projected point of collision with precision when

---

*A photographic illustration of this point is given in Regan and Beverley, 1982, p. 195.

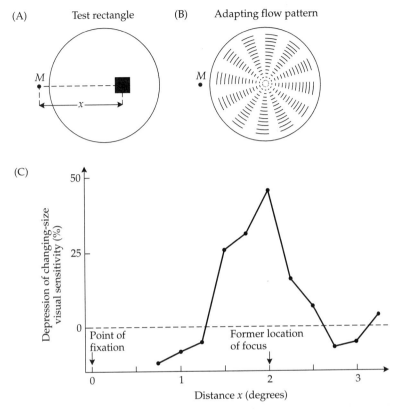

I.3 Effects of adapting to a radial expansion pattern. The observer's task was to detect changes in the size of a test rectangle (part A) after adapting to a radially expanding/contracting pattern of contours (part B). (C) Adaptation depressed visual sensitivity to size changes, but only at locations close to the former location of the focus of expansion. After Regan and Beverley (1979b).

the simulated fence was curved in depth. When approaching an object that is curved in depth, the retinal image contains at least one local maximum of div **V** that, in our experiment, observers were able to locate.

Hypotheses, Experiments, Serendipity, Journals, and Grants

[Niels H. D.] Bohr never trusted a purely formal or mathematical argument. "No, no," he would say, "You are not thinking; you are just being logical."

O. R. Frisch, *What Little I Remember* (1979; cited in Glen, 1994)

What Is It Like to Be a Researcher?

Not many active researchers have provided for the beginning researcher a frank account of what it feels like to do scientific research, one that also offers advice and inspires. Medawar (1981, 1996) and Cajal (1999) are helpful and informative. Another helpful book was written by Kolb (1996). I also have found that the writing of some historians illuminates the nature of research (e.g., Carr, 1990; Cantor, 1991). Elton (1984) is especially revealing on the purpose of the Ph.D. degree in the life of a future researcher.

On "how to do it," who better to turn to than the Nobel Laureate Sir Ernest Rutherford, whose Cavendish Laboratory has so far produced 22 Nobel Prizes?

One of the quantities that Rutherford conveyed to his pupils was the importance of alertness in noticing and exploring the unexpected. At Montreal he had noticed that opening and shutting the door of his laboratory produced effects that led him to the discovery of the thorium emanation, of crucial importance in developing his theory of radioactivity as due to the spontaneous disintegration of atoms. . . Speaking in his later years Blackett felt that though theory was becoming extremely sophisticated, discovery by accident was still very important. It was as vital then as it was in Rutherford's time to keep one's eyes open for something new, whenever doing an experiment. (Crowther, 1974, p. 216)

> Psychology researchers who delegate the "running of experiments" to others choose to forgo this opportunity for discovery.

W. L. Bragg, quoted in Crowther (1974, pp. 275–277), stated that,

> Britain like the United States, Germany, Holland and Scandinavia was a "physicist-producing country." . . . It was hard to understand how the British physicist held his own, especially in competition with the wealth of knowledge, mathematical ability, power of philosophical generalization and industry possessed particularly by the German student . . . [Bragg] thought that the compensating advantage of the British physicist was a curious kind of horse-sense, which made him distrust the too rigorous application of logic to his experimental observations, that gave him a good sense of proportion in what to accept and what to reject. It was like Tolstoy's repeated theme of the superiority of peasant directness over clever brilliance . . . He thought that Shaw's criticism of the traditional academic system in the words of Undershaft in *Major Barbara* was bitterly correct. If a student shows the least ability, he is fastened on by schoolmasters; trained to win scholarships like a racehorse; crammed with secondhand ideas; dulled and disciplined in docility and what they call good taste; and lamed for life so that he is fit for nothing but teaching. . . . If the origin of a valuable research development was traced, it was nearly always found that it had arisen from a chance remark made in a scientific discussion, or from reading another man's paper. If we were preoccupied with details of administration, the muse of inspiration would be prevented from visiting us. The most important factor in research was that researchers should have *brain waves*. . . . [T]here should also be a good store of material, and especially of *junk*. The latter was a priceless source of oddments, which could be used constructively in rapidly devising a first rough apparatus for trying out a new idea.

I end with a note published by P. M. S Blackett on *The Craft of Experimental Physics*, published in 1933. Although he is talking about what it took to be an experimental physicist in the Cavendish Lab in the 1930s, the spirit of his words applies equally well to the experimental psychophysicist of today.

> The experimental physicist is a Jack-of-All-Trades, a versatile but amateur craftsman. He must blow glass and turn metal, though he could not earn his living as a glass-blower nor even be classed as a skilled mechanic; he must carpenter, photograph, wire electric circuits and be a master of gadgets of all kinds; he may find invaluable a training as an engineer and can profit always by utilizing his gifts as a mathematician. In such activities he will be engaged for three-quarters of his working day. During the rest he must be a physicist, that is, he must cultivate an intimacy with the behavior of the physical world. . . The experimental physicist must be enough of a theorist to know what experiments

are worth doing and enough of a craftsman to do them. He is only pre-eminent in being able to do both. (Crowther, 1974, p. 218)

What Is Science?

The equating of science with FACTS and of the humane arts with IDEAS is one of the shabby genteelisms that bolster up the humanist's self-esteem. (Medawar, 1996, pp. 60–61)

To some research students it is a surprise to find that there is, as it were, no generally accepted instruction manual on how to do science, and indeed no agreed definition of what science is. Philosophers have attempted to provide a formal definition of science, but the student is chagrined to be offered not one, but several conflicting definitions. Maxwell (1985) provides a succinct overview.

A not-uncommon reaction to this confusion is to adopt the working definition that science is what creative and successful scientists do. But the formalized style of the typical research publication can convey a quite misleading impression of the mental strategy that led to the scientific advance being described. Beneath the tidy facade of journal articles the inquiring student discovers that the mental and experimental strategy of practicing scientists seems to be as much a craft as a formal system; more of an art than a rote methodology; more like a competitive sport than a bookkeeping exercise; and that equally creative scientists have quite different personal styles.*

One school of thought asserts that science begins with observations and experiment, and that theoretical knowledge is then derived from these data by inductive reasoning.

> Taken to its extreme, this approach carries the risk of clogging the scientist's mind with an accumulation of experimental data, most of which is devoid of theoretical importance.

On this point Medawar (1996, p. 30) cites Claude Bernard, "A hypothesis is the obligatory starting point of all experimental reasoning. Without it no investigation would be possible, and one would learn nothing: one could only pile up barren observations"; and Medawar adds that scientists are not hunting for facts nor are they busy formulating "laws." "Scientists are building explanatory structures, *telling stories* which are scrupulously tested to see if they are stories about real life."

---

* One reason why graduate students and postdoctoral fellows compete so fiercely to work in the leading laboratories is the realization that close-range experience of how outstanding and creative scientists think and act when doing science, and the atmosphere of a world-ranking laboratory, can convey an intuitive understanding of an effective scientific style that cannot be obtained from reading books or hearing lectures. Just what is passed on in this way may be difficult to express in words, even for the scientist whose example provides the lesson.

Rather than piling fact upon fact to create a mindless edifice, a scientist's focus is on persuading research peers to take serious note of his or her ideas and hopefully to accept them, rejecting previously held ideas. This is more of a "hearts and minds" exercise than the building of an edifice of facts. Indeed, scientific progress involves demolition. On encountering and attempting to evaluate a new finding it is no bad thing to ask oneself, So what? In other words, How does this new finding impact the theories that comprise my current understanding?

Popper's view is that only the *falsification* of scientific hypotheses leads to scientific discovery (Popper, 1934/1965, 1983). For Popper, an essential requirement of a scientific hypothesis is that it should in principle be falsifiable. (Whether any given hypothesis can be conclusively falsified by experiment is, he notes, a different matter altogether.) The claim that a theory can be *verified* is quite unacceptable and is strongly attacked by Popper, who also shows that a theory may be falsified without any other (nontrivial) theory being ipso facto verified.*

> But at a practical level we can feel confident that, in rationally planned research, at least, the value of a formal experiment is determined mainly by the quality of the hypothesis it is designed to test.

The Role of Scientific Hypothesis

Facts are stupid things.

Ronald Reagan

According to Medawar (1996, p. 18), "In the modern professional vocabulary a hypothesis is an imaginative pre-conception of *what might be true* in the form of a declaration with verifiable deductive consequences." For the experimental researcher the role of the scientific hypothesis is to provide guidance for selecting one from the indefinitely large number of possible experiments.

All hypotheses eventually die. The merit of a hypothesis lies less in the length of its life than in the quality of its life. For example, the average physics student of today is expected not only to understand Bohr's hypothesis of the atom, but also to criticize its limitations—all within one or two lecture periods. It is puzzling to reflect that the Bohr atom was conceived by one of this century's most distinguished physicists after a long period of conflict with other distinguished physicists. Can this mean that the average physics student of today is the intellectual equal of Bohr, in much the same way that Roger Bannister's four-minute mile is now no more than a rather impressive high-school level of achievement?

---

* Popper's view of science seems to exclude several kinds of activity that most working scientists accept as genuine science such as, for example, the endeavor to measure physical constants with greater and greater precision. According to Harré, the sharpest conflict between Popper's views and what working scientists actually do is in the matter of existential statements such as assertions that bacteria, genes, viruses and so on, exist.

Not at all! The significance of Bohr's concept of the atom is that, in its lifetime, it guided human experimental research on the nature of matter. The relegation of the Bohr atom to a one-hour lecture in the present-day physics undergraduate curriculum detracts from Bohr's achievement no more than the modern tourist, sitting comfortably in a Boeing 747 flying over Antarctica, detracts from the achievements of the 1915 Shackleton expedition (see Worseley, 1977).

Where Do Hypotheses Come From?

Some philosophers of science seem to assume that one always starts off with a hypothesis. They seem concerned chiefly with the differences between scientific and unscientific hypotheses (e.g., falsifiability), with the distinctions between hypotheses of higher and lower quality, and with the logic of testing and refuting hypotheses (e.g., Popper, 1934/1965, 1983). An important question receives comparatively little attention: *Where do hypotheses come from?* This omission may well be a delicate recognition of our comparative ignorance of how one sets about generating an original idea, let alone a creative and fruitful hypothesis. The proliferation of books and papers on the nature of hypotheses and hypothesis testing can cause one to overlook the fact that one first needs a hypothesis to test.

Many experimenters find that pure analytic thought is not enough when working toward creating a hypothesis. They find it helpful to carry out exploratory empirical forays that at times resemble play. This probing search can trigger lines of thought, spark creative analogies, and somehow lead to hypotheses that can be tested formally. The aim of such informal experimentation is to create testable hypotheses, and as such it is quite different from the formal experimental testing of a hypothesis that already exists.

It is true that students preparing for formal examination are helped by a textbook that logically organizes past and current scientific hypotheses and reviews them with clarity.

> But perhaps this very logic and clarity can insidiously misrepresent one reality of original research by giving the impression that the creation of good rather than sterile hypotheses is other than a mystery.

The beginning experimental scientist should not be too hasty in relegating the role of experimental work to "hypothesis testing" at best and "searching in the dark" at worst. Experimental work can also play an important role in the creation of hypotheses.

According to Medawar (1996, p. 25), "[T]here is a clear distinction between the acts of mind involved in discovery and in proof. The generative or elementary act of discovery is 'having an idea' or proposing a hypothesis. Although one can put oneself in the right frame of mind for having ideas and can abet the process, the process itself is outside logic and cannot be made the subject of logical rules." Kolb (1996, p. x) states: "It is my experience that the scientific method is easily confused with the scientific process. . . . [T]he process of developing new ideas in science is a very human endeavor. As with any enterprise involving people, the process is very personal. . . . The process of science involves heroic ideas as well as its share of stupidity." On the scientific method, Medawar (1996, p. 25) adds, "Hypothesis must be tested. These tests take the form of finding out whether or not the deductive consequences of the hypothesis or systems of hypothesis are statements that correspond to reality."

Where Do Good Hypotheses Come From?

It is just as true in the life sciences as it is in physics that, if a hypothesis is to advance our understanding of phenomena, the hypothesis should amount to more than a mere generalized description of observations or of empirical correlations between observations. Rather, the hypothesis should state principles that are not immediately given by the empirical data, and also predict that previously unknown events will occur under a new set of experimental conditions. The prediction may then be disproved by experiment. On the other hand it may be consistent with the data so that the hypothesis survives for another day.

With sufficient hindsight it is easy to judge the quality of a hypothesis. The passage of years shows which hypotheses take their creators along blind alleyways, and which lead to experimental discoveries that in turn lead to new concepts, and even create new branches of science. But to recognize at once that a hypothesis has lasting value is a clarity of vision that is granted as sparingly as the gift of great artistic or athletic ability.

For the general run of scientists, (notional) betting odds can provide a useful rule of thumb in assessing one's own and others' hypotheses. If you would offer 5 to 1 that experimental test would not refute the prediction of a particular hypothesis, then the hypothesis is uninteresting because it does little more than state the obvious. On the other hand, if the hypothesis seems logically sound and is based on accepted data, then the realization that one would offer even betting that the hypothesis will be experimentally refuted makes the hypothesis interesting indeed.

"Fishing Expeditions" and the Role of Luck

> Chance favors only the prepared mind.
> Louis Pasteur (quoted in Geison, 1995)

A researcher sometimes makes an important discovery that leads to important fresh insights by stumbling across it while looking for something else. There are some famous examples. This has been called serendipity. But the reviewers of grants do not look kindly on what they regard as "fishing expeditions," putting them in the category of providing a bunch of monkeys with typewriters in the hope that they will eventually type out the collected works of Shakespeare and then go on to add more of equal quality. Why this seeming blindness to the role of serendipity in research?

There are several reasons, one of which is that there is more to serendipitous discovery than good luck. To a not inconsiderable extent a researcher, like a sports player, makes his or her own luck. To have placed oneself in the mental territory where the "good luck" occurs implies a good "nose" for where the unexpected gold nuggets might be found—even though one cannot articulate what this "nose" picks up. And a researcher who cannot write a grant proposal that is far from dull and is methodologically sound, surmises our notional grant reviewer, is unlikely to get into the experimental zone where the fruitfully unexpected happens. Grant reviewers seem to believe that, for every researcher who is mentally capable of making a serendipitous discovery of importance, there are many others who might come face to face with the same finding and not recognize its true significance. A useful aid to serendipitous discovery in a particular area is a good critical understanding of the theories and hypotheses current in that area (as distinct from a memorized mass of undigested facts).

Can a Researcher Be Disadvantaged by Having an Encyclopedic and Up-to-date Knowledge of His or Her Research Area?

But there is another side to this last point. At one time, the large British chemical firm I.C.I had a small division, distinct from its large research divisions, whose purpose was to generate lines of research that were not expected to become profitable for one or two decades. Many of the researchers in this division had no Ph.D. and indeed no training in chemistry whatsoever. The firm recruited individuals who had, during their time as undergraduates, read intellectually demanding subjects such as Classical Greek and Latin, philosophy, or Medieval history, and had demonstrated outstanding intellectual ability.

> The rationale behind this adventurous kind of research appointment was the suspicion that a too-detailed knowledge of modern chemistry and especially many years devoted to absorbing and regurgitating (in written examinations) currently popular theories and attitudes can hinder the kind of thinking that would render current theories obsolete.

For the vision researcher too, it is no bad idea to venture outside what one imagines to be one's area of expertise. The worst that can happen is to be made to feel a fool—and that comes with the job.

Journal Articles Give a Misleading Impression of How Scientists Operate

In response to his own question, "Is the scientific paper a fraud?" Medawar (1996, p. 33) stated: "The scientific paper in its orthodox form does embody a totally mistaken conception, even a travesty, of the nature of scientific thought." He added (p. 29) that it is not possible to learn what scientists do by reading journal articles, "for they not merely conceal but actively misrepresent the reasoning that goes into the work they describe. If scientific papers are to be accepted for publication they must be written in the inductive style. The spirit of John Stuart Mill glares out the eyes of every editor of a Learned Journal."

What is this *inductive style*? The conception that underlies this style of scientific writing is that scientific discovery is an inductive process. In other words, the formulation of a scientific theory starts with simple observation (data collection), and out of this empirical evidence, Medawar (1996, p. 34) says: "generalizations will grow up and take shape almost as if some process of crystallization or condensation were taking place. Out of a disorderly array of facts, an orderly theory, an orderly general statement, will somehow emerge. This conception of scientific discovery in which the initiative comes from the unembroidered evidence of the senses was mainly the work of a great and wise, but in this context, I think, very mistaken man—John Stuart Mill."

Drawing a distinction between the natural sciences and what he calls the unnatural sciences, Medawar (1996, p. 144) states that a distinguishing mark of the latter is "that their practitioners try most painstakingly to initiate what they believe—quite wrongly, alas for them—to be the distinctive manners and observances of the natural sciences." Among those are:

"1. The belief that measurement and numeration are intrinsically praiseworthy activities
2. The whole discredited farrago of inductionism
3. [F]aith in the efficacy of statistical formulae, particularly when processed by a computer—the use of which is interpreted as a mark of scientific manhood."

Grants

I have refereed very many grant proposals over the last 35 years and have also written a few. The following comments are based on that experience and are intended to help you in your first encounter with a grant proposal package.

1. Choose the right grant-giving body. If in doubt, ask several experienced colleagues, and if any doubt remains, telephone the grant-giving body.
2. Read the instructions. Read every word very carefully. Follow the instructions in every detail, no matter how tiny.

Whoever wrote the instructions may or may not have taken them seriously. But your proposal will be pre-filtered by nonscientists who *do* take them seriously. If there is any deviation from the instructions (even as to type size and font) your proposal will likely never be seen by a scientist and will not reach the peer review committee. Every year a surprising proportion of proposals fail because the writer did not follow the instructions.

Next, I discuss factors that become important for proposals that reach the peer review committee. Your chance of being funded is improved if, when writing your proposal, your first priority is to get your proposal funded. This may call for some self-questioning and soul-searching on your part. *Bear in mind that a first priority is unique. You can have only one first priority.* A surprising number of grant applicants seem to have something else in mind. For example, do not give the impression that you are a researcher of such merit it is the nation's duty to support your research. Do not give the impression that grant funding is included among your human rights. Also, it is better to express yourself clearly than to try to stun the reviewer with your erudition. Remove all typos. Typos give a bad impression. Do not try to be witty or funny.

As to the scientific content of your proposal. Some pilot data can enhance your chances. (But not too much. I was present when a proposal was turned down because, so it was said, there was so much pilot data that the proposed research had already been done.)

I recommend that you start writing at least three months before the due date. Expect to go through several drafts. When you have achieved what you would like to think of as your final draft, ask someone who has been on a grant review committee to look it over. (Do not try this with your first effort.)

If your proposal is turned down, ask for copies of the reviewers' comments, take them seriously, and try again. Very good applications are turned down at one meeting of a committee that might well be recommended for funding at another meeting. There is a random element. And remember: If you do not try, you are 100% certain not to be funded.

If the government-funded granting agencies turn you down, find a book that lists the enormous number of private funding agencies. And keep trying.*

---

* E. B. Chain joined the faculty of Imperial College in the late 1950s. At afternoon tea one day he told me of his disenchantment with the peer review system. Some years previously the Medical Research Council had decided that his grant proposal was of insufficient scientific merit and turned it down. But he found another source for the small amount requested and with Florey carried out the work that was later recognized by the award of a Nobel Prize and by the gratitude of the many millions who were saved from death and ghastly diseases by antibiotics. MacFarlane (1979) provides an insider's account of how antibiotic drugs came to be.

References

Adelson, E. H. & Bergen, J. R. (1985). Spatio-temporal energy models for the perception of motion. *Journal of the Optical Society of America, 2,* 284–299.

Adini, Y. & Sagi, D. (1992). Parallel processes within the "spotlight" of attention. *Spatial Vision, 6,* 61–77.

Ahissar, M. & Hochstein, S. (1993). Attentional control of early perceptual learning. *Proceedings of the National Academy of Science, U.S.A., 90,* 5718–5722.

Ahnelt, P. K., Kolb, H. & Pflug, R. (1987). Identification of a subtype of cone photo-receptor likely to be blue sensitive in the human retina. *Journal of Comparative Neur-ology, 255,* 18–34.

Albrecht, D. G. & De Valois, R. L. (1981). Striate cortex responses to periodic patterns with and without the fundamental harmonics. *Journal of Physiology, 219,* 497–514.

Albrecht, D. G., Farrar, S. B. & Hamilton, D. B. (1984). Spatial contrast adaptation characteristics of neurones recorded in the cat's visual cortex. *Journal of Physiology, 347,* 713–739.

Allman, J., Miezin, F. & McGuiness, E. (1985). Stimulus specific responses from beyond the classical receptive field. *Annual Review of Neuroscience, 8,* 407–430.

Allusi, E. A. (1970). Information and uncertainty: The metrics of communications. In K. B. DeGreene (Ed.), *Systems psychology.* New York: Holt, Rinehart & Winston.

Anderson, C. H. & Van Essen, D. C. (1987). Shifter circuits: A computational strategy for dynamic aspects of visual processing. *Proceedings of the National Academy of Sciences, U. S. A., 84,* 6297–6301.

Anderson, S. J. & Burr, D. C. (1985). Spatial and temporal selectivity of the human motion detection system. *Vision Research, 25,* 1147–1154.

Anderson, S. J. & Burr, D. C. (1987). Receptive field size of human motion detection units. *Vision Research, 27,* 621–635.

Andrews, D. P. (1965). Perception of contours in the central fovea. *Nature, 205,* 1218–1220.

Andrews, D. P. (1967). Perception of contour orientation in the central fovea. Part I: Short lines. *Vision Research, 7,* 1975–1977.

Andrews, D. P., Butcher, A. K. & Buckley, B. R. (1973). Acuities for spatial arrangement in line figures: Human and ideal observers compared. *Vision Research, 13,* 599–620.

Anstis, S. M. (1970). Phi movement as a subtraction process. *Vision Research, 10,* 1411–1430.

Anstis, S. M. (1980). The perception of apparent movement. *Philosophical Transactions of the Royal Society of London, B, 290,* 153–168.

Anstis, S. M. (1989). Kinetic edges become displaced, segregated and invisible. In D. M. K. Lam (Ed.), *Neural mechanisms of visual perception* (pp. 247–260). Houston: Portfolio Press.

Anstis, S. M. (1997). Experiments on motion aftereffects. In M. Jenkin & L. Harris (Eds.). *Computational and Psychophysical Mechanisms of Visual Coding* (pp. 61–73). Cambridge: Cambridge University Press.

Anstis, S. M. & Cavanagh, P. (1983). A minimum motion technique for judging equiluminance. In J. D. Mollen & L. T. Sharpe (Eds.) (pp. 155–166). *Color vision.* New York: Academic Press.

Anstis, S. M. & Harris, J. P. (1974). Movement aftereffect contingent on binocular disparity. *Perception, 3,* 153–168.

Apkarian, P., Tijssen, R., Spekreijse, H. & Regan, D. (1987). Origin of notches in the CSF: optical or neural? *Investigative Ophthalmology and Visual Science, 28,* 607–612.

Arnulf, A. & Dupuy, O. (1960). La transmission des contrastes par le systeme optique de l'oeil et les seuils des contrasts retiniens. *Comptes Rend. Aca. Science, Paris, 250,* 2757–2759.

Aseltine, J. A. (1958). *Transform methods in linear systems analysis.* New York: McGraw–Hill.

Aslin, R. N. & Li, A. (1993). Multiple mechanisms of contrast adaptation. *Investigative Ophthalmology and Visual Science,* Supplement 34, p. 1362.

Atkin, A., Wolkstein, M., Bodis-Wollner, I., Anders, M., Kels, B. & Podos, S. M. (1980). Interocular comparison of contrast sensitivites in glaucoma patients and suspects. *British Journal of Ophthalmology, 64,* 858–862.

Attneave, F. (1954). Some informational aspects of visual perception. *Psychological Reviews, 61,* 183–193.

Attneave, F. (1959). *Applications of information theory to psychology.* New York: Holt, Rinehart & Winston.

Averbach, E. & Sperling, G. (1961). Short-term storage of information in vision. In C. Cherry (Ed.), *Fourth London Symposium on Information Theory.* London: Butterworth.

Ayama, M. & Ikeda, M. (1989). Dependence of the chromatic valence function on chromatic standards. *Vision Research, 29,* 1233–1244.

Badcock, D. R. (1984a). Spatial phase or luminance profile description? *Vision Research, 24,* 613–623.

Badcock, D. R. (1984b). How do we discriminate relative spatial phase? *Vision Research, 24,* 1847–1857.

Badcock, D. R. (1988). Discrimination of spatial phase changes: Contrast and position codes. *Spatial Vision, 3,* 305–322.

Badcock, D. R. & Derrington, A. M. (1985). Detecting the displacement of periodic patterns. *Vision Research, 25,* 1253–1258.

Badcock, D. R. & Derrington, A. M. (1987). Detecting the displacements of spatial beats: A monocular capability. *Vision Research, 27,* 793–797.

Badcock, D. R. & Derrington, A. M. (1989). Detecting the displacement of spatial beats: no role for distortion products. *Vision Research, 29,* 731–739.

Badcock, D. R. & Schor, C. M. (1985). Depth–increment detection function for individual spatial channels. *Journal of the Optical Society of America, A, 2,* 1211–1216.

Badcock, D. R. & Westheimer, G. (1985). Spatial locations and hyperacuity: Flank position within the centre and surround zones. *Spatial Vision, 1,* 3–11.

Baker, C. L. & Braddick, O. J. (1985). Temporal properties of the short-range process in apparent motion. *Perception, 14,* 181–192.

Banks, M. S., Geisler, W. S. & Bennett, P. J. (1987). The physical limits of grating visibility. *Vision Research, 37,* 1915–1924.

Barker, P. (1998). *Another World.* London: Penguin.

Barlow, H. B. (1972). Single units and sensation: A neuron doctrine for perceptual psychology? *Perception, 1,* 371–394.

Barlow, H. B. (1974). Inductive inference, coding, perception and language. *Perception, 3,* 123–134.

Barlow, H. B., Blakemore, C. & Pettigrew, J. D. (1967). The neural mechanism of binocular depth discrimination. *Journal of Physiology, 193,* 327–337.

Barlow, H. B., Narasimban, R. & Rosenfeld, S. (1972). Visual pattern analyzers in machines and animals. *Science, 177,* 567–575.

Barlow, R. B., Boudreau, E. A, Moore, D. C., Huckins, S. C., Linstrom, A. M & Farell, B. (1997). Glucose and time of day modulate human contrast sensitivity and (MRI signals from visual cortex. *Investigative Ophthalmology and Vision Science,* Supp., *38,* S735.

Bassi, C. J. & Powers, M. K. (1986). Daily fluctuations in the detectability of dim lights by humans. *Physiology and Behaviour, 38,* 871–877.

Baylor, D. A., Nunn, B. J. & Schnapf, J. L. (1987). Spectral sensitivity of cones of the monkey Macaca fasicularis. *Journal of Physiology (London), 390,* 145–160.

Beauchamp, K. G. (1975). *Walsh functions and their applications.* New York: Academic Press, p.153.

Beck, J. (1966a). Effect of orientation and of shape similarity on perceptual grouping. *Perception and Psychophysics, 1,* 300–302.

Beck, J. (1966b). Perceptual grouping produced by changes in orientation and shape. *Science, 154,* 538–540.

Beck, J. (1967). Perceptual grouping produced by like figures. *Perception and Psycho-physics, 2,* 491–495.

Beck, J. (1972). Similarity grouping and peripheral discriminability under uncertainty. *American Journal of Psychology, 85,* 1–19.

Beck, J. (1982). Textural segmentation. In J. Beck (Ed.), *Organization and representation in perception.* Hillsdale, N.J.: Erlbaum.

Beck, J., Prazdny, K. & Rosenfeld, A. (1983). A theory of texture segregation . In Beck, J., Hope, B. & Rosenfeld, A. (Eds.), *Human and machine vision.* New York: Academic Press.

Beck, J., Sutter, A. & Ivry, R. (1987). Spatial frequency channels and perceptual grouping in texture segmentation. *Computational Vision, Graphics and Image Processing, 37,* 299–325.

Beeler, G. W, Fender, D. H., Nobel, P. S. & Evans, C. R. (1964). Perception of pattern and color in the stabilized retinal images. *Nature, 203,* 1200.

Beery, K. (1968). Estimation of angles. *Perceptual and Motor Skills, 26,* 11–14.

Békésy, G. von. (1947). A new audiometer. *Acta Otolaryngology, 35,* 441–422.

Bell, A. J. & Sejnowski, T. J. (1997). The "independent components" of natural scenes are edge filters. *Vision Research, 37,* 3327–3338.

Bennett, P. J. & Banks, M. S. (1987). Sensitivity loss in odd–symmetric mechanisms and phase anomalies in peripheral vision. *Nature, 326,* 873–876.

Benton, A. L. & Hecean, N. H. (1970). Stereoscopic vision in patients with unilateral cerebral damage. *Neurology, 20,* 1084–1088.

Bergen, J. R. (1991). Theories of visual texture perception. In D. Regan, (Ed.), *Spatial vision* (pp. 114–134). London: Macmillan.

Bergen, J. R. & Adelson, E. (1988). Early vision and texture perception. *Nature* (London), *333,* 363–364.

Bergen, J. R. & Julesz, B. (1983). Rapid discrimination visual patterns. IEEE Transaction Systems, *Man and Cybernetics, 13,* 857–863.

Berkeley, M. A., Kitterle, F. & Watkins, D. W. (1975). Grating visibility as a function of orientation and retinal eccentricity. *Vision Research, 15,* 239–245.

Berkson, J. (1951) Why I prefer logits to probits. *Biometrics, 7,* 327–339.

Berkson, J. (1953). A statistically precise and relatively simple method estimating the bio-assay with quantal response based on the logistic function. *Journal of the American Statistical Association, 48,* 565–599.

Berkson, J. (1955a). Maximum likelihood and minimum chi–squared estimates of the logistic function. *Journal of the American Statistical Association, 50,* 130–162.

Berkson, J. (1955b). Estimate of the integrated normal curve by minimum normal chi–square with particular reference to bio–assay. *Journal of the American Statistical Association, 50,* 529–549.

Berkson, J. (1957). Tables for use in estimating the normal distribution function by normit analysis *Biometrika, 44,* 441–453.

Berkson, J. (1960). Nomograms for fitting the logistic function by maximum likelihood. *Biometrica, 47,* 121–141.

Beverley, K. I. & Regan, D. (1973). Evidence for the existence of neural mechanisms selectively sensitive to the direction of movement in space. *Journal of Physiology, 235,* 17–29.

Beverley, K. I. & Regan, D. (1974a). Temporal integration of disparity information in stereoscopic perception. *Experimental Brain Research, 19,* 228–232.

Beverley, K. I. & Regan, D. (1974b). Visual sensitivity to disparity pulses: evidence for directional selectivity. *Vision Research, 14,* 357–361.

Beverley, K. I. & Regan, D. (1975). The relation between discrimination and sensitivity in the perception of motion in depth. *Journal of Physiology, 249,* 387–398.

Beverley, K. I. & Regan, D. (1979a). Separable aftereffects of changing–size and motion–in–depth: Different neural mechanisms? *Vision Research, 19,* 727–732.

Beverley, K. I. & Regan, D. (1979b). Visual perception of changing-size: The effect of object size. *Vision Research, 19,* 1093–1104.

Beverley, K. I. & Regan, D. (1980a). Visual sensitivity to the shape and size of a moving object: Implications for models of shape perception. *Perception, 9,* 151–160.

Beverley, K. I. & Regan, D. (1980b). Temporal selectivity of changing-size channels. *Journal of the Optical Society of America, 11,* 1375–1377.

Beverley, K. I. & Regan, D. (1980c). Device for measuring the precision of eye–hand coordination while tracking changing size. *Aviat. Space Environ. Med., 51,* 688–693.

Birch, J. (1991). Colour-vision tests: General classification. In D. H. Foster (Ed.), *Inherited and acquired colour vision deficiencies: Fundamental aspects and clinical studies* (pp. 215–234). Boca Raton, Fla.: CRC Press.

Birch, J. (1993). *Diagnosis of defective colour vision.* New York: Oxford University Press.

Blakemore, C. (1970). The range and scope of binocular depth discrimination in man. *Journal of Physiology, 211,* 599–622.

Blakemore, C. (1990) (Ed.). *Vision: Coding and efficiency.* Cambridge: Cambridge University Press.

Blakemore, C. & Campbell, F. W. (1969). On the existence of neurons in the human visual system selectively sensitive to the orientation and size of retinal images. *Journal of Physiology, 203,* 237–260.

Blakemore, C., Muncey, J. P. J. & Ridley, R. M. (1971). Perceptual fading of a stabilized cortical image. *Nature, 233,* 204–205.

Blakemore, C., Muncey, J. P. J. & Ridley, R. M. (1973). Stimulus specificity in the human visual system. *Vision Research, 13,* 1915–1931.

Blakemore, C. & Nachmias, J. (1971). The orientational specificity of two visual aftereffects. *Journal of Physiology, 213,* 157–174.

Blakemore, C. & Over, R. (1974). Curvature detectors in human vision? *Perception, 3,* 3–7.

Blakemore, C. & Sutton, P. (1969). Size adaptation: A new aftereffect. *Science, 166,* 245–247.

Blaquière, A. (1966) *Nonlinear systems analysis.* New York: Academic Press.

Bloch, M. (1968). *Strange defeat.* New York: Norton.

Bodis-Wollner, I. (1972). Visual acuity and contrast sensitivity in patients with cerebral lesions. *Science, 178,* 769–771.

Bodis-Wollner, I. & Diamond, S. (1976). The measurement of spatial contrast sensitivity in cases of blurred vision associated with cerebral lesions. *Brain, 99,* 695–710.

Bodis-Wollner, I., Ghilardi, M. F. & Mylin, L. H. (1986). The importance of stimulus detection in VEP practice. In R. Q. Cracco & I. Bodis-Wollner (Eds.), *Evoked potentials* (pp. 15–27). New York: A. R. Liss.

Bodis-Wollner, I., Hendley, C. D., Mylin, L. H. & Thornton, J. (1978). Visual evoked potentials and the visuogram in multiple sclerosis. *Annals of Neurology, 5,* 40–47.

Bodis-Wollner, I., Marx, M. S., Mitra, S., Bobak, P., Mylin, L. & Yahr, M. (1987). Visual dysfunction in Parkinson's disease–loss in spatiotemporal contrast sensitivity. *Brain, 110,* 1675–1698.

Bodis-Wollner, I. & Regan, D. (1991). Spatiotemporal contrast vision in Parkinson's disease and MPTP–treated monkeys: The role of dopamine. In D. Regan (Ed.), *Spatial vision.* London: Macmillan.

Bonds, A. B. (1989). Role of inhibition in the specification of orientation selectivity of cells in the cat striate cortex. *Visual Neuroscience, 2,* 41–55.

Bonds, A. B. (1991). Temporal dynamics of contrast gain in single cells of the cat striate cortex. *Visual Neuroscience, 6,* 239–255.

Born, M. & Wolf, E. (1959). *Principles of optics: Electromagnetic theory of propagation, interference and diffraction of light.* London: Pergamon Press.

Bowen, R. W. (1977). Latencies for chromatic and achromatic visual mechanisms. *Vision Research, 17,* 1457–1466.

Bowen, R. W., Pokorny, J. & Cacciato, D. (1977). Metacontrast masking depends on luminance transients. *Vision Research, 17,* 971–976.

Bowmaker, J. K. & Dartnell, J. J. A. (1980). Visual pigments of rods and cones in the human retina. *Journal of Physiology, 298,* 501–511.

Bown, S. F. (1990). Contrast discrimination cannot explain spatial frequency, orientation or temporal frequency discrimination. *Vision Research, 30,* 449–461.

Boycott, B. B. & Wässle, H. (1974). The morphological types of ganglion cell in the domestic cat's retina. *Journal of Physiology, 240,* 397–419.

Boynton, R. M. (1973). Implications of the minimally distinct border. *Journal of the Optical society of America, 63,* 1037–1043.

Boynton, R. M. (1978). Ten years of research with the minimally distinct border. In C. E. Carterette and M. P. Freidman (Eds.), *Handbook of perception.* New York: Academic Press.

Boynton, R. M. & Kaiser, P. K. (1978). The additivity law made to work for heterochromatic photometry with bipartite fields. *Science, 161,* 366–368.

Bracewell, R. (1965). *The Fourier transform and its applications.* New York: McGraw–Hill.

Braddick, O. J. (1974). A short–range process in apparent motion. *Vision Research, 14,* 519–527.

Braddick, O. J. (1980). Low–level and high–level processes in apparent motion. *Philosophical Transactions of the Royal Society of London, B, 290,* 137–151.

Braddick, O. J., Campbell, F. W. & Atkinson, J. (1978). Channels in vision: Basic aspects. In R. Held, H. Leibowitz, and H. L. Teuber (Eds.), *Handbook of Sensory Physiology,* Vol. VIII. Berlin: Springer.

Bradley, A. & Scottun, B. C. (1984). The effects of large orientation and spatial frequency differences on spatial discriminations. *Vision Research, 241,* 1889–1896.

Bradley, A. & Scottun, B. C. (1987). Effects of contrast and spatial frequency on Vernier acuity. *Vision Research, 27,* 1817–1824.

Bradley, A., Scottun, B. C., Ohzawa, I., Sclar, G. & Freeman, R. D. (1985). Neurophysio-logical evaluation of the differential response model for orientation and spatial frequency discrimination. *Journal of the Optical Society of America, A2,* 1607–1610.

Bradley, A., Switkes, E. & DeValois, K. K. (1988). Orientation and spatial frequency selectivity of adaptation to color and luminance patterns. *Vision Research, 28,* 841–856.

Bradley, A., Zhang, X. & Thibos, L. N. (1991). Achromatising the human eye. *Optometry and Vision Science, 68,* 608–616.

Bradley, A., Zhang, X. & Thibos, L. N. (1992). Failures of isoluminance caused by ocular chromatic aberration. *Applied Optics, 31,* 3657–3667.

Brain, W. R. & Walton, J. N. (1969). *Brain's diseases of the nervous system.* London: Oxford University Press.

Bravo, M. J. & Blake, R. (1992). The contributions of figure and ground to texture segregation. *Vision Research, 32,* 1793–1800.

Brigham, E. D. (1974). *The fast Fourier transform.* New Jersey: Prentice–Hall.

Brilloulin, L. (1962). *Science and information theory* (2nd ed.). New York: Academic Press.

Brindley, G. S. (1970). *Physiology of the retina and visual pathway.* London: Edward Arnold.

Brown, P. K. & Wald, G. (1964). Visual pigments in single rods and cones of human retina. *Science, 144,* 45–52.

Bryam, G. M. (1944). The physical and photochemical basis for visual resolving power. Part 2. Visual acuity and the photochemistry of the retina. *Journal of the Optical Society of America, 34,* 718–738.

Bulens, C., Meerwaldt, F. D. & Van der Wildt, G. J. (1988). Effect of stimulus orientation on contrast sensitivity in Parkinson's disease. *Neurology, 36,* 76–81.

Bulens, C., Meerwaldt, F. D., Van der Wildt, G. J. & Kreemink, C. (1986). Contrast sensitivity in Parkinson's disease. *Neurology, 36,* 1121–1125.

Bulens, C., Meerwaldt, F. D., Van der Wildt, G. J. & van Deursen, J. B. P. (1987). Effect of levodopa treatment on contrast sensitivity in Parkinson's disease. *Annals of Neurology, 22,* 365–369.

Bullock, T. H. (1976). In search of principles of neural integration. In J. C. Fentress (Ed.), *Simple networks and behaviour* (pp. 52–60). Sunderland, Mass: Sinauer.

Burbeck, C. A. (1987). Position and spatial frequency in large scale judgements. *Vision Research, 27,* 417–427.

Burbeck, C. A. & Pizer, S. M. (1995). Object representation by cores: identifying and representing primitive spatial regions. *Vision Research, 35,* 1917–1930.

Burbeck, C. A, Pizer, S. M., Morse, B. S., Ariely, D, Zauberman, G. L & Rolland, J. P. (1996). Linking object boundaries at scale: a common mechanism for size and shape judgements. *Vision Research, 36,* 361–372.

Burbeck, C. A. & Regan, D. (1983a). Independence of orientation and size in spatial discriminations. *Journal of the Optical Society of America, 73,* 1691– 1694.

Burbeck, C. A. & Regan, D. (1983b). Temporal factors in color discrimination. *Investigative Ophthalmology and Visual Science, 24,* Supp. 3, 205.

Burbeck, C. A. & Zauberman, G. S. (1997). Across–object relationships in perceived object orientation. *Vision Research, 37,* 879–884.

Burgess, A. (1985). Visual signal detection. III. On Bayesian use of prior knowledge and cross–correlation. *Journal of the Optical Society of America, A, 2,* 1498–1507.

Burgess, A. & Ghandeharian, H. (1984). Visual signal detection. I. Ability to use phase information. *Journal of the Optical Society of America, A, 1*, 900–910.

Burns, S. A., Elsner, A. E., Pkorny, J. & Smith, V. C. (1984). The Abney effect: chromaticity coordinates of unique and other constant hues. *Vision Research, 24*, 479–489.

Burr, D. (1980). Sensitivity to spatial phase. *Vision Research, 20*, 391–396.

Burr, D., Morrone, C. & Maffei, L. (1981). Intra-cortical inhibition prevents simple cells from responding to textured visual patterns. *Experimental Brain Research, 43*, 455–458.

Burr, D., Morrone, C. & Vaina, I. M. (1998). Large receptive fields for optic flow detection in humans. *Vision Research, 38*, 1731–1743.

Burr, D. C., Ross, J. & Morrone, M. C. (1985). Local regulation of luminance gain. *Vision Research, 25*, 717–727.

Burr, D. C., Ross, J. & Morrone, M. C. (1986). A spatial illusion from motion rivalry. *Perception, 15*, 59–66.

Burt, P. & Sperling, G. (1981). Time distance and feature trade-offs in visual apparent motion. *Psychophysical Reviews, 88*, 171–195.

Burton, G. J. (1973). Evidence for non–linear response processes in the human visual system from measurements on the thresholds of spatial beat frequencies. *Vision Research, 13*, 1211–1225.

Caelli, T. (1985). The processing characteristics of visual segregation. *Spatial Vision, 1*, 19–30

Cajal, S. R. (1999). *Advice for a young investigator.* Translated by N. Swanson & L. W. Swanson. Cambridge, Mass.: MIT Press. Originally published in Spanish (1897).

Camisa, J. M., Blake, R. & Lema, S. (1977). The effects of temporal modulation on the oblique effect in humans. *Perception, 6*, 165–171.

Campbell, F. W. (1957). The depth of field of the human eye. *Optica Acta, 4*, 157–164.

Campbell, F. W. & Green, D. G. (1965). Optical and retinal factors affecting visual resolution. *Journal of Physiology, 181*, 576–593.

Campbell, F. W. & Gubisch, R. W. (1966). Optical quality of the human eye. *Journal of Physiology, 186*, 558–578.

Campbell, F. W. & Kulikowski, J. J. (1966). Orientation selectivity of the human visual system. *Journal of Physiology, 187*, 437–445.

Campbell, F. W., Nachmias, J. & Jukes, J. (1970). Spatial frequency discrimination in human vision. *Journal of the Optical Society of America, 60*, 555–559.

Campbell, F. W. & Robson, J. G. (1968). Application of Fourier analysis to the visibility of grating. *Journal of Physiology, 197*, 551–566.

Cannon, M. W. & Fullenkamp, S. C. (1991). Spatial interactions in apparent contrast: Inhibitory effects among grating patterns of different spatial frequencies, spatial positions and orientation. *Vision Research, 31*, 1985–1998.

Cantor, N. F. (1991). *Inventing the Middle Ages.* New York: William Morrow.

Carlson, C. R. & Klopfenstein, R. W. (1985). Spatial frequency model for hyperacuity. *Journal of the Optical Society of America, A2*, 1747–1751.

Carmon, A. & Becholdt, H. P. (1969). Dominance of the right cerebral hemisphere for stereopsis. *Neuropsychologia, 1*, 29–40.

Carney, T. & Klein, S. (1989). Parameter free prediction of bisection threshold. *Investigative Ophthalmology and Visual Science*, Supp., 30, 453.

Carney, T. & Klein, S. (1997). Resolution acuity is better than Vernier acuity. *Vision Research, 37*, 525–539.

Carney, L. G., Liubinas, J. & Bowman, K. J. (1981). The role of corneal distortion in the occurrence of monocular diplopia. *Acta Ophthalmolgia, 59*, 271–281.

Carney, T., Silverstein, D. A. & Klein, S. A. (1995). Vernier acuity during image rotation and translation: Visual performance limits. *Vision Research, 35,* 1951–1964.

Carpenter, R. S. H. & Blakemore, C. (1973). Interactions between orientations in human vision. *Experimental Brain Research, 18,* 287–303.

Carr, E. H. (1990). *What is history?* London: Penguin.

Carson, J. R. (1922). Notes on the theory of modulation. *Proceedings of the Institute of Radio Engineers, 10,* 57–65.

Cavanagh, P. (1989). Multiple analyses of orientation in the visual system. In D. Lam (Ed.), *Neural mechanisms of visual perception* (pp. 25–43). Woodlands, Tex.: Portfolio Publishing.

Cavanagh, P., Anstis, S. M. & McLeod, D. I. A. (1987). Equiluminance: Spatial and temporal factors and the contribution of blue–sensitive cones. *Journal of the Optical Society of America, A, 4,* 1428–1438.

Cavanagh, P. & Mather, G. (1989). Motion: The long and the short of it. *Spatial Vision, 4,* 103–130.

Cavanagh, P., Tyler, C. W. & Favreau, O. (1984). Perceived velocity of moving chromatic gratings. *Journal of the Optical Society of America, A, 1,* 893–899.

Chamberlain, T. C. (1965). The method of multiple working hypothesis. *Science, 148,* 754–759.

Chang, J. J. & Julesz, B. (1985). Cooperative and non-cooperative processes of apparent movement of random-dot cinematograms. *Spatial Vision, 1,* 39–46.

Chaparro, A., Stromeyer, C. F. III, Kronauer, R. E. & Eskew, R. T. Jr. (1994). Separable red–green and luminance detectors for small flashes. *Vision Research, 34,* 751–762.

Charman, W. H. (1991). Limits on visual performance set by the eye's optics and the retinal cone mosaic. In J. J. Kulikowsky, V. Walsh & I. J. Murray (Eds.), *Limits of Vision* (pp. 81–96). Boca Raton, Fla.: CRC Press.

Chen, S. & Levi, D. M. (1996). Angle judgements: Is the whole the sum of the parts? *Vision Research, 36,* 1721–1735.

Chua, F. K. (1990). The processing of spatial frequency and orientation information. *Perception and Psychophysics, 47,* 79–86.

Chubb, C. & Landy, M. S. (1991). *Orthogonal distribution analysis: A new approach to the study of texture perception.* In M. S. Landy, and J. A. Movshon (Eds.), *Computation models of visual processing.* Cambridge, Mass: MIT Press.

Chubb, C. & Sperling, G. (1988). Drift–balanced random stimuli: A general basis for studying non-Fourier motion. *Journal of the Optical Society of America, A,* 1986–2007.

Chung, S. H., Raymond, S. A. & Lettvin, J. Y. (1970). Multiple meaning in single visual units. *Brain, Behaviour and Evolution, 3,* 72–101.

Chung, S. T. K., Levi, D. M. & Bedell, H. E. (1996). Vernier in motion: What accounts for the threshold elevation? *Vision Research, 36,* 2395–2410.

Clark, M. & Bovik, A. C. (1989). Experiments in segmenting texton patterns using localized spatial filters. *Pattern Recognition, 6,* 707–717.

Cleary, R. & Braddick, O. J. (1990a). Directional discrimination for band–pass filtered random dot kinematograms. *Vision Research, 30,* 303–316.

Cleary, R. & Braddick, O. J. (1990b). Masking of low frequency information in short–range apparent motion. *Vision Research, 30,* 317–328.

Clowes, M. B. (1962). A note on colour discrimination under conditions of retinal image constraint. *Optica Acta, 9,* 65–68.

Clynes, M. (1969). (Ed.). Symposium on rein control, or unidirectional rate sensitivity, a fundamental dynamic and organizing function in biology. *Annals of the New York Academy of Science, 156,* 627–698.

Cole, G. R., Hine, T. & McHagga, W. (1993). Detection mechanisms in L-, M-, and S-cone contrast space. *Journal of the Optical Society of America, A, 10,* 38–51.

Collewijn, H., Steinman, R. M., Erkelens, C. J. & Regan, D. (1991). Binocular fusion, stereopsis and stereoacuity with a moving head. In D. Regan (Ed.), *Binocular vision*. London: Macmillan.

Conrady, A. E. (1957). *Applied optics and optical design*. New York: Dover.

Cooper, G. R. & McGillem, C. D. (1967). *Methods of signal and system analysis*. New York: Holt, Rinehart & Winston.

Cooper, L. A. & Shepard, R. N. (1973*)*. Chronometric studies of the rotation of mental images. In W. G. Chase (Ed.), *Visual information processing* (pp. 75–176). New York: Academic Press.

Cormack, L. K., Stevenson, S. B. & Schor, C. M. (1993). Disparity-tuned channels of the human visual system. *Visual Neuroscience, 10*, 585–596.

Craik, K. J. W. (1960). *The nature of psychology*. Cited in Braddick et al., 1978.

Crawford, B. H. (1947). Visual adaptation in relation to brief conditioning stimuli. *Proceedings of the Royal Society (London), B134*, 283–302.

Creed, R. S. (1935). Observations on binocular fusion and rivalry. *Journal of Physiology, 84*, 381–392.

Critchley, M. (1953). *The parietal lobes*. London: Edward Arnold.

Crone, R. A. (1973). *Diplopia*. New York: Elsevier.

Crosby, A. W. (1997). *The measure of reality: Quantification and Western society 1250–1600*. Cambridge: Cambridge University Press.

Crowther, J. G. (1974). *The Cavendish Laboratory 1874–1974*. New York: Neale Watson Academic Publications.

Curcio, C. A., Allen, K. A., Sloan, K. R., Lerea, C. L., Hurley, J. B., Klock, I. B. & Milam, A. H. (1991). Distribution and morphology of human cone receptors stained with anti–blue opsin. *Journal of Comparative Neurology, 312*, 610–624.

Curcio, C. A. & Sloan, K. R. (1992). Packing of human cone receptors: variation with eccentricity and evidence of local anisotrophy. *Visual Neuroscience, 9*, 169–180.

Cynader, M. & Regan, D. (1978). Neurones in cat parasite cortex sensitive to the direction of motion in three-dimensional space. *Journal of Physiology, 274*, 549–569.

Cynader, M. & Regan, D. (1982). Neurons in cat visual cortex tuned to the direction of motion in depth: Effect of positional disparity. *Vision Research, 22*, 967–982.

Daintith, J. & Nelson, R. D. (1989) (Eds.). *Dictionary of mathematics*. London: Penguin.

Damasio, A., Yamada, Y., Damasio, H., Corbett, J. & McKee, J. (1980). Central achromatopsia: Behavioural anatomic and physiological aspects. *Neurology, 30*, 1064–1071.

Dartnell, H. J. A., Bowmaker, H. K. & Mollon, J. D. (1983). Human visual pigments: Microspectrophotometric results from the eyes of seven persons. *Proceedings of the Royal Society (London), B, 220*, 115–130.

Darwin, C. (1859). *On the origin of species by means of natural selection, or The preservation of favoured races in the struggle for life*. London: John Murray. (A reprint is published by Penguin Books.)

Daugman, J. G. (1980). Two-dimensional spectral analysis of cortical receptive field profiles. *Vision Research, 25*, 671–684.

Daugman, J. G. (1988). Complete discrete 2–D Gabor transforms by neural networks for image analysis and compression. IEEE Transactions on *Acoustics, Speech, and Signal Processing, 36*, 1169–1179.

Daugman, J. G. & Downing, C. J. (1995). Demodulation, predictive coding and spatial vision. *Journal of the Optical Society of America, 12A*, 641–660.

Davidson, M. L. (1968). Perturbation approach to spatial brightness interaction in human vision. *Journal of the Optical Society of America, 58*, 1300–1309.

Dealy, R. S. & Tolhurst, D. J. (1974). Is spatial adaptation an after-effect of prolonged inhibition? *Journal of Physiology*, *241*, 261–270.

DeLange, H. Dzn. (1952). Experiments on flicker and some calculations on an electrical analogue of the foveal systems. *Physics, 18*, 935.

DeLange, H. Dzn. (1954). Relationship between critical flicker frequency and a set of low frequency characteristics of the eye. *Journal of the Optical Society of America, 44*, 380–385.

DeLange, H. Dzn. (1957). *Attenuation characteristics and phase shift characteristics of human foveal–cortex systems in relation to flicker fusion phenomena.* Thesis, Technische Hogeschool, Delft.

DeLange, H. Dzn. (1958). Research into the dynamic nature of the human fovea–cortex systems with intermittent and modulated light. I. Attenuation characteristics with white and colored lights. *Journal of the Optical Society of America, 48*, 777–784.

DeMonastrario, F. M. & Gouras, P. (1975). Functional properties of ganglion cells of the rhesus monkey retina. *Journal of Physiology, 251*, 167–195.

Derenfeldt, G. (1991). Colour appearance systems. In P. Gouras (Ed.), *The perception of color* (pp. 218–261). Boca Raton, Fla.: CRC Press.

Derrington, A. R. & Badcock, D. R. (1985). Separate detectors for simple and complex grating patterns? *Vision Research, 25*, 1869–1878.

Derrington, A. R. & Badcock, D. R. (1986). Detection of spatial beats: Nonlinearity or contrast increment detection? *Vision Research, 26*, 343–348.

Desimone, R., Schein, S. J., Moran, J. & Ungerleider, L. G. (1985). Contour, color and shape analysis beyond the striate cortex. *Vision Research, 25*, 441–452.

DeValois, K. K. (1978). Interactions among spatial frequency channels in the human visual system. In S. J. Cool & E. L. Smith (Eds.), *Frontiers in visual science.* New York: Springer-Verlag.

DeValois, K. K. & Switkes, E. (1982). Simultaneous masking interactions between chromatic and luminance gratings. *Journal of the Optical Society of America, 73*, 11–18.

DeValois, K. K. & Tootel, R. (1983). Spatial-frequency-specific inhibition in cat striate cortical cells. *Journal of Physiology, 336*, 359–376.

DeValois, R. L., Albrecht, D. G. & Thorell, L. G. (1982). Spatial frequency selectivity of cells in macaque visual cortex. *Vision Research, 22*, 545–559.

DeValois, R. L. & DeValois, K. K. (1980). Spatial vision. *Annual Review of Psychology, 31*, 309–341.

DeValois, R. L. & DeValois, K. K. (1991). Vernier acuity with stationary moving Gabors. *Vision Research, 31*, 1619–1626.

DeValois, R. L. & Switkes, E. (1983). Simultaneous masking interactions between chromatic and luminance gratings. *Journal of the Optica Society of America, 73*, 11–18.

DeValois, R. L., Yund, E. W. & Hepler, N. (1982). The orientation and direction selectivity of cells in macaque visual cortex. *Vision Research, 22*, 531–544.

De Yoe, E. A. & Van Essen, D. C. (1985). Segregation of efferent connections and receptive field properties in visual area V2 of the macaque. *Nature, 317*, 58–61.

DiStefano, J. J., Stubberud, A. R. & Williams, I. J. (1967). *Feedback and control systems.* New York: McGraw–Hill, Schaum's Outline Series.

Ditchburn, R. W. (1976). *Light.* London: Academic Press.

Ditchburn, R. W. & Ginsberg, B. L. (1952). Vision with a stabilized retinal image. *Nature, 170*, 36–37.

Domenici, L., Trimarchi, C., Piccolino, M., Fiorentini, A. & Maffei, L. (1985) Dopaminergic drugs improve human visual contrast sensitivity. *Human Neurobiology, 4*, 195–197.

Dorfman, D. And Alf, A. S. (1969). Maximum likelihood estimation of parameters of signal-detection theory and determination of confidence intervals–rating–method data. *Journal of Mathematical Psychology, 6*, 487–496.

Dowling, J. E. (19XX). The retina: An approachable part of the brain. Cambridge, Mass.: Belknap Press of the Harvard University Press.

Drum, B. (1983). Short–wavelength cones contribute to achromatic sensitivity. *Vision Research, 12,* 1433–1439.

Duffieux, P. M. (1946). *L'Intergrade de Fourier es ses applications a l'optique.* Printed privately at Besancon. English version. *The Fourier transform and its application to optics.* (1983). New York: Wiley.

Durnford, M. & Kimura, D. (1971). Right hemisphere specialization for depth perception reflected in visual field differences. *Nature, 231,* 394–395.

Durr, D. (1980). Sensitivity to spatial phase. *Vision Research, 20,* 391–396.

Eagle, R. A. (1998). Upper displacement limits for spatially broadband patterns containing bandpass noises. *Vision Research, 38,* 1775–1787.

Efron, R. (1957). Stereoscopic vision: I. Effect of temporal summation. *British Journal of Ophthalmology, 41,* 709–630.

Ehinger, B. (1985). Retinal circuitry and clinical ophthalmology. *Biological Bulletin, 168,* 333–349.

Eisenhardt, L. P. (1960). *Riemannian Geometry.* Princeton: Princeton University Press.

Eisner, A. & MacLeod, D. I. A. (1980). Blue sensitive cones do not contribute to luminance. *Journal of the Optical Society of America, 70,* 121–123.

Elliot, D. B. & Bullimore, M. A. (1993). Assessing the reliability discriminative ability and validity of disability glare tests. *Investigative ophthalmology and visual science, 34,* 108–119.

Ellis, B., Burrell, G. J., Wharf, J. H & Hawkins, T. D. F. (1975). Independence of channels in colour contrast perception. *Nature, 254,* 691–692.

Elton, G. R. (1984). *The practice of history.* London: Fontana.

Erkelens, C. J. & Collewijn, H. (1985a). Motion perception during dichoptic viewing of moving random–dot sterograms. *Vision Research, 25,* 583–588.

Erkelens, C. J. & Collewijn, H. (1985b). Eye movements and stereopsis during dichoptic viewing of moving random–dot stereograms. *Vision Research, 25,* 1689–1700.

Eskew, R. T. Jr., Stromeyer, C. F. III, Picotte, C. J. & Kronauer, R. E. (1991). Detection uncertainty and the facilitation of chromatic detection by luminance contours. *Journal of the Optical Society of America, A, 8,* 394–403.

Fahle, M. (1997). Specificity of learning curvature, orientation and Vernier discrimination. *Vision Research, 37,* 1885–1895.

Fahle, M. & Harris, J. P. (1992). Visual memory for Vernier offsets. *Vision Research, 32,* 1033–1042.

Fahle, M. & Morgan, M. (1996). No transfer of perceptual learning between similar stimuli in the same retinal position. *Current Biology, 6,* 292–297.

Farrell, B. & Krauskopf, J. (1988). Influence of chromatic content on Vernier thresholds. ARVO abstract, *Investigative Ophthalmology and Visual Science, 29,* 371.

Favreau, O. E. & Cavanagh, P. (1981). Color and luminance: Independent frequency shifts. *Science, 212,* 831–832.

Fechner, G. T. (1860). *Elemente der Psychophysik.* Leipzig: Breitkopf & Härtel.

Felton, T. B., Richards, W. & Smith, R. A. Jr. (1972). Disparity processing of spatial frequencies in man. *Journal of Physiology, 225,* 349–362.

Ferraro, M. & Foster, D. H. (1986). Discrete and continuous modes of curved line discrimination controlled by effective stimulus duration. *Spatial Vision, 1,* 219–230.

Field, D. (1987). Relations between the statistics of natural images and the response properties of cortical cells. *Journal of the Optical Society of America, A, 4,* 2379–2394.

Fincham, E. F. (1963). Monocular diplopia. *British Journal of Ophthalmology, 47,* 705–714.

Findlay, J. M. (1973). Feature detectors and Vernier acuity. *Nature, 241,* 135–137.

Fink, D. G. (Ed.) (1975). *Electronic engineers' handbook*, Sec. 13-7. New York: McGraw–Hill, Section 13–7).

Finney, D. J. (1971). *Probit analysis*. Cambridge: Cambridge University Press.

Fiorentini, A., Pirchio, M. & Spinelli, D. (1983). Electrophysiological evidence for spatial frequency selective mechanisms in adults and infants. *Vision Research, 23,* 119–127.

Fisher, G. (1969). An experimental study of linear inclination. *Quarterly Journal of Psychology, 21,* 356–366.

Flamant, F. (1955). Étude de la répartition de lumière dans l'image rétienne d'une fente. *Rev. Opt. (théor. instrum.), 34,* 433–459.

Flitcroft, D. I. (1989). The interactions between chromatic aberration, defocus and stimulus chromaticity: Implication for visual physiology and colorimetry. *Vision Research, 29,* 349–360.

Fogel, I. & Sagi, D. (1989). Gabor filters as texture discriminators. *Biological Cybernetics, 61,* 103–113.

Foley, J. M. (1994). Human luminance pattern-vision mechanisms: Masking experiments require a new model. *Journal of the Optical Society of America, 11,* 1710–1719.

Foley, J. M. & Chen, C. C. (1997). Analysis of the effect of pattern adaptation on pattern pedestal effects: A two process model. *Vision Research, 37,* 2779–2788.

Foley, J. M. & Legge, G. E. (1981). Contrast detection and near- hreshold discrimination in human vision. *Vision Research ,21,* 1041–1053.

Foley-Fisher, J. A. (1977). Contrast, edge - gradient and target line width as factors in Vernier acuity, *Optica Acta, 24,* 179–218.

Foley-Fisher, J. A. & Ditchburn, R. W. (1986). Effect of imposed retinal image movements on color vision at a heterochromatic boundary in a stabilized retinal image. *Ophthalmic and Physiological Optics, 6,* 377–384.

Foster, D. H. (1980). A description of discrete internal representation schemes for visual pattern discrimination. *Biological Cybernetics, 38,* 151–157.

Foster, D. H. & Ward, P. A. (1991). Asymmetries in oriented-line detection indicate two orthogonal filters in early vision. *Proceedings of the Royal Society (Lond.) B, 243,* 75–81.

Fox, R., Patterson, R. & Lehmkuhle, S. (1982). Effect of depth position on the motion aftereffect. *Investigative Ophthalmology and Visual Science, 22* (ARVO abstracts), 144.

Fraser, G. MacDonald (1992). *Quartered Safe Out Here*. London: Harvill. Trade paperback ed., 1995. London: Harper Collins.

Fredericksen, R. E., Verstraten, F. A. J. & van der Grind, W. A. (1997). Pitfalls in estimating motion detector receptive field geometry. *Vision Research, 37,* 99–119.

Freeman, R. D., Mitchell, D. E. & Millodot, M. (1972). A neural effect of partial visual deprivation in humans. *Science, 175,* 1384–1386.

Freeman, R. D. & Thibos, L. N. (1973). Electrophysiological evidence that early visual experience can modify the human brain. *Science, 180,* 876–878.

Frisén, L. & Frisén, M. (1981). How good is normal visual acuity? *Albrecht v. Graefes Arch. Klin. Ophthal., 215,* 149–157.

Frome, F. S., Levinson, J. Z., Danielson, J. T. & Clavadetscher, J. E. (1979). Shift in perception of size after adaptation to gratings. *Science, 206,* 1327–1329.

Frost, B. J. & Nakayama, K. (1983). Single visual neurons code opposing motion independent of direction. *Science, 220,* 744–745.

Frost, B. J., Scilley, P. L. & Wong, S. C. P. (1981). Moving background patterns reveal double-opponency of directionally specific pigeon tectal neurons. *Experimental Brain Research, 43,* 173–185.

Fry, G. A., Bridgman, C. S. & Ellerbrock, V. J. (1949). The effect of atmospheric scattering on binocular depth perception. *American Journal of Optometry, 26,* 9–15.

Gabor, D. (1946). Theory of communication. *Journal of the Institute of Electrical and Electronic Engineers, 93,* 429–456.

Galambos, R. (1986). Identification of the newborn with hearing disorder using the auditory brainstem response (ABR). In R. Q. Cracco & I. Bodis-Wollner (Eds.), *Evoked potentials* (pp. 463–470). New York: A. R. Liss.

Galvin, R. J., Regan, D., & Heron, J. R. (1976). A possible means of monitoring the progress of demyelination in multiple sclerosis: Effect of body temperature on visual perception of double light flashes. *Journal of Neurology, Neurosurgery, and Psychiatry, 39,* 861–865.

Ganz, L. (1966). Mechanism of the figural after–effects. *Psychological Reviews, 73,* 128–150.

Ganz, L. & Day, R. H. (1965). An analysis of the satiation-fatigue mechanism in figural after-effects. *American Journal of Psychology, 78,* 345–361.

Gaskell, J. D. (1978). *Linear systems, Fourier transforms and optics.* New York: Wiley.

Geisler, W. S. (1984). Physical limits of acuity and hyperacuity. *Journal of the Optical Society of America, A, 1,* 775–782.

Geisler, W. S. (1989). Sequential ideal-observer analysis of visual discriminations. *Psychological Review, 96,* 267–314.

Geisler, W. S. & Albrecht, D. G. (1992). Cortical neurons: Isolation of contrast gain control. *Vision Research, 32,* 1409–1410.

Geisler, W. S. & Davila, K. D. (1985). Ideal discriminators in spatial vision: Two point stimuli. *Journal of the Optical Society of America, A, 2,* 1483–1497.

Geison, G. L. (1995). *The private science of Louis Pasteur.* Princeton, N.J.: Princeton University Press.

Georgeson, M. (1985). The effect of spatial adaptation on perceived contrast. *Spatial Vision, 1,* 103–112.

Georgeson, M. (1991). Over the limit: Encoding contrast above threshold in human vision. In J. J. Kulikowski, V. Walsh, & I. J. Murray (Eds.), *Limits of vision* (pp. 106–119). Boca Raton, Fla.: CRC Press.

Georgeson, M. & Harris, M. G. (1984). Spatial selectivity of contrast adaptation: Models and data. *Vision Research, 24,* 729–741.

Georgeson, M. & Sullivan, G. D. (1975). Contrast constancy: Deblurring in human vision by spatial frequency channels. *Journal of Physiology, 252,* 627–656.

Gerrits, H. J. M. (1967). *Observations with stabilized retinal images and their neural correlates.* Ph.D. thesis, Catholic University of Nijmegen. Rotterdam: Bronder-Offset.

Giaschi, D., Lang, A. & Regan, D. (1997). Reversible dissociation of sensitivity to dynamic stimuli in Parkinson's disease: Is magnocellular function essential to reading motion-defined letters. *Vision Research, 37,* 3531–3534.

Giaschi, D., Regan, D., Kothe, A. C., Hong, X. H. & Sharpe, J. A. (1992). Motion-defined letter detection and recognition in patients with multiple sclerosis. *Annals of Neurology, 31,* 621–628.

Gibson, E. J. (1969). *Principles of perceptual learning and development.* New York: Appleton-Century-Crofts.

Gibson, J. J. (1933). Adaptation, aftereffect, and contrast in the perception of curved lines. *Journal of Experimental Psychology, 16,* 1–31.

Gibson, J. J. (1950). *The perception of the visual world.* Boston: Houghton Mifflin.

Gibson, J. J. (1966). *The senses considered as perceptual systems.* Boston: Houghton Mifflin.

Gibson, J. J. (1979). *The ecological approach to visual perception.* Boston: Houghton Mifflin.

Gilbert, C. D. (1994). Comments. In G. R. Bock and J. A. Goode (Eds.), *Higher order processing in the visual system* (p. 261). New York: Wiley.

Gilbert, C. D., Hirsch, J. A. & Weisel, T. N. (1990). Lateral interactions in visual cortex. *Cold Spring Harbor Symposium on Quantitative Biology, 55,* 663–667.

Gilbert, C. D. & Kelly, J. P. (1975). The projection of cells in different layers of the cat's visual cortex. *Journal of Comparative Neurology, 163,* 81–106.

Gilbert, C. D. & Wiesel, T. N. (1985). Intrinsic connectivity and receptive field properties in visual cortex. *Vision Research, 25,* 365–374.

Gilbert, C. D. & Wiesel, T. N. (1990). The influence of contextual stimuli on the orientation selectivity of cells in the primary visual cortex of the cat. *Vision Research, 30,* 1689–1701.

Gilinsky, A. S. (1968). Orientation-specific effects of adapting light on visual acuity. *Journal of the Optical Society of America, 58,* 13–18.

Ginsburg, A. P. (1978). *Visual information processing based upon spatial filters constrained by biological data.* Ph.D. dissertation, Cambridge University (England). Reprinted as AFAMRL Technical Report 78–129. Library of Congress 79–600156.

Ginsburg, A. P. (1981). Spatial filtering and vision: Implications for normal and abnormal vision. In L. M. Proenza, J. M. Enoch & A. Jampolsky (Eds.), *Clinical applications of visual psychophysics* (pp. 70–106). Cambridge: Cambridge University Press.

Glazier, V. D, Ivanoff, V. A. & Tscherbach, T. (1973). Investigation of complex and hypercomplex receptive fields of visual cortex of the cat as spatial frequency filters. *Vision Research, 13,* 1875–1904.

Glen, W. (1994). *The mass extinction debates: How science works in a crisis.* Stanford, Calif.: Stanford University Press.

Glennerster, A. (1998). dmax stereopsis and motion in random dot displays. *Vision Research, 38,* 925–935.

Glennerster, A. & Parker, A. J. (1997). Computing stereo channels from masking data. *Vision Research, 37,* 2143–2152.

Glovinsky, Y., Quigley, H. A. & Dunkelberger, G. R. (1991). Retinal ganglion cell loss is size dependent in experimental glaucoma. *Investigative Ophthalmology and Visual Science, 32,* 484–491.

Godel, C. L. & Lawson, R. B. (1973). The effects of time interval duration between disparity stimuli upon stereoscopic depth perception. *Psychological Review, 23,* 243–248.

Gogol, W. C. (1965). Equidistance tendency and its consequences. *Psychological Bulletin, 64,* 153–163.

Gogol, W. C. & Tietz, J. D. (1973). Absolute motion parallax and the specific distance tendency. *Perception and Psychophysics, 13,* 284–292.

Goldsmith, T. H. (1991). The evolution of visual pigments and colour vision. In P. Gouras (Ed.), *The perception of color* (pp. 62–89). Boca Raton, Fla.: CRC Press.

Golomb, B., Andersen, R. A., Nakayama, K., MacLeod, D. I. A. & Wong, A. (1985). Visual thresholds for shearing motion in monkey and man. *Vision Research, 25,* 813–820.

Gonzalez, F., Krause, F., Perez, R., Alonzo, J. M. & Acuna, C. (1993). Binocular matching in monkey visual cortex: Single cell responses to correlated and uncorrelated dynamic random dot stereograms. *Neuroscience, 52,* 933–939.

Goodman, J. W. (1968). *Introduction to Fourier optics.* San Francisco: McGraw–Hill.

Gordon, D. A. (1965). Static and dynamic visual fields in human space perception. *Journal of the Optical Society of America, 55,* 1296–1303.

Gordon, J. & Shapley, R. M. (1989). Spectral sensitivity of achromatic visual mechanisms. *Investigative Ophthalmology & Vision Science, Supp., 30,* 128.

Gorea, A. & Papathomas, T. V. (1991a). Extending a class of motion stimuli to study multi-attribute texture perception. *Behavioural Research Methods, Instruments & Computers, 23,* 5–8.

Gorea, A. & Papathomas, T. V. (1991b) Texture segregation by chromatic and achromatic visual pathways: An analogy with motion processing. *Journal of the Optical Society of America, A, 8,* 386–393.

Gorea, A. & Papathomas, T. V. (1993). Double opponency as a generalized concept in texture segregation illustrated with stimuli defined by color, luminance and orientation. *Journal of the Optical Society of America, A10,* 1450–1462.

Gottlieb, M. D., Fugate-Wentzek, L. A., & Wallman, J. (1988). Different visual deprivations produce different ametropias and different eye shapes. *Investigative Ophthalmology and Visual Science, 28,* 1225–1235.

Gould, S. J. & Lewontin, R. C. (1979). The spandrels of San Marco and the Panglossian paradigm. *Proceedings of the Royal Society (London), B,* 205, 581–598.

Gouras, P. (1991a). The history of color vision. In P. Gouras (Ed.), *The perception of color* (pp.1–9). Boca Raton, Fla.: CRC Press.

Gouras, P. (1991b). Precortical physiology of color vision. In P. Gouras (Ed.), *The perception of color* (pp. 163–178). Boca Raton, Fla.: CRC Press.

Gouras, P. (1991c). Cortical mechanisms of color vision. In P. Gouras (Ed.), *The perception of color* (pp. 179–197). Boca Raton, Fla.: CRC Press.

Gouras, P. & Zrenner, E. (1981). Colour coding in primate retina. *Vision Research, 21,* 1591–1598.

Graeme, J. G., Tobey, G. E. & Huelsman, L. P. (1971). *Operational amplifiers, Parts 1–3,* New York: McGraw-Hill.

Graham, C. H. (1965). Visual form perception. In C. H. Graham (Ed.), *Vision and visual perception* (pp. 548–574). New York: Wiley.

Graham, M. E. & Rogers, B. J. (1982). Simultaneous and successive contrast effects in the perception of depth from motion–parallax and stereoscopic information. *Perception, 11,* 247–262.

Graham, N. (1989). *Visual pattern analyzers.* New York: Oxford University Press.

Graham, N. & Nachmias, J. (1971). Detection of grating patterns containing two spatial frequencies: A comparison of single–channel and multiple–channel models. *Vision Research, 11,* 251–259.

Graham, N. & Robson, J. G. (1987). Summation of very close spatial frequencies: The importance of spatial probability summation. *Vision Research, 27,* 1997–2007.

Granger, E. M. & Heurtley, J. C. (1973). Visual chromaticity modulation transfer functions. *Journal of the Optical Society of America, 63,* 1173–1174.

Gratton-Guiness, I. (1972). *Joseph Fourier 1768–1830.* Cambridge, Mass.: MIT Press.

Gray, R. & Regan, D. (1996). Accuracy of reproducing angles: Is a right angle special? *Perception, 25,* 531–542.

Gray, R. & Regan, D. (1997). Vernier step acuity and bisection acuity for texture-defined form. *Vision Research, 37,* 1713–1723.

Gray, R. & Regan, D. (1998a). Spatial frequency discrimination and detection characteristics for gratings defined by orientation texture. *Vision Research, 38,* 2601–2617.

Gray, R. & Regan, D. (1998b). Accuracy of estimating time to collision based on binocular and monocular information. *Vision Research, 38,* 499–512.

Gray, R. & Regan, D. (1999a). Estimating time to collision with a rotating non-spherical object. *Vision Research, 40,* 49.

Gray, R. & Regan, D. (1999b). Motion in depth: Adequate and inadequate simulation. *Perception and Psychophysics, 61,* 236–245.

Green, D. M. & Luce, R. D. (1975). Parallel psychometric functions from a set of independent detectors. *Psychological Review, 82,* 483–486.

Green, D. M. & Swets, J. A. (1974). *Signal detection theory and psychophysics.* New York: Wiley.

Green, G. J. & Lessell, S. (1977). Acquired cerebral dyschromatopsia. *Archives of Ophthalmology, 95,* 121–128.

Greenlee, M. W. (1990). Dimensionality of the neuronal representation of visual images. *Perception, 20,* A40.

Greenlee, M. W., Georgeson, M. A., Magnussen, S. & Harris, J. P. (1991). The time course of adaptation to spatial contrast. *Vision Research, 31,* 223–236.

Greenlee, M. W. & Thomas, J. P. (1992). Effect of pattern adaptation on spatial frequency discrimination. *Journal of the Optical Society of America, A, 9,* 857–862.

Gregory, R. L. (1974). *Concepts and mechanisms of perception* (pp. 475–481). London: Duckworth.

Gregory, R. L. (1977). Vision with isoluminant color contrast: I. A projection technique with observations. *Perception, 6,* 113–119.

Gregory, R. L. & Heard, P. (1979). Border locking and the café wall illusion. *Perception, 8,* 365–380.

Grinberg, D. L. & Williams, D. R. (1985). Stereopsis with chromatic signals from the blue sensitive mechanism. *Vision Research, 25,* 531–537.

Grunau, M. von, & Frost, B. J. (1983). Double-opponent-process mechanism underlying RF-structure of directionally-specific cells of cat lateral suprsylvian visual area. *Experimental Brain Research, 49,* 84–92.

Guidarelli, S. (1972). Off–axis imaging in the human eye. *Atti. Fond. G. Ronchi, 27,* 407–415.

Guild, J. (1926). A trichromatic colorimeter suitable for standardization work. *Transactions of the Optical Society of London, 27,* 106–128.

Guild, J. (1931). The colorimetric properties of the spectrum. *Philosophical Transactions of the Royal Society of London,* 230A, 149–187.

Gurnsey, R. & Browse, R. A. (1987). Micropattern properties and presentation conditions influencing visual texture discrimination. *Vision Research, 41,* 239– 252.

Gwiazda, J., Bauer, J., Thorn, F. & Held, R. (1986). Meridional amblyopia does result from astigmatism in early childhood. *Clinical Vision Science, 1,* 145–152.

Gwiazda, J., Brill, S., Mohindra, I. & Held, R. (1980). Preferential looking acuity in infants from two to fifty–eight weeks of age. *American Journal of Optometry and Physiological Optics, 57,* 428–432.

Hagedorn, P. (1982). *Nonlinear oscillations.* Oxford: Oxford University Press.

Hall, J. L. (1981). Hybrid adaptive procedure for estimation of psychometric functions. *Journal of the Acoustical Society of America, 69,* 1763–1769.

Halpern, D. L. & Blake, R. R. (1988). How contrast affects stereoacuity. *Perception, 17,* 483–495.

Hamstra, S. J. (1994). *Effects of adaptation and disparity on shape discrimination for cyclopean form.* Ph. D. thesis, York University, North York, Ontario, Canada.

Hamstra, S. J. & Regan, D. (1995). Orientation discrimination in cyclopean vision. *Vision Research, 35,* 365–374.

Hansen, R. M. & Skavenski, A. A. (1977). Accuracy of eye position information for motor control. *Vision Research, 17,* 919–926.

Harmon, L. D. & Julesz, B. (1973). Masking in visual recognition: Effect of two–dimensional filtered noise. *Science, 180,* 1194–1197.

Hartline, H. K. (1938). The responses of single optic nerve fibers of the vertebrate eye to illumination of the retina. *American Journal of Physiology, 121,* 400–415.

Hartridge, H. (1947). The visual perception of fine detail. *Philosophical Transactions of the Royal Society of London, 232,* 519–581.

Hartridge, H. (1950). *Recent Advances in the Physiology of Vision* (p. 401). London: Churchill.

Hartridge, H. (1992). Visual acuity and the resolving power of the eye. *Journal of Physiology, 57,* 52–67.

Hayashi, C. (1964). *Nonlinear Oscillation in Physical Systems.* New York: McGraw-Hill.

Hayhoe, M. M, Benimoff, N. I. & Hood, D. C. (1987). The time–course of multiplicative and subtractive adaptation processes. *Vision Research, 27,* 1981–1996.

Heeger, D. J. (1992). Normalization of cell responses in cat striate cortex. *Visual Neuroscience, 9,* 181–197.

Heeley, D. W & Buchanan-Smith, H. M. (1994). Evidence for separate, task-dependent noise processes in orientation and size perception. *Vision Research, 34,* 2059–2069.

Heeley, D. W., Buchanan-Smith, H. M. & Heywood, S. (1993). Orientation acuity for sinewave gratings with random variations of spatial frequency. *Vision Research, 33,* 2509–2513.

Heeley, D. W. & Timney, B. (1988). Meridional anisotropies of orientation discrimination for sinewave gratings. *Vision Research, 28,* 337–344.

Heeley, D. W. & Timney, B. (1989). Spatial frequency discrimination at different orientations. *Vision Research, 29,* 1221–1228.

Held, R. (1991). The development of binocular vision and stereopsis. In D. Regan (Ed.), *Binocular vision.* London: Macmillan.

Helmholtz, H. von. (1962). *Handbook of physiological optics* (pp. 295–296). Translated by J. P. C. Southall. New York: Dover. (Work first published 1866.)

Henning, G. B, Hertz, B. G, & Broadbent, D. E. (1975). Some experiments bearing on the hypothesis that the visual system analyzes spatial patterns in independent bands of spatial frequency. *Vision Research, 15,* 887–897.

Hering, E. (1920). *Grundzüge der Lehre vom Lichten.* Berlin: Springer-Verlag. *(Outlines of a theory of the light sense.* Translated by L. M. Hurvich & D. Jameson. Cambridge, Mass.: Harvard University Press [1964].)

Herzog, M. H. & Fahle, M. (1997). The role of feedback in learning a Vernier discrimination task. *Vision Research, 37,* 2133–2141.

Hess, R. F. & Baker, C. L. (1984). Human pattern-evoked electroretinogram. *Journal of Neurophysiology, 51,* 939–951.

Hess, R. F. & Plant, G. T. (1983). The effect of temporal frequency variation on threshold contrast sensitivity deficits in optic neuritis. *Journal of Neurology Neurosurgery and Psychiatry, 46,* 322–330.

Hess, R. F. & Plant, G. T. (1986). The psychophysical loss in optic neuritis: Spatial and temporal aspects. In R. F. Hess & G. T. Plant (Eds.), *Optic neuritis* (pp. 109–151). Cambridge: Cambridge University Press.

Hess, R. F. & Pointer, J. S. (1987). Evidence for spatially local computations underlying discrimination of periodic patterns in fovea and periphery. *Vision Research, 27,* 1343–1360.

Heydt, R. von der, Peterhans, E. & Baumgartner, G. (1984). Illusory contours and cortical neuron responses. *Science, 224,* 1260–1262.

Heywood, C. A., Wilson, B. & Cowey, A. (1987). A case study of cortical colour blindness with relatively intact achromatic discrimination. *Journal of Neurology Neurosurgery and Psychiatry, 50,* 22–29.

Hildreth, E. C. (1998) (Ed.). *Models of recognition.* Special edition of *Vision Research, 38,* No. 15/16.

Hiltz, R. & Cavonius, C. R. (1974). Functional organization of the peripheral retina: Sensitivity to periodic stimuli. *Vision Research, 14,* 1333–1343.

Hines, M. (1976). Line spread function variation near the fovea. *Vision Research, 16,* 567–572.

Hirsch, J. (1985). Comment on "Line separation discrimination curve in the human fovea: Smooth or segmented?" *Journal of the Optical Society of America, A,* 477–478.

Hirsch, J. & Curcio, C. A. (1989). The spatial resolution capacity of human foveal retina. *Vision Research, 29,* 1095–1102.

Hirsch, J. & Hylton, R. (1982). Limits of spatial frequency discrimination as evidence of neural interpolation. *Journal of the Optical Society of America, A, 2,* 1170–1190.

Hirsch, J. & Hylton, R. (1984a). Orientation dependence of visual hyperacuity contains a component with hexagonal symmetry. *Journal of the Optical Society of America, A, 1,* 300–308.

Hirsch, J. & Hylton, R. (1984b). Quality of the primate photoreceptor lattice and limits of spatial vision. *Vision Research, 24,* 347–356.

Hirsch, J. & Miller, W. H. (1987). Does cone positional disorder limit resolution? *Journal of the Optical Society of America, A, 4,* 1481–1492.

Hirsch, M. & Smale, S. (1974). *Differential equations, dynamical systems and linear algebra.* New York: Academic Press.

Hochstein, S. & Shapley, R. M. (1976). Linear and nonlinear spatial subunits in Y cat retinal ganglion cells. *Journal of Physiology, 262,* 265–284.

Hoffman, D. D. & Richards, W. (1984). Parts of recognition. *Cognition, 18,* 65–96.

Hogervorst, M. A., Bradshaw, M. F. & Eagle, R. A. (1998). Evidence for independent channels in the perception of motion–parallax–defined surfaces. *Perception, 27* (Supp.), 113.

Hogervorst, M. A., Bradshaw, M. F. & Eagle, R. A. (2000). Spatial frequency tuning for 3D corrugations from motion parallax. *Vision Research,* in press.

Holmes, G. & Horax, G. (1919). Disturbances of spatial orientation and visual attention, with loss of stereoscopic vision. *Archives of Neurobiology and Psychiatry, 1,* 385–407.

Hong, X. & Regan, D. (1989). Visual field defects for unidirectional and oscillatory motion in depth. *Vision Research, 29,* 809–819.

Hopkins, H. H. (1950). *Wave theory of aberrations.* Oxford: Clarendon Press.

Hopkins, H. H. (1955). The frequency response of a defocused optical system. *Proceedings of the Royal Society of London, Series A, 231,* 91–103.

Hopkins, H. H. (1956). The frequency response of optical systems. *Proceedings of the Physical Society UK, Series B, 69,* 562–576.

Hopkins, H. H. (1962). The application of frequency response techniques in optics. *Proceedings of the Physical Society (London), 79,* 889–919.

Howard, I. P. & Rogers, B. J. (1995). *Binocular vision and stereopsis.* New York: Oxford University Press.

Howard, J. H. & Richardson, K. H. (1988). Absolute phase uncertainty in sinusoidal grating detection. *Perception and Psychophysics, 43,* 38–44.

Hoyle, F. (1957). *The black cloud.* London: Heinemann. Republished 1960. London: Penguin Books.

Hsu, H. P. (1970). *Fourier analysis.* New York: Simon & Schuster.

Hu, Q., Klein, S. & Carney, T. (1993). Can sinusoidal Vernier acuity be predicted by contrast discrimination? *Vision Research, 33,* 1241–1258.

Hubel, D. H. (1988). *Eye, Brain and Vision.* Scientific American Library. New York: W. H. Freeman.

Hubel, D. H. & Wiesel, T. N. (1962). Receptive fields, binocular interaction and functional architecture in the cat's striate cortex. *Journal of Physiology, 160,* 106–154.

Hubel, D. H. & Wiesel, T. N. (1968). Receptive fields and functional architecture of monkey striate cortex. *Journal of Physiology, 195,* 215–243.

Hubel, D. H. & Wiesel, T. N. (1970). Cells sensitive to binocular depth in area 18 of the macaque monkey cortex. *Nature, 255,* 41–42.

Hubel, D. H., Wiesel, T. N. & Stryker, M. P. (1978). Anatomical demonstration of orientation columns in macaque monkey. *Journal of Comparative Neurology, 177,* 361–380.

Hudspeth, A. J. (1983). Transduction and tuning by vertebrate hair cells. *Trends in Neuroscience, 6,* 366–369.

Hughes, A. (1986). The schematic eye comes of age. In J. D. Pattigrew, K. J. Sanderson & W. R. Levick (Eds.), *Visual neuroscience.* Cambridge: Cambridge University Press.

Humanski, R. A. & Wilson, H. R. (1992). Spatial frequency mechanisms with short-wavelength-sensitive cone inputs. *Vision Research, 32,* 549–560.

Humphreys, G. W. & Bruce, V. (1989). *Visual cognition..* Hove, U.K.: Lawrence Erlbaum.

Hurvich, L. M. (1981). *Color vision.* Sunderland, Mass.: Sinauer.

Hurvich, L. M. & Jameson, D. (1955). Some quantitative aspects of an opponent-colors theory. II. Brightness, saturation and hue in normal and dichromatic vision. *Journal of the Optical Society of America, 45,* 602–616.

Hurvich, L. M. & Jameson, D. (1957). An opponent-process theory of color vision. *Psychological Review, 64,* 384–404.

Ingling, C. R., Jr. (1991). Psychophysical correlates of parvo channel function. In A. Valberg & B. B. Lee (Eds.), *From pigments to perception* (pp. 413–424). New York: Plenum Press.

Ingling, C. R. & Martinez, E. (1983a). The relationship between spectral sensitivity and spatial sensitivity for the primate r-g X channel. *Vision Research, 23,* 1495–1500.

Ingling, C. R. & Martinez, E. (1983b). The spatiochromatic signal of the r-g channel. In J. D. Mollon & R. T. Sharpe (Eds.), *Colour vision* (pp. 433–444). New York: Academic Press.

Ingling, C. R., Tsou, B. H., Gast, T. J., Burns., S. A., Emerick, J. O. & Risenberg, L. (1978). The achromatic channel. I. The nonlinearity of minimally distinct border and flicker matches. *Vision Research, 18,* 379–390.

Irwin, D. (1991). Information integration across saccadis movements. *Cognitive Psychology, 23,* 420–456.

Ivanoff, A. (1947). Les aberrations de chromatisme et de sphericitie de l'oeil. *Rev. Opt. Theor. Instrumen., 26,* 145–171.

Jameson, D. & Hurvich, L. M. (1955). Some quantitative aspects of an opponent–colors theory. I. Chromatic responses and spectral saturation. *Journal of the Optical Society of America, 45,* 546–552.

Jastrow, J. (1892). On the judgement of angles and positions of lines. *American Journal of Psychology, 5,* 214–248.

Jenkins, F. A. & White, H. E. (1957). *Fundamentals of optics.* New York: McGraw–Hill.

Jenkins, G. M. & Watts, D. G. (1968). *Spectral analysis.* Oakland, Calif.: Holden-Day.

Jennings, J. A. M. & Charman, W. N. (1981). Off-axis image quality in the human eye. *Vision Research, 21,* 445–455.

Jones, R. V. (1978). *Most secret war.* London: Hamish Hamilton; reprinted 1998 by Wordsworth Editions Ltd., Ware, U.K. (Published in the United States as *The wizard war.* New York: Coward, McCann & Geoghegan.)

Jordon, J., Geisler, W. & Bovik, A. (1990). Color as a source of information in the stereo correspondence process. *Vision Research, 30,* 1955–1970.

Joseph, S. & Victor, J. D. (1994). A continuum of non-Gaussian self–similar image ensembles with white power spectra. *Spatial Vision, 8,* 503–513.

Julesz, B. (1960). Binocular depth perception of computer-generated patterns. *Bell System Technical Journal, 39,* 1125–1162.

Julesz, B. (1971). *Foundations of cyclopean perception.* Chicago: University of Chicago Press.

Julesz, B. (1975). Experiments in the visual perception of texture. *Scientific American, 232,* 34–43.

Julesz, B. (1981). Textons: The elements of texture perception and their interactions. *Nature, 290,* 91–97.

Julesz, B. (1983). Towards an axiomatic theory of preattentive vision. In G. M. Edelman, W. Einar Gall, & M. W. Cowan (Eds.), *Dynamic aspects of neocortical function.* New York: Wiley.

Julesz, B. (1984). A brief outline of the texton theory of human vision. *Trends in Neuroscience, 7,* 41–45.

Julesz, B. (1991). Early vision and focal attention. *Reviews of Modern Physics, 63,* 735–772.

Julesz, B., Gilbert, E. N. & Victor, J. D. (1978). Visual discrimination of textures with identical third-order statistics. *Biological Cybernetics, 31,* 137–140.

Julesz, B. & Krose, B. (1988). Visual texture perception: Features and spatial filters. *Nature, 333,* 302–303.

Julesz, B. & Miller, J. E. (1975). Independent spatial-frequency-tuned channels in binocular fusion and rivalry. *Perception, 4, 125,* 143.

Kaiser, P. K. (1971). Minimally distinct border as a preferred psychophysical criterion in visual heterochromatic photometry. *Journal of the Optical Society of America, 61,* 966–971.

Kaiser, P. K. (1984). Photometric measurements. In C. J. Bartleson & F. Grum (Eds.), *Optical radiation measurements.* New York: Academic Press.

Kaiser, P. K. (1988). Sensation luminance: A new name to distinguish CIE luminance from luminance dependent on an individual's spectral sensitivity. *Vision Research, 29,* 445–456.

Kaiser, P. K. & Boynton, R. M. (1996). *Human color vision.* Washington, D. C.: Optical Society of America.

Kankeo, C. R. S. (1980). A practical approach to understanding central pattern generators. *Behavioural and Brain Sciences, 3,* 554.

Karni, A. & Sagi, D. (1991). Where practice makes perfect in texture discrimination: Evidence for primary visual cortex plasticity. *Proceedings of the National Academy of Science, U. S. A., 88,* 4966–4970.

Kashi, R. S., Papathomas, T. V., Gorea, A. & Julesz, B. (1996). Similarities between texture grouping and motion perception: The role of color, luminance and orientation. *International Journal of Imaging Systems and Technology, 7,* 85–93.

Kaufman, L. (1974). *Sight and mind.* New York: Oxford University Press.

Keesey, U. (1972). Flicker and pattern detection: A comparison of thresholds. *Journal of the Optical Society of America, 62,* 446–448.

Kelly, D. H. (1960). J_0 stimulus patterns for vision research. *Journal of the Optical Society of America, 50,* 1115–1116.

Kelly, D. H. (1966). Frequency doubling in visual responses. *Journal of the Optical Society of America, 56,* 1628–1633.

Kelly, D. H. (1976). Pattern detection and the two-dimensional Fourier transform. *Vision Research, 16,* 277–287.

Kelly, D. H. (1977). Visual contrast sensitivity. *Optica Acta, 24,* 107–129.

Kelly, D. H. (1983). Spatiotemporal variation of chromatic and achromatic contrast thresholds. *Journal of the Optical Society of America, 73,* 742–750.

Kelly, D. H. (1989). Opponent–color receptive fields profiles determined from large–area psychophysical measurements. *Journal of the Optical Society of America, A, 6,* 784–793.

Kelly, D. H. (1996). Frequency doubling in visual responses. *Journal of the Optical Society of America, 56,* 1628–1633.

Kelly, D. H. & Burbeck, C. A. (1984). Critical problems in spatial vision CRC. *Critical Reviews of Biomedical Engineering, 10,* 125–177.

Kelley, D. H. & Magnuski, H. S. (1975). Pattern detection and the two-dimensional Fourier transform: Circular targets. *Vision Research, 15,* 911–915.

Kelly, D. H. & van Norren, D. (1977). Two band model of heterochromatic flicker. *Journal of the Optical Society of America, 67,* 1081–1091.

King-Smith, P. E. & Carden, D. (1976). Luminance and opponent–color contributions to visual detection and adaptation to temporal and spatial integration. *Journal of the Optical Society of America, 66,* 709–717.

Kingdom, F. A. A., Keeble, D. & Mouldon, B. (1994). Sensitivity to orientation modulation in micropattern–based textures. *Vision Research, 35,* 79–91.

Kingdom, F. A. A. & Mouldon, B. (1992). A multi–channel approach to brightness coding. *Vision Research, 32*, 1565–1582.

Kingslake, R. (1978). *Lens design fundamentals.* New York: Academic Press.

Kittel, C. (1953). *Introduction to solid state physics.* New York: Wiley.

Klatzky, R. L. (1980). *Human memory.* San Francisco: Freeman.

Klein, S., Stromeyer, C. F., III & Ganz, L. (1974). The simultaneous frequency shift: A dissociation between the detection and perception of gratings. *Vision Research, 14*, 1421–1432.

Klein, S. A. (1985). Double–judgement psychophysics: Problems and solutions. *Journal of the Optical Society of America, 2A*, 1560–1585.

Klein, S. A. (1989). Visual multipoles and the assessment of visual sensitivity to displayed images. In B. E. Rogowitz (Ed.), *Human vision, visual processing and digital display* (pp. 83–92). Proc. SPIE, 1077.

Klein, S. A. (1992). Channels: Bandwidth, channel independence, detection vs. discrimination. In B. Blum (Ed.), *Channels in the visual nervous system: Neurophysiology, psychophysics and models* (pp. 11–27). London: Freund.

Klein, S. A., Casson, E. & Carney, T. (1990). Vernier acuity as line and dipole detection. *Vision Research, 30*, 1703–1719.

Klein, S. A. & Levi, D. M. (1985). Hyperacuity thresholds of 1 sec.: Theoretical interpretations and empirical validation. *Journal of the Optical Society of America, A2*, 1170–1190.

Klein, S. A. & Levi, D. M. (1987). Positional sense in the peripheral retina. *Journal of the Optical Society of America, A*, 1543–1553.

Kling, J. W. & Riggs, L. A. (1971). (Eds.), *Woodworth & Schlosberg's Experimental psychology.* London: Methuen.

Knierim, J. J. & Van Essen, D. C. (1992). Neuronal responses to static texture patterns in area V1 of the alert macaque monkey. *Journal of Neurophysiology, 67*, 961–980.

Koenderink, J. J. (1972). Contrast enhancement and the negative afterimage. *Journal of the Optical Society of America, 62*, 685–689.

Koenderink, J. J., Bouman, M. A., de Mesquita, A. E. & Slappendal, S. (1978a). Perimetry of contrast detection thresholds of moving spatial sinewave patterns. 1. The near peripheral visual field. *Journal of the Optical Society of America, 68*, 845–849.

Koenderink, J. J., Bouman, M. A., de Mesquita, A. E. & Slappendal, S. (1978b). Perimetry of contrast detection thresholds of moving spatial sinewave patterns. 2. The far peripheral visual field. *Journal of the Optical Society of America, 68*, 850–854.

Koenderink, J. J. & Richards, W. (1988). Two-dimensional curvature operators. *Journal of the Optical Society of America, A, 5*, 1136–1141.

Koenderink, J. J. & van Doorn, A. J. (1976). Local structure of movement parallax of the plane. *Journal of the Optical Society of America, 66*, 717–723.

Koenderink, J. J. & van Doorn, A. J. (1979). The structure of two-dimensional scalar fields with applications to vision. *Biological Cybernetics, 33*, 151–158.

Koenderink, J. J. & van Doorn, A. J. (1981). Exterospecific components of the motion parallax field. *Journal of the Optical Society of America, 71*, 953–957.

Koenderink, J. J. & van Doorn, A. J. (1986). Representations of local geometry in the visual system. *Biological Cybernetics, 55*, 1–9.

Koffka, K. (1935). *Principles of gestalt psychology.* New York: Harcourt, Brace & World.

Köhler, W. & Wallach, H. (1944). Figural after–effects: An investigation of visual processes. *Proceedings of the American Philosophical Association, 88*, 269–357.

Kohly, R. P. & Regan, D. (1998). Independent encoding of speed and displacement for a moving cyclopean grating. *Investigative Ophthalmology and Visual Science, 39*, S462.

Kohly, R. P. & Regan, D. (1999a). Evidence for a mechanism sensitive to the speed of cyclopean form. *Vision Research, 39,* 1011–1024

Kohly, R. P. & Regan, D. (1999b). Coincidence detectors with outputs labelled with orientation difference and mean orientation. *Investigative Ophthalmology and Visual Science, 40,* Supp. 4, S222.

Kohly, R. P. & Regan, D. (1999c). Three-task discrimination of the speed, displacement and temporal frequency of moving cyclopean gratings. *Vision Research* (under review).

Kohly, R. P. & Regan, D. (2000). Long-distance interactions in cyclopean vision. *Vision Research* (submitted).

Kolb, E. W., "Rocky" (1996). *Blind watchers of the sky.* New York: Addison–Wesley.

Kolers, P. A. (1972). *Aspects of motion perception.* New York: Pergamon Press.

Kontsevich, L. L. & Tyler, C. W. (1998) How much of a visual object is used in estimating its position? *Vision Research, 38,* 3025–2039.

Korenberg, M. J. & Hunter, I. W. (1986). The identification of nonlinear biological systems: LNL cascade models. *Biological Cybernetics, 55,* 125–134.

Korn, G. A & Korn, T. M. (1968) *Mathematical handbook for scientists and engineers* (2nd ed.). New York: McGraw-Hill.

Kothe, A. C. & Regan, D. (1990). The component of gaze selection/control in the development of visual acuity in children. *Optometry and Vision Science, 67,* 770–778.

Kranz, D. H. (1975). Color measurement and color theory. II. Opponent–colors theory. *Journal of Mathematical Psychology, 12,* 304–327.

Krauskopf, J. (1962). Light distribution in human retinal images. *Journal of the Optical Society of America, 52,* 1046–1050.

Krauskopf, J. (1976). The effect of contrast and target width on Vernier acuity. *Bell Laboratories Technical Memo, 76,* 1222–1223.

Kruk, R. & Regan, D. (1983). Visual test results compared with flying performance in telemetry-tracked aircraft. *Aviation, Space and Environmental Medicine, 54,* 906–911.

Kruk, R., Regan, D., Beverley, K. I. & Longridge, T. (1981). Correlations between visual test results and flying performance on the Advanced Simulator for Pilot Training (ASPT). *Aviation, Space and Environmental Medicine, 52,* 455–460.

Kruk, R., Regan, D., Beverley, K. I. & Longridge, T. (1983). Flying performance on the Advanced Simulator for Pilot Training and laboratory tests of vision. *Human Factors , 25,* 457–466.

Kulikowski, J. J. (1971). Effects of eye movement on the contrast sensitivity of spatio–temporal patterns. *Vision Research, 11,* 261–273.

Kulikowski, J. J. & King-Smith, P. E. (1973). Spatial arrangement of line, edge and grating detector revealed by subthreshold summation. *Vision Research, 13,* 1455–1478.

Kulikowski, J. J. & Tolhurst, D. J. (1973). Psychophysical evidence for sustained and transient detectors in human vision. *Journal of Physiology, 232,* 149–162.

Kupersmith, M. J., Nelson, J. I., Seiple, W. H., Carr, R. E. & Weiss, P. A. (1983). The 20/20 eye in multiple sclerosis. *Neurology, 33,* 1015–1020.

Kupersmith, M. J., Seiple, W. H., Nelson, J. I. & Carr, R. E. (1984). Contrast sensitivity loss in multiple sclerosis. *Investigative Ophthalmology and Visual Science, 25,* 632–639.

Kupersmith, M. J., Shakn, E., Siegel, I. M. & Lieberman, A. (1982). Visual system abnormalities in patients with Parkinson's disease. *Archives of Neurology, 39,* 284–286.

Kurtenbach, W. & Magnussen, S. (1981). Inhibition, disinhibition and summation among orientation detectors in human vision. *Experimental Brain Research, 43,* 193–198.

Kwan, L. & Regan, D. (1998). Orientation-tuned spatial filters for texture-defined form. *Vision Research, 38,* 3849–3855.

Laband, J. (1992). *Kingdom in crisis: The Zulu response to the British invasion of 1879.* Natal, South Africa: University of Natal Press.

Lages, M. & Treisman, M. (1998). Spatial frequency discrimination: Visual long-term memory or criterion setting? *Vision Research, 38,* 557–572.

Land, E. H., Hubel, D. H., Livingstone, M. S., Perry, S. H. & Burns, M. M. (1983). Colour-generating interactions across the corpus callosum. *Nature (London), 303,* 616–618.

Land, M. F. & Fernald, R. D (1992). The evolution of eyes. *Annual Review of Neuroscience, 15,* 1–29.

Landy, M. S & Bergen, J. R. (1991). Texture segregation and orientation gradient. *Vision Research, 31,* 679–691.

Lánský, P., Yakimoff, N. & Radil, T. (1988). Influence of local orientation cues on estimating the tilt of two-dimensional patterns. *Spatial Vision, 3,* 9–13.

Lasley, D. J. & Cohn, T. E. (1981). Why luminance discrimination may be better than detection. *Vision Research, 21,* 273–278.

Lawden, M. C. (1983). An investigation of the ability of the human visual system to encode spatial phase relationships. *Vision Research, 12,* 1451–1463.

Lee, B. B. & Harris, J. (1996). Contrast transfer characteristics of visual short–term memory. *Vision Research, 36,* 2159–2166.

Lee, B. B., Martin, P. R. & Valberg, A. (1988).The physiological basis of hetero-chromatic flicker photometry demonstrated in the ganglion ccells of the macaque retina. *Journal of Physiology. (London) 404,* 323–347.

Lee, B. B., Martin, P. R. & Valberg, A. (1989). Nonlinear summation of M- and L-cone input to phasic retinal ganglion cells of the macaque. *Journal of Neuroscience, 9,* 1433–1442.

Lee, B. B. & Rogers, B. (1997). Disparity modulation sensitivity for narrow–band–filtered stereograms. *Vision Research, 37,* 1769–1777.

Lee, D. N. (1976). A theory of visual control of braking based on information about time to collision. *Perception, 1976,* 437–459.

Lee, J. & Stromeyer, C. F. III (1989). Contribution of human short–wave cones to luminance and motion detection. *Journal of Physiology (London), 413,* 563–593.

Lee, T. S. (1988). A framework for understanding texture segmentation in the primary visual cortex. *Vision Research, 18,* 2643–2657.

Legge, G. E. (1980) A power law for contrast discrimination. *Vision Research, 21,* 457–467.

Legge, G. E. & Foley, J. M. (1980). Contrast masking in human vision. *Journal of the Optical Society of America, 70,* 1458–1471.

Legge, G. E. & Gu, Y. (1989). Stereopsis and contrast. *Vision Research, 29,* 989–1004.

LeGrand, Y. (1937). La formation des image retiniennes. Sur un mode de vision éliminant les defauts optiqeus de l'oeil. *2e Réunion de l'Institute d'Optique, Paris.*

LeGrand, Y. & El Hage, S. G. (1980). *Physiological optics.* Berlin: Springer Verlag.

Leguire, L. E. (1991). Do letter charts measure contrast sensitivity? *Clinical Vision Science, 6,* 391–400.

Lehmann, D. & Julesz, B. (1978). Lateralized cortical potentials evoked in human by dynamic random–dot stereograms. *Vision Research, 18,* 1265–1271.

Lennie, P., Pokorny, J. & Smith, V. C. (1993). Luminance. *Journal of the Optical Society of America, A, 10,* 1283–1293.

Leuwenberg, E. L. J. & Buffart, H. F. J. M (1978) (Eds.). *Formal theories of visual perception.* New York: Wiley.

Levi, D. M. (1991). Spatial vision in amblyopia. In D. Regan (Ed.), *Spatial vision* (pp. 212–238). London: Macmillan.

Levi, D. M. & Klein, S. (1982). Differences in Vernier discrimination for gratings between strabismic and anisometropic amblyopes. *Investigative Ophthalmology and Visual Science, 23,* 398–407.

Levi, D. M. & Klein, S. A. (1983). Spatial localization in normal and amblyopic vision. *Vision Research, 23,* 1005–1017.

Levi, D. M. & Klein, S. A. (1989). Both separation and eccentricity can limit precise positional judgements: A reply to Morgan and Watt. *Vision Research, 29,* 1463–1469.

Levi, D. M. & Klein, S. A. (1990). The role of separation and eccentricity in encoding position. *Vision Research, 30,* 557–585.

Levi, D. M., Klein, S. A. & Yap, Y. L. (1988). "Weber's Law" for position: Unconfounding the role of separation and eccentricity. *Vision Research, 28,* 597–603.

Levinson, E. & Sekular, R. (1980). A two-dimensional analysis of direction-specific adaptation. *Vision Research, 20,* 103–108.

Levinson, J. Z. & Frome, F. S. (1979). Perception of size of one object among many. *Science, 206,* 1425–1426.

Levitt, H. (1967). Testing for sequential dependencies. *Journal of the Acoustical Society of America, 43,* 65–69.

Levitt, H. (1971). Transformed up–down methods in psychoacoustics. *Journal of the Acoustical Society of America, 49,* 467–477.

Li, A. & Aslin, R. N. (1992). Contrast adaptation and perceptual "filling in" at specific retinal locations. *Investigative Ophthalmology and Visual Science (Supp. 33),* S1256.

Li, W. & Westheimer, G. (1997). Human discrimination of the implicit orientation of simple symmetrical patterns. *Vision Research, 37,* 565–572.

Lieberman, H. R. & Penland, A. P (1982). Computer technology: Microcomputer-based estimation on psychophysical thresholds: The best PEST. *Behavior Research Methods and Instrumentation, 14,* 21–25.

Liebman, P. A. & Entine, G. (1964). Sensitive low–level microspectrophotometer: Detection of photo sensitive pigments of retinal cones. *Journal of the Optical Society of America, 54,* 1451–1459.

Liebmann, S. (1927). Über des Verhalten farbiger Formen bei Helligkeitsgleichieit von Figur und Grund. *Psychologisches Forschung, 9,* 300–353.

Lillestæter, O. (1993). Complex contrast, a definition for structured targets and backgrounds. *Journal of the Optical Society of America, A, 10,* 2453–2457.

Lin, L. M. & Wilson, H. R. (1996). Fourier and non-Fourier pattern discrimination compared. *Vision Research, 36,* 1907–1918.

Linberg, P. (1954). Measurement of contrast transmission characteristics in optical image formation. *Optica Acta, 1,* 80–87.

Linfoot, E. H. (1964). *Fourier methods of optical image evaluation.* London: Focal Press.

Lit, A., Finn, J. P., & Vicars, W. M. (1972). Effect of target background luminance contrast on binocular depth discrimination at photopic levels of illumination. *Vision Research, 12,* 1241–1251.

Livingstone, M. S. & Hubel, D. H. (1984). Anatomy and physiology of a color system in the primate visual cortex. *Journal of Neuroscience, 4,* 309–356.

Llewellyn, K. R. (1971). Visual guidance of locomotion. *Journal of Experimental Psychology, 91,* 245–261.

Longuet–Higgins, H. C. & Prazdny, K. F. (1980). The interpretations of a moving retinal image. *Proceedings of the Royal Society of London, B, 268,* 285–297.

Losada, M. A. & Mullen, K. T. (1994). The spatial tuning of chromatic mechanisms identified by simultaneous masking. *Vision Research, 34,* 331–341.

Lotze, H. (1885). *Microcosmos.* Translated by E. Hamilton and E. E. Constance–Jones. Edinburgh: T. & T. Clark (cited in White et al., 1992).

Ludvigh, E. (1953). Direction sense of the eye. *American Journal of Ophthalmology, 36,* 139–142.

Lueck, C. J., Zeki, S. M., Fronton, K. J., Deicer, M-P., Cope, P., Cunningham, V. J., Lammertsma, A. A., Kennard, C. & Frackowiack, R. S. J. (1989). The colour centre in the cerebral cortex of man. *Nature (London), 340,* 386–389.

Lumsden, C. E. (1970). In P. J. Vinker & G. W. Bruyn (Eds.), *Handbook of clinical neurology*, Vol.9 (pp. 235–258). Amsterdam: North Holland.

MacFarlane, G. (1979). *Howard Florey*. Oxford: Oxford University Press.

Machiavelli, N. (1981). *The prince*. (Translated by G. Bull). London: Penguin Classics.

MacKay, D. M. (1950). Complementary measures of scientific information–content. *Proceedings of the First London Conference on Information Theory, Methodos, 8*, 63–89.

MacKay, D. M. (1956). Towards an information–flow model of human behaviour. *British Journal of Psychology, 57*, 30–43.

MacKay, D. M. (1965). Cerebral organization and the conscious control of action. In *Semaine d'étude sur cerveau et expérience consciente* (pp. 1–29). Rome: Pontificiae Academiae Scientiarum Scripta Varia, Vol. 30.

MacLean, I. & Stacey, B. (1971). Judgement of angle size: An experimental appraisal. *Perception and Psychophysics, 9*, 499–504.

Macmillan, N. A. & Creelman, C. D. (1991). *Detection theory: A user's guide*. Cambridge: Cambridge University Press.

MacRae, A. & Loh, H. (1981). Constant errors occur in matched reproduction of angles even when likely biases are eliminated. *Perception and Psychophysics, 30*, 341–346.

Madigan, R. & Williams, D. (1987). Maximum likelihood procedures in two–alternative forced choice. Evaluation and recommendations. *Perception and Psychophysics, 42*, 240–249.

Magnussen, S., Greenlee, M. W., Asplund, R. & Dyrnes, S. (1990). Perfect visual short–term memory for periodic patterns. *European Journal of Cognitive Psychology, 2*, 345–362.

Magnussen, S., Landro, N. I. & Johnson, T. (1985). Visual half–field symmetry in orientation perception. *Perception, 14*, 265–273.

Mahowald, M. A. & Mead, C. (1991). The silicon retina. *Scientific American, 264(5)*, 76–82.

Malik, J. & Perona, P. (1990). Preattentive texture discrimination with early visual mechanisms. *Journal of the Optical Society of America, A7*, 923–932.

Marc, R. E. & Sperling, H. G. (1977). Chromatic organization of primate cones. *Science, 196*, 454–456.

Marceltja, S. (1980). Mathematical descriptions of the responses of simple cortical cells. *Journal of the Optical Society of America, 70*, 1297–1300.

Marimont, D. H. & Wandell, B. A. (1994). Matching color images: The effects of axial chromatic aberration. *Journal of the Optical Society of America, A, 11*, 3113–3122.

Marks, L. E. & Bornstein, M. H. (1973). Spectral sensitivity by constant CFF: Effect of chromatic adaptation. *Journal of the Optical Society of America, 63*, 220–226.

Marks, W. B, Dobelle, W. H. & MacNichol, M. F. Jr. (1964). Visual pigments of single primate cones. *Science, 143*, 1181–1183.

Marmarelis, P. Z. & Marmarelis, V. Z. (1978). *Analysis of physiological systems: The white noise approach*. New York: Plenum Press.

Marr, D. (1976). Early processing of visual information. *Philosophical Transactions of the Royal Society of London, B, 275*, 483–524.

Marr, D. (1982). *Vision*. San Francisco: W. H. Freeman.

Marr, D. & Hildreth, E. C. (1980). A theory of edge detection. *Proceedings of the Royal Society of London, B, 207*, 187–217.

Marr, D. & Nishihara, H. K. (1978). Representation and recognition of the spatial organization of three-dimensional shapes. *Proceedings of the Royal Society (London), B, 200*, 269–294.

Marr, D. & Poggio, T. (1976). A cooperative computation of stereo disparity. *Science, 194*, 283–287.

Marr, D. & Poggio, T. (1979). A computational theory of human stereo vision. *Proceedings of the Royal Society of London, B*, 204– 301–328.

Marr, D., Ullman, S., & Poggio, T. (1979). Bandpass channels, zero crossings, and early visual information processing. *Journal of the Optical Society of America*, 69, 914–916.

Marrocco, R. T. & McClurkin, J. W. (1985). Evidence for spatial structure in the cortical input to the monkey lateral geniculate nucleus. *Experimental Brain Research*, 59, 50–56.

Matin, L. (1972). Eye movements and perceived visual direction. In D. Jameson and L. M. Hurvich (Eds.), *Visual psychophysics* (pp. 331–380). New York: Springer Verlag.

Matthews, P. B. C. (1964). Muscle spindles and their motor control. *Physiological Review*, 44, 219–388.

Maudarbocus, A. Y. & Rudduck, K. M. (1973). Nonlinearity of visual signals in relation to shape–sensitive adaptation responses. *Vision Research, 13*, 1713–1737.

Maunsell, J. H. R. (1995). The brain's visual world: Representations of visual targets in cerebral cortex. *Science, 270*, 764–769.

Maunsell, J. H. R. & Newsome, W. T. (1987).Visual processing in monkey extrastriate cortex. *Annual Review of Neuroscience, 10*, 363–401.

Maxwell, J. C. (1860). On the theory of compound colours and the relations of the colours of the spectrum. *Philosophical Transactions of the Royal Society of London, 150*, 57–68.

Maxwell, N. (1985). Methodological problems in neuroscience. In D. Rose & V. G. Dobson (Eds.), *Models of the visual cortex* (pp. 11–21). New York: Wiley.

Mayhew, J. E. W. & Frisby, J. P. (1976). Rivalrous texture stereograms. *Nature, 264*, 53–56.

McAlpine, D., Lumsden, C. E. & Acheson, E. D. (1965). *Multiple sclerosis*. Edinburgh: Livingstone.

McCree, K. J. (1960). Colour confusion produced by voluntary fixation. *Optica Acta, 7*, 281–290.

McDonald, W. I. (1974). Pathophysiology in multiple sclerosis. *Brain, 97*, 179–196.

McGhee, G. R. J. (1966). *The Late Devonian mass extinction* (pp. 1–5). New York: Columbia University Press.

McKee, S. M. (1981). A local mechanism for differential velocity detection. *Vision Research, 21*, 491–500.

McKee, S. P., Klein, S. A. & Teller, D. Y. (1985). Statistical properties of forced–choice psychometric functions: Implications of probit analysis. *Perception and Psychophysics, 37*, 286–298.

McKee, S. P. & Westheimer, G. (1978). Improvement in Vernier acuity with practice. *Perception and Psychophysics, 24*, 258–262.

McLauchlan, N. W. (1961). *Bessel functions for engineers*. London: Oxford University Press.

Medawar, P. B. (1981). *Advice to a young scientist*. New York: Basic Books.

Medawar, P. B. (1996). *The strange case of the spotted mice*. New York: Oxford University Press.

Medjbeur, S. & Tulunay-Kessey, U. (1985). Spatio-temporal responses of the visual system in demyelinating diseases. *Brain, 108*, 123–138.

Merigan, W. H., Byrne, C. E. & Maunsell, J. H. R. (1991b). Does primate motion perception depend on the magnocellular pathways? *Journal of Neuroscience, 11*, 3422–3429.

Merigan, W. H., Katz, L. M. & Maunsell, J. H. R. (1991a). The effects of parvocellular lateral geniculate lesions on the acuity and contrast sensitivity of macaque monkeys. *Journal of Neuroscience, 11*, 994–1001.

Merigan, W. H. & Maunsell, J. H. R. (1990). Macaque vision after magnocellular lateral geniculate lesions. *Vis. Neuroscience, 5*, 347–352.

Metcalf, H. (1965). Stiles-Crawford apodisation. *Journal of the Optical Society of America, 55*, 72–74.

Milsum, J. H. (1966). *Biological control systems analysis*. New York: McGraw–Hill

Mitchell, D. E. (1966). Retinal disparity and diplopia. *Vision Research, 6*, 441–451.

Mitchell, D. E. (1969). Qualitative depth localization with diplopic images of dissimilar shape. *Vision Research, 9,* 991–994.

Mitchell, D. E. (1970). Properties of stimuli eliciting vergence eye movements and stereopsis. *Vision Research, 10,* 145–162.

Mitchell, D. E., Freeman, R. D., Millodot, M., & Haegerstrom, G. (1973). Meridional amblyopia: Evidence for modification of the human visual system by early visual experience. *Vision Research, 13,* 535–558.

Mitchell, D. E. & Wilkinson, F. (1974). The effect of early astigmatism on the visual resolution of gratings. *Journal of Physiology (London), 243,* 739–756.

Mohler, S. R. & Johnson, B. H. (1971). *Wiley Post, his Winnie Mae and the world's first pressure suit.* Washington, D. C.: Smithsonian Institute Press.

Mohn, G. & Van Hof-Van Duin, J. (1991). Development of spatial vision. In D. Regan (Ed.), *Spatial vision* (pp. 179–211). London: Macmillan.

Mollon, J. D. (1982). A taxonomy of tritanopes. *Documenta Ophthalmolgia, Proceedings Series, 33,* 87–101.

Mollon, J. D. (1989). The uses and origins of primate colour vision. *Journal of Experimental Biology, 146,* 21–38.

Mollon, J. D., Newcombe, F., Polden, P. G. & Ratcliff, G. (1980). On the presence of three cone mechanisms in a case of total achromatopia. In G. Verriest (Ed.), *Colour vision deficiencies* (pp. 130–135). Bristol: Adam Hilger.

Moreland, J. D. (1982). Spectral sensitivity measured by motion photometry. *Documenta Ophthalmolgia, Proceedings Series., 33,* 61–66.

Morgan, M. J. (1986a). The detection of spatial discontinuities: interactions between contrast and spatial contiguity. *Spatial Vision, 1,* 291–303.

Morgan, M. J. (1986b). Positional acuity without monocular cues. *Perception, 15,* 157–162.

Morgan, M. J. (1991). Hyperacuity. In D. Regan (Ed.), *Spatial vision* (pp.87–113). London: MacMillan.

Morgan, M. J. (1992). On the scaling of size judgements by orientational cues. *Vision Research, 32,* 1433–1445.

Morgan, M. J., Adam, A. & Mollon, J. D. (1992). Dichromats detect colour-camouflage objects that are not detected by trichromats. *Proceedings of the Royal Society (London), B,* 291–295.

Morgan, M. J. & Aiba, T. S. (1985a). Vernier acuity predicted from changes in the light distribution of the retinal image. *Spatial Vision, 1,* 151–171.

Morgan, M. J. & Aiba, T. S. (1985b). Positional acuity with chromatic stimuli. *Vision Research, 25,* 689–695.

Morgan, M. J. & Fahle, M. (1992). Effects of pattern element density upon displacement limits for motion detection in random binary luminance patterns. *Proceedings of the Royal Society (London), B, 248,* 189–198.

Morgan, M. J. & Mather, G. (1994). Motion discrimination in two-frame sequences with differing spatial frequency content. *Vision Research, 34,* 197–208.

Morgan, M. J. & Regan, D. (1987). Opponent model for line interval discrimination: Interval and Vernier performance compared. *Vision Research, 27,* 107–118.

Morgan, M. J., Ross, J. & Hayes, A. (1991). The relative importance of local phase and local amplitude in patchwise image reconstruction. *Biological Cybernetics, 65,* 113–119.

Morgan, M. J. & Ward, R. M. (1985). Spatial and spatial-frequency primitives in spatial-interval discrimination. *Journal of the Optical Society of America, A, 2,* 1205–1210.

Morgan, M. J. & Watt, R. J. (1982). The modulation transfer function of a display oscilloscope. *Vision Research, 22,* 1083–1085.

Morgan, M. J. & Watt, R. J. (1983a). On the failure of spatio-temporal interpolation: A filtering model. *Vision Research, 23,* 997–1003.

Morgan, M. J. & Watt, R. J. (1983b). Mechanisms of interpolation in human spatial vision. *Nature, 299,* 553–555.

Morgan, M. J. & Watt, R. J. (1984). Spatial frequency interference effects and interpolation in Vernier acuity. *Vision Research, 24,* 1911–1919.

Morgan, M. J. & Watt, R. J. (1989). The Weber relation for position is not an artifact of eccentricity. *Vision Research, 29,* 1457–1462.

Morgan, M. J. & Watt, R. J. (1997). The combination of filters in early spatial vision: a retrospective analysis of the MIRAGE model. *Perception, 26,* 1073–1088.

Morgan, M. J., Watt, R. J. & McKee, S. P. (1983). Exposure duration affects the sensitivity of Vernier acuity to target motion. *Vision Research, 23,* 541–546.

Morrone, M. C. & Burr, D. (1986). Evidence for the existence and development of visual inhibition in humans. *Nature, 321,* 235–237.

Morrone, M. C., Burr, D. & Maffei, L. (1982). Functional implications of cross-orientation inhibition of cortical visual cells: I. Neurophysiological evidence. *Proceedings of the Royal Society, B, 216,* 335–354.

Morrone, M. C., Burr, D. & Vaina, L. M. (1995). Two stages of visual processing for radial and circular motion. *Nature, 376,* 507–509.

Mountcastle, V. B. (1979). An organizing principle for cerebral functions: The unit module and the distributed system. In F. O. Schmitt & F. G. Worden (Eds.) *The neurosciences: Fourth study program* (pp. 21–42). Cambridge, Mass.: MIT Press.

Mountcastle, V. B. (1995). The evolution of ideas concerning the neocortex. *Cerebral Cortex, 5,* 289–295.

Mountcastle, V. B. (1997). The columnar organization of the neocortex. *Brain, 120,* 701–722.

Mountcastle, V. B. (1998). *Perceptual neuroscience.* Cambridge, Mass.: Harvard University Press.

Mullen, K. T. (1985). The contrast sensitivity of human colour vision to red–green and blue–yellow chromatic gratings. *Journal of Physiology, 359,* 381–400.

Mullen, K. T. & Boulton, J. C. (1992). Absence of smooth motion perception in color vision. *Vision Research, 32,* 483–488.

Mullen K. T. & Losada, M. A. (1994). Evidence for separate pathways for color and luminance mechanisms. *Journal of the Optical Society of America, A, 11,* 3136–3151.

Mulligan, J. B. & Krauskopf, J. (1983). Vernier acuity for chromatic stimuli. *Investigative Ophthalmology and Visual Science, 24,* 276.

Murakami, I. & Shimojo, S. (1996). Assimilation-type and contrast-type bias of motion induced by the surround in a random-dot display: Evidence for center-surround interaction. *Vision Research, 36,* 3629–3639.

Mustillo, P., Francis, E., Oross, S., Fox, R. & Orban, G. A. (1988). Anisotropies in global stereoscopic orientation discrimination. *Vision Research, 28,* 1315–1321.

Nachmias, J. (1981). On the psychometric function for contrast detection. *Vision Research, 21,* 215–223.

Nachmias, J. & Rogowitz, B. E. (1983). Masking by spatially–modulated gratings. Vision Research, 23, 1621–1629.

Nachmias, J. & Sansbury, R. V. (1974). Grating contrast: discrimination may be better than detection. *Vision Research, 14,* 1039–1042.

Nachmias, J., Sansbury, R. V., Vassilev, A. & Weber, A. (1973). Adaptation to square-wave gratings: In search of the elusive third harmonic. *Vision Research, 13,* 1335–1342.

Nachmias, J. & Weber, A. (1975). Discrimination of simple and complex gratings. *Vision Research, 15,* 217–224.

Naka, K. I. & Rushton, W. A. H. (1966). S-potentials from luminosity units in the retina of fish (cyprinidae). *Journal of Physiology, 185,* 587–599.

Nakayama, K. (1990). The iconic bottleneck and the tenuous link between early visual processing and perception. In C. Blakemore (Ed.). *Vision: Coding and efficiency* (pp. 411–422). Cambridge: Cambridge University Press.

Nakayama, K. & Loomis, J. M. (1974). Optical velocity patterns, velocity- sensitive neurons, and space perception: A hypothesis. *Perception, 3*, 63–80.

Nakayama, K. & Silverman, G. H. (1985). Detection and discrimination of sinusoidal grating displacements. *Journal of the Optical Society of America, A*, 2, 267–274.

Nakayama, K. & Tyler, C. W. (1981). Psychophysical isolation of movement sensitivity by removal of familiar position cues. *Vision Research, 21*, 427–433.

National Highway Traffic Safety Administration (NHTSA). *Traffic safety facts 1996*. Washington, D. C.: NHTSA.

Nelson, J. I. & Frost, B. (1978). Orientation selective inhibition from beyond the classic visual receptive field. *Brain Research, 139*, 359–365.

Nelson, J. I., Seiple, W. H., Kupersmith, M. J. & Carr, R. E. (1984). A rapid evoked potential index of cortical adaptation. *Investigative Ophthalmology and Visual Science, 59*, 454–464.

Nelson, R., Famiglietti, E. V. Jr & Kolb, H. (1978). Intracellular staining reveals different levels of stratification for on- and off-center cells in cat retina. *Journal of Neurophysiology, 41*, 472–483.

Nielson, K. R. K., Watson, A. B. & Ahumada, A. J. (1985). Application of a computable model of human spatial vision to phase discrimination. *Journal of the Optical Society of America, A2*, 1600–1606.

Nikara, T., Bishop, P. O. & Pettigrew, J. D. (1968). Analysis of retinal correspondence by studying receptive fields of binocular single neurons in cat cortex. *Experimental Brain Research, 6*, 353–363.

Nishihara, H. K. (1987). Practical real-time imaging stereo matcher. In M. A. Fischler & O. Firschein (Eds.). *Readings in computer vision* (pp. 63–72). Los Altos, Calif.: Kauffman.

Noorlander, C., Heuts, M. J. G & Koenderink, J. J. (1981). Sensitivity to spatiotemporal combined luminance and chromaticity contrast. *Journal of the Optical Society of America, 71*, 453–459.

Noorlander, C. & Koenderink, J. J. (1983). Spatial and temporal discrimination ellipsoids in color space. *Journal of the Optical Society of America, 73*, 1533–1543.

Norcia, A. M., Sutter, E. F. & Tyler, C. W. (1985). Electrophysiological evidence for the existence of coarse and fine disparity mechanisms in human. *Vision Research, 25*, 1603–1611.

Norcia, A. M. & Tyler, C. W. (1985). Spatial frequency sweep VEP: Visual acuity during the first year of life. *Vision Research, 25*, 1399–1408.

Norcia, A. M., Tyler, C. W. & Allen, D. (1986). Electrophysiology assessment of contrast sensitivity in human infants. *American Journal of Optometry and Physiological Optics, 63*, 12–15.

Norcia, A. M., Tyler, C. W. & Hammer, R. D. (1988). High visual contrast sensitivity in the young human infant. *Investigative Ophthalmology and Visual Science, 29*, 44–49.

Nothdurft, H. C. (1985a). Orientation sensitivity and texture segmentation in patterns with different line orientation. *Vision Research, 25*, 551–560.

Nothdurft, H. C. (1985b). Sensitivity for structure gradient in texture discrimination tasks. *Vision Research, 25*, 1957–1968.

Nothdurft, H. C. (1990). Texture segregation by associated differences in global and local luminance distribution. *Proceedings of the Royal Society London, B, 239*, 295–320 (erratum, *B*, 249–250).

Nothdurft, H. C. (1991a). Texture segmentation and pop-out from orientation contrast. *Vision Research, 31*, 1073–1078.

Nothdurft, H. C. (1991b). Different effects from spatial frequency masking in texture segregation and texture detection tasks. *Vision Research, 31*, 299–320.

Nothdurft, H. C. (1992). Feature analysis and the role of similarity in preattentive vision. *Perception and Psychophysics, 52*, 355–375.

Nothdurft, H. C. (1994). Common properties of visual segmentation. In G. R. Bock and J. A. Goode (Eds.), *Higher-order processing in the visual system* (pp. 245–268). Chichester: Wiley.

Nothdurft, H. C. (1997). Different approaches to the coding of visual segmentation. In L. Harris & M. Jenkins (Eds.), *Computational and psychophysical mechanisms of visual coding* (pp. 20–43). New York: Cambridge University Press.

Nothdurft, H. C., Gallant, J. L. & Van Essen, D. C. (1992). Neural responses to texture borders in macaque area V1. *Society for Neuroscience* (abstracts), 18(2), 1275.

Obergfell, J., Greenlee, M. W. & Magnussen, S. (1989). Short-term memory for motion: Temporal–frequency discrimination of drifting gratings. *Perception, 18*, A38.

Ogle, K. N. (1953). Precision and validity of stereoscopic depth perception from double images. *Journal of the Optical Society of America, 43*, 906–913.

Ogle, K. N. (1963). Stereoscopic depth perception and exposure delay between images to the two eyes. *Journal of the Optical Society of America, 53*, 1296–1304.

Ogle, K. N. (1964). *Researchers in binocular vision*. New York: Hafner.

Ohzawa, I., Sclar, G & Freeman, R. D. (1982). Contrast gain control in the cat visual cortex. *Nature, 289*, 266–268.

Ohzawa, I., Sclar, G. & Freeman, R. D. (1985). Contrast gain control in the cat's visual system. *Journal of Neurophysiology, 54*, 651–667.

Olsen, R. K. & Attneave, F. (1970). What variables produce similarity grouping? *American Journal of Psychology, 83*, 1–21.

Olzak, L. A. & Thomas, J. P. (1991). When orthogonal orientations are not processed independently. *Vision Research, 31*, 51–57.

Olzak, L. A. & Thomas, J. P. (1992). Configural effects constrain Fourier models of pattern discrimination, *Vision Research, 32*, 1885–1898.

Olzak, L. A. & Thomas, J. P. (1996). Characteristics of third-stage mechanisms in pattern vision. *Investigative Ophthalmology and Visual Science, 37*, S1148.

Oppenheim, A. V. & Lim, J. S. (1981). The importance of phase in signals. *Proceedings of the IEEE, 69*, 529–541.

Optican, L. M. & Richmond, B. J. (1987). Temporal encoding of two-dimensional patterns by single units in primate inferior temporal cortex. 3. Information theoretic analysis. *Journal of Neurophysiology, 57*, 162–178.

O'Regan, J. K., Rensink, R. A. & Clark, J. J. (1999). Change-blindness as a result of "mudsplashes." *Nature, 398*, 34.

O'Shea, R. P., Blackburn, S. G. & Ono, H. (1994). Contrast as a depth cue. *Vision Research, 34*, 1595–1604.

O'Toole, C. (1995). *Alien empire*. London: BBC Books.

Pantle, A. (1973a). Flicker adaptation. I. Effect on visual sensitivity to temporal fluctuations of light intensity. *Vision Research, 13*, 943–952.

Pantle, A. (1973b). Visual effects of sinusoidal components of complex gratings: Independent or additive? *Vision Research, 13*, 2195–2205.

Pantle, A. (1992). Immobility of some second-order stimuli in human peripheral vision. *Journal of the Optical Society of America, A, 9*, 863–867.

Pantle, A. & Sekuler, R. (1968). Size detecting mechanisms in human vision. *Science, 162*, 1146–1148.

Papathomas, T. V. & Gorea, A. (1990). The role of visual attributes in texture perception. *SPIE, 1249*, 395–403.

Papathomas, T. V., Kashi, R. S. & Gorea, A. (1997). A human vision based computational model for chromatic texture segregation. *IEEE Transactions on Systems, Man and Cybernetics, 27*, 428–440.

Papoulis, A. (1962). *The Fourier integral and its applications*. New York: McGraw-Hill.

Parish, D. H. & Sperling, G. (1991). Object spatial frequencies, retinal spatial frequencies, noise, and the efficiency of letter discrimination. *Vision Research, 31*, 1399–1415.

Parker, A. & Hawken, M. J. (1985). Capabilities of monkey cortical cells in spatial resolution tasks. *Journal of the Optical Society of America, A2*, 1101–1114.

Parker, A. & Hawken, M. J. (1988). Two-dimensional spatial structure of receptive fields in monkey striate cortex. *Journal of the Optical Society of America, A5*, 598–605.

Patel, A. S. (1966). Spatial resolution by the human visual system. *Journal of the Optical Society of America, 56*, 689–694.

Patterson, R. D. (1976). Auditory filter shapes derived with noise stimuli. *Journal of the Acoustical Society of America, 59*, 640–654.

Pearlman, A. L., Birch, J. & Meadows, J. C. (1978). Cerebral colour blindness, an acquired defect in hue discrimination, *Annals of Neurology, 5*, 253–261.

Pelah, A. (1997). The vision of natural and complex images. *Vision Research, 37*, No.23, complete edition.

Pelli, D. G. (1984). Uncertainty explains many aspects of visual contrast detection and discrimination. *Journal of the Optical Society of America, A2*, 1508–1531.

Pelli, D. G. (1990). Contrast in complex images. *Journal of the Optical Society of America, A, 7*, 2032–2040.

Pelli, D. G. (1996). Contrast of slightly complex patterns. *SPIE: Human Vision and Electronic Imaging, 2657*, 166–174.

Pelli, D. G., Robson, J. G. & Wilkins, A. J. (1988). The design of a new letter chart for measuring contrast sensitivity. *Clinical Vision Sciences, 2*, 187–199.

Pentland, A. (1980). Maximum likelihood estimation: The best PEST. *Perception and Psychophysics, 28*, 377–379.

Pfungst, O. (1911/1965). *Clever Hans: The horse of Mr. Von Osten*. New York: Henry Holt. Reprinted in 1965 by Holt, Rinehart & Winston Inc., New York.

Phillips, G. C. & Wilson, H. R. (1984). Orientation bandwidths of spatial mechanisms measured by masking. *Journal of the Optical Society of America, A1*, 226–232.

Phillips, W. A. (1983). Short–term visual memory. *Philosophical Transactions of the Royal Society of London, B, 302*, 295–309.

Piéron, H. (1931). La sensation chromatique donne sur la latence propre et l'etablissement des sensations du couleur. *Année Psychologique, 32*, 1–29.

Plant, G. T. (1991). Temporal properties of normal and abnormal spatial vision. In D. Regan (Ed.), *Spatial vision* (pp. 43–63). London: Macmillan.

Platt, J. R. (1964). Strong inference. *Science, 146*, 347–353.

Plomp, R. (1976). *Aspects of tone sensation*. New York: Academic Press.

Poggio, G. F. (1991). Physiological basis of stereoscopic vision. In D. Regan (Ed.). *Binocular vision* (pp. 224–238). London: Macmillan.

Poggio, T., Fahle, M. & Edelman, S. (1992). Fast perceptual learning in visual hyperacuity. *Science, 256*, 1018–1021.

Poggio, G. F. & Fischer, B. (1997). Binocular interaction and depth sensitivity in striate cortical neurons of behaving rhesus monkey. *Journal of Neurophysiology, 40*, 1392–1405.

Poggio, G. F., Gonzalez, F. & Krause, F. (1988). Stereoscopic mechanisms in monkey visual corex. Binocular correlation and disparity selectivity. *Journal of Neuroscience, 8*, 4531–4550.

Poggio, G. F., Motter, B. C., Squatrito, S.& Trotter, Y. (1985). Responses of neurons in visual cortex (V1 and V2) of the alert macaque to dynamic random–dot stereograms. *Vision Research, 25*, 397–406.

Poggio, G. F. & Talbot, W. H. (1981). Neural mechanisms of static and dynamic stereopsis in foveal cortex of rhesus monkey. *Journal of Physiology, 315*, 469–492.

Pohlmann & Sorkin, (1976) Simultaneous three-channel signal detection. *Perception and Psychophysics, 20*, 179–186.

Poirson, A. B. & Wandell, B. A. (1993). Appearance of colored patterns: pattern–color separability. *Journal of the Optical Society of America, A, 10*, 2458–2470.

Pokorny, J., Bowen, R. W., Williams, D. T. & Smith, V. C. (1979). Duration thresholds for chromatic stimuli. *Journal of the Optical Society of America, 69*, 103–106.

Pokorny, J., Shevell, S. K. & Smith, V. C. (1991). Colour appearance and colour constancy. In P. Gouras (Ed.), *The perception of colour* (pp.43–61). Boca Raton: CRC Press.

Pokorny, J., Smith, V. C. & Lutze, M. (1989). Heterochromatic modulation photometry. *Journal of the Optical Society of America, A, 6*, 1618–1623.

Polat, U. & Sagi, D. (1993). Lateral interactions between spatial channels: Suppression and facilitation revealed by lateral masking-experiments. *Vision Research, 33*, 993–999.

Polat, U. & Sagi, D. (1994). Spatial interactions in human vision: From near to far via experience-dependent cascades of connections. *Proceedings of the National Academy of Science, U. S. A., 91*, 1206–1209.

Pollen, D. A., Lee, J. R. & Taylor, J. H. (1971). How does the striate cortex begin the reconstruction of the visual world. *Science, 173*, 74–77.

Pollen, D. A. & Taylor, J. H., (1974). The striate cortex and the spatial analysis of visual space. *The neurosciences. Third study program* (pp.239–247). Cambridge, Mass.: MIT Press.

Popper, K. S. (1934/1965). *The logic of scientific discovery*. New York: Harper & Row. (In German, 1934. English version 1965).

Popper, K. S. (1983). *Realism and the aim of science*. London: Hutchinson, Rowman & Littlefield.

Portfors, C. V. & Regan, D. (1997). Just–noticeable difference in the speed of cyclopean motion in depth and of cyclopean motion within a frontoparallel plane. *Journal of Experimental Psychology: Human Perception and Performance, 23*, 1074–1086.

Portfors-Yeomans, C. V. & Regan, D. (1996). Cyclopean discrimination thresholds for the direction and speed of motion in depth. *Vision Research, 36*, 3265–3279.

Pulliam, K. (1981). Spatial frequency analysis of three–dimensional vision. SPIE 303, *Visual Simulation and Image Realism, II*, 71–77.

Quam, L. H. (1987). Hierarchial warp stereo. In M. A. Fischler & O. Firschein (Eds.), *Readings in computer vision* (pp. 80–86). Los Altos, California: Kauffman.

Quick, R. F. (1974). A vector magnitude model of contrast detection. *Kybernetik, 16*, 65–67.

Quigley, H. A. (1999). Neuronal death in glaucoma. *Progress in Retinal Eye Research, 1*, 39–57.

Quigley, H. A., Dunkelberger, G. R.& Green, W. R. (1988). Chronic human glaucoma causing a selectively greater loss of large optic nerve fibres. *Ophthalmology, 95*, 357–363.

Quigley, H. A., Sanchez, R. M., Dunkelberger, G. R., L'Hernault, N. L. & Baginski, T. A. (1987). Chronic glaucoma selectively damages large optic nerve fibres. *Investigative Ophthalmology and Visual Science, 28*, 913–920.

Quine, W. V. (1987) *Quiddities* (pp.72–73). Cambridge, Mass.: Harvard University Press.

Ramachandran, V. S. & Anstis, S. M. (1983). Displacement thresholds for coherent apparent motion in random dot–patterns. *Vision Research, 23*, 1719–1724.

Ramachandran, V. S. & Anstis, S. M. (1990). Illusory displacement of equiluminant kinetic edges. *Perception, 19*, 611–616.

Ramirez, R. W. (1985). *The FFT: Fundamentals and concepts*. Englewood Cliffs, N. J.: Prentice-Hall.

Rao, A. R. & Lohse, G. L. (1996). Towards a texture naming system. Identifying relevent dimensions of texture. *Vision Research, 36*, 1649–1669.

Records, R. E. (1980). Monocular diplopia. *Survey of Ophthalmology, 24*, 303–308.

Reed, S. K. (1973). *Psychological processes in pattern recognition.* New York: Academic Press.

Regan, D. (1964). A study of the visual system by the correlation of light stimuli and evoked electrical responses. Ph.D. thesis, Imperial College.

Regan D. (1966). Some characteristics of average steady-state response. *Electroenceph-alography and Clinical Neurophysiology, 20,* 238–248.

Regan, D. (1968). Evoked potentials and sensation. *Perception and Psychophysics,* 4, 347–350.

Regan, D. (1970). Objective method of measuring the relative spectral–luminosity curve in man. *Journal of the Optical Society of America, 60,* 856–859.

Regan, D. (1972). *Evoked potentials in psychology, sensory physiology and clinical medicine.* New York: Wiley.

Regan, D. (1973a). Rapid objective refraction using evoked brain responses. *Investigative Ophthalmology, 12,* 669–679.

Regan, D. (1973b). Evoked potentials specific to spatial patterns of luminance and colour. *Vision Research, 13,* 2381–2402.

Regan, D. (1974). Electrophysiological evidence for colour channels in human pattern vision. *Nature, 250,* 437–439.

Regan, D. (1975a). Recent advances in electrical recording from the human brain. *Nature , 253,* 401–407.

Regan, D. (1975b). Color coding of pattern responses in man investigated by evoked potential feedback and direct plot techniques. *Vision Research, 15,* 175–183.

Regan, D. (1977). Speedy assessment of visual acuity in amblyopia by the evoked potential method. *Ophthalmolgia, 175,* 159–164.

Regan, D. (1979). Electrical responses evoked from the human brain. *Scientific American, 241*(1), 134–146.

Regan, D. (1982). Visual information channeling in normal and disordered vision. *Psychological Review, 89,* 407–444.

Regan, D. (1983). Spatial frequency mechanisms in human vision investigated by evoked potential recording. *Vision Research, 23,* 1401–1408.

Regan, D. (1985a). Masking of spatial frequency discrimination. *Journal of the Optical Society of America, A2,* 1153–1159.

Regan, D. (1985b). Storage of spatial-frequency information and spatial-frequency discrimination. *Journal of the Optical Society of America, 2A,* 619– 621.

Regan, D. (1986a). Form from motion parallax and form from luminance contrast: Vernier discrimination. *Spatial Vision, 1,* 305–318.

Regan, D. (1986b). Visual processing of four kinds of relative motion. *Vision Research, 26,* 127–145.

Regan, D. (1988). Low contrast letter charts and sinewave grating tests in ophthalmological and neurological disorders. *Clinical Vision Science, 2,* 235–250.

Regan, D. (1989a). *Human brain electrophysiology.* New York: Elsevier.

Regan, D. (1989b). Orientation discrimination for objects defined by relative motion and objects defined by luminance contrast. *Vision Research, 29,* 1389–1400.

Regan, D. (1991a). A brief review of some of the stimuli and analysis methods used in spatiotemporal vision research. In D. Regan (Ed.), *Spatial vision* (pp. 1–42). London: Macmillan.

Regan, D. (1991b). Detection and spatial discriminations for objects defined by colour contrast, binocular disparity and motion parallax. In D. Regan (Ed), *Spatial vision* (pp. 135–178). London: Macmillan.

Regan, D. (1991c). Specific tests and specific blindness: keys, locks and parallel processing. *Optometry and Vision Science, 68,* 489–512.

Regan, D. (1991d). Depth from motion and motion–in–depth. In D. Regan (Ed.) *Binocular Vision.* London: Macmillan.

Regan, D. (1992). Visual judgements and misjudgements in cricket and the art of flight. *Perception, 21,* 91–115.

Regan, D. (1995a). Orientation discrimination for bars defined by orientation texture. *Perception, 24,* 1131–1138.

Regan, D. (1995b). Spatial orientation in aviation: Visual contributions. *Journal of Vestibular Research, 5,* 455–471.

Regan, D. (1998). Visual factors in catching and hitting. *Journal of Sports Sciences, 15,* 533–558.

Regan, D., Bartol, S., Murray, T. J. & Beverley, K. I. (1982). Spatial frequency discrimination in normal vision and in patients with multiple sclerosis. *Brain, 105,* 735–754.

Regan, D. & Beverley, K. I. (1973a). The dissociation of sideways movement and movement in depth: Psychophysics. *Vision Research, 13,* 2403–2415.

Regan, D. & Beverley, K. I. (1973b). Disparity detectors in human depth perception: Evidence for directional selectivity. *Science. 181,* 877–879.

Regan, D. & Beverley, K. I. (1973c). Electrophysiological evidence for the existence of neurones sensitive to the direction of depth movement. *Nature, 246,* 504–506.

Regan, D. & Beverley, K. I. (1973d). Some dynamic features of depth perception. *Vision Research, 13,* 2369–2379.

Regan, D. & Beverley, K. I. (1978a). Looming detectors in the human visual pathway. *Vision Research, 18,* 415–421.

Regan, D. & Beverley, K. I. (1978b). Illusory motion in depth: Aftereffect of adaptation is changing size. *Vision Research, 18,* 209–212.

Regan, D. & Beverley, K. I. (1979a). Binocular and monocular stimuli for motion in depth: changing-disparity and changing-size feed the same motion-in-depth stage. *Vision Research, 19,* 1331–1342.

Regan, D. & Beverley, K. I. (1979b). Visually guided locomotion: psychophysical evidence for a neural mechanism sensitive to flow patterns *Science, 205,* 311–313.

Regan, D. & Beverley, K. I. (1979c). Separable aftereffects of changing-size and motion-in-depth. Different neural mechanisms? *Vision Research, 19,* 727–732.

Regan, D. & Beverley, K. I. (1980). Visual responses to changing size and to sideways motion for different directions of motion in depth: Linearization of visual responses. *Journal of the Optical Society of America, 70,* 1289–1296.

Regan, D. & Beverley, K. I. (1981). Motion sensitivity measured by a psychophysical linearizing technique. *Journal of the Optical Society of America, 71,* 958–65.

Regan, D. & Beverley, K. I. (1982). How do we avoid confusing the direction we are looking with the direction we are moving? *Science, 215,* 194–196.

Regan, D. & Beverley, K. I. (1983a). Spatial frequency discrimination and detection: comparison of postadaptation thresholds. *Journal of the Optical Society of America, 73,* 1684–1690.

Regan, D. & Beverley, K. I. (1983b). Visual fields described by contrast sensitivity, by acuity and by relative sensitivity to different orientations. *Investigative Ophthalmology and Vision Science, 24,* 754–759.

Regan, D. & Beverley, K. I. (unpublished data 1983). Postadaptation spatial frequency discrimination and the Blakemore–Sutton aftereffect. (Rejected by different journals in 1983, 1984, 1986, 1988).

Regan, D. & Beverley, K. I. (1984). Figure ground segregation by motion contrast and by luminance contrast. *Journal of the Optical Society of America, A1,* 433–442.

Regan, D. & Beverley, K. I. (1985a). Postadaptation orientation discrimination. *Journal of the Optical Society of America, A 2,* 147–155.

Regan, D. & Beverley, K. I. (1985b). Visual responses to vorticity and the neural analysis of optic flow. *Journal of the Optical Society of America, A, 2,* 280–283.

Regan, D., Beverley, K. I. & Cynader, M. (1979). The visual perception of motion in depth. *Scientific American*, 24(6), 135–151.

Regan, D. & Cynader, M. (1982). Neurons in cat visual cortex tuned to the direction of motion in depth: Effect of stimulus speed. *Investigative Ophthalmology and Visual Science, 22*, 535–543.

Regan, D., Erkelens, C. J. & Collewijn, H. (1986a). Necessary conditions for the perception of motion in depth. *Investigative Ophtahlmology and Visual Science, 27*, 584–597.

Regan, D., Erkelens, C. J. & Collewijn, H. (1986b). Visual field defects for vergence eye movements and for stereomotion perception. *Investigative Ophthalmology and Vision Science, 27*, 806–19.

Regan, D., Frisby, J., Poggio, G., Schor, C. & Tyler, C. W. (1990). The perception of stereodepth and stereomotion: cortical mechanisms. In L. A. Spillman & J. S. Werner (Eds.), *The neurophysiological foundations of visual perception* (pp. 317–347). New York: Academic Press.

Regan, D., Giaschi, D. & Fresco, B. (1993a). Measurement of glare susceptibility in cataract patients using low-contrast letter charts. *Ophthalmic and Physiological Optics, 13*, 115–123.

Regan, D., Giaschi, D. & Fresco, B. (1993b). Measurement of glare susceptibility using low–contrast letter charts. *Optometry and Vision Science, 70*, 969–975.

Regan, D., Giaschi, D., Kraft, S. & Kothe, A. C. (1992a). Method for identifying amblyopes whose reduced line acuity is caused by defective selection and/or control of gaze. *Ophthalmic and Physiological Optics, 12*, 425–432.

Regan, D., Giaschi, D., Sharpe, J. A. & Hong, X. H. (1992b). Visual processing of motion- defined form: Selective failure in patients with parieto-temporal lesions. *Journal of Neuroscience, 12*, 2198–2210.

Regan, D., Gray, R. & Hamstra, S. J. (1996a). Evidence for a neural mechanism that encodes angles. *Vision Research, 36*, 323–330.

Regan, D., Gray, R., Portfors, C. V., Hamstra, S. J., Vincent, A., Hong, X. H., Kohly, R. & Beverley, K. I. (1998). Catching, hitting and collision avoidance. In L. Harris & M. Jenkin (Eds.),*Vision and Action* (pp. 171–209). New York: Cambridge University Press.

Regan, D., Hajdur, L. V. & Hong, X. H. (1996). Two-dimensional aspect ratio discrimination and one-dimensional width and height discriminations for shape defined by orientation texture. *Vision Research, 36*, 3695–3702.

Regan, D. & Hamstra, S. J. (1991). Shape discrimination for motion-defined and contrast-defined form: Squareness is special. *Perception, 20*, 315–336.

Regan, D. & Hamstra, S. J. (1992a). Shape discrimination and the judgement of perfect symmetry: dissociation of shape from size. *Vision Research, 32*, 1655–1666.

Regan, D. & Hamstra, S. J. (1992b). Dissociation of orientation discrimination from form detection for motion–defined bars and luminance–defined bars: effects of dot lifetime and presentation duration. *Vision Research, 32*, 1655–1666.

Regan, D. & Hamstra S. J.(1993). Dissociation of discrimination thresholds for time to contact and for rate of angular expansion. *Vision Research, 33*, 447–462.

Regan, D. & Hamstra, S. J. (1994). Shape discrimination for rectangles defined by disparity alone, disparity plus luminance and by disparity plus motion. *Vision Research, 34*, 2277–2291.

Regan, D. & Hong, X. H. (1990). Visual acuity for optotypes made visible by relative motion. *Optometry and Vision Science, 67*, 49–55.

Regan, D. & Hong, X. H. (1994). Recognition and detection of texture-defined letters. *Vision Research, 34*, 2403–2407.

Regan, D. & Hong, X. H. (1995). Two models of the recognition and detection of texture-defined letters compared. *Biological Cybernetics, 72*, 389–396.

Regan, D., Kaiser, P. K. & Nakano, Y. (1993). Dissociation of chromatic and achromatic processing of spatial form by the titration method. *Journal of the Optical Society of America, A10,* 1314–1323.

Regan, D., Kaufman, L.& Lincoln, J. (1986). Motion in depth and visual acceleration. In K. R. Boff, L. Kaufman & J. P. Thomas (Eds.), *Handbook of perception and human performance* pp. 19-1–19-46). New York: Wiley.

Regan, D. & Kaushal, S. (1994). Monocular judgement of the direction of motion in depth. *Vision Research, 34,* 163–177.

Regan, D., Kothe, A. C. & Sharpe, J. A. (1991). Recognition of motion-defined shapes in patients with multiple sclerosis and optic neuritis. *Brain, 114,* 1129–1115.

Regan, D. & Lee, B. B. (1993). A comparison of the human 40 Hz response with the properties of macaque ganglion cells. *Visual Neuroscience, 10,* 439–445.

Regan, D. & Maxner, C. (1986). Orientation-dependent loss of contrast sensitivity for pattern and flicker in multiple sclerosis. *Clinical Vision Sciences, 1,* 1–23.

Regan, D. & Maxner, C. (1987). Orientation-selective visual loss in patients with Parkinson's disease. *Brain, 110,* 239–271.

Regan, D., Milner, B. A. & Heron, J. R. (1976). Delayed visual perception and delayed evoked potentials in the spinal form of multiple sclerosis and in retrobulbar neuritis. *Brain, 99,* 43–66.

Regan, D. & Neima, D. (1983). Low-contrast letter charts as a test of visual function. *Ophthalmology, 90,* 1192–1200.

Regan, D. & Neima, D. (1984a). Balance between pattern and flicker sensitivities in the visual fields of neurological patients. *British Journal of Ophthalmology, 68,* 310–315.

Regan, D. & Neima, D. (1984b). Low contrast letter charts in early diabetic retinopathy, ocular hypertension, glaucoma, and Parkinson's disease. *British Journal of Ophthalmology, 68,* 885–889.

Regan, D. & Price, P. (1986). Periodicity in orientation discrimination and the unconfounding of visual information. *Vision Research, 26,* 1299–1302.

Regan, D., Raymond, J., Ginsburg, A. P. & Murray, T. J. (1981). Contrast sensitivity, visual acuity and the discrimination of Snellen letters in multiple sclerosis. *Brain, 104,* 333–350.

Regan, D. & Regan, M. P. (1986). Spatial frequency tuning, orientation tuning, and spatial discrimination investigated by nonlinear analysis of pattern evoked potentials. Abstracts, Third International Evoked Potential Symposium, Berlin.

Regan, D. & Regan, M. P. (1987). Nonlinearity in human visual responses to two-dimensional patterns and a limitation of Fourier methods. *Vision Research, 27,* 2181–2183.

Regan, D. & Regan, M. P. (1988). Objective evidence for phase-independent spatial frequency analysis in the human visual pathway. *Vision Research, 28,* 187–191.

Regan, D. & Regan, M. P. (1999). The visual processing of chromatic contrast: an hypothesis. *Vision Research,* in preparation.

Regan, D., Schellart, N. A. M., Spekreijse, H. & van den Berg, T. J. T. P. (1975). Photometry in goldfish by electrophysiological recording: comparison of criterion response method with heterochromatic flicker photometry. *Vision Research, 15,* 799–807.

Regan, D., Silver, R. & Murray, T. J. (1977). Visual acuity and contrast sensitivity in multiple sclerosis-hidden visual loss. *Brain, 100,* 563–579.

Regan, D. & Simpson, T. L. (1995). Multiple sclerosis can cause visual processing deficits specific to texture-defined form. *Neurology. 45,* 809–815.

Regan, D. & Spekreijse, H. (1970). Electrophysiological correlate of binocular depth perception in man. *Nature, 255,* 92–94.

Regan, D. & Spekreijse, H. (1974). Evoked potential indications of colour blindness. *Vision Research, 14,* 89–95.

Regan, D. & Spekreijse, H. (1986). Evoked potentials in vision research: 1961–1985. *Vision Research, 26*, 1461–1480.

Regan, D. & Sperling, H. (1971). A method of evoking contour–specific scalp potentials by chromatic checkerboard patterns. *Vision Research, 11*, 173–176.

Regan, D. & Tyler, C. W. (1971a). Wavelength–modulated light generator. *Vision Research, 11*, 43–56.

Regan, D. & Tyler, C. W. (1971b). Some dynamic features of color vision. *Vision Research, 11*, 1307–1321.

Regan, D. & Tyler, C. W. (1971c). Temporal summation and its limit for wavelength changes: An analog of Bloch's law for color vision. *Journal of the Optical Society of America, 61*, 1414–1421.

Regan, D. & Vincent A (1995). Visual processing of looming and time to contact throughout the visual field. *Vision Research, 35*, 1845–1857.

Regan, D., Whitlock, J., Murray, T. J. & Beverley, K. I. (1980). Orientation-specific losses of contrast sensitivity in multiple sclerosis. *Investigative Ophthalmology and Visual Science, 19*, 324–328.

Regan, M. P. (1994). A method for calculating the spectral response of a hair cell to a pure tone. *Biological Cybernetics, 71*, 13–16.

Regan, M. P. (1996). Half-wave linear rectification of a frequency modulated sinusoid. Journal of Applied Mathematics and Computation, *79*, 137–162.

Regan, M. P. & Regan, D. (1988). A frequency domain technique for characterizing nonlinearities in biological systems. *Journal of Theoretical Biology, 133*, 293– 317.

Regan, M. P. & Regan, D. (1989a). Objective investigation of visual function using a nondestructive zoom–FFT technique for evoked potential analysis. *Canadian Journal of Neurological Science, 16*, 1–12.

Regan, M. P. & Regan, D. (1989b). Nonlinear interactions between responses to different spatial frequencies. *Investigative Ophthalmology and Vision Research* (Suppl.), *30*, 515.

Regan, M. P. & Regan, D. (1993). Nonlinear terms produced by passing amplitude modulated sinusoids through Corey & Hudspeth's hair cell transducer function. *Biological Cybernetics, 69*, 439–446.

Reichardt, W. (1961). Autocorrelation, a principle for the evaluation of sensory information by the central nervous system. In W. Rosenblith (Ed.), *Sensory communication* (pp. 160-175). New York: Wiley.

Reichardt, W. (1986). Processing of optical information by the visual system of the fly. *Vision Research, 26*, 113–126.

Reichardt, W. & Poggio, T. (1981) (Eds.). *Theoretical approaches in neurobiology.* Cambridge, Mass: MIT Press.

Reichardt, W., Poggio, T. & Hausen, K. (1983a). Figure–ground discrimination by relative movement in the fly. Part II. *Biological Cybernetics, 46*, 1–15.

Reichardt, W., Poggio, T. & Hausen, K. (1983b). Figure–ground discrimination by relative movement in the fly. Part III. Towards the neural circuitry. *Biological Cybernetics, 46*, 81–100.

Reichardt, W. & Schlögl, R. W. (1988). A two-dimensional field theory for motion computation. *Biological Cybernetics, 60*, 23–35.

Reichardt, W., Schlögl, R. W. & Egelhaaf, M. (1988). Movement detectors provide sufficient information for local computation of 2–D velocity field. *Naturwissenschaften, 75*, 313–315.

Rentschler, I. & Fiorentini, A. (1974). Meridional anisotropy of psychophysical spatial interactions. *Vision Research, 14*, 1467–1473.

Rentschler, I. & Treutwein, B. (1985). Loss of spatial phase relationships in extrafoveal vision. *Nature, 313*, 308–310.

Richards, W. (1970). Stereopsis and stereoblindness. *Experimental Brain Research, 10*, 380–388.

Richards, W. (1971a). Motion detection in man and other animals. *Brain, Behaviour and Evolution, 4*, 162–1181.

Richards, W. (1971b). Anomalous stereoscopic depth perception. *Journal of the Optical Society of America, 61*, 410–414.

Richards, W. (1975). Visual space perception. In E. C. Carterette & M. P. Friedman (Eds.), *Handbook of perception* (pp.351–386). New York: Academic Press.

Richards, W. (1977). Stereopsis with and without monocular contours. *Vision Research, 17,* 967–969.

Richards, W. (1979). Quantifying sensory channels: Generalizing colorimetry to orientation and texture, touch and tones. *Sensory Processes, 3,* 207–209.

Richards, W., Dawson, B. & Whittington, D. (1986). Encoding contour shape by curvature extrema. *Journal of the Optical Society of America, A, 3,* 1483–1491.

Richards, W, Koenderink, J. J. & Hoffman, D. D. (1987). Inferring three-dimensional shapes from two-dimensional silhouettes. *Journal of the Optical Society of America, A4,* 1168–1175.

Richards, W. & Lieberman, H. R. (1982). Velocity blindness during shearing motion. *Vision Research, 22,* 97–100.

Richards, W. & Polit, A. (1974). Texture matching. *Kybernetik, 16,* 155–162.

Richards, W. & Regan, D. (1973). A stereo field map with implications for disparity processing. *Investigative Ophthalmology, 12,* 904–909.

Richmond, B. J., Optican, L. M., Podell, M. & Spitzer, H. (1987). Temporal encoding of two-dimensional patterns by single units in primate inferior temporal cortex. 1. Response characteristics. *Journal of Neurophysiology, 57,* 132–146.

Richter, E. R. & Yager, D. (1984). Spatial frequency difference thresholds for central and peripheral vision. *Journal of the Optical Society of America, A, 1,* 1136–1139.

Riddoch, G. (1917). Dissociation of visual perceptions due to occipital injuries with especial reference to appreciation of movement. *Brain, 40,* 15–57.

Rijsdijk, J. P., Kroon, J. N. & Wildt, G. J. von der (1980). Contrast sensitivity as a function of position on the retina. *Vision Research, 20,* 235–242.

Ritchie, A. (1975). *King of the road: An illustrated history of cycling.* Berkeley, California: Ten Speed Press.

Rivest, J. & Cavanagh, P. (1996). Localizing contours defined by more than one attribute. *Vision Research, 36,* 53–66.

Rivest, J., Intriligator, J., Suzuki, S. & Warner, J. (1998). A shape distortion effect that is size invariant. *Investigative Ophthalmology and Visual Science* (ARVO abstracts), *38,* S853.

Rivest, J., Intriligator, J., Warner, J. & Suzuki, S. (1997). Color and luminance combine at a common neural site for shape distortions. *Investigative Ophthalmology and Visual Science* (ARVO abstracts), *38,* S1000.

Robinson, J. O. (1972). *The psychology of visual illusion.* London: Hutchinson Education.

Robson, J. G. (1966). Spatial and temporal contrast sensitivity functions of the human eye. *Journal of the Optical Society of America, 56,* 1141–1150.

Robson, J. G. (1975). Receptive fields: Neural representation of the spatial and intensive attributes of the visual image. In E. C. Carterette and M. P. Friedman (Eds.), *Handbook of perception* (pp. 82–116). New York: Academic Press.

Robson, J. G. (1983). Frequency domain visual processing. In O. Braddick & A. Sleigh (Eds.), *Physical and biological processing of images.* New York: Springer–Verlag.

Robson, J. G. & Graham, N. (1981). Probability summation and regional variation in contrast sensitivity across the visual field. *Vision Research, 21,* 409–418.

Rock, W. J., Drance, S. M. & Morgan, R. W. (1972). A modification of the Armaly visual field screen technique for glaucoma. *Canadian Journal of Ophthalmology, 7,* 283–292.

Rodieck, R. W. (1965). Quantitative analysis of cat retinal ganglion cell responses to visual stimuli. *Vision Research, 5,* 583–601.

Rodieck, R. W. & Stone, J. (1965a). Responses of cat retinal ganglion cells to moving visual patterns. *Journal of Neurophysiology, 28,* 819–832.

Rodieck, R. W & Stone, J. (1965b). Analysis of receptive fields of cat retinal ganglion cells. *Journal of Neurophysiology, 28*, 833–849.

Rogers, B. J. & Graham, M. E. (1979). Motion parallax as an independent cue for depth perception. *Perception, 8*, 125–134.

Rogers, B. J. & Graham, M. E. (1982). Similarities between motion parallax and stereopsis in human depth perception. *Vision Research, 22*, 261–270.

Rogers, B. J. & Graham, M. E. (1983). Anisotropies in the perception of three-dimensional form. *Science, 221*, 1409–1411.

Rohaly, A. M. & Buchsbaum, G. (1988). Inference of global spatiochromatic mechanisms from contrast sensitivity functions. *Journal of the Optical Society of America, A5*, 572–576.

Rohaly, A. M. & Buchsbaum, G. (1989). Global spatiochromatic mechanism accounting for luminance variations in contrast sensitivity functions. *Journal of the Optical Society of America, A, 6*, 312–317.

Rohaly, A. M. & Wilson, H. R. (1993). Nature of coarse-to-fine constraints on binocular fusion. *Journal of the Optical Society of America, A*, 2433–2441.

Rohaly, A. M. & Wilson, H. R. (1999). The effects of contrast on perceived depth and depth discrimination. *Vision Research, 39*, 9–18.

Ross, D. (1976). Time delay in estimation of angles. *Perceptual and Motor Skills, 42*, 625–626.

Ross, J. (1983). Disturbance of stereoscopic vision in patients with unilateral stroke. *Behavioural Brain Research, 7*, 99–112.

Ross, J. (1992). How adaptation and masking alter contrast gain control. *Perception, 21*, Suppl. 2, 60.

Ross, J. & Speed, H. D. (1991). Contrast adaptation and contrast masking in human vision. *Proceedings of the Royal Society, B, 246*, 61–69.

Ross, J. & Speed, H. D. (1996). Perceived contrast following adaptation to gratings of different orientations. *Vision Research, 36*, 1811–1818.

Ross, J., Speed, H. D. & Morgan, M. J. (1993). The effects of adaptation and masking on incremental thresholds for contrast. *Vision Research, 33*, 2051–2056.

Rouse, M. W., Tittle, J. S. & Braunstein, M. L. (1989). Stereoscopic depth perception by static stereo-deficient observers in dynamic displays with constant and changing disparity. *Optometry and Vision Science, 66*, 355–362.

Roy, J. P., Konatsu, H. & Wurtz, R. H. (1992). Disparity sensitivity of neurons in monkey extrastriate area MST. *Journal of Neuroscience, 12*, 2478–2492.

Rubenstein, B. S. & Sagi, D. (1990). Spatial variability as a limiting factor in texture-discrimination tasks: Implications for performance asymmetries. *Journal of the Optical Society of America, A7*, 1632–1643.

Ruddock, K. H. (1991). Psychophysics of inherited colour vision deficiencies. In D. H. Foster (Ed.), *Inherited and acquired color vision deficiencies: Fundamental aspects and clinical studies* (pp. 4–37). Boca Raton, Fla.: CRC Press.

Russell, B. (1961). *History of Western Philosophy*. London: Allen & Unwin.

Russell, P. W. (1979). Chromatic input to stereopsis. *Vision Research, 19*, 831–834.

Sachs, M. B., Nachmias, J. & Robson, J. G. (1971). Spatial–frequency channels in human vision. *Journal of the Optical Society of America, 61*, 1176–1186.

Sachtler, W. L. & Zaidi, Q. (1992). Chromatic and luminance signals in visual memory. *Journal of the Optical Society of America, A, 9*, 877–894.

Sagi, D. (1990). Detection of an orientation singularity in Gabor textures: Effect of signal density and spatial frequency. *Vision Research, 30*, 1377–1388.

Sagi, D. & Hochstein, S. (1985). Lateral inhibition between spatially adjacent spatial frequency channels? *Perception and Psychophysics, 37*, 215–322.

Sagi, D. & Julesz, B. (1985). Fast noninterial shifts of attention. *Spatial Vision, 1*, 141–150.

Sagi, D. & Julesz, B. (1987). Short-range limitations on detection of feature differences. *Spatial Vision, 2,* 39–49.

Saleh, B. E. A. (1982). Optical information processing and the human visual system. In *Applications of the optical Fourier transform* (pp. 431–465). New York: Academic Press.

Sankeralli, M. & Mullen, K. T. (1996). Estimation of the L-, M-, and S-cone weights of the postreceptoral detection mechanisms. *Journal of the Optical Society of America, A, 13,* 906–915.

Scarff, L. W. & Geisler, W. L. (1992). Stereopsis at isoluminance in the absence of chromatic aberrations. *Journal of the Optical Society of America, A, 9,* 868–876.

Schade, O. H. (1948) Electro-optic characteristics of television systems. *RCA Review, 9,* 5–37, 245–286, 490–530, 653–686.

Schade, O. (1956). Optical and photoelectric analog of the eye. *Journal of the Optical of America, 46,* 721–739.

Schade, O. H. (1958). On the quality of color-television images and the perception of color detail. *Journal of the Society of Motion Picture and Television Engineers, 67,* 801–819.

Schaeffel, F., Glasser, A. & Howland, H. C. (1988). Accommodation, refractive error and eye growth in chickens. *Vision Research, 28,* 630–657.

Schaeffel, F., Troilo, D., Wallman, J.& Howland, H. C. (1990). Developing eyes that lack accommodation grow to compensate for imposed defocus. *Visual Neuroscience, 4,* 177–183.

Scharff, L. V. & Geisler, W. S. (1992). Stereopsis at isoluminance in the absence of chromatic aberrations. *Journal of the Optical Society of America, A, 9,* 868–876.

Schey, H. M. (1973). *Div, grad, curl, and all that.* New York: Norton.

Schiller, P. H. (1986). The central visual system. *Vision Research, 26,* 1351–1386.

Schiller, P. H. (1993). The effects of V4 and middle temporal (MT) area lesions on visual performance in the monkey. *Visual Neuroscience, 10,* 717–746.

Schiller, P. H. & Colby, C. L. (1983). The responses of single cells in the lateral geniculate nucleus of the rhesus monkey to color and luminance contrast. *Vision Research, 23,* 1631–1641.

Schiller, P. H. & Lee, K. (1991). The role of extrastriate area V4 in vision. *Science, 251,* 1251–1253.

Schiller, P. H, Sandell, J. H. & Maunsell, J. H. R. (1986). Functions of the ON and OFF channels of the visual system. *Nature, 322,* 824–828.

Schnapf, J. L., Kraft, T. W. & Baylor, D. A. (1987). Spectral sensitivity of human cone photoreceptors. *Nature, 325,* 439–441.

Schor, C. M., Heckman, T. & Tyler, C. W. (1989). Binocular fusion limits are independent of contrast, luminance gradient and component phases. *Vision Research, 29,* 821–835.

Schor, C. M. & Howarth, P. A. (1986). Suprathreshold stereo–depth matches as a function of contrast and spatial frequency. *Perception, 15,* 249–258.

Schumer, R. A. & Ganz, L. (1979). Independent stereoscopic channels for different extents of spatial pooling. *Vision Research, 19,* 1303–1314.

Schwartz, S. H. & Loop, M. S. (1982). Evidence for transient luminance and quasi–sustained color mechanisms. *Vision Research, 22,* 445–447.

Scott, G. I. (1957). *Traquair's clinical perimetry.* London: Kimpton.

Scottun, B. C., Bradley, A., Sclar, G., Ohzawa, I. & Freeman, R. D. (1987). The effect of contrast on visual orientation and spatial frequency discrimination: A comparison of single cells and behaviour. *Journal of Neurophysiology, 57,* 733–786.

Sekiguchi, N., Williams, D. R. & Brainard, D. H. (1993a). Aberration–free measurements of the visibility of isoluminant gratings. *Journal of the Optical Society of America, A, 10,* 2105–2117.

Sekiguchi, N., Williams, D. R. & Brainard, D. H. (1993b). Efficiency in detection of isoluminant and isochromatic interference fringes. *Journal of the Optical Society of America, A, 10,* 2118–2133.

Selverston, A. I. (1980) Are central pattern generators understandable? (with peer commentary). *Behaviour and Brain Sciences, 3*, 535–571.

Shannon, C. E. & Weaver, W. (1949). *The mathematical theory of communication.* Urbana, Ill.: University of Illinois Press.

Shapley, R. M. & Enroth-Cugell, C. (1984). Visual adaptation and retinal gain control. In N. N. Osbourne & G. J. Chader (Eds.). *Progress in retinal research, Vol.3* (pp. 263–343). Oxford: Pergamon.

Shapley, R. M. & Kaplan, E. (1989). Responses of magnocellular LGN neurons and M retinal ganglion cells to drifting heterochromatic gratings. *Investigative Ophthalmology and Vision Science, 30* (Suppl.), 323.

Shapley, R. M., Kaplan, E. & Soodak, R. E. (1981). Spatial summation and contrast sensitivity of X- and Y-cells in the lateral geniculate nucleus of the macaque. *Nature, 292,* 543–545.

Shapley, R. M. & Tolhurst, D. J. (1973). Edge detectors in human vision. *Journal of Physiology, 279,* 165–183.

Sharpe, L. T., Stockman, A., Jägle, H. & Nathans, J. (1999). Opsin genes, cone photopigments, color vision and color blindness. In K. Gegenfurter & L. T. Sharpe (Eds.), *Color vision: From genes to perception* (pp. 1–87). New York: Cambridge University Press.

Shepard, R. N. & Metzler, J. (1971). Mental rotation of 3-D objects. *Science, 171,* 701–705.

Sherk, H. (1986). The claustrum and the cerebral cortex. In Jones, E. G. & Peters A (Eds.), *Cerebral cortex, Vol. 5* (pp. 467-499). New York: Plenum.

Shiori, S. & Cavanagh, P. (1992). Visual persistence of figures defined by relative motion. *Vision Research, 32,* 943–951.

Simpson, T. & Regan, D. (1995). Test–retest variability and correlations between tests of texture processing, motion processing, visual acuity and contrast sensitivity. *Optometry and Vision Science, 72,* 11–16.

Singer, W. (1977). Control of thalamic transmission by corticofugal and ascending reticular pathways in the visual system. *Physiological Reviews, 57,* 386–420.

Smallman, H. S., MacLeod, D. T. A., He, S. & Kentridge, R. W. (1996). Fine grain of the neural representation of human spatial vision. *Journal of Neuroscience, 16,* 1852–1859.

Smirnov, M. S. (1962). Measurement of the wave aberration of the human eye. *Biofizika, 6,* 687–703.

Smith, R. A. (1970). Adaptation of visual contrast sensitivity to specific temporal frequencies. *Vision Research, 10,* 275–279.

Smuts, J. C. (1926). *Holism and evolution.* New York: Macmillan. Reprinted 1973 by Greenwood, Westport, Conn..

Smuts, J. C. Jr. (1952). *Jan Christian Smuts.* Capetown: Heineman & Cassell.

Snowden, R. J. & Hammett, S. T. (1992). Subtractive and divisive adaptation in the human visual system. *Nature, 355,* 248–250.

Snowden, R. J. & Hammett, S. T. (1996). Spatial frequency adaptation: Threshold elevation and perceived contrast. *Vision Research, 36,* 1797–1809.

Snyder, A. W., Bossomaier, T. J. R. & Hughes, A. (1986). Photoreceptor diameter and spacing for highest resolving power. *Journal of the Optical Society of America, 67,* 696–698.

Spekreijse, H. (1966). *Analysis of EEG responses in man.* Thesis. The Hague: Junk Publishers.

Spekreijse, H. (1969). Rectification in the goldfish retina: analysis by sinusoidal and auxiliary stimulation. Vision Research, *9,* 1461–1473.

Spekreijse, H. & Norton, A. L. (1970). The dynamic characteristics of color-coded S-potentials. *Journal of General Physiology, 56,* 1–15

Spekreijse, H. & Oosting, H. (1970). Linearizing, a method for analyzing and synthesizing nonlinear systems. *Kybernetic, 7,* 23–31.

Spekreijse, H. & Reits, D. (1982). Sequential analysis of the visual evoked potential system in man: Nonlinear analysis of a sandwich system. *Annals of the New York Academy of Science, 388*, 72–97.

Spekreijse, H. & van der Tweel, L. H. (1965). Linearization of evoked responses to sine wave modulated light by noise. *Nature, 205*, 913.

Spekreijse, H., van der Tweel, L. H. & Regan, D. (1972). Interocular sustained suppression: correlations with evoked potential amplitude and distribution. *Vision Research, 12*, 521–526.

Spekreijse, H., van Norren, D.& van den Berg, T. J. (1971). Flicker responses in monkey lateral geniculate nucleus and human perception of flicker. *Proceedings of the National Academy of Sciences U.S.A., 68*, 2802–2805.

Sperling, G. (1960). The information available in brief presentations. *Psychological Monographs, 74*, No. 498.

Sperling, G. (1965). Temporal and spatial visual masking. I. Masking by impulse flashes. *Journal of the Optical Society of America, 55*, 541–559.

Sperling, H. (1980). Blue receptor distribution in primates from intense light and histochemical studies. In G. Verriest (Ed.), *Color vision deficiencies* (pp.30–44). Bristol: Hilger.

Sperling, H. G. & Harwerth, R. S. (1971). Red–green cone interaction in the increment-threshold spectral sensitivity of primates. *Science, 172*, 180–184.

Sperry, R. (1980). Mind–brain interaction: Mentalism, yes; dualism, no. *Neuroscience, 5*, 195–206.

Spileers, W., Orban, G. A., Gulyás, B. & Maes, H. (1990). Selectivity of cat area 18 neurons for direction and speed in depth. *Journal of Neurophysiology, 63*, 936–954.

Stampfer, K. A. & Tredici, T. J. (1975). Monocular diplopia in flying personnel. *American Journal of Ophthalmology, 80*, 769–765.

Steinman, R. M. & Collewijn, H. (1980). Binocular retinal image motion during active head rotation. *Vision Research, 20*, 415–429.

Steinman, R. M., Levinson, J. Z., Collewijn, H. & Steen, J. (1985). Vision in the presence of known retinal image motion. *Journal of the Optical Society of America, A2*, 226–232.

Stockman, A., MacLeod, D. I. A. & Lebrun, S. J. (1993). Faster than the eye can see: Blue cones respond to rapid flicker. *Journal of the Optical Society of America, A, 10*, 1396–1402.

Stoker, J. J. (1950). *Nonlinear vibrations*. New York: Wiley Interscience.

Stone, J. (1983). *Parallel Processing in the Visual System*. New York: Plenum.

Stromeyer, C. F. III, Cole, G. R. & Kronauer, R. E. (1985). Second–site adaptation in the red–green chromatic pathways. *Vision Research, 25*, 219–237.

Stromeyer, C. F. III & Julesz, B. (1972). Spatial frequency in vision: Critical bands and spread of masking. *Journal of the Optical Society of America, 62*, 1221–1232.

Stromeyer, C. F. III. & Klein, S. (1974). Spatial frequency channels in human vision as an asymmetric (edge) mechanism. *Vision Research, 14*, 1409–1420.

Stromeyer, C. F. III & Klein, S. (1975). Evidence against narrow-band spatial frequency channels in human vision: the detectability of frequency modulated gratings. *Vision Research, 15*, 899–910.

Stromeyer, C. F. III, Kronauer, R. E., Madsen, J. C. & Klein, S. A. (1984). Opponent-movement mechanisms in human vision. *Journal of the Optical Society of America, A, 1*, 876–884.

Stuart, R. D. (1961). *An introduction to Fourier analysis*. London: Methuen. New York: Wiley.

Sullivan, G. D., Oatley, K. & Sutherland, N. S. (1972). Vernier acuity is affected by target length and separation. *Perception and Psychophysics, 12*, 438–444.

Sutherland, N. S. (1961). Figural aftereffects and apparent size. *Quarterly Journal of Experimental Psychology, 13*, 222–228.

Sutherland, N. S. (1968). Outline of a theory of visual pattern recognition in animals and man. *Proceedings of the Royal Society (London), B, 171,* 297–317.

Sutherland, N. S. (1973). Object recognition. In E. C. Carterette & M. P. Friedman (Eds.) *Handbook of Perception,* vol. 3 (pp. 157–185). New York: Academic Press.

Sutter, A., Beck, J. & Graham, N. (1989). Contrast and spatial variables in texture segregation: Testing a simple spatial-frequency channels model. *Perception and Psychophysics, 46,* 312–332.

Suzuki, S. & Cavanagh, P. (1998). A shape-contrast aftereffect for briefly presented stimuli. *Journal of Experimental Psychology: Human Perception and Performance, 24,* 1315–1341.

Suzuki, S. & Rivest, J. (1998). Interactions among "aspect ratio channels." *Investigative Ophthalmology and Visual Science* (ARVO abstracts), *38,* 51000.

Swets, J. A. (1973). The relative operating characteristics in psychology *Science,* 182, 990–1000.

Swift, D. J. & Smith, R. A. (1982). An action spectrum for spatial frequency adaptation. *Vision Research, 22,* 235–246.

Switkes, E., Bradley, A. & DeValois, K. K. (1988). Contrast dependence and mechanisms of masking interactions among chromatic and luminance gratings. *Journal of the Optical Society of America,* A5, 1149–1162.

Szentagothai, J. (1978). The local neuronal apparatus of the cerebral cortex. In P. Buser, and A. Rougeul-Buser (Eds.), *Cerebral Correlates of Conscious Experience* (pp. 131–138). Amsterdam: Elsevier.

Tadmore, Y. & Tolhurst, D. J. (1992). Both the phase and the amplitude spectrum may determine the appearance of natural images. *Vision Research, 31,* 141–145.

Tadmore, Y. & Tolhurst, D. J. (1994). Discrimination of changes in the second order statistics of natural and synthetic images. *Vision Research, 34,* 541–554.

Tadmore, Y. & Tolhurst, D. J. (1995). The contrasts in natural scenes and their representation by mammalian retinal geniculate neurones. In M. Burrows, T. Matheson, P. L. Newland & H. Schuppe (Eds.) *Nervous Systems and Behaviour. Proceedings of the Fourth International Congress of Neuroethology.* New York: Thieme.

Takeuchi, T. (1997). Visual search of expansion and contraction. *Vision Research, 37,* 2083–2090.

Tanaka, Y. & Sagi D. (1998). Long-lasting, long-range detection facilitation. *Vision Research, 38,* 2591–2599.

Tayler, H. R. (1981). Racial variations in vision. *American Journal of Epidemiology,* 113, 62–80.

Taylor, M. M. (1963). Visual discrimination and orientation. *Journal of the Optical Society of America, 53,* 763–765.

Taylor, M. M. & Creelman, C. D. (1967) PEST: Efficient estimates on probability functions. *Journal of the Acoustical Society of America, 41,* 782–787.

Taylor, S. (1994). *Shaka's children: A history of the Zulu people.* London: Harper-Collins.

Teller, D. Y. (1979). The forced–choice preferential–looking procedure: a psychophysical technique for use with human infants. *Infant Behaviour and Development,* 2, 135–153.

Teller, D. Y. & Lindsey, D. T. (1993). Motion at isoluminance: motion dead zones in three–dimensional color space. *Journal of the Optical Society of America, A, 16,* 1324–1331.

Teller, D. Y. & Movshon, J. A. (1986). Visual development. *Vision Research, 26,* 1483–1506.

Terborgh, J. (1992). *Diversity and the tropical rain forest.* New York: Scientific American Library.

Teuber, H. L. (1963). Space perception and its disturbance after brain injury in man. *Neuropsychologia, 1,* 47–57.

Thomas, J. P. (1968). Linearity of spatial integrations involving inhibitory interactions. *Vision Research, 8,* 49–60.

Thomas, J. P. (1970). Model of the function of receptive fields in human vision. *Psychological Review, 77,* 121–134.

Thomas, J. P. (1983). Underlying psychometric function for detecting gratings and identifying spatial frequency. *Journal of the Optical Society of America, 73,* 751–758.

Thomas, J. P. & Gille, J. (1979). Bandwidths of orientation channels in human vision. *Journal of the Optical Society of America, 69,* 652–660.

Thomas, J. P., Gillie, J. & Barker, R. A. (1982). Simultaneous detection and identification: Theory and data. *Journal of the Optical Society of America, 72,* 1642–1651.

Thomas, J. P. & Olzak, L. A. (1990). Cue summation in spatial discriminations. *Vision Research, 30,* 1865–1875.

Thomas, J. P. & Olzak, L. A. (1996). Uncertainty experiments support the roles of second-order mechanisms in spatial frequency and orientation discriminations. *Journal of the Optical Society of America, A13,* 689–696.

Thornton, J. E. & Pugh, E. N. Jr. (1983a). Red/green color opponency at detection threshold. *Science, 219,* 191–193.

Thornton, J. E. & Pugh, E. N. Jr. (1983b). Relationships of opponent–colours cancellation measures to cone-antagonistic signals deduced from increment threshold data. In J. D. Mollon & L. T. Sharpe (Eds.). *Colour vision.* London: Academic Press.

Thrane, N. (1979). *Zoom FFT.* Technical Review 2–1980. Naerum, Denmark: Bruel & Kjaer.

Thrane, N. (1980). *Discrete Fourier transform and FFT analysis.* Technical Review 1–1979. Naerum, Denmark: Bruel & Kjaer.

Tigges, J. & Tigges, M. (1985). Subcortical sources of direct projections to visual cortex. In A. Peters and E. G. Jones (Eds.), *Cerebral Cortex,* Vol. 3 (pp. 351–378). New York: Plenum Press.

Timney, B. N. & Muir, D. W. (1976). Orientation anistropy: Incidence and magnitude in Caucasian and Chinese subjects. *Science, 193,* 673–677.

Toet, A. & Koenderink, J. J. (1987). Two–point resolution near detection threshold. *Journal of the Optical Society of America, A1,* 1448–1454.

Toet, A., van Eekhout, H. L., Simons, J. J. & Koenderink, J. J. (1987). Scale invariant features of differential spatial displacement discrimination. *Vision Research, 27,* 441–452.

Tolhurst, D. J. (1972a). On the possible existence of edge detector neurones in the human visual system. *Vision Research, 12,* 797–804.

Tolhurst, D. J. (1972b). Adaptation to squarewave grating: Inhibition between spatial frequency channels in the human visual system. *Journal of Physiology, 236,* 231–248.

Tolhurst, D. J. (1973). Separate channels for the analysis of the shape and the movement of a moving visual stimulus. *Journal of Physiology, 231,* 385–402.

Tolhurst, D. J. (1975). Sustained and transient channels in human vision. *Vision Research, 15,* 1151–1156.

Tolhurst, D. J. & Barfield, L. (1978). Interactions between spatial frequency channels. *Vision Research, 18,* 951–958.

Tolhurst, D. J. & Dealy, R. S (1975). The detection and identification of lines and edges. *Vision Research, 15,* 1367–1372.

Tolhurst, D. J. & Tadmor, Y. (1997a). Band–limited contrast in natural images explains the detectability of changes in the amplitude spectra. *Vision Research, 37,* 3203–3215.

Tolhurst, D. J. & Tadmor, Y. (1997b). Discrimination of changes in the slopes of the amplitude spectra of natural images: band–limited contrast and psychometric functions. *Perception, 26,* 1011–1025.

Tolhurst, D. J., Tadmore, Y. & Arthurs, G. (1996). The detection of changes in the amplitude spectra of natural images is explained by a band-limited local-contrast model. *SPIE—Human Vision and Electronic Imaging,* No. 2657, 154–165.

Tolhurst, D. J., Tadmore, Y. & Chao, T. (1992). The amplitude spectra of natural images. *Ophthalmic and Physiological Optics, 12,* 229–232.

Tolhurst, D. J. & Thompson, I. D. (1981). On the variety of spatial frequency selectivities shown by neurones in area 17 of the cat. *Proceedings of the Royal Society of London, B, 213,* 183–199.

Tolhurst, D. J. & Thomson, P. G. (1975). Orientation illusions and aftereffects: Inhibition between channels. *Vision Research, 15,* 967–972.

Tomita, T., Kaneko, A., Murakami, M. & Paulter, E. L. (1967). Spectral response curves of single cones in carp. *Vision Research, 7,* 519–531.

Townsend J. T., Hu, G. G. & Evans, R. J. (1984). Modeling feature perception: I. Brief displays. *Perception and Psychophysics, 36,* 35–49.

Toyama, K., Kimura, M. & Tanaka, K. (1981). Organization of cat visual cortex as investigated by cross-correlation techniques. *Journal of Neurophysiology, 46,* 202–214.

Treisman, A. (1996). The binding problem. *Current Opinion in Neurobiology, 6,* 171–178.

Treisman, M. & Falkner, A. (1984). The setting and maintenance of criteria representing levels of confidence. *Journal of Experimental Psychology: Human Perception and Performance, 10,* 119–139.

Treisman, M. & Falkner, A. (1985). Can decision criteria exchange locations? Some positive evidence. *Journal of Experimental Psychology: Human Perception and Performance, 11,* 187–208.

Treisman, M. & Williams, T. C. (1984). A theory of criterion setting with an application to sequential dependencies. *Psychological Review, 91,* 68–111.

Troy, J. B. (1983). Spatio-temporal interactions in neurons of the cat's dorsal lateral geniculate nucleus. *Journal of Physiology, 344,* 419–432.

Tsotsos, J. K. (1993). An inhibitory beam for attentional selection. In L. Harris & M. Jenkin (Eds). *Spatial Vision in Humans and Robots* (pp. 313–331). Cambridge: Cambridge University Press.

Turner, M. R. (1986). Texture-discrimination by Gabor functions. *Biological Cybernetics, 55,* 71–82.

Tyler, C. W. (1973). Stereoscopic vision: Clinical limitations and a disparity scaling effect. *Science, 181,* 276–278.

Tyler, C. W. (1974). Depth perception in disparity gratings. *Nature, 251,* 140–142.

Tyler, C. W. (1975). Stereoscopic tilt and size aftereffects. *Perception, 4,* 187–309.

Tyler, C. W. (1983). Sensory processing of binocular disparity. In C. M. Schor, and K. J. Cuiffreda (Eds.), *Vergence Eye Movements* (pp. 199–295). Boston , Mass.: Butterworth.

Tyler, C. W. (1991). Cyclopean vision. In D. Regan (Ed.) , *Binocular Vision* (pp.38–74). London: Macmillan.

Tyler, C. W. (1995). Cyclopean riches: cooperativity, neurontropy, hysteresis, stereoattention, hyperglobality, and hypercyclopean processes in random-dot stereopsis. In T. V. Papathomas, C. Chubb, A. Gorea, and E. Kowler (Eds.), *Early vision and beyond.* Cambridge, Mass.: MIT Press.

Tyler, C. W., Barghout, L. & Kontsevich, L. L. (1996). Computational reconstruction of the mechanisms of human stereopsis. *SPIE Proceedings, 2054,* 52–68.

Tyler, C. W. & Julesz, B. (1980). On the depth of the cyclopean retina. *Experimental Brain Research, 40,* 196–202.

Ungerleider, L. G. (1995). Functional brain imaging studies of cortical mechanisms for memory. *Science, 270,* 769–775.

Ungerleider, L. G. & Mishkin, M. (1982). Two cortical visual systems. In D. J. Ingle, M. A. Goodale & R. J. W. Mansfield (Eds.), *Analysis of visual behavior* (pp. 549–586). Cambridge, Mass.: MIT Press.

Van der Horst, G. J. C. (1969). Chromatic flicker. *Journal of the Optical Society of America, 59,* 1213–1217.

Van der Horst, G. J. C. & Bouman, M. A. (1969). Spatiotemporal chromaticity discrimination. *Journal of the Optical Society of America, 59,* 1482–1488.

Van der Horst, G. J. C., deWeert, C. M. M. & Bouman, M. A. (1967). Transfer of spatial chromaticity contrast at detection threshold in the human eye. *Journal of the Optical Society of America, 57,* 1260–1266.

Van der Schaaf, A. & van der Hateren, J. H. (1996). Modelling the power spectra of natural images: statistics and information. *Vision Research, 36,* 2759–2770.

Van der Tweel, L. H. (1961). Some problems in vision regarded with respect to linearity and frequency response. *Annals of the New York Academy of Science, 89,* 829–856.

Van der Tweel, L. H. (1964). Relation between psychophysics and electrophysiology of flicker. *Documenta Ophthalmologica, 18,* 287–304.

Van der Tweel, L. H. & Lunel, H. F. E. (1965). Human visual responses to sinusoidally modulated light. *Electroencephalography and Clinical Neurophysiology, 18,* 587–598.

Van der Tweel, L. H. & Reits, D. (1998). Systems analysis in vision. *Eye, 12,* 85–101.

Van der Tweel, L. H. & Spekreijse, H. (1969). Signal transport and rectification in the human evoked response system. *Annals of the New York Academy of Science, 156,* 678–695.

Van der Zwan, R. & Wenderoth, P. (1995). Mechanisms of purely subjective contour tilt aftereffects. *Vision Research, 35,* 2547–2557.

Van Dijk, B. W. & Spekreijse, H. (1983). Nonlinear versus linear opponency in vertebrate retina. In J. D. Mollon & L. D. Sharpe (Eds.), *Colour vision.* London: Academic Press.

Van Doorn, A. J., Koenderink, J. J. & Bouman, M. A. (1972). The influence of retinal inhomogeneity on the perception of spatial patterns. *Kybernetik, 10,* 233–245.

Van Essen, D. C. (1985). Functional organization of primate visual cortex. In A. Peters & E. G. Jones (Eds.), *Cerebral Cortex,* Vol. 3, 259–329. New York: Plenum.

Van Essen, D. C., Felleman, D. J., De Yoe, E. A., Olavarria, J. & Knierim, J. (1990). Modular and hierarchical organization of extrastriate visual cortex in the macaque. In *The Brain,* Vol. 15, 679696. Cold Spring Harbor, N.Y.: Cold Spring Harbor Laboratory.

Van Essen, D. C. & Maunsell, J. H. RA. J(1983). Hierarchical organization and functional streams in the visual cortex. *Trends Neurosci., 6,* 370375.

Van Meeteran, A. (1974). Calculations on the optical transfer function of the human eye for white light. *Optica Acta, 21,* 395–412.

Van Nes, F. L. & Bouman, M. A. (1967). Spatial modulation transfer in the human eye. *Journal of the Optical Society of America, 57,* 401–406.

Van Nes, F. L., Koenderink, J. J., Nas, H. & Bouman, M. A. (1967). Spatiotemporal modulation transfer in the human eye. *Journal of the Optical Society of America, 57,* 1082–1088.

Van Santen, J. P. H. & Sperling, G. (1984). A temporal covariance model of motion perception. *Journal of the Optical Society of America, A1,* 451–473.

Van Santen, J. P. H. & Sperling, G. (1985). Elaborated Reichardt detectors. *Journal of the Optical Society of America, A2,* 300–321.

Verstraten, F. A. J., Verlinde, R., Fredericksen, R. E. & van der Grind, W. A. (1994). A transparent motion aftereffect contingent on binocular disparity. *Perception, 23,* 1181–1188.

Victor, J. D. (1988). Models for preattentive texture discrimination: Fourier analysis and local feature processing in a unified framework. *Spatial Vision, 3,* 263–280.

Victor, J. D. (1994). Images, statistics and textures. *Journal of the Optical Society of America, A, 11,* 1680–1684.

Victor, J. D. & Brodie, S. E. (1978). Discriminable textures with identical Buffonneedle statistics. *Biological Cybernetics, 31,* 231–234.

Victor, J. D. & Conte, M. M (1991). Spatial organization of nonlinear interactions in form perception. *Vision Research, 31,* 1457–1488.

Victor, J. D. & Conte, M. M. (1996). The role of high-order correlations in texture processing. *Vision Research, 36,* 1615–1631.

Victor, J. D., Maiese, K., Shapley, R., Sidtis, J. & Gazzaniga, M. S. (1989). Acquired central dyschromatopsia: Analysis of a case with preserved colour discrimination. *Clinical Vision Sciences, 4,* 183–196.

Victor, J. D., Purpura, K. & Mao, B. (1994). Population encoding of spatial frequency, orientation, and color in macaque V1. *Journal of Neurophysiology, 72,* 2151–2166.

Victor, J. D. & Shapley, R. M. (1979). Receptive fields of cat X and Y retinal ganglion cells. *Journal of General Physiology, 74,* 275–298.

Vimal, R. L. P. (1988). Spatial frequency discrimination: Inphase and counterphase photopic conditions compared. *Investigative Ophthalmology and Visual Science, 29,* 448.

Vincent, A. & Regan, D. (1995). Parallel independent encoding of orientation, spatial frequency and contrast. *Perception, 24,* 491–499.

Vogels, R. & Orban, G. A. (1986). Decision processes in visual discrimination of line orientation. *Journal of Experimental Psychology: Human Perception and Performance, 12,* 115–132.

Vogels, R. & Orban, G. A. (1987). Illusory contour orientation discrimination. *Vision Research, 27,* 543–567.

Von Frisch, O. (1973). *Animal Camouflage.* New York. Franklin Watts.

Von Grünau, M., Dubé, S. & Kwas, M. (1993). The effect of disparity on motion coherence. *Spatial Vision, 7,* 227–241.

Von Grünau, M. & Frost, B. J. (1983). Double–opponent–process mechanism underlying RF–structure of directionally specific cells of cat lateral supersylvian visual area. *Experimental Brain Research, 49,* 84–92.

Walker, A. & Shipman, P. (1996). *The Wisdom of Bones.* London: Weidenfeld and Nicolson.

Walker, J. S. (1988). *Fourier analysis.* New York: Oxford University Press.

Wallman, J. & Adams, J. (1987). Developmental aspects of experimental myopia in chicks: susceptibility, recovery and relation to emmetropization. *Vision Research, 27,* 1139–1163.

Walls, G. L. (1942). *The vertebrate eye and its adaptive radiation.* Bloomington Hills, Mich.: Cranbrook Institute. Reprinted 1963, New York: Hafner.

Walls, G. L. (1956). The G. Palmer story (Or what it's like, sometimes, to be a scientist). *Journal of the History of Medicine and Allied Sciences, 11,* 66–96.

Walraven, P. (1962). *On the mechanisms of colour vision.* Ph.D. thesis, University of Utrecht. Published by the Institute of Perception, RVO–TNO, Soesterberg, The Netherlands.

Walsh, J. W. T. (1953). *Photometry.* London: Constable.

Walters, J. S. (1988). *Fourier analysis.* New York: Oxford University Press.

Wandell, B. A. (1982). Measurement of small color differences. *Psychological Review, 89,* 281–302.

Wandell, B. A. & Marimont, D. (1992). Axial chromatic aberration and cone-isolation. *Investigative Ophthalmology, 33,* 770.

Watson, A. B. (1983). Detection and recognition of simple spatial forms. In O. J. Braddick, and A. C. Sleigh (Eds.), *Physical and biological processing of images* (pp. 100–114). New York: Springer-Verlag.

Watson, A. B. & Pelli, D. G. (1983). QUEST: A Bayesian adaptive psychometric method. *Perception and Psychophysics, 33,* 113–120.

Watson, A. B. & Robson, J. G. (1981). Discrimination at threshold: labeled detectors in human vision. *Vision Research, 21*, 1115–1122.

Watt, R. J. (1984a). Towards a general theory of the visual acuities for shape and spatial arrangement. *Vision Research, 24*, 1377–1386.

Watt, R. J. (1984b). Further evidence concerning the analysis of curvature in human foveal vision. *Vision Research, 24*, 251–253.

Watt, R. J. & Andrews, D. P (1981). APE: Adaptive probit estimates of psychometric functions. *Current psychophysical Reviews, 1*, 205–214.

Watt, R. J. & Andrews, D. P. (1982). Contour curvature analysis: hyperacuities in the discrimination of detailed shape. *Vision Research, 22*, 449–460.

Watt, R. J. & Morgan, M. J. (1983a). The recognition and representation of edge blur: evidence for spatial primitives in vision. *Vision Research, 23*, 1465–1477.

Watt, R. J. & Morgan, M. J. (1983b). Mechanisms responsible for the assessment of visual location: theory and evidence. *Vision Research, 23*, 97–109.

Watt, R. J. & Morgan, M. J. (1984). Spatial filters and the localization of luminance changes in human vision. *Vision Research, 24*, 1387–1397.

Watt, R. J. & Morgan, M. J. (1985). A theory of the primitive spatial code in human vision. *Vision Research, 25*, 1661–1674.

Watt, R. J., Morgan, M. J. & Ward, R. M. (1983). The use of different cues in vernier acuity. *Vision Research, 23*, 991–995.

Waugh, S. J., Levi, D. M. & Carney, T. (1993). Orientation, masking and vernier acuity for line targets. *Vision Research, 33*, 1619–1638.

Weale, R. A. (1957). Trichromatic ideas in the seventeenth and eighteenth centuries. *Nature, 179*, 648–651.

Weale, R. A. (1960). *The eye and its function.* London: Lewis.

Weale, R. A. (1963). *The aging eye.* London: Lewis.

Weale, R. A. (1968). *From sight to light.* London: Oliver & Boyd.

Weberman, H. R. & Penland, H. P. (1982). Computer technology: Microcomputer-based estimation of psychophysical thresholds: The best PEST. *Behaviour Research Methods and Instrumentation, 14*, 21–25.

Webster, M. A., DeValois, K. K. & Switkes, E. (1990). Orientation and spatial frequency discrimination for luminance and chromatic gratings. *Journal of the Optical Society of America, A7*, 1034–1049.

Webster, M. A. & Mollon, J. D. (1993). Contrast adaptation dissociates different measures of luminous efficiency. *Journal of the Optical Society of America, A, 10*, 1332–1340.

Webster, W. R., Panthradil, J. T. & Conway, D. M. (1998). A rotating stereoscopic 3–dimensional movement aftereffect. *Vision Research, 38*, 1745–1752.

Weingarten, F. S. (1972). Wavelength effects on visual latency. *Science, 176*, 682–684.

Wenderoth, P. (1994). The salience of vertical symmetry. *Perception, 23*, 221–236.

Wenderoth, P. & Van der Zwan, R. (1991). Local and global mechanisms of one- and two-dimensional orientation illusions. *Perception and Psychophysics, 50*, 321–332.

Wenderoth, P., Van der Zwan, R, & Williams, M. (1993). Direct evidence for competition between local and global mechanisms of two–dimensional orientation illusion. *Perception, 22*, 273–286.

Wenderoth, P. & White, D. (1979). Angle–matching illusions and perceived line orientation. *Perception, 8*, 565–575.

Westheimer, G. (1960). Modulation thresholds for sinusoidal light distributions on the retina. *Journal of Physiology (London), 152*, 67–74.

Westheimer, G. (1967). Spatial interaction in human cone vision. *Journal of Physiology (Lond.), 190*, 139–154.

Westheimer, G. (1975). Visual acuity and hyperacuity. *Investigative Ophthalmology and Visual Science, 14,* 570–572.

Westheimer, G. (1977). Spatial frequency and light–spread descriptions of visual acuity and hyperacuity. *Journal of the Optical Society of America, 67,* 207–212.

Westheimer, G. (1979). The spatial sense of the eye. *Investigative Ophthalmology and Visual Science, 18,* 893–912.

Westheimer, G. (1981). Visual hyperacuity. In D. Ottoson et al. (Eds). *Progress in sensory physiology,* Vol.1 (pp.1–30). New York: Springer.

Westheimer, G. (1984). Line separation discrimination curve in the human fovea: Smooth or segmented? *Journal of the Optical Society of America, A1,* 1683–1684.

Westheimer, G. (1985). Reply to comment on "Line separation discrimination curve in the human fovea: Smooth or segmented?". *Journal of the Optical Society of America, A2,* 477–478.

Westheimer, G. (1986). Physiological optics during the first quarter-century of *Vision Research. Vision Research, 26,* 1513.

Westheimer, G. (1996). Location and line orientation as distinguishable primitives in spatial vision. *Proceedings of the Royal Society, B, 263,* 503–508.

Westheimer, G. (1998). Lines and Gabor functions compared as spatial visual stimuli. *Vision Research, 38,* 487–491.

Westheimer, G. & Campbell, F. W. (1962). Light distribution in the image formed by the living human eye. *Journal of the Optical Society of America, 52,* 1040–1045.

Westheimer, G. & Li, W. (1996). Classifying illusory contours by means of orientation discrimination. *Journal of Neurophysiology, 75,* 523–528.

Westheimer, G. & McKee, S. P. (1975). Visual acuity in the presence of retinal image motion. *Journal of the Optical Society of America, 65,* 847–850.

Westheimer, G. & McKee, S. P. (1977a). Spatial configurations for visual hyperacuity. *Vision Research, 17,* 941–947.

Westheimer, G. & McKee, S. P. (1977b). Integration regions for visual hyperacuity. *Vision Research, 17,* 89–93.

Westheimer, G., Shimamura, K. & McKee, S. P. (1976). Interference with line orientation sensitivity. *Journal of the Optical Society of America, 66,* 332–338.

Westheimer, G. & Tanzman, I. J. (1956). Qualitative depth localization with diplopic images. *Journal of the Optical Society of America, 46,* 116–117.

Wetherill, G. B. (1966). *Sequential methods in statistics.* London: Chapman and Hall. New York: Wile (Halsted)

Wetherill, G. B. & Levitt, H. (1965). Sequential estimation of points on a psychometric function. *British Journal of Mathematical and Statistical Psychology, 18,* 1–10.

Wheatstone, C. (1838). Contributions to the physiology of vision. *Philosophical Transactions of the Royal Society, 13,* 371–394.

White, H. J. & Tauber, S. (1969). *Systems analysis.* Philadelphia: W. B. Saunders.

White, J. M., Levi, D. M. & Aitsebaomo, A. P. (1992). Spatial localization without visual references. *Vision Research, 32,* 513–526.

Wickelgren (1967). Strength theories of disjunctive visual detection. *Perception & Psychophysics, 2,* 331–337.

Wicks, B. (1989a) *The day they took the children.* Toronto: Stoddart.

Wicks, B. (1989b). *No time to wave good-bye.* London: Bloomsbury Publishing.

Wilcox, L. M. & Hess, R. F. (1998). When stereopsis does not improve with increasing contrast. *Vision Research, 38,* 3671–3679.

Wildsoet, C. & Wallman, J. (1995). Choroidal and scleral mechanisms of compensation for spectacle lenses in chicks. *Vision Research, 35,* 1175–1194.

Williams, D. R. (1985). Aliasing in human foveal vision. *Vision Research, 25,* 195–205.

Williams, D. R., Brainard, D. H., McMahon, M. J. & Naverro, R. (1994). Double-pass and interferometric measures of the optical quality of the eye. *Journal of the Optical society of America, A, 11,* 3123–3135.

Williams, D. R. & Collier, R. (1983). Consequences of spatial sampling by a human photoreceptor mosaic. *Science, 221,* 385–387.

Williams, D. R., Collier, R. J. & Thompson, B. J., (1983). Spatial resolution of the short–wavelength mechanism. In J. D. Mollon & L. T. Sharpe (Eds.) *Colour Vision.* London: Academic Press, pp. 487–503.

Williams, D. R., MacLeod, D. I. A. & Hayhoe, M. M (1981). Foveal tritanopia. *Vision Research, 21,* 1341–1356.

Williams, D. R., Tweten, S. & Sekuler, R. (1991). Using metamers to explore motion perception. *Vision Research, 31,* 275–286.

Williams, R. A., Enoch, J. M. & Essock, E. A. (1984). Optic and photoelectric analog of the eye. *Journal of the Optical Society of America, 46,* 721–739.

Williamson, S. J. & Cummings, H. Z. (1983). *Light and color in nature and art.* New York: Wiley.

Wilson, H. R. (1975). A synaptic model for spatial frequency adaptation. *Journal of Theoretical Biology, 50,* 327–352.

Wilson, H. R. (1978). Quantitative characterization of two types of line-spread function near the fovea. *Vision Research, 18,* 971–981.

Wilson, H. R. (1980). A transducer function for threshold and suprathreshold human vision. *Biological Cybernetics, 38,* 171–178.

Wilson, H. R. (1985). Discrimination of contour curvature: Data and theory. *Journal of the Optical Society of America, A, 2,* 1191–1199.

Wilson, H. R.(1986). Responses of spatial mechanisms can explain hyperacuity. *Vision Research, 26,* 453–469.

Wilson, H. R. (1991a). Pattern discrimination, visual filters and spatial sampling irregularity. In M. S. Landy & J. A. Movshon (Eds.), *Computational models of visual processing.* Cambridge, Mass: MIT Press.

Wilson, H. R. (1991b). Psychophysical models of spatial vision and hyperacuity. In D. Regan (Ed.), *Spatial vision* (pp. 64–86). London: Macmillan.

Wilson, H. R. & Bergen, J. R. (1979). A four mechanism model for threshold spatial vision. *Vision Research, 19,* 19–32.

Wilson, H. R., Blake, R. & Halpern, D. L. (1991). Coarse spatial scales constrain the range of binocular fusion on fine scales. *Journal of the Optical Society of America, A, 8,* 229–236.

Wilson, H. R., Blake, R. & Pokorny, J. (1988). Limits of binocular fusion in the short wave sensitive ("blue") cones. *Vision Research, 28,* 555–562.

Wilson, H. R. & Gelb, D. J. (1984). Modified line element theory for spatial frequency and width discrimination. *Journal of the Optical Society of America, A1,* 124–131.

Wilson, H. R. & Humanski, R. (1993). Spatial frequency adaptation and contrast gain control. *Vision Research, 33,* 1133–1149.

Wilson, H. R. & Kim, J. (1988). Dynamics of a divisive gain control in human vision. *Vision Research, 38,* 2735–2741.

Wilson, H. R., McFarlane, D. K. & Phillips, G. C. (1983). Spatial frequency tuning of orientation selective units estimated by oblique masking. *Vision Research, 23,* 873–882.

Wilson, H. R. & Regan, D. (1984). Spatial frequency adaptation and grating discrimination: predictions of a line-element model. *Journal of the Optical Society of America, A1,* 1091–1096.

Wilson, H. R. & Richards, W. A. (1989). Mechanisms of contour curvature discrimination. *Journal of the Optical Society of America, A, 6,* 106–115.

Wilson, H. R. & Wilkinson, F. (1997). Evolving concepts of spatial channels in vision: From independence to non-linear interactions. *Perception, 26,* 939–960.

Wolfson, S. S. & Landy, M. S. (1995). Discrimination of orientation–defined texture edges. *Vision Research, 35,* 2863–2877.

Wolfson, S. S. & Landy, M. S. (1998) Examining edge–and region–based texture analysis mechanisms. *Vision Research, 38,* 439–446.

Wolpert, D. M., Miall, R. C & Kawato, M. (1988). Internal models in the cerebellum. *Trends in Cognitive Science, 2,* 338–347.

Woodford, F. P. (1967). Sounder thinking through clearer writing. *Science, 156,* 743–745.

Woods, R. L., Bradley, A. & Atchison, D. A. (1996). Consequences of monocular diplopia for the contrast sensitivity function. *Vision Research, 36,* 3587–3596.

Woodward, M., Ettinger, E. R. & Yager, D. (1985). The spatial frequency discrimination function at low contrasts. *Spatial Vision, 1,* 13–17.

Worsley, F. A. (1977). *Shackleton's boat journey.* New York: Norton.

Wright, W. D. (1928). A trichromatic colorimeter with spectral primaries. *Transactions of the Optical Society of London, 29,* 225–241.

Wright, W. D. (1928–29). A re-determination of the mixture curves of the spectrum. *Transactions of the Optical Society of London, 30,* 141–164.

Wright, W. D. (1946). *Researches on normal and defective color vision.* London: Henry Kimpton.

Wright, W. D. (1952). The characteristics of Tritanopia. *Journal of the Optical Society of America, 42,* 509–521.

Wright, W. D. (1953). The convergence of the tritanopic confusion loci and the derivation of the fundamental response functions. *Journal of the Optical Society of America, 43,* 890–894.

Wright, W. D. (1970). The origins of the 1931 C. I. E. system. *Journal of the Color Group, 15,* 166–177.

Wright, W. D. (1991). The measurement of colour. In P. Gouras (Ed.), *The perception of color* (pp. 10–21). Boca Raton, Fla.: CRC Press.

Wright, W. D. & Pitt, F. H. G. (1934a). Hue discrimination in normal color vision. *Proceedings of the Physical Society (London), 46,* 459–468.

Wright, W. D. & Pitt, F. H. G. (1934b). The color vision characteristics of two trichromats. *Proceedings of the Physical Society (London), 47,* 207–208.

Wyszecki, G. & Stiles, W. S. (1967). *Color science.* New York: Wiley.

Yamamoto, T. S. & DeValois, K. K. (1996). Chromatic-spatial selectivity for luminance-varying patterns. *Investigative Opthalmology and Visual Science, 37* (Supp.), S1064.

Yang, Y. & Blake, R. (1991). Spatial frequency tuning of human stereopsis. *Vision Research, 31,* 1177–1189.

Yang, Y. & Blake, R. (1994). Broad tuning for spatial frequency of neural mechanisms underlying visual perception of coherent motion. *Nature, 371,* 793–796.

Yang, J. & Makous, W. (1995a). Zero frequency masking and a model of contrast sensitivity. *Vision Research, 35,* 1965–1978.

Yang, J. & Makous, W. (1995b) Modeling pedestal experiments with amplitude instead of contrast. *Vision Research, 35,* 1979–1989.

Yap, Y. L., Levi, D. M. & Klein, S. A.(1987a). Peripheral hyperacuity: 3-dot bisection scales to a single factor from 0 to 10 deg. *Journal of the Optical Society of America, A, 4,* 1554–1561.

Yap, Y. L., Levi, D. M. & Klein, S. A.(1987b). Peripheral hyperacuity: Isoeccentric bisection is better than radial bisection. *Journal of the Optical Society of America, A, 4,* 1562–1567.

Yeh, S. L., Chen, I. P., DeValois, K. K. & DeValois, R. L. (1992). Figural aftereffects with isoluminant gaussian blobs. *Investigative Ophthalmology and Visual Science* (Suppl.) *33*, 704.

Young, F. A. & Leary, G. A. (1991). Refractive error in relation to the development of the eye. In W. N. Charman (Ed.) *Visual optics and visual instrumentation.* London: Macmillan

Yujiri, A., Ejima, Y., Alita, H. & Noguchi, T. (1980). Spatial frequency selectivity of human color vision mechanism. *Investigative Ophthalmology and Visual Science* (Suppl.), *21*, 217.

Zeki, S. M. (1973). Colour coding in rhesus monkey prestriate cortex. *Brain Research, 53*, 422–427.

Zeki, S. M. (1977). The third visual complex of rhesus monkey prestriate cortex. *Journal of Physiology, 277*, 245–272.

Zeki, S. M. (1980). The representation of colours in the cerebral cortex. *Nature, 284*, 412–418.

Zeki, S. M. (1990). A century of cerebral achromatopsia. *Brain, 113*, 1721–1777.

Zemany, L., Stromeyer, C. F. III, Chaparro, A. & Kronauer, R. E. (1998). Motion detection on flashed stationary pedestal gratings: Evidence for an opponent–motion mechanism. *Vision Research, 38*, 795–812.

Zhang, J. (1995). Motion detectors and motion segregation. *Spatial Vision, 9*, 261–273.

Zhang, X., Bradley, A. & Thibos, L. N. (1993). Experimental determination of the chromatic difference of magnification for the human eye and the location of the anterior nodal point. *Journal of the Optical Society of America, A, 10*, 213–220.

Zhang, X., Thibos, L. N. & Bradley, A. (1991). Relationship between the chromatic difference of focus and the chromatic difference of magnification for the reduced eye. *Optometry and Vision Science, 68*, 456–458.

Zimmern, R. L., Campbell, F. W. & Wilkinson, I. M. S. (1979). Subtle disturbances of vision after optic neuritis elicited by studying contrast sensitivity. *Journal of Neurology, Neurosurgery and Psychiatry, 42*, 407–412.

Zrenner, E. & Krüger, C. J. (1981). Ethambutol mainly affects the functions of red/green opponent neurons. *Documenta Ophthalmolgia, 27*, 13–26.

Illustration Credits

Unless cited below, full bibliographic information for all copyrighted illustrations, tables, and photographs can be found in the References. We are grateful to the following publishers for their permission to adapt or reprint copyrighted material.

From Cambridge University Press: Fig. 2.11.

From HarperCollins: Fig. 1.1, © 1995 Christopher O'Toole.

From *Science*: copyright American Association for the Advancement of Science and reprinted with permission: Figs. 1.16, Panel A © 1969, Panels B–E © 1979; 5.17, © 1973; F.5, © 1973; I.3, © 1979.

From *Journal of Neuroscience*, copyright Elsevier Science and reprinted with permission: Fig. 5.18.

From *Vision Research*, copyright Elsevier Science and reprinted with permission: Figs. 2.9, © 1988; 2.10, © 1988; 2.12, © 1983; 2.13, © 1983; 2.14, © 1983; 2.18, © 1977; 2.31, © 1986; 2.32, © 1997; 2.33, © 1997; 2.34, © 1996; 2.37, © 1996; 2.40, © 1982; 2.41, © 1982; 2.43, © 1983; 2.47, © 1985; 2.51, © 1997; 2.52, © 1997; 2.53, © 1987; 2.54, © 1987; 2.55, © 1987; 2.58, © 1975; 2.59, © 1975; 2.60, © 1992; 2.62, © 1992; 3.1, © 1973; 3.7, © 1971; 3.8, © 1971; 3.9, © 1971; 3.15, © 1973; 4.2, © 1991; 4.3, Panel A © 1998, Panel B © 1996, Panel C © 1997; 4.4, © 1998; 4.5, © 1998; 4.6, © 1998; 4.7 Panel B, © 1996; 4.8, © 1997; 4.9, © 1998; 4.13, © 1998; 5.5, © 1986; 5.6, © 1981; 5.7, © 1981; 5.13 Panels A,B, © 1989; 5.20, © 1979; 5.21, © 1979; 6.1 lower half, © 1994; 6.3 Panel B, © 1973; 6.7, © 1973; 6.10, Panels A, B © 1995, Panels C, D © 1994; B.9, © 1976; E.1, © 1982; F.3, © 1985; F.4, © 1985; F.6, © 1985; F.7, © 1988; F.8, © 1988; F.9, © 1989; F.10, © 1985.

Index

563